Health and Fitness for Life

Development Edition

Raschel Larsen

Health and Fitness for Life

ISBN: 978-1-943536-44-3
Development Edition 0.9 (Fall 2018)

Chemeketa Press

Chemeketa Press is a nonprofit publishing endeavor at Chemeketa Community College that works with faculty, staff, and students to create affordable and effective alternatives to commercial textbooks. All proceeds from the sales of this textbook go toward the development of new textbooks. To learn more, visit www.chemeketapress.org.

Publisher: Tim Rogers
Director: Steve Richardson
Managing Editor: Brian Mosher
Instructional Editor: Stephanie Lenox
Manuscript Editors: Catherine Shride and Chris Cottrell
Design Editor: Ronald Cox IV
Cover Design: Ronald Cox IV
Interior Design: Mackenzie Allen, Noah Barerra, Shaun Jaquez, Casandra Johns, Jess Kolman, Faith Martinmaas, Keyiah McClain, Erica Meyer, Michael Ovens, Matt Sanchez
Cover photo by Jennifer Birdie Shawker is in the public domain (https://unsplash.com/photos/jz4EyFcTcBc).

Acknowledgments appear on pages 366 to 373 and constitute an extension of the copyright page.

Contents

About Development Editions

Chemeketa Press uses a software development model to publish textbooks that are more affordable and more effective than commercial textbooks. This means that we first publish books like this textbook when they are fully functional and *mostly* finished, like an early release of a new software program. We then work with the faculty and students who are using the development edition — you, for example — to make improvements, correct errors, and thus prepare the book for its final publication in about a year. Because this is still a work in progress, we've reduced the price to you by 20%.

You can join Chemeketa Press in its mission to make textbooks affordable again by helping us finish this textbook. Do you have any suggestions for how we can make this book more effective for you and others? Have you found any errors within chapters? If so, let us know. You can either tell your professor, who will tell us, or you can contact us directly at collegepress@chemeketa.edu. Thanks for your help!

Chapter 1
Introduction to Health and Wellness

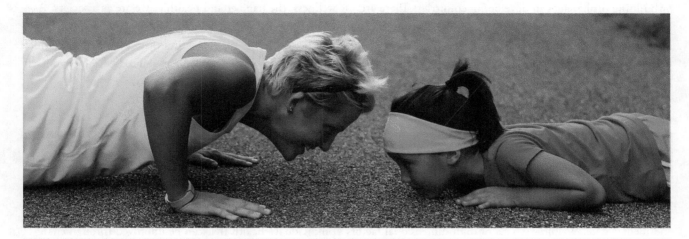

Learning Objectives

1. Describe the dimensions of wellness.

2. Identify the major health problems in the US today and discuss their causes.

3. Describe the behaviors that are part of a fit and well lifestyle.

4. Identify the factors that influence your wellness behaviors.

5. Develop a personalized plan for successful behavior change, including appropriate goals and strategies for overcoming behaviors.

Have you ever thought about what it means to be healthy? We hear a lot about exercise, diet, weight, and illness when we talk about health, but the word "healthy" often makes us think about being "unhealthy." The same is true about being "well." When a friend asks you "How are you?" and you respond with "I'm well, thank you," what are you really saying? Does it just mean not sick? Or does it mean that you feel great and highly functional in your daily routine, that you have a high quality of life?

Sure, in comparison to your friend Chuck who eats fast food from the comfort of his recliner each day, you *do* seem healthy. Yesterday you heard him rationalize his lifestyle by saying, "life is short," you have to "live life to the fullest." He sees denying himself what he wants as not enjoying life. Chuck may be enjoying those onion rings and his recliner, but you'd hardly consider his life full and are likely concerned about his longevity. When friends ask him to hike up to the top of Multnomah Falls to see the view, will he go? Can *you* make it to the top (Figure 1)?

Why would someone say no? It's easy to just say that it doesn't interest you. Who really wants to see the sunrise peeking through white, fluffy clouds above the Columbia River while listening to the water plunge down the side of a mountain as the birds sing anyway? Maybe witnessing something majestic like this isn't enjoyable to you, or maybe the truth is that you're not sure if you can make it to the top.

Can you do all the things you truly want to do? Let's forget about the waterfalls and hikes. Can you get through your work or school day giving everything your best effort? If your answer is no, your health is impacting your quality of life.

This doesn't just happen overnight. The little choices you make each day add up over the course of your lifetime—good or bad. They can make the difference not only in how long you live but also in what you are able to do with that time. Your friend Chuck in the recliner probably made a series of choices that have now impacted his quality of life. Imagine if that had been a series of healthy choices, even small choices, over the course of a year. Instead of sitting in the recliner, he might be hiking the Pacific Crest Trail with his friends or getting a promotion due to his efforts at work. He could have been helping in his local community or building orphanages in developing countries. There are short- and long-term payoffs when we make decisions that impact our health and wellness.

You can use the terms "health" and "wellness" in relation to society or to an individual, but what do they really mean? This chapter will define and explain health and wellness, show why wellness is so important, and describe a basic goal-setting method for improving individual behaviors associated with wellness.

The more individuals who take charge of their health or wellness, the happier and healthier we are as a society. As a whole, our goal should be to spend less of our energy treating illnesses and more on preventing them by making healthier choices. This book will encourage you to be healthy yourself and to focus on your personal wellness.

What Are Health and Wellness?

Health and wellness are linked in definition and so are often used interchangeably. While **health** refers to the general condition of our bodies and minds, **wellness** can be considered a deliberate effort to actually be healthy. Health is a person's physical and mental state. Wellness is a set of multidimensional factors of individuals' health that can be improved through changes in behavior. Public health refers to the health condition in a group of people, and is linked to life expectancy, disease, and general wellness.

These three terms are wrapped up in one another. To improve public health, individuals must make choices that improve their own health and wellness. That's all you have control over. You can't make Chuck put down the junk food and take a walk, but you can make sure that you don't end up trapped in your own recliner.

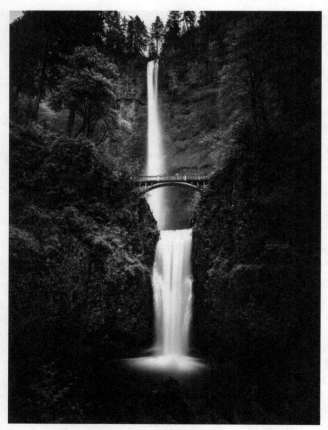

Figure 1. Do physical challenges keep you from enjoying life?

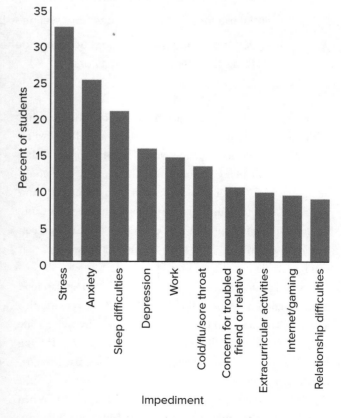

Figure 2. Top 10 problems students report that affect their academic performance (Source: American College Health Association).

The term "health" has evolved since Hippocrates (circa 460 BC), one of the most noted medical practitioners in ancient Greece, began teaching people ways to fight diseases and to look at the body as a whole unit. In 1948, the **World Health Organization (WHO)** defined health as "a state of complete physical, mental, and social well-being, and not merely the absence of disease or infirmity," a definition they still use today. What both have in common is the idea that health is not just about being free from sickness, but also about the holistic nature of the body and its capability to keep us thriving in life.

Wellness is a work in progress in the US, and its importance comes down to keeping people alive longer and maintaining or improving quality of life. Our population's average life expectancy, our likelihood of developing disease and disability, and the average amounts of physical activity we perform are all used to measure how healthy we are as a nation. These measurements help determine public policies that can lead to a healthier population.

The US still struggles with certain health-related issues, but we've made a lot of progress since Hippocrates. Much of this is due to advances in medical care and programs that bring awareness to individuals about the importance of health and wellness. As a student, the stresses of life can be overwhelming (Figure 2). But even now, you can make changes to your lifestyle to help you live a longer, happier life and avoid disease. If enough people pursue improved wellness, the status of our public health can improve with it. Those changes happen within the dimensions of wellness.

Dimensions of Wellness

Wellness is an active process. Each dimension of wellness factors into individual wellness, and each well person contributes to the public health of their community. All people are somewhere on a continuum with wellness at one end and illness at the other, and every action they take causes them to shift their position on that continuum, either toward illness or wellness (Figure 3).

Wellness includes seven dimensions of an individual's well-being. Each dimension has its own important qualities but should be thought of as an interactive web where each overlaps and intersects with others in different ways. The whole group of seven dimensions makes up overall wellness (Figure 4). The dimensions all have this in common: they are equal parts recognition of the dimension's importance and acting on that knowledge.

Physical wellness is the complete physical conditioning and functioning of the body. It includes physical fitness, eating habits, sleeping habits, and choices that affect your risk

of illness or injury, such as substance use/abuse, sexual habits, safe-driving habits, and other self-care practices like getting regular check-ups and recognizing symptoms of disease. It gets more complicated to care of yourself as you age (Figure 5). Physically well individuals recognize the difference between healthy habits and destructive habits and then make choices that help rather than hurt their longevity. Part of the work is knowing which habits lead to physical wellness. Actions make up the rest.

Emotional wellness is the ability to cope with the challenges of daily life. An emotionally well person acknowledges that difficulties are normal. They tend to embrace and share the ups and downs in life equally. They handle their emotions with a generally positive outlook. They have control of their behavioral response to strong feelings. They know stress is bound to occur, so they learn to manage and cope with it as it happens.

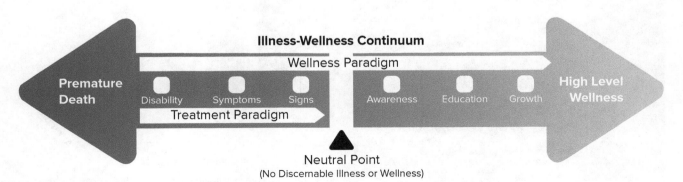

Figure 3. Your health is related to where you fall on the illness-wellness continuum.

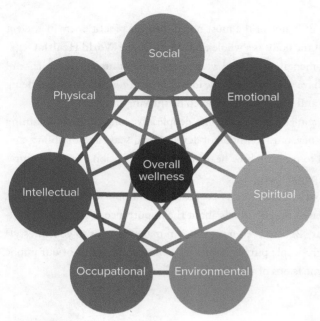

Figure 4. The seven dimensions of wellness.

Students experience high stress levels, and without emotional wellness, they are open to potentially damaging effects (Figure 6). People with emotional wellness often share certain traits, such as optimism, trust, enthusiasm, self-confidence, self-acceptance, resiliency, and self-esteem. You can already begin to see how these dimensions overlap and intersect with each other. A physically well person may achieve emotional wellness easier without health concerns. Someone with a positive outlook, likewise, might not see challenges to physical wellness as difficult to overcome.

Intellectual wellness describes the ability to use logic and problem-solving to respond to experiences and continue to learn throughout life. An intellectually well person applies this open-mindedness—a willingness to think things through—to their own decisions, their interactions with

others, and the improvement of their community. They want to learn about new things. They want to improve their sense of self, build upon their skills, and challenge themselves to see life in new ways.

Social wellness describes the ability to interact and connect with others in your family, your community, and the world around you, developing and nurturing positive relationships. Social wellness is about more than just spending time with others. It's about taking an active role in establishing and fostering positive contact with the people in your life (Figure 7). Socially well people confide in and communicate with others respectfully, support others in different social interactions, and receive love openly and willingly.

Spiritual wellness may be less concrete than the other dimensions but is just as important. A spiritually well person has a sense of meaning and purpose in their life. They can identify their important values, such as compassion, forgiveness, altruism, tolerance, and capacity for love. They can then connect their values with their actions. There are many ways a person can experience spiritual wellness. Some find it through religion. Others practice it through volunteering, spending time in nature, being creative, meditating, or contributing to a greater cause (Figure 8).

Environmental wellness describes the ability to take responsibility for the quality of our surroundings. An environmentally well person understands that individual choices have an impact on the safety of the air, water, land and, by extension, people's health. They find ways to have a net positive impact on that safety. This dimension of wellness can be experienced at both local and global levels by participating with others in networks of environmental wellness (Figure 9).

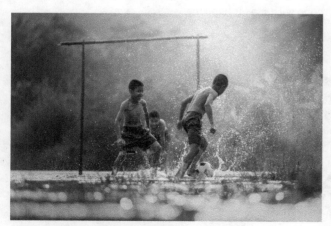

Figure 5. Physical activity is important at all ages.

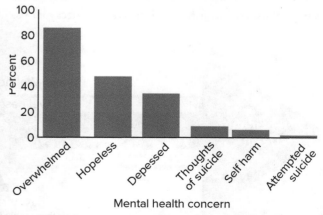

Figure 6. US college students mental health concerns in the past 12 months (Source: American College Health Association).

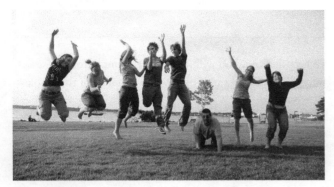

Figure 7. Social wellness includes being part of a community.

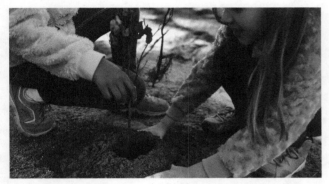

Figure 8. Interacting with nature builds environmental wellness.

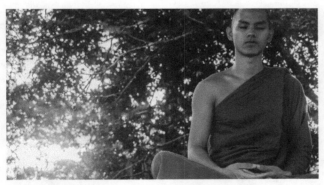

Figure 9. Spiritual wellness helps create peace in your life.

Occupational wellness describes the ability to take pride in the jobs and career fields that we pursue while balancing the demands of our work and home life. A person who is occupationally well contributes to their career with the desire to have a positive impact on the organization or people they work with. They also maintain a healthy balance between that contribution, not working too much or too little. Being able to recognize what this balance looks like for you is critical to your occupational wellness. This enables you to grow at work and still feel satisfied.

Each dimension of wellness needs attention, and many dimensions overlap with one another and can be improved with a single action. For example, some types of exercise, like biking instead of driving to work, can positively impact your physical, emotional, social, and environmental wellness. But some areas of wellness require attention before you can address others.

According to psychologist Abraham Maslow's theory on human's needs, we have to have our basic needs met—like food, water, and sleep—before we can pay attention to any "higher level" needs like intellectual satisfaction. Wellness works the same way. Focusing on your emotional wellness by improving your relationships isn't really possible if you haven't met your physiological need to feel safe at home (Figure 10). When proper attention is paid to each dimension of wellness, your life can be more fulfilling and even be extended by the habits you build.

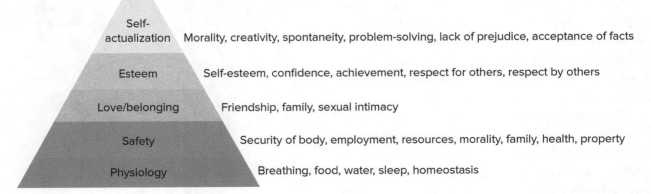

Figure 10. Needs at the bottom of Maslow's hierarchy of needs must be met before you can give attention to needs closer to the top.

Health Challenges in the US

Medical and technological advancements have improved areas of health in the US like life expectancy, but we still have improvements to make. Let's look at how some of the measurable factors of health—including causes of death and health care costs—have changed over the last 100 years.

Causes of Death

The leading causes of death have shifted over the years due to advances in science, medical technology, and public health initiatives. In 1900, the leading causes of death were infectious diseases including pneumonia, influenza, and tuberculosis. We have much lower rates of infectious disease today. The creation of vaccines and antibiotics, and improvements in food safety and environmental conditions, are some of the major factors that have reduced the death rate in the US (Figure 11). Infectious diseases and injuries are still a public health concern, and you can find more information about infectious diseases in Chapter 10.

In 2015, the leading causes of death were chronic diseases such as heart disease, cancer, chronic lower respiratory diseases, and cerebrovascular disease (stroke). In fact, nearly half of Americans have at least one chronic disease. Approximately 70% of all deaths in the US are caused by chronic diseases (Figure 12). Other common serious health concerns among Americans today include obesity, unintentional injuries (drug overdose, motor vehicle accidents, unintentional falls), suicide, Alzheimer's disease, depression, anxiety, and other mental health issues.

The leading causes of death vary by age and gender. Adults in the US age 15–24 are more likely to die from unintentional injuries, homicide and suicide, while those age 25–44 have higher death rates from cancer and heart disease. In fact, heart disease is the leading cause of death for both men and women in the US, followed by cancer. Men, however, have a higher risk for prostate cancer, while women have higher rates of breast cancer. Men experience higher rates of death from unintentional injury, suicide, and chronic liver disease. Women experience higher death rates from stroke, Alzheimer's disease, and septicemia (bloodstream infections).

This information might seem a bit scary, but knowledge is power. You can avoid many chronic diseases, prevent obesity and lessen your risk of injuries and infections with healthy lifestyle behaviors. It's possible to stop or slow their development with good physical activity, healthy nutrition, and low tobacco

and alcohol use. You will learn more about chronic diseases, nutrition, and substance use in later chapters of this book.

Life Expectancy

Life expectancy is the expected number of years an average person will live. This number has risen significantly during the last century. In 1901, the average American could expect

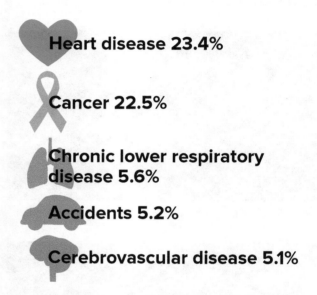

Heart disease 23.4%

Cancer 22.5%

Chronic lower respiratory disease 5.6%

Accidents 5.2%

Cerebrovascular disease 5.1%

Figure 11. Leading causes of death in the US (Source: CDC).

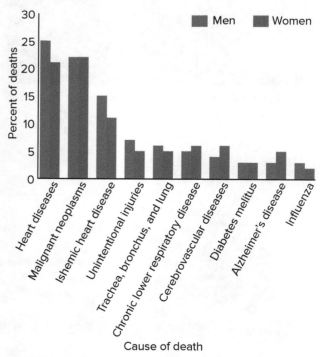

Figure 12. Causes of death by gender (Source: CDC).

to live 49.3 years. In other words, most Americans died before their 50th birthday. In 2010, the average life expectancy in the US was 78.8 years, an increase of almost 30 years. That's a huge difference!

Healthy living isn't just about how long we live, but how many of those years are lived in good health. This is our **healthy life expectancy, our** expected years of life free of disability or chronic disease. Your friend Chuck, for example, might live to be 70. But he could spend the last 20 of those 70 years with a chronic illness like heart disease, cancer, or diabetes related to his lack of physical activity and nutrition. The WHO indicated in 2015 that the healthy life expectancy for an average person in the US was 69.1 years of age, just behind the United Kingdom at 71.4 years.

Life expectancy in the US varies based on gender, ethnicity, and geography. For example, women have a life expectancy of 81.2 years, and men have a life expectancy of 76.3 years, according to the Centers for Disease Control (CDC). The average life expectancy for white Americans is 79 years, while the average life expectancy of African Americans is 75.6 years and Hispanic Americans is 81 years (Figure 13).

The dramatic increase in life expectancy from 1901 to today can be attributed to changes in public policy, such as community education, immunization programs, and the availability of health care, as well as advances in science and technology. Basically, the new ideas in the late 1800s and early 1900s about germ theory and disease led to better health infrastructure and personal behavior. This led to major life-saving scientific innovations like vaccines and medical procedures like surgery and transplants. All of these factors have contributed to the rising life expectancy not just in the US but in developed countries around the world (Figure 14).

Health Care Costs

Public health experts also use the cost of health care to measure health in a given population. The total dollar amount spent on treating health problems indicates two things: the frequency and seriousness of health conditions in that population throughout life and the relative cost of treatment in their area (Figure 15). This isn't the best way to determine health because it doesn't give a complete picture of health. If the cost of health care in one population is high and the number of health problems are low, the amount spent on health care might still be the same as a population where costs are lower but problems are higher.

However, as a tool for measuring health, cost is an example of how health and wellness intersect. Take the example above. If costs are high and health problems are low, the relative burden on an individual's expenses for health care causes greater stress in other areas of their lives. They may even have to choose between paying for health care and, say, paying their college tuition. In this scenario, the population's health status (ill or healthy) is relatively positive, but

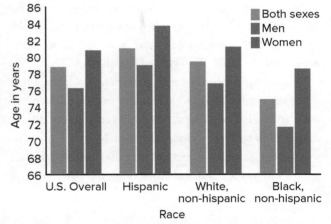

Figure 13. Life expectancy by race and gender (Source: CDC).

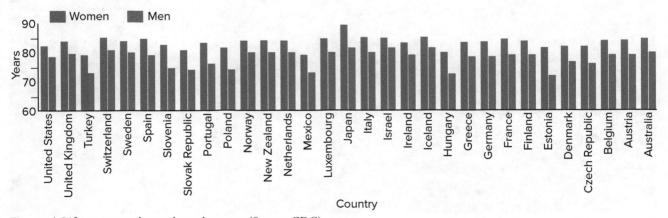

Figure 14. Life expectancy by gender and country (Source: CDC).

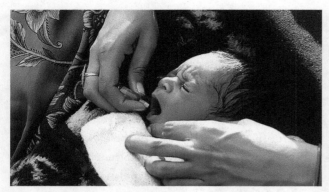

Figure 15. Infants receive some vaccines orally.

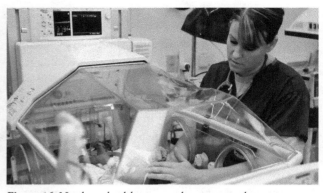

Figure 16. Newborn health care can be very complex.

the cost of care negatively impacts the population's wellness. On the other hand, many individuals may choose to put their other expenses before their health, increasing costs to themselves or the community later on or even spreading illness as a result.

Health Disparities and Inequalities

Life expectancy may have increased over time, but there are still too many people who die at a younger-than-average age because of factors beyond their control (Figure 16). An important thing to consider when describing public health challenges is the unequal way those challenges affect different groups of people. This is called **health disparity.**

Health disparities and inequalities are avoidable, unfair differences in health status that occur within and between populations. For example, differences in contracting chronic disease rates by age, receipt of preventative vaccinations by socioeconomic status, or occurrence of risky behaviors by race are all examples of health disparities (Figure 17). According to

the WHO, the social determinants of health—the conditions in which persons are born, grow, live, work, and age—are mostly responsible for health inequalities.

Let's say, for example, that you and your cousin Mary both have asthma. You have health insurance and live in a quiet, suburban neighborhood. You visit your health care provider once each year and your asthma is well controlled. You almost never visit the emergency room . Mary lives in a congested, urban neighborhood of Pittsburgh, Pennsylvania. Her apartment is in a smoggy area on a busy street not far from an industrial plant. She has been forced to make eight trips to the emergency room in the past year. Her asthma is not well-controlled, but she can't afford to move to an area with better air quality. Mary also can't afford health insurance that covers medications and better preventative care. If the air quality were better (something Mary has no control over) and better insurance were less expensive (another thing Mary has no control over), her need for care would decrease and she would spend less.

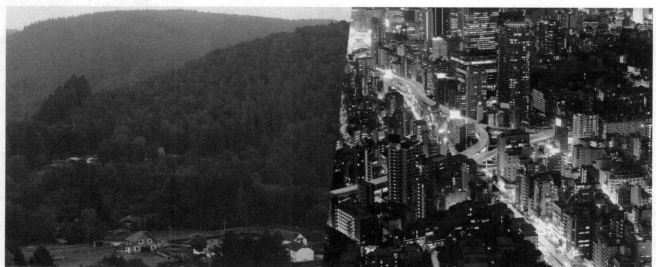

Figure 17. Health outcomes and health care options often differ by geographic location.

Let's look at some examples of health disparities from a Centers for Disease Control report published in 2013 based on two tools of measurement—mortality and morbidity.[1]

The **mortality rate** is the statistical odds for when a person will die. When a person dies, basic identifying information about them—age, ethnicity, sex, geographic location, cause of death—is collected in a database. The total numbers of death, sorted into these categories, form mortality rates for those segments of a population. Basic data is widely available

on the rate of different causes of death (Figure 18), but you may find more specific details quite surprising. For example, most people would be surprised to learn that based on past data

- Blacks are more likely to die before the age of 75 from stroke and heart disease than whites

- Black infants are more likely to die before their first birthday than white infants

- Men are over 200% more likely to be homicide victims than women

- Blacks, Hispanics, and Native Americans are far more likely to be homicide victims than whites or Asians (Figure 19)

- Men are more likely to die in an auto accident than women, with Native Americans having a higher rate of death in this category than other ethnicities

- Suicide rates are higher for whites and Native Americans than other ethnicities (Figure 20)

Morbidity is the rate people contract infectious or chronic diseases. It is measured like mortality, by tracking categories of information when people are sick. The information can be used to determine an individual's statistical odds of contracting a disease if they are a member of a given population. For example, based on prior data:

- Women and whites have a significantly greater life expectancy and healthy life expectancy than males or blacks

- Asthma attacks are more common for children than adults, people below the federal poverty level (FPL), and people in the US who in the South and West

- Approximately 50% of people under 30 years have some form of gum disease, especially older adults, those with lower household incomes, those who did not finish high school, and current smokers

- In the first part of the century, obesity rates have increased among males and disparities continue to exist based upon race/ethnicity, sex, and education

- Diabetes occurs more often among males, senior citizens, blacks and those of mixed race, Hispanics, people who did not finish high school, people who are poor, and people with a disability

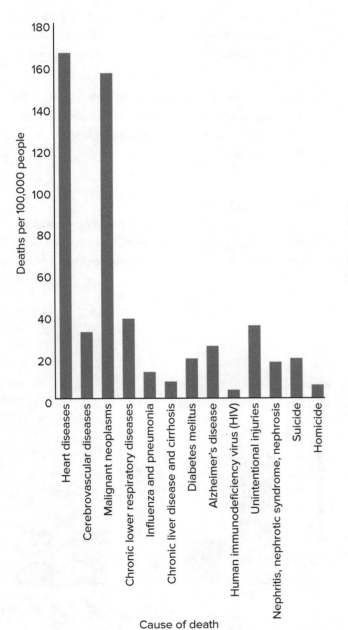

Figure 18. Mortality rate by cause of death (Source: CDC).

[1] For the data in the remainder of this chapter, the terms "blacks" and "whites" refer to those of non-Hispanic origin and the term "Native American" includes both American Indian and Alaskan natives unless otherwise indicated.

Health Care Access and Preventive Health Services

Many Americans do not have access to proper health care services to treat and prevent illness. This disparity may be linked to morbidity rates. When people don't have easy access to health care, they're less likely to seek care when they need it or advice to avoid illnesses. For example:

- In 2010, 64.5% of the US population aged 50–75 years met the US Preventive Services Task Force's criteria for up-to-date colon cancer screening. Screening increased with age, education level, and household income but varied by insurance status and race/ethnicity.

- Influenza vaccination coverage for children increased from the 2009–2010 to the 2010–2011 flu season. Among adults aged 65 years and older, coverage increased for Hispanics but decreased for non-Hispanic whites.

Behavioral Risk Factors

You are the biggest challenge when it comes to health and wellness. Some behaviors put you at greater risk for morbidity and mortality. The statistical likelihood of this can be tracked as well. If more people in a given population engage in risky behaviors, that population is said to be at risk for those behaviors and the consequences that potentially accompany them. Consider this:

- Binge drinking is more common among people aged 18–34, men, whites, and people with higher household incomes. Binge drinkers aged 65 and older report the highest binge drinking frequency, and those 18–24, along with Native Americans, report the highest binge drinking intensity.

- Teen pregnancy rates among blacks and Hispanics remain approximately double those of whites and Asian/Pacific Islanders. This is despite an 18% decrease in these rates overall during 2007–2010.

- Little progress has been made in reducing cigarette smoking among persons of low socioeconomic status despite improvements in racial/ethnic groups in recent years (Figure 21).

Environmental Hazards

Your buddy Chuck may never have to worry about whether his environment is posing a direct risk to his health, unless his recliner becomes infested. But many people experience health

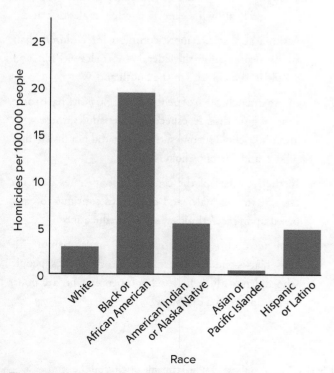

Figure 19. Homicide rate by race (Source: CDC).

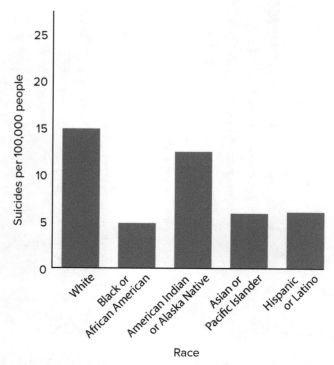

Figure 20. Suicide rate by race (Source: CDC).

Smoking Status	Total (285)	White (82)	Black/African American (119)	Hispanic (84)
Current Cigarette Smoker	77% (219)	72% (59)	86% (102)	69% (58)
Former Cigarette Smoker	23% (66)	28% (23)	14% (17)	31% (26)

Figure 21. Chances of quitting smoking are affected by race (Source: International Journal of Environmental Research and Public Health.)

challenges because of where they work or live. We mentioned environmental pollutants a bit earlier in this chapter and they will be covered again at other points in the book. It's easy to imagine how smog, poor water quality, and toxins are an environmental hazard, but there are others. Police officers and firefighters have obvious dangers in their professions, and many other risks exist in jobs and neighborhoods that we may not be aware of.

Government agencies track risks associated with hazardous living, working, and air quality conditions using the number of deaths and injuries resulting from those conditions, and comparing them to the categories of people in those environments. For example:

- Racial and ethnic minorities, foreign-born people, and people who speak a non-English language at home were

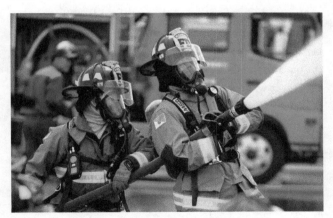

Figure 22. Firefighters have a hazardous job.

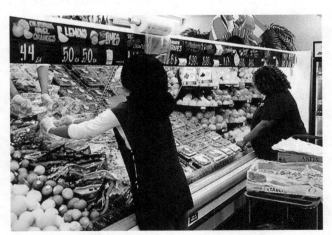

Figure 23. Healthy food retailers aren't always available.

more likely to be living near major highways in 2010, suggesting increased exposure to traffic-related air pollution and an elevated risk for adverse health outcomes.

- The likelihood of working in a high-risk occupation—an occupation with an elevated injury and illness rate—is greatest for those who are Hispanic, are low wage earners, were born outside of the US, have no education beyond high school, or are male (Figure 22).

- Work-related death rates are highest for those who are Hispanic, foreign-born, or are male and that work-related homicide rates were highest for blacks, Native Americans, and Asian/Pacific Islanders.

Social Determinants of Health

By now you can likely see a link between the "health disparity and inequalities" challenge and many of the other health challenges we face in the US. Social determinants are a significant reason for this. Some disparities result from social factors, such as unemployment, poor or incomplete education, and living area. These factors increase morbidity and mortality based on the social impact they have on individual health:

Unemployment—The prevalence of unemployment was much higher among blacks, Hispanics, and Native Americans than among whites in 2006 and 2010. In 2010, unemployed adults were much less likely than employed adults to report their health as excellent or very good.

Education—Hispanics, people with income less than 1.9% of the federal poverty level, those with a disability, or those who are foreign born are less likely to complete high school.

Living Area—Many people live in areas that lack access to services, such as those living in rural census tracts, or those living in areas with a higher percentage of senior citizens. Data show they more often lacked at least one healthy food retailer nearby (within a half-mile of the tract boundary) compared with persons living in other census tracts (Figure 23).

What Can Be Done about Health Disparities?

The goal of public health initiatives—and of looking at health challenges and disparities in general—is to achieve health equity and improve the health of all Americans. The future health of the nation will be determined, to a large extent, by how effectively government and private agencies and organizations work to eliminate disparities that cause disease, disability, and death. The CDC and its partners can use the information they collect to stimulate action on lessening disparities in the US (Figure 24).

The multiple, complex causes of health disparities can be fully addressed only with the involvement of many people and organizations in fields that influence health such as housing, transportation, education, and business.

Understanding Our Role

It's important to understand the barriers and challenges many face in the US and do our best to be part of the solution. Sometimes, that begins at home. Some barriers to healthy behaviors that come from social disparities can also occur among any group of people, even those without the socioeconomic risk factors listed above. We are all products of our environment, to some extent. Chuck may have been raised by parents who valued the relative safety of their recliners, just as he does. Junk food may have been a main staple in his diet as a child. If we have unhealthy behaviors keeping us from pursuing wellness, the behavioral change we need might take some hard work.

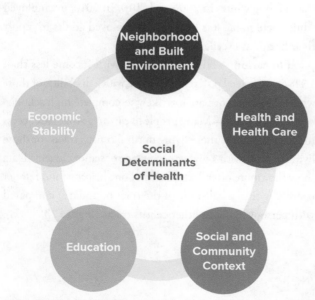

Figure 24. Social categories impact individual and group health.

Issues with a lack of motivation, knowledge, resources, willpower, energy, and support can frequently arise from inside the home and from the examples surrounding us in our families and neighborhoods. A tendency to procrastinate or have a negative attitude toward change can be hard-wired into us from an early age. Experiences with public health programs like the ones in public schools can give us knowledge and a desire to improve wellness, but without support at home or in your community, relapsing into poor behaviors after a positive change is common. We must consider how our behaviors are reinforced and enabled by people around us, how we reinforce and enable others, and use that knowledge to break the cycle of bad behavior.

Reinforcing

If you've ever spent time with a toddler or trained a pet, then you know what it means to reinforce actions. A toddler might throw herself, kicking and screaming, on the grocery store floor store because she wants a candy bar. No one likes a scene and, let's face it – they smell fear! But, if you panic and give her the treat, you are reinforcing her negative behavior. The next time she wants a candy bar at the store, the tantrum might be her first approach. It worked as a strategy to get what she wanted before, so why not try it again? When a puppy learns to sit on command, you give him a dog treat or ask him "Who's a good boy?" in that silly, high-pitched voice we all use (you know you do it), motivating him to want to follow instructions. The treat reinforces his positive behavior.

Adult humans are more complex, of course, and our behaviors can be harder to reinforce. Why? First, our experience with toddlers and puppies makes it so we know when reinforcing is happening. We are not so easy to please. Second, we have more control over our situation. If we don't perform to get our "treat," we can often get it ourselves, even if we didn't earn it. Third, our learned behaviors may have become habits after years of bad choices. It may take a lot of the right kind of reinforcement to change them. That doesn't mean we can't do it. It just means that we need to remind ourselves who is in control and choose reinforcements that makes sense for us.

Chuck once spent three months trying to lose weight. He got up from his recliner, took walks, and ate a fairly healthy diet. Each time he lost a few pounds he treated himself to an abundance of his old favorite foods. It took him a few days to get back on track after these episodes and he never really lost weight. Instead, he reinforced the same behavior that caused him to gain weight in the first place.

For Chuck, a reward like a new pair of jeans might have done more to reinforce his positive changes in a healthy way. Chuck could have called some friends to go hiking or shoot pool. They would probably have noticed and praised his efforts. Both the time spent with friends and their encouraging words would have reinforced his positive behavior change.

Enabling

Certain factors in our environment enable us to slip backward into old habits. Say, for example, that your partner has been instructed by their health care provider to cut sugar out of their diet. It has been your habit to bake homemade cookies each week. It's really hard for you to give that up, so you continue to do so (you're proud of your baking skills).

You tell them that one little cookie won't hurt them – after all, they've had a hard day and earned it. As if on cue, they can't seem to turn down it down. This makes you an enabler of the negative behavior they need to change.

Enabling can be positive, too. Maybe you and a friend have both decided to hit the gym together, but you're really struggling to get motivated. Each time you make an excuse not to go to the gym, your friend shows up in your driveway. She is enabling your success. We can set ourselves up for success when we surround ourselves with positive enablers. You may not always be in a supportive environment that offers positive reinforcement or enables your success but forming new support systems to offset unhelpful ones can make a huge difference. It doesn't mean you have to stop baking for your spouse. How about finding a sugar-free cookie recipe?

Improving Health and Wellness

Part of the reason textbooks like this one exist is to help solve challenges to public health. If public health is seen as a problem worth solving, then working toward better public health is everyone's responsibility. The rest of this chapter looks first at how communities are taking action, then provides guidance for how individuals can assess their health status, create a plan for improvement, and effectively take action.

Public Health Initiatives and Programs

The Centers for Disease Control are leading multiple initiatives that address each of the challenges to public health listed above and more. These initiatives range from "action plans" to "strategies," and offer road maps to elimination of targeted problems. These initiatives represent the majority of public health programming at the federal governmental level.

One major initiative is the program Healthy People 2020. This is a nationwide set of goals and objectives bringing together many individuals' and organizations' efforts. It is a 10-year program — begun in 2010 and updated in 2012 and 2014 — with objectives that align with measurable improvements to health across the country. These objectives strive to:

- Attain high-quality, longer lives free of preventable disease, disability, injury, and premature death

- Achieve health equity, eliminate disparities, and improve the health of all groups

- Create social and physical environments that promote good health for all

- Promote quality of life, healthy development, and healthy behaviors across all life stages

The initiative began when CDC data revealed that chronic diseases such as heart disease, cancer, and diabetes are responsible for seven out of every ten deaths in the US each year, and that their treatment accounts for 75% of the nation's health spending. Preventing these diseases from occurring in the first place is the primary challenge facing the Department of Health and Human Services, according to a Healthy People 2020 press release.

Healthy People 2020 published a list of objectives that target specific areas of public health. Each area below has its own set of goals that must be met for the initiative to claim improvements in that area (Figure 25).

As progress is made in each objective area, the Healthy People 2020 initiative has adjusted their targets based on continuous tracking of the health indicators. Changes were proposed in 2012 and 2014 to adapt to improvements to most objectives and to worsening trends in a few categories.

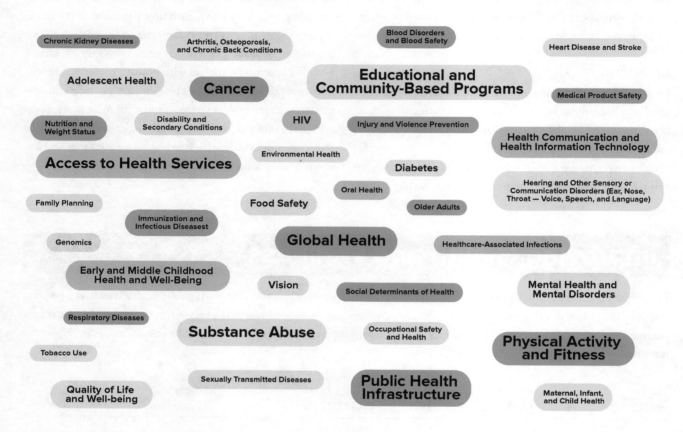

Figure 25. Healthy People 2020 have targeted all these public health areas as objectives to improve.

Assessments of Health and Determinants of Wellness

There are many factors that contribute to public health and individual wellness. You can assess your own health and wellness by investigating the aspects of your life that impact health. The following influences on health and wellness can help you see things you can do every day and long-term habits that can help you maintain a healthy lifestyle.

Be Physically Active

The amount and intensity of recommended physical activity varies for adults and children based on a variety of factors, but the basic guidelines from the US Department of Health and Human Services recommend aerobic activity and strength training for all individuals. At least 150 minutes of moderate activity or 75 minutes of vigorous activity per week is recommended for adults, spread out over several days during a given week. Additional benefits occur with higher levels of activity. Adults should also perform strengthening exercises of moderate or high-intensity at least twice a week with all major muscle groups (Figure 26).

You can find more information on physical activity in Chapters 2, 3, 4, and 5.

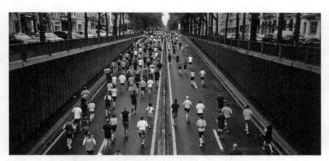

Figure 26. Marathon running is a common way to stay active.

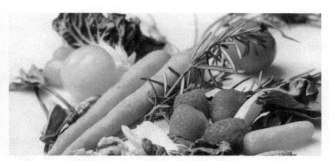

Figure 27. Healthy food choices include fruits and vegetables.

Choose a Healthy Diet to Maintain a Healthy Body Weight

A healthy diet gives you the energy and nutrients you need and can help prevent future health problems. Several of the leading causes of disease are connected to nutrition, and choosing healthful foods can help improve your quality of life and overall wellness. According to the *Dietary Guidelines for Americans 2015–2020*, a healthy eating plan:

- Emphasizes fruits, vegetables, whole grains, and fat-free or low-fat milk and milk products (Figure 27)

- Includes lean meats, poultry, fish, beans, eggs, and nuts

- Is low in saturated fats, trans fats, cholesterol, salt (sodium), and added sugars

- Stays within your daily calorie needs

You can find more information on body composition and nutrition in Chapters 6 and 7.

Manage Stress

Stress is a normal psychological and physical reaction to the ever-increasing demands of life. Some days by the time we make it to work or school we've already argued with our roommate, spilled coffee on our shirt, been stuck in traffic, and arrived 20 minutes late with the phrase "I'm so stressed" on the tip of our tongue. And those are only the small stressors, the insignificant ones that only matter because they accumulate. Larger stressors, like job loss, illness, or financial worries can pose an even stronger reaction. None of us are immune to it. Surveys show that many Americans experience challenges with stress at some point during the year (Figure 28).

That's why learning how to handle it is so important. Your body can respond to stress like it's a fire alarm, and stress management gives you a range of tools to reset your alarm system (Figure 29). Over time, high levels of stress can lead to serious health problems as your body adapts to being on high alert. Don't wait until stress has a negative impact on your health, relationships, or quality of life to start practicing a range of stress management techniques. You can start today.

You can find more information about stress management techniques in Chapter 8.

Get Adequate Sleep

This is one piece of advice that most of us would love to follow though we often struggle to do so. What isn't commonly known is that insufficient sleep is associated with many chronic diseases and conditions—such as diabetes, cardiovascular disease, obesity, and depression—which

Stressor	Examples
Environmental Stressors	Hypo- or hyper-thermic temperatures, elevated sound levels, over-illumination, overcrowding
Daily Stress Events	Traffic, lost keys, quality and quantity of physical activity
Life Changes	Divorce, death of loved ones, career change, moving homes
Workplace Stressors	High job demand vs. low job control, repeated or sustained exertions, forceful exertions, extreme postures
Chemical Stressors	Tobacco, alcohol, drugs, caffeine
Social Stressors	Social expectations, family demands, politics, required events, fun events

Figure 28. Stress is normal, but you should learn to manage your stress levels as you experience these common stressors.

threaten our nation's health. Inadequate sleep is also responsible for motor vehicle and machinery-related crashes, causing substantial injury and disability each year (Figure 30). In testing done on sleep-deprived individuals using a driving simulator, the participants often performed the same or worse than a person who was intoxicated. Some Americans have become so accustomed to functioning while sleep deprived that they don't even realize the toll it takes on their minds and bodies—it just becomes a new, riskier version of normal.

Often, this lack of sleep is self-inflicted and well within our control. How many times have you stayed up late bingeing a television series, playing a game on your laptop, or checking social media? How often have you put off writing an essay for a class until 2:00 a.m. the day it is due? You knew you would be tired the next day, but you may not have known how dangerous it might be to you or those around you. That is because many of us have allowed ourselves to accept being tired as a part of life.

Over 25% of the US population report occasionally not getting enough sleep, while nearly 10% experience chronic insomnia. However, new methods for assessing and treating sleep disorders bring hope to the millions suffering from insufficient sleep. For those of us who miss out on adequate sleep due to poor planning or poor choices, it's time for a "wake up call." Getting sufficient sleep is not a luxury—it is a necessity—and should be thought of as a "vital sign" of good health.

Avoid Tobacco

Tobacco use leads to disease and disability and harms nearly every organ of the body. More than 16 million Americans are living with a disease caused by smoking. For every death caused by smoking, at least 30 more people live with a serious smoking-related illness. Diseases like cancer, heart disease, stroke, lung diseases, diabetes, and chronic obstructive pulmonary diseases including emphysema and chronic bronchitis are just a few of the diseases caused by smoking, and the list goes on.

Smoking even causes harm to those who don't smoke. Secondhand smoke exposure contributes to approximately 41,000 deaths among nonsmoking adults and 400 deaths in infants each year (Figure 31). It increases the risk of stroke, lung cancer, and coronary heart disease in adults. Children who are exposed to secondhand smoke are at increased risk for sudden infant death syndrome, slowed lung growth, and a host of other medical issues.

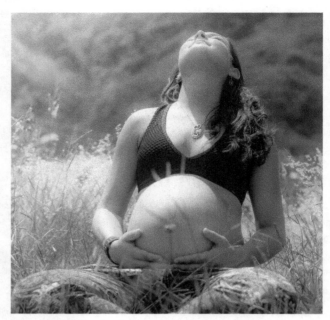

Figure 29. Meditation is just one stress management tool.

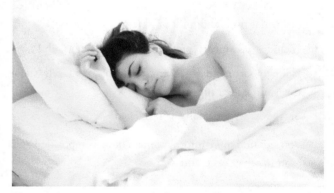

Figure 30. Not getting enough sleep can affect your health.

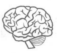 Second hand smoke impairs a child's ability to learn, and high levels of exposure are associated with deficits in reading, math, and spatial reasoning.

 Children who breathe second hand smoke are at an increased risk for ear infections.

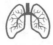 Children who breathe second hand smoke are more likely to suffer from pneumonia, bronchitis, asthma, and other lung diseases.

 Pets in smoking households have a 60% higher risk of developing lung cancer.

Figure 31. Second hand smoke affects those around you, even animals.

After Quitting for	Results
20 Minutes	Circulation improves in the hands and feet.
2 Hours	Pulse, heartbeat, and blood pressure normalize.
8 Hours	Carbon monoxide is reduced and no longer stops oxygen from reaching the blood cells.
24 Hours	Your risk of heart attack drops.
48 Hours	Nicotine is completely eliminated from your body.
1 Week	Blood pressure falls.
3 Months	On average lung capacity rises by 39 percent.
3 to 9 Months	Smokers cough and susceptibility to infections are reduced.
12 Months	The risk of cardiovascular disease is halved.
5 Years	The risk of stomach, mouth, throat, esophageal, and lung cancer is halved.
10 Years	Cell and tissue that were precancerous have largely been replaced.
15 Years	Your risk of cancer is the same amount as that of a nonsmoker.

Figure 32. The benefits of quitting smoking begin almost immediately and continue for several years.

The good news is that people who use tobacco can quit, and their body is able to recover from much of the damage, especially if a person stops using tobacco while a young adult (Figure 32).

You can find more information about the dangers of tobacco and strategies for quitting in Chapter 11.

Limit Alcohol Consumption

Excessive alcohol use, including underage drinking and binge drinking (drinking 5 or more drinks on an occasion for men or 4 or more drinks on an occasion for women), can lead to an increased risk of health problems such as injuries, violence, liver disease, and cancer. Excessive alcohol use was responsible for approximately 88,000 deaths and 2.5 million years of potential life lost (the amount of expected life left after early deaths) each year in the US from 2006–2010, shortening the lives of those who died by an average of 30 years.

In addition to injury and death, excessive alcohol use has immediate effects that increase your risk for many harmful conditions. Alcohol poisoning, violence, sexual assault or risky sex, miscarriages, pregnancy, and other problems can occur while binge drinking.

Over time, excessive alcohol use can lead to the development of chronic diseases and other serious problems including:

- High blood pressure, heart disease, stroke, liver disease, and digestive problems

- Cancer of the breast, mouth, throat, esophagus, liver, and colon

- Learning and memory problems, including dementia and poor school performance

- Mental health problems, including depression and anxiety

- Social problems, including lost productivity, family problems, and unemployment

- Alcohol dependence or alcoholism

By limiting alcohol consumption, you can reduce the risk of these short and long-term health risks. You can find more information about alcohol abuse and treatment in Chapter 11.

Protect Yourself from Infectious Diseases

Everyone is exposed to germs on a regular basis. You can't help it. Even Chuck, with his love of the indoors, will encounter them on the bags of his carry-out goodies. Some can live on surfaces like door handles and ATM buttons for up to 24 hours, making it easy for them to spread from person to person. Some may be the common cold virus, while others, like bacterial meningitis, can be dangerous and cost you a stay in the hospital or even your life.

While you may have heard that it is good to challenge your immune system on occasion, there are steps you can take to avoid being constantly bombarded by infectious agents.

Stopping the spread of disease can be as simple as regular, effective handwashing. To wash your hands adequately, follow these steps:

1. Wet your hands with running water — either warm or cold

2. Apply liquid, bar, or powder soap

3. Lather well

4. Rub your hands vigorously for at least 20 seconds

5. Remember to scrub all surfaces, including the backs of your hands, wrists, between your fingers and under your fingernails

6. Rinse well

7. Dry your hands with a clean or disposable towel or air dryer

8. If possible, use a towel or your elbow to turn off the faucet

In addition to frequent, thorough hand washing, you can often prevent illness or lessen its effects by taking good care of yourself in general. A healthy diet and adequate sleep can keep your body ready to fight what comes its way. Your body doesn't have what it takes to do the job when you're fatigued or malnourished.

Protect Yourself from Injuries

We like to think we should laugh in the face of danger – after all, we can't predict everything that can happen to us. We want to enjoy our lives. Most of us look at caution or warning signs and think, "It won't happen to me," right? Instead of considering why certain guidelines exist and being respectful of them, we take that extra step up the ladder, or stupidly dive head-first into the shallow end of the pool.

Some injuries are more avoidable than others, of course, but special attention should be paid in many situations. For example, be especially careful concerning poisonous household products, playing in or around water, prescription and over-the-counter drug storage, fire safety, motor vehicle and bicycle safety, pedestrian safety, and caring for older adults and children. And, please, listen to the warning labels. If the dosage instructions are to take two tablets of acetaminophen every 4 to 6 hours, do that rather than assuming more is better because you're 6 feet tall. If the box says to "Keep away from small children," you should probably do that — every time.

Apply Critical Thinking Skills as a Health Consumer

Many people avoid a trip to their health care provider like it's a luxury rather than a necessity, but getting regular preventative care and prompt emergency care should be part of your lifestyle. It is important to know your body's limits and understand when you need to seek professional medical help rather than waiting too long. This is an essential part of maintaining personal health and striving toward wellness. Schedule regular check-ups to find hidden problems before they begin to affect your life.

In the twenty-first century, most people who recognize a problem with their health — maybe an unexpected pain or discomfort — visit one of the many health websites on the Internet to seek advice. These websites are a great place to learn introductory information about different conditions. But they can be alarming to naïve users who go looking for the cause of the pain in their foot, and come away thinking it "could be cancer!" This jump to an extreme conclusion seems to happen all the time, and there's no wonder, since most health

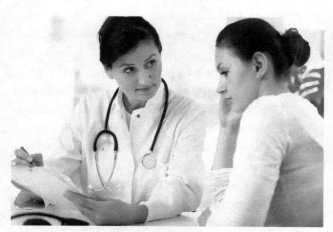

Figure 33. Always carefully consider your health care choices..

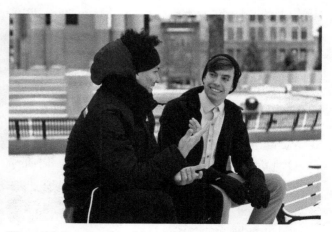

Figure 34. Fostering friendships is key to social wellness.

Isolation and Social Withdrawal	Defining spirituality as a connection to the sacred, and encouraging trauma survivors to seek supportive, healthy communities can directly address these symptoms.
Guilt and Shame	Though not part of the diagnostic criteria for PTSD, guilt and shame are recognized as important clinical issues. Spirituality may lead to self-forgiveness and an emphasis on compassion toward self.
Anger and Irritability	Beliefs and practices related to forgiveness can address anger and chronic hostile attitudes that lead to social isolation and poor relationships with others.
Hypervigilance, Anxiety, and Physiological Arousal	Inwardly-directed spiritual practices such as mindfulness, meditation, and prayer may help reduce hyperarousal.
Foreshortened Future and Loss of Interest in Activities	Rediscovery of meaning and purpose in one's life may potentially have enormous impact on these symptoms.

Figure 35. Social problems can be improved by focusing on spiritual wellness. This can have physical effects, too.

information seems so foreign to most readers. And, let's face it, everyone on the Internet has an opinion, informed or not. It's an easy trap to fall into, so thinking critically about health advice from a website should be your first line of defense against alarmist cancer fears.

You should always apply your critical thinking skills when researching health information on your own, but this same attitude is helpful when you see advertisements for prescription medication, pick up a health-related brochure, or even when speaking with a health care professional (Figure 33). You don't always need a "second opinion," but being equipped with the knowledge that other opinions are out there can be really useful when a serious situation — like high treatment costs or dangers in a procedure — comes up. Some level of critical thinking is essential in all interactions regarding our health.

Cultivate Relationships and Social Support

Consider all the songs and movies written about friendship – don't you get by with a little help from your friends? Social interactions are some of the most impactful life experiences you will have. Without overstating it, your relationships help define who you are, what your interests are, how you spend your time, and how much enjoyment you get out of life. Nourishing these relationships is a key ingredient to wellness, and represents a significant investment in your health.

Don't overlook or take for granted the people in your life who encourage you to improve and grow, show you loyalty, honesty, and companionship (Figure 34). Do the same for them in return. Responsibility to others is a mark of good citizenship, and becoming a thoughtful and involved member of your community—whatever its size—creates meaningful bonds. Those bonds may come and go, but the experience of growing together and apart is essential to being supported by and supportive of others.

Nourish Your Spiritual Side

As mentioned earlier in this chapter, spirituality takes many forms, not just religion and belief in a "higher power." The simplest way to describe spiritual wellness is an alignment between personal values and the purpose of one's life (Figure 35). The idea of spirituality is not that different today than what some in the nineteenth century called "transcendentalism," or the belief that all of humanity and nature held a divine connection. Today, we might see this universal energy as a god or deity, or we may see it as a deep understanding of our self, our values, our connection to the world and everything in it – even a higher purpose.

We often undervalue spiritual wellness because it can seem intangible and abstract. But the emotional and physical benefits we can obtain from it can be seen and experienced. Many emotional challenges occur at different points in our lives, but these can be improved if we work on this dimension.

Setting Goals and Understanding How Changes Happen

Wellness, with all its dimensions, may always be a work in progress for many of us. You may need to change certain behaviors to better strive toward wellness, and there are strategies you can use to increase your chances of success. Two of those strategies are goal-setting and becoming aware of the stages you will likely encounter as you make these changes.

Your goals should be short- and long-term. Don't be tempted to have just one humongous goal, like "lose weight," for example. Having a long-term goal is okay, but you should fill the space between the present and future with many more short-term goals that you can celebrate meeting along the way (Figure 36). Behavior change is not always an easy process and can be a bit like learning to ride a bike. You probably fell a lot when you first got on a bike. You may have even gotten scraped up pretty bad, cried, and even changed your mind about learning to ride a few times. To avoid as many of those falls as possible, you should be SMART about the goals you set.

SMART Goals

For your goals to be effective, they should represent SMART thinking. SMART goals are:

- **S—Specific**. Choose goals that target particular actions or behavior. For example, if you want to eat healthier, select a specific nutritional issue. "Eat healthier" is too general and vague. Instead, say that you will eat more vegetables or prepare more meals at home to be more specific.

- **M—Measurable**. Be sure you can measure your completion and your progress along the way. Creating a nutrition goal to eat more vegetables is specific but not measurable. Include a way to measure the amount of vegetables you eat, such as aiming for three servings per day. Establish a number for how many meals you will cook at home, such as eight per week. Chances are you won't be certain if you're meeting your goals if you're not measuring them and may be disappointed.

- **A—Achievable**. Set goals that you can actually complete. You may want to lose 20 pounds by next month, but you can't do it safely, if at all, and will be setting yourself up for failure. It's important to set meaningful goals that are within your limits in order to achieve them. As you achieve one short-term goal, you can add another. For example, Chuck once decided to become a vegetarian – cold turkey (or, better yet, tofurky)! He lasted just a few weeks before he declared it impossible. A better approach would have been to eat three servings of vegetables each day and two meatless meals a week for a few weeks, hitting several short-term goals on his way to becoming a vegetarian.

- **R—Relevant**. Set goals that are relevant to your life. Each person has different behaviors they'd like to change or goals they want to achieve based on their own needs. Make sure that the goals you set put you on a path to that change, and that meeting your goal will let you see progress. Realistic goals are all about meaning. You need to believe they are important and will have a positive impact.

- **T—Time-based**. Your goals should have a limit and be based on some kind of deadline system. Otherwise, you may never reach them. Imagine yourself as an archer with your bow and arrow. You have a target, a bullseye to hit. Aim at nothing and you may hit nothing.

We often need to make adjustments to our goals and change the plan over time. It could be that your goals need to be more challenging or more reasonable. Some goals require more lifestyle changes than others and might require more adjustments. It can help to focus on process goals (what you

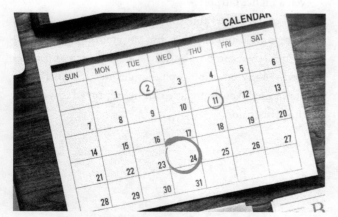

Figure 36. Smaller goals can help you avoid getting discouraged.

are doing) rather than outcome goals (where you want to be).

For example, you may initially have been trying to lose 15 pounds over a 4-month period, but it was more difficult than expected. Try focusing on process, the behaviors you need to change in order to lose the weight. Maybe one goal is to always pack your lunch for school or work so that you don't eat fast food. This process goal can help you adjust your behavior over time and reach your goal.

Keep your approach flexible. Sometimes things happen beyond our control that can force us to modify our goals. Adjust them to better suit your situation. This is fine as long as you are still progressing toward your goals. No matter what changes you may need to make along the way, SMART goals can help you stay encouraged and move forward.

Stages of Change Model

One model for how behavior change happens is the Stages of Change, or Transtheoretical model. It includes six different stages of change individuals must go through on their way to changing their behavior: pre-contemplation, contemplation, preparation, action, maintenance, and termination. The model suggests that each of us is in one of the different stages for any given behavior. It can be hard to identify whether you've actually changed your behavior or not, so this model can be helpful as you see your progress from one stage to the next. It is also helpful to identify the current stage you are in so that you can develop strategies to help you move to the next stage.

The main idea behind the Stages of Change model is that all the stages are normal parts of changing your behavior. Lapses and relapses are common. Most of the time, people don't fall all the way back to pre-contemplation from action. People can learn through their mistakes and moving through the stages can help a person know what success feels like. Even slow progress can lead to improved self-efficacy and motivation, so we shouldn't feel too discouraged with some amount of backwards movement (Figure 37).

During the **pre-contemplation** stage, you haven't thought about any changes to your behavior, but you might be noticing unpleasant feelings or conditions that could be connected to the behavior you end up changing. At this stage, you don't intend to start the healthy behavior in the near future (within 6 months), and are unaware of the need to change. You might have tried to change in the past but were unsuccessful, and you now feel frustrated or discouraged. You might be more focused on the reasons not to change than the reasons to change. You may be like Chuck, who is still parked in his recliner but is starting to notice that his energy level is deteriorating, wondering if he'll ever get to go windsurfing in Hawaii. He hasn't yet connected his feelings to a behavior, but something is starting to simmer in the back of his mind.

During the **contemplation** stage, you start to think that your behavior is problematic and that you might want to make a change in your life (within the next 6 months). You might fantasize about what that change would take or the pros and cons of making it. You might even start researching ways of taking action. No actions have happened yet, but the wheels are turning in your mind. People in this stage learn about the kind of person they could be if they changed their behavior and learn more from people who behave in healthy ways. Others can influence and help you at this stage by encouraging you to increase the list of pros and reduce the list of cons you made for changing your behavior. Chuck wants to exercise more, but he worries that it will make him even more tired. His friend, Roy, encourages him by saying that when he exercises it gives him more energy, not less.

During the **preparation** stage, you're ready to start taking action within the next 30 days. You take small steps that you believe can help make healthier behavior a part of your life. Chuck might tell his friends and family that he wants to be more active and has started doing a bit of research on diet and exercise. People in this stage should be encouraged to seek support from friends they trust, tell people about their plan to

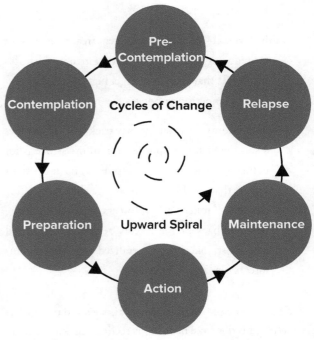

Figure 37. Every behavioral change goes through stages.

change the way they act, and think about how they would feel if they behaved in a healthier way. Their number one concern is: when they act, will they fail? They learn that the better prepared they are, the more likely they are to keep progressing.

During the **action** stage, you have changed your behavior within the last 6 months and need to work hard to keep moving ahead. Above all, you need to learn how to strengthen your commitments to change and to fight urges to slip back. People in this stage progress by learning techniques for keeping up their commitments, such as replacing activities related to the unhealthy behavior with more positive ones, rewarding themselves for taking steps toward changing, and avoiding people and situations that tempt them to behave in unhealthy ways:

Self-Management — Employment of behavior analytic interventions to the behavior of oneself; requires the desired change in the behavior

Self-Monitoring — Procedure in which a person observes his/her own behavior systematically and records occurrence or nonoccurrence of behavior

Self-Instruction — Self generated verbal responses, covert or overt, that function as response prompts for desired behavior; often used to guide a person through a behavior change

Massed Practice — Forcing oneself to perform an undesired behavior repeatedly; occasionally this strategy may decrease behavior

Habit Reversal — A multi-component treatment package for reducing unwanted habits that involves identifying events that precede a target behavior and engaging in competing responses

Token Economy — A contingency package that includes a specified list of responses to reinforce, tokens for exhibiting the specified responses, back-up reinforcers that can be purchased with the token; effectiveness of tokens as reinforcers depends upon the power of back-up reinforcers; response cost is used with most; tokens are generalized conditioned reinforcers for target responses

Chuck has been taking brisk walks each day and has been letting his dog take naps in his recliner, making it more

difficult to get comfortable in it. He has bought a Hawaiian shirt as a reward for positive behavior and is saving his money for a vacation to Maui.

During the **maintenance** stage, you changed your behavior at least 6 months ago. You have to be aware of situations that may tempt you to slip back into doing the unhealthy behavior — particularly stressful situations. The maintenance stage never ends for some people. They have to continually choose to engage in healthy behaviors. People in this stage benefit when they seek support from friends and talk with people they trust, spend time with people who behave in healthy ways, and engage in healthy activities to cope with stress. Chuck walks his dog with a neighbor every day, practices surfing balance techniques when he watches TV, and swims laps at the pool 3 days a week. He watches airline prices every week for a cheap ticket to Maui.

Termination is the sixth stage that may be reached. This is where people have exited the cycle of change and are no longer tempted to fall into their old behavior. They have developed ways of coping with behaviors and mastered those mechanisms. This may or may not be possible with certain behaviors. Chuck knows his weaknesses. He has replaced his favorite recliner with a chair that is comfortable enough to watch a bit of television from but not comfy enough for meals and naps. Now instead of burrowing into his recliner with a large bag of candy when he's stressed, he goes for a run with his dog, watches just one old episode of *The Three Stooges*, or calls up a friend to go have coffee. The trip to Maui last fall was a blast, and he has the photos to prove it. He now tries to plan at least one trip every year.

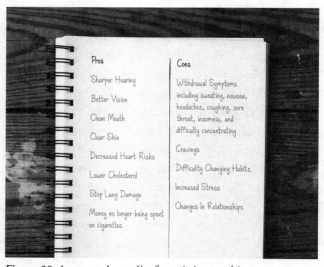

Figure 38. A pros and cons list for quitting smoking.

Relapse is not necessarily a stage in itself, but is a return from the action or maintenance stages to an earlier stage. The word "relapse" is most often associated with addictive behaviors, but is very common in other unhealthy behaviors, as well. A long-term behavior change often requires ongoing support from family members, a health coach, a health care provider, supportive literature, or another motivational source.

Decisional Balance and Self Efficacy

It's common for humans to evaluate important things and large decisions based on their merits. This is true with behaviors as well. Individuals go through a process known as decisional balance, where they weigh the pros and cons of the change (Figure 38). The balance factor of this process is how the number or importance of pros and cons must shift over time as a person gets closer to changing their behavior. The cons of changing outweigh the pros in the pre-contemplation stage. The pros meet or surpass the cons in the middle stages. The pros outweigh the cons in the action stage. Think about how Chuck adjusted his pros and cons.

Your self-efficacy is your belief in your own ability to succeed in certain situations or under certain influences that may or may not be within your control. This can impact how we approach behavior change and the goals we've set for ourselves. We measure our self-efficacy by how confident we are in high-risk situations that may trigger relapse or present temptation to veer away from our goals.

Let's say, for example, that you are trying to lose weight. Your sister Karen is coming to visit. The two of you typically spend your time trying out new bars and restaurants in Portland and making late-night runs to Voodoo Doughnut. This presents some serious temptation. Your level of confidence that you can keep your calorie intake reasonable is your degree of self-efficacy.

During the first two stages of change, pre-contemplation and contemplation, the temptation to relapse may be stronger than our ability to refrain from the negative behavior. While we are in the preparation stage and moving to the action stage, the gap between temptation and feelings of self-efficacy closes, and we make a behavior change. Relapse occurs when your self-efficacy is not as great as the temptation in front of you.

Motivation

Motivation is the reason someone has for acting or behaving a certain way or their desire to complete the action. People who decide to make a behavioral change must be motivated to do so by something in their life. That motivation to change can come from yourself or from others. The source of your motivation can impact your decision making. Internal motivation can be more personally fulfilling, but it lacks the accountability that an external motivation source can provide (e.g., your health care provider asking if you've been eating better or your trainer measuring your percentage of body fat).

Your motivation is often impacted by whether you believe you have control over your behavior or not. If you believe you have control over your personal outcomes, it is known as an **internal locus of control** (control is located inside you). An internal locus suggests changes occur as a result of effort on your part, and your commitment to change will result in positive changes.

If you believe your ability to change is out of your control, it is known as an **external locus of control** (control is outside

Internal — **Locus of Control** — **External**

The consequences of my behavior are under my control	The consequences of my behavior are outside my control
Better academic achievement	Resigned to conditions "as they are"
Better interpersonal relations	Lower efforts to deal with health
Greater efforts to learn	Change only happens through luck
Positive attitudes to exercise	Lower sense of satisfaction
Lower cigarette smoking	Pessimism about improvement

Figure 39. Internal and external locus of control.

of you). People with an external locus believe any behavioral change can only result from luck or chance. People who believe they control changes to their behavior (internal) are more likely to pursue those changes than people who think they have no control over their behavior (Figure 39).

Be honest with yourself – this can often help you find an internal locus of control. People are great at making excuses for why they can't make a change or find reasons why their problem is caused by someone or something else. Let's face it—it's easier that way. It's much harder to admit the reality that you haven't yet chosen your health as a priority over the gratification you gain from a particular behavior.

For example, it's easy to say that you can't lose weight because the people around you aren't helping. But maybe if you tracked what you ate during the day, you would find that you consumed way more than what is recommended for healthy weight loss. Yes, it's often true that weight loss is more difficult for some people than others due to their gender, a genetic predisposition, or environmental factors.

But people in those situations can still set realistic goals that they can achieve.

For most people, it comes down to honesty and acceptance of their unique reality. Be honest with yourself about your limitations and strengths and what that means for you as you are setting goals.

Consider all the things you could gain by achieving your goals compared to the things you may be missing out on by staying the same. Is the candy you snacked on last night or the pack of cigarettes you smoked yesterday worth lost years with your family? Do you want to look back on your life and wonder if you could have controlled your behavior, or do you want to do something about it now? Do you believe that you are responsible for changing your behavior? If the answer is yes, then you believe you have the power to make positive changes, an internal locus, that can help you as you work toward your goals. Chuck found his internal locus and so can you.

Conclusion

This introductory chapter gives you some critical tools and techniques to learn about public and personal health. We described:

- Definitions of health and wellness dimensions that prepare you to discuss health topics with a community and individual scope
- Challenges to public and personal health as defined by health agency guidelines
- Objectives of several public health initiatives to improve public health and quality of life
- Basic frameworks for assessing your fitness and health status
- SMART goals to help you improve your health status
- Stages of Change model of behavior modification

As you can see from this chapter, learning about health and fitness is not just about defining the terms health scientists use to talk about their field, but applying those terms to your own life to improve your own health. The best thing about studying health and wellness is that it can make an actual difference in people's lives. The following chapters each focus on particular improvement areas, encourage assessment along with SMART goal setting and planning, and recommend training for each area.

Reflection Questions

1. How has the definition of "health" evolved over the years?

2. What is an example of how one dimension of wellness can influence another dimension?

3. Which dimension of wellness do you see the greatest strengths in at this point in your life? Which dimension of wellness would you develop more?

4. What is the difference between life expectancy and healthy life expectancy?

5. What are some of the differences between the leading causes of death between men and women in the US?

6. What is a health disparity? Identify a health disparity that concerns you and explain your reasoning.

7. What is the purpose of Healthy People 2020?

8. Identify one of the areas targeted in Healthy People 2020. What impact do you think this area has on health in the US?

9. Identify a dimension of wellness you would like to improve and select a specific target behavior. What are some SMART goals for the behavior you have selected?

10. What are the stages in the Stages of Change model?

11. Why is self-efficacy an important aspect of behavior change?

12. What is the difference between internal and external locus of control? Do you think your locus of control tends to be internal or external? Do you notice that it changes depending on the situation?

Chapter 2
Fitness and Exercise

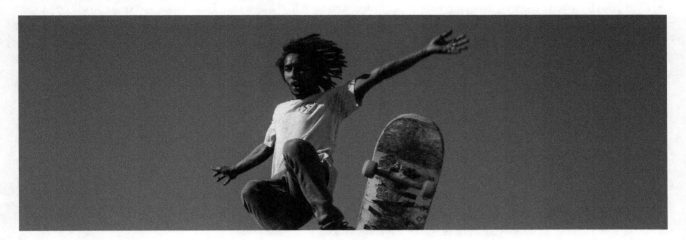

Learning Objectives

1. Describe how much physical activity is recommended for developing health and fitness.

2. Identify the health-related components of physical fitness and the way each component affects wellness.

3. Describe the principles involved in designing a well-rounded exercise program.

4. Discuss the steps that can be taken to make an exercise program safe, effective, and successful.

5. Explain the best ways to prevent weather-related exercise injuries.

One of the most important aspects of health and wellness is fitness. Fitness is one of the components of the physical dimension of wellness, and several chapters in this book address how fitness plays a role in other dimensions of wellness. Most Americans today begin learning the importance of physical fitness as early as elementary school, yet many of us are not fit and not doing enough to meet the recommended levels of physical activity established by the US Department of Health and Human Services.

In the past, physical fitness was frequently part of the work that people did for their jobs. Today, fitness is something we usually need to make time for. Technological advancements have erased the physical aspect of work for many people, as productivity, communication, and many other areas of work become digitized or automated. If you think about it, many Americans cruise through life from behind a computer screen or from a smartphone in the palm of their hand.

This chapter will define and explain the differences between fitness, physical activity, and exercise and show why it is important to implement a fitness plan. You will also learn how to create a safe, effective exercise plan. A lifestyle that includes physical activity can have a positive impact on social, intellectual, emotional, and physical wellness that can improve your overall quality of life.

What Does It Mean to Be Fit?

Fitness is the ability to conduct your daily life without undue fatigue. When you are young and naturally more active, you rarely think about your energy after tying your shoes or walking up a flight of stairs. Things like that never made you tired. But as you get older or you become less physically active, the fatigue that can come from these simple tasks might surprise you (Figure 1). Climbing stairs, doing laundry, shopping, or playing with your children and pets should be easy, but for many Americans with a sedentary lifestyle, routine physical activity can become a struggle, even something to dread.

Fitness enables you to do the things you want to do without worrying about being too tired. It sounds easy – maybe you would already call yourself "fit." But consider what might happen if what you want to do and what you're able to do don't quite align. Imagine that you've arranged to take a vacation to Arizona. The first day, your family decides to go on a walking tour of Phoenix, but you know you won't be able to keep up with the group. You decide to skip it. You spend your afternoon playing Sudoku on your phone in the hotel lobby. The next day, they book a bus tour to the balancing rocks of the Chiricahua mountains. You ride along, but when it's time to hike through the misty rock fields, you stay on the bus and resume your Sudoku. At the end of the trip, you're late for your flight, and everyone must run to get to the gate in time. Can you make it?

True fitness is really a type of freedom. It means you have more energy and agility and fewer physical limitations (Figure 2). It means being able to go where you want as fast and as far as you want or need to.

Defining Fitness

The freedom that comes with fitness starts with an understanding of how movement affects your body. We commonly use the terms, "physical activity," "exercise," and "physical fitness" as if they are the same, but the terms are not interchangeable. Students of health need to know the difference.

Physical activity is any body movement that expends energy. Just getting through your day requires physical activity. This could be as gentle as walking to class, pulling weeds in your garden, or brushing your teeth. It could be as intense as running a half-marathon, biking to work, shoveling snow, or swimming laps in the pool at your gym. Different activities have a different activity level, defined by the amount of energy the activity requires. For example, you will expend more energy swimming laps than while planting flowers.

The energy is measured by calories, which are units of heat that are burned during our movements. The number of calories burned varies based on the intensity of the activity and on each person's physical makeup (Figure 3). Swimming at high intensity for ten minutes would result in more energy spent than if you tread water for the same amount of time. Additionally, someone with greater muscle mass may burn more calories during the same swim.

We often think that if we are busy during the day, then we are "getting exercise," particularly if the activity makes

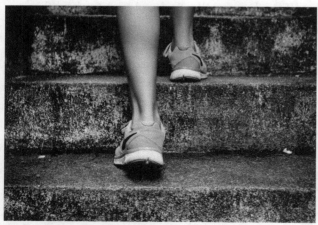

Figure 1. Staying fit means regular physical activity.

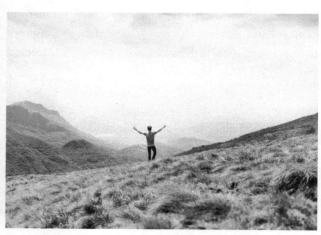

Figure 2. Some people find freedom through fitness.

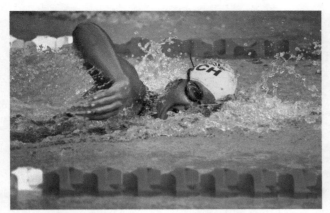

Figure 3. Physical activity can take many different forms.

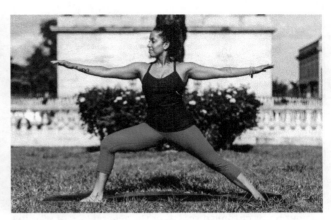

Figure 4. Be sure to choose activities you enjoy.

us tired. Most of our routine physical activities, however, are considered "baseline" rather than "health-enhancing." As we move around doing dishes, folding clothes, or walking the occasional flight of stairs, we are participating in baseline activities that will burn fewer calories than the health-enhancing ones we perform when we exercise.

Exercise is sustained and planned physical activity that results in improvements to your fitness. You may engage in a great deal of physical activity in your day-to-day life. This is great and certainly much better than nothing, but it may not have the same impact on your health as an exercise routine. A routine might include walking, running, swimming, aerobics, or weight training. As long as it's sustained, it's exercise. These activities have regular sessions, adjustable goals, and intervals, all of which are the result of a plan. A pizza delivery job may keep you moving from place to place rather than sitting, but your day-to-day physical activity is probably not intense enough to count as real exercise, so it doesn't contribute significantly to your physical fitness.

Physical fitness is the result of planned exercise. It is a set of attributes we obtain related to health, many of which can be measured. Our cardiorespiratory (heart and lung) endurance, muscular endurance, muscle strength, flexibility, and body composition (weight and body fat percentage) can all be assessed and evaluated to determine just how fit we are and what we need to do to improve our fitness and overall health. Each of these areas of fitness are covered in much more detail in Chapters 3, 4, 5, and 6.

Benefits of Physical Fitness

People have praised the numerous benefits that consistent exercise has on our health for many years. This can be seen throughout western history, but it wasn't until the 1950s that we had the scientific data to prove what we seem to have known for so long—maintaining a healthy fitness level helps us physically and psychologically.

According to the Centers for Disease Control (CDC), one of the greatest physical benefits of exercise is lowering your risk of developing chronic diseases. About half of all Americans are living with at least one chronic disease, such as Type 2 diabetes, heart disease, stroke, high blood pressure, and osteoporosis. These issues can often be lessened or avoided if a person is physically fit. You can find more information about chronic disease in Chapter 1 and Chapter 9.

Some of the less obvious benefits might surprise you. For example, exercise reduces our risk of developing Alzheimer's disease, reduces symptoms of premenstrual syndrome, and even helps women manage menopausal symptoms. Even the risk of developing colon, breast, and endometrial cancer can be reduced. The bike ride you take in the morning, the run with your dog after dinner, and the time you spend on the yoga mat trying to achieve the perfect warrior pose all help to strengthen your bones and muscles, improve your stamina, control your weight, and increase your life expectancy (Figure 4).

Regular exercise helps your mental health, as well. We tend to sleep better after regular exercise,. and improvements to mood and self-confidence lower the risk of depression and anxiety. Even in people who suffer from these mental health issues, exercise can help make their symptoms more manageable. It even improves cognition, helping our ability to learn, think critically and creatively, and make decisions sharply. Think about the times in your life you've been sick. The lack of energy, fatigue, mental fogginess, and side effects of taking cold or flu medicines tend to have a negative impact on your mood, right? The same things can result from excess weight

Mental	Physical
Fights depression	Lowers cholesterol levels
Relieves stress	Builds stronger bones, joints, and ligaments
Boosts confidence	Boosts energy levels
Improves memory	Improves sleeping habits
Lengthens attention span	Postpones fatigue

Figure 5. Exercise has many mental and physical benefits.

Activity Levels Based on Steps Per Day	
Steps Per Day	**Lifestyle Activity Level**
Under 5000	Sedentary
5000 to 7499	Low Active
7500 to 9999	Somewhat Active
10000 to 12499	Active
More than 12500	Highly Active

Figure 6. Step trackers help you determine your activity level.

on your body, chronic diseases, or the general lack of stamina related to poor physical fitness. It can feel similar to being sick, or even worse. It's no wonder that we are happier when we are fit.

Scientists continue to research the nature and significance of the benefits of physical activity and exercise. We're still learning about the full impact on different health concerns, both physical and mental. It's a safe bet at this point that, with the information currently available, future studies will likely show even more benefits to fitness (Figure 5).

How Much Exercise Do You Need?

In their 2008 Physical Activity Guidelines, the US Department of Health and Human Services (DHHS) recommends adults complete a minimum of 150 minutes of moderate-intensity physical activity or 75 minutes of vigorous-intensity physical activity. This should be done each week to experience health benefits. Studies suggest that the benefits increase as the minutes increase. The greatest possible improvements are seen when a person goes from sedentary to active.

Individuals focused on weight loss or wanting additional fitness in general should increase to 300 minutes of moderate-intensity activity or 150 minutes of vigorous-intensity (or a combination of both). The DHHS strongly promotes adding muscle-strengthening activities of moderate or high intensity at least two days per week to improve results even more. More information on muscular endurance is available in Chapter 4.

One way to gauge your activity level is by steps per day (Figure 6). Are you sedentary? Active? Pull that smartphone out of your pocket for a moment. It has probably been tracking your steps and is ready to tell you just what category you fall into.

Children and adolescents today have it better and worse than past generations. The increase in technology-based forms of play and social communication has enabled and encouraged many young people to maintain a more sedentary lifestyle. They don't have to leave the house, or even their bedroom,

to spend time with their friends. We also see many public schools moving to shorter recesses and less physical education (in some states) to allow more classroom time. We may be raising a generation at higher risk for chronic diseases, and at younger ages than ever before.

The good news is that young people today are still being encouraged to join sports, dance, gymnastics, and many other competitive programs. This, too, is happening at younger ages and with greater variety and better access to these programs across the country.

The DHHS Physical Activity Guidelines recommend at least 60 minutes of physical activity each day for people under 18 years. This should include aerobic activity of moderate- or vigorous-intensity, muscle-strengthening, and bone-strengthening at least 3 days each week. Muscle-strengthening activities can be unstructured, like climbing on playground equipment or playing tug-of-war, or they can be structured, like weight lifting or resistance training. Bone-strengthening activities put force on the bones to encourage growth and strength. Running, jumping, and sports like tennis, football, and basketball all meet this standard. Any activities of this nature during the day count toward the minimum 60 minutes.

Senior citizens have their own set of challenges as well. Medical improvements have led to older people living longer than previous generations. This is great, of course, but it can be especially difficult for older adults to stay healthy and maintain a good quality of life. Physical activity plays a large role in this. Inactivity at this age can begin a downward slide in abilities that can be difficult to reverse. Older adults vary widely in the level of deterioration of their bodies, affecting what they are capable of doing. Most people over 65 years have at least one chronic condition, making regular exercise even harder.

The DHHS Physical Activity Guidelines for adults over 65 years are the same as for other adults as far as aerobic and muscle-strengthening exercises, with the added category of balance training activities. Older adults are more at risk for

	Key Guidelines for Health	Additional Benefits	Additional Exercise
Children and Adolescents	Most of the 60 or more minutes per day should be either moderate- or vigorous-intensity aerobic physical activity and should include vigorous-intensity physical activity at least 3 days per week.	It is important to encourage young people to participate in physical activities that are appropriate for their age, that are enjoyable, and that offer variety.	As part of their 60 or more minutes of daily physical activity, children and adolescents should include muscle-strengthening physical activity on at least 3 days per week.
Adults	For substantial health benefits, adults should do at least 150 minutes (2 hours and 30 minutes) a week of moderate-intensity, or 75 minutes (1 hour and 15 minutes) a week of vigorous-intensity aerobic physical activity, or an equivalent combination of moderate- and vigorous intensity aerobic activity.	For additional and more extensive health benefits, adults should increase their aerobic physical activity to 300 minutes (5 hours) per week of moderate intensity, or 150 minutes per week of vigorous intensity aerobic physical activity, or an equivalent combination of moderate- and vigorous-intensity activity.	Adults should also do muscle-strengthening activities that are moderate or high intensity and involve all major muscle groups on 2 or more days per week.
Older Adults	When older adults cannot do 150 minutes of moderate-intensity aerobic activity per week because of chronic conditions, they should be as physically active as their abilities and conditions allow.	Older adults should do exercises that maintain or improve balance.	Older adults with chronic conditions should understand whether and how their conditions affect their ability to do regular physical activity safely.

Figure 7. Exercise guidelines change based on age. Additional exercise can provide additional benefits for most people.

injuries from falling than any other demographic. Their bones are more brittle than younger people, so even a small accident can result in a serious injury (e.g. hip fractures) that could potentially have irreversible effects.

Balance exercises include walking on your toes and heels, walking backwards and side-to-side, and standing from a sitting position. This might sound pretty easy, but seniors may need to begin doing these activities with assistance before they can progress to doing them unsupported.

The sooner in life you begin making true physical fitness a priority, the better. Yes, it is true that some exercise is always better than none. However, the guidelines suggest that we don't see and feel significant results until we are consistently meeting or surpassing the recommended minutes for physical activity (Figure 7).

Now that you have a better understanding of what we consider "exercise" vs. "physical activity," let's get back to

tracking those steps for a moment. There is recent emphasis on the importance of moving throughout the day, not just during an exercise session, so we don't want to downplay it. You may have noticed that many of our "smart" devices—our phones, watches, and even special gadgets we wear like bracelets—now also function as pedometers that track how many steps we take, miles we walk, or flights of stairs we climb during the day. These can be used to track activity both when we are exercising and as we are moving during our daily activities, helping us avoid being sedentary for too long. Healthy adults can reasonably target 8,000–10,000 steps each day.

Tracking your steps can be especially helpful if you are time-constrained and are trying to build more physical activity into your lifestyle. Determine how many steps you normally take, and then try increasing your step count by about 500 to 1000 every few weeks to safely make progress.

The Health-Related Components of Exercise

There are many types of exercises, each with distinct benefits and guidelines. The types you choose to do should be enjoyable to you, but they should also push you to improve. This progressive thinking appears differently in different types of exercise, so look at later chapters for more detailed information on each type.

Cardiorespiratory exercise moves your large muscles for a sustained period and gets your heart pumping at a faster rate. This strengthens your cardiorespiratory system, which is really a couple of systems that work together — the cardiovascular and respiratory systems, which include the heart, lungs, and blood vessels. Over time, the heart is able to pump more blood with each beat and your resting heart rate often lowers. The lungs become more efficient, taking in more oxygen with each breath and increasing their ability to deliver oxygen and remove carbon dioxide in the blood.

Your heart rate should be elevated for at least ten minutes during this type of exercise to be most effective. Ideally, your 150 minutes of cardiorespiratory exercise will be 20–60 minutes per day, 3–5 days per week, depending upon intensity. Many common exercises are aerobic (Figure 8).

Any combination of moderate- and vigorous-intensity exercise is helpful. You may choose to bike for 40 minutes one day and swim laps for 20 minutes the next day. Maybe your dog looks forward to his 30-minute run every morning and his brisk, 20-minute walk after dinner. No matter the exercise, a good rule to remember is to consider two minutes of moderate activity as the equivalent of one minute of vigorous activity. Short on time? Consider increasing the intensity to compensate if your fitness level and ability allows.

So how do we determine if an activity is light, moderate, or vigorous? We measure it. **Absolute intensity** refers to the amount of energy expended per minute during the activity. Vigorous activity uses 6 times the amount of energy that you expend when you are at rest, moderate 3.0–5.9 times, and light 1.1–2.9 times.

A simpler way to determine intensity is by measuring **relative intensity**. Moderate intensity exercise, to a fit person, may qualify as vigorous intensity for someone who is not regularly active. You can estimate relative intensity using a scale of 0–10. Zero is at rest and 10 is the maximum level of effort we are capable of. Moderate intensity would be approximately a 5 or 6 on this scale, and vigorous intensity would be a 7 or 8.

Your friend Kendal is a track star who can run a 6-minute mile without breaking a heavy sweat. It is moderate to her. She might rate her relative intensity as a 5. You, on the other hand, find that running a mile in just 6 minutes requires vigorous activity. It causes you to exert much more effort than you are used to. By the end, you are breathing heavy, your heart is racing, and your legs feel like rubber. You might rate your relative intensity as an 8 or 9. Regular exercise from training to run on a track team like Kendal, has increased her cardiorespiratory fitness to the point where a mile is literally no sweat. For more information on cardiorespiratory fitness see Chapter 3.

Muscle strengthening and endurance activities that are moderate or high intensity should be done two or more days each week. **Muscular strength** refers to your muscles' ability to exert force against resistance — how much weight you can lift, for example. **Muscular endurance** refers to the length of time the muscle can sustain or repeat the action (Figure 9).

The goal in muscle strengthening and endurance is to

Moderate Intensity		Vigorous Intensity	
Walking briskly (3 mph or faster but not race-walking)	200 cal/hr	Running	600–1000 cal/hr
Water aerobics	250–300 cal/hr	Swimming laps	400–700 cal/hr
Tennis (doubles)	280 cal/hr	Aerobics	350–500 cal/hr
Bicycling (10 mph or less)	400 cal/hr	Tennis (singles)	500–600 cal/hr
Ballroom dancing	200–400 cal/hr	Bicycling (over 10 mph)	500–800 cal/hr
General gardening	200–400 cal/hr	Heavy gardening (continuous digging/hoeing with elevated heart rate)	400–600 cal/hr
Race-walking, jogging, or running	300 cal/hr	Hiking (uphill or with heavy backpack)	500– cal/hr

Figure 8. Physical activity guidelines for different exercises from the DHHS.

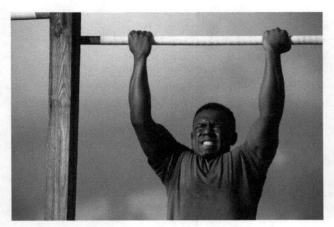

Figure 9. Pull-ups test muscular endurance.

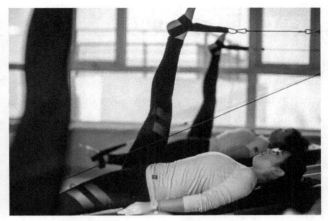

Figure 10. Some exercises require good flexibility.

challenge your muscles, particularly the major muscle groups (chest, arms, legs, abdomen, shoulders, back, and hips), at times pushing them beyond what they are used to. To do this, you should repeat the muscle movement until you reach a point where you think you can't do another repetition. The next time you exercise that muscle, you should be able to do at least one more repetition, getting better each time. Good examples of activities that strengthen muscles include working with weights or resistance bands, doing calisthenics, or using your body for resistance (e.g. push-ups and pull-ups). For more information about muscle strength and endurance, see Chapter 4.

Flexibility is the capacity of a joint or muscle to reach the full extent of its range of motion. These types of activities are an important part of any exercise program. Certain physical activities require a person to be more flexible and have a greater range of motion than others. This can be very helpful in certain professions and hobbies where your ability to bend and move is important to your performance. Athletes and dancers obviously need to be flexible, but so do firefighters and house painters, who often stretch to get the job done. Many jobs call for more flexibility than you might imagine. Ask your Aunt Marge, a pre-school teacher, how many times she gets up and down off the floor or bends over to tie a tiny shoe during the day.

Your job and hobbies may not be physically demanding, but the ability to reach that upper cabinet in your kitchen, touch your toes, or get up off the ground without hanging on to a chair can contribute to your overall quality of life, particularly as you age. The American College of Sports Medicine recommends doing flexibility exercises (e.g. stretching or lunges) two or more days each week. For variety, consider activities such as yoga or Pilates, which also work your muscles

and improve your balance at the same time they improve your flexibility (Figure 10). For more information on flexibility, see Chapter 5.

Body composition, the relative amounts of muscle, fat, bone and other vital body tissues, plays an important role in our exercise goals. Body composition is one of the indicators used to assess fitness level and health risk. As you will read in Chapter 6, the amount of fat on your body impacts how your body functions, as well as your life expectancy.

The next three chapters in this book focus on how well you can move your body and how well our internal organs and bodily systems function, but they all relate in some way to body composition. The frequency, intensity, time, and type of your exercises—the FITT formula, featured in each chapter on fitness—may change based on your body composition. Each fitness component is measurable and can be targeted different ways, depending on your goals, interests, and abilities.

Your Aunt Marge, for example, has recently had her percentage of body fat measured and learned that it is too high for good health. She knew this, however, even before the trainer measured it. She had been having trouble keeping up with the preschoolers she teaches and was getting fatigued much easier than she used to. She knew she had gained some weight, but it wasn't until one of the adorable little cherubs at the preschool asked her if she was having a baby (she isn't) that she realized her weight had gotten a bit out of hand (it had). Don't you love the honesty of children? Marge added more aerobic exercise—and a bit of yoga for strength, balance, and flexibility—to her daily activities to start lowering her body composition. She also assessed her nutrition to identify possible areas of improvement. For more information on nutrition, see Chapter 7.

Are You Fit Enough?

Aunt Marge makes it sound easy, but the hard reality is that this kind of change is tough for most people to do. Unfortunately, most people in the US don't meet the recommended amounts of activity or exercise. According to the CDC, only 20 percent of adults meet the federal recommendations for both aerobic and muscle strengthening activity, though nearly half meet the guidelines for aerobic alone. This number is slightly higher among people aged 18–24 at close to 60 percent meeting aerobic guidelines, but it declines gradual-

ly with the age of the population. Among college students, approximately 46% meet the aerobic guidelines. Women are even less likely to meet the guidelines than men of their same age.

Though some of the statistics seem a bit bleak, the CDC's data shows that the numbers have risen since the federal guidelines were updated, indicating that we are doing better. Over the last few years, however, the numbers have been fairly stagnant, suggesting our progress as a nation has begun to slow.

Improving Your Fitness

So, what can you do to avoid being part of the population that isn't physically fit? The data is clear and the information is at your fingertips. You now know that fitness can help you avoid chronic diseases and improve your quality of life. You just need to take the necessary steps to be on the positive side of the statistics. To do this, it is important to assess your current level of fitness, plan your improvements, and follow a training program.

Assessing Your Current Activity Level

You must first assess your current activity level and set goals for improvements. There are a few common methods for assessing your cardiorespiratory fitness level and establishing a baseline from which to plan, such as the **Physical Activity Readiness Questionnaire** (PAR-Q).

The PAR-Q helps you determine any risk factors that may need to be discussed with your health care provider prior to beginning an exercise program or physical assessment. It presents a series of questions related to how you feel when you exercise, your medical history, medications, and general questions about your lifestyle. This should be done first to rule out any issues that could arise during physical activity. Individuals with chronic pain or injuries (such as back or knee problems), illness or diseases (such as heart disease or high blood pressure), who are pregnant, or who experience pain or dizziness during exercise are examples of those who may need medical clearance before beginning an exercise program. A sample PAR-Q form can be found on pages 36-37.

Fitness-Related Goals

Setting goals is an important step when developing a fitness plan. These goals can involve improvement to health or skill. The Surgeon General states that while many Americans often begin an exercise program with excitement and good intentions, they frequently abandon their efforts. How many times have you decided to get up early to exercise before work and found yourself hitting the snooze button on your alarm? Or maybe you set a goal of completing a two-mile run each day only to realize that you didn't have the stamina (you hadn't even walked briskly in several months) and ended up consoling yourself with a cold bowl of ice cream and a warm bath. Setting SMART

goals (specific, measurable, achievable, relevant, and time bound) that fit with your lifestyle and current fitness level can help you avoid this pitfall, helping you stay encouraged and keeping you focused. For more information on SMART goals, see Chapter 1.

Goals for Improved Health

We discussed in Chapter 1 how important it is to set goals, without which we may never see significant improvements. Health-related goals can be measured in 5 areas—improvements in cardiorespiratory health, muscular endurance, muscular strength, flexibility, and body composition.

You've already learned a few of the many significant benefits to improving your cardiorespiratory health. You can measure your cardiorespiratory capacity using a test like the Rockport Walking Test, and set a goal that directly affects your health (see Chapter 3). You can see the benefits and adjust your goals each time you perform at a more intense level, such as running farther or faster.

The same applies to muscular endurance and strength. You can assess these initially by seeing how much weight you can lift, how many repetitions you can complete, or how long you can run (see Chapter 4). Then you can set SMART goals and reassess along the way. The same is true with body composition—the amount of fat your body has in comparison to the amount of muscle and bone (see Chapter 6)—and with the flexibility of your muscles and joints (see Chapter 5). For many of us, our health-related goals are even more specific. We may want to lower our blood pressure, improve our cholesterol levels, or decrease your blood-sugar, all things that can be measured and improved with goals adapted to suit our current needs.

Goals for Improved Skills

In addition to the more obvious health benefits, improvements to your skill levels can be valuable in your day-to-day life. Setting goals in this area could lead to a real difference in how you function. They might include improvements in:

- **Agility**—your ability to change positions quickly
- **Balance**—your ability to maintain equilibrium
- **Coordination**—your ability to conduct physical tasks smoothly
- **Power**—your ability to use force based on strength and speed
- **Reaction time**—your ability to respond quickly to a given situation
- **Speed**—your ability to move within a certain period of time

Most skill improvements can be measured, particularly if part of a sport. A high jumper, for example, can accurately gauge progress in the power of their vertical leap (Figure 11). However, a person will most likely notice the change in how they are able to move and respond when presented with daily tasks. Remember the vacation to Arizona we imagined earlier

in the chapter? A stronger cardiorespiratory system certainly helps you catch that flight you were about to miss, but so does your speed and response time. That hike to balancing rocks your family wanted to take? Your agility, balance, and coordination skills help you navigate that uneven terrain. Your life starts to become more manageable and enjoyable with improvements in these areas. Your lifestyle, age, current fitness level, and how you need or want to use your body will help you determine what goals you set. Keeping them SMART will keep them reasonable and you'll be more likely to achieve them.

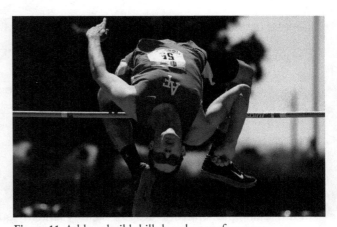

Figure 11. Athletes build skills based on performance of a particular task.

Creating a Fitness Plan

Your fitness plan should be concerned with helping you meet your goals. One prominent type of fitness plan is the **FITT Principle**. FITT stands for Frequency, Intensity, Time, and Type, which focus on exercise strategies:

Frequency refers to how often a particular physical activity is completed. Completing a cardiorespiratory activity at least 3 times each week can condition your body and reduce the risk of injury and excess fatigue from exercise. For strengthening and flexibility exercises, such as weight lifting, 2 to 3 days per week is a good guideline.

ARE YOU READY FOR EXERCISE?

Physical activity and exercise have several benefits to individuals' health and wellness. Some of those benefits include improved cardiorespiratory function, decreased risk for chronic diseases, effective weight management, and improved body strength and capabilities.

If you are healthy, there is no reason to consider physical activity and exercise to be negative for your health because most exercise activities are safe and effective. However, before you start a physical activity and exercise program, you should evaluate your medical history. If any health problems or concerns are identified, it is advised that you consult with your doctor before participating in any type of exercise.

Read each statement and select the appropriate answer.

	Yes	No
I have been diagnosed with a heart disease.		
I have experienced chest pain during times of rest.		
I have experienced pain in my chest, neck, jaw, or arms during physical activity.		
I have high blood pressure.		
I have experienced dizziness or loss of consciousness.		
I have asthma.		
I have diabetes.		
I have arthritis.		
I have experienced shortness of breath with mild exertion, when resting, or when lying down.		
I have lower back pain.		
I have a bone, joint, or muscle injury.		
I experience lower leg pain when I walk.		
I am taking prescriptions drugs that may limit my activity.		
I have a medical reason not to exercise.		

If you selected yes for any of the statements, you should talk with your doctor before you engage in a physical activity or exercise program. If you selected no for each of the statements, you can start participating in a physical activity or exercise program. Remember to start slowly and increase the time and intensity gradually, as needed, or as recommended by your doctor or fitness trainer.

Most health experts suggest that you consult with your doctor before participating in a physical activity or exercise program if any of the following apply

- You have a heart condition
- You have asthma
- You have diabetes
- You have arthritis
- You are obese
- You have any signs or symptoms of heart or other condition that might be serious, including
  - Pain in your chest, neck, jaw, or arms when exercising
  - You have experienced fainting or dizziness when exercising
  - You experience shortness of breath when resting, lying down, or with mild exertion
  - You have an irregular heartbeat
  - You have high blood pressure or high cholesterol

Intensity, as mentioned earlier in the chapter, refers to how much energy a person exerts during the exercise—how hard he or she works (e.g. moderate or vigorous). Each different fitness component measures intensity differently, which will be discussed in future chapters.

Time refers to the duration of the exercise. This varies depending upon the activity, the intensity, and/or part of the body being targeted. This is generally measured in minutes for cardiorespiratory exercise, repetitions and sets for muscular strength and endurance, and seconds and repetitions for flexibility.

Type, or specificity, refers to the particular activity a person chooses to complete. For example, a person wanting to target their cardiovascular system and burn calories might choose to run or bike. Someone wanting to tone or gain strength in their arms may use weights or use tension bands to target their biceps and triceps.

Training can be organized around how your chosen training will address each of the FITT principles (Figure 12). There are many considerations that must be taken into account when developing a training plan, some general and some personal. Each person will take their own fitness level, goals, interests, and lifestyle into account when developing their plan.

Applying Fitness Planning Techniques

You've assessed your fitness level (where you are) and probably have some goals in mind for what you want to achieve (where you want to be). Your fitness plan can help you get from point A to point B and so on. Some general planning techniques to help you move from goal point to goal point are overload, progression, specificity, reversibility, and recovery.

Overload is when we place a more intense level of stress on the body than it is used to, causing it to adapt and improve. When we do aerobic activities, our heart, lungs, and muscles are stressed and must work harder to do their job, increasing their overall efficiency. The same is true for exercises that impact muscle or bone strength. The effort taxes them and makes them stronger.

The amount of overload depends upon the person. Someone with very strong legs, for example, will not see much progression if they add just 5 squats to their training. Someone new to a fitness program or that particular type of training may find adding 5 squats to be helpful. It is important to increase based on your own needs. If your goal was to do 30 squats, you've reached it, and are happy with the results, continuing to do 30 squats will enable you to maintain that level. You will need to overload the body part you're working if you want to improve.

Progression goes along with overload (often called progressive overload). Once our body is accustomed to the added intensity (the overload), we gradually increase it to cause the body to adapt again, gaining more benefits from the exercise. For example, you may find your brisk, one-mile walk tiring initially, but after a week or two, you will notice that your breathing is easier and your leg muscles are not as tired. This is when progressive overload comes into play (Figure 13). You may choose to turn your walk into a jog or increase the distance to overload again.

It is important for the progression to be applied gradually

	Cardiorespiratory	**Flexibility**	**Muscular Endurance**	**Muscular Strength**
Frequency	3–5 days per week	2–3 days per week	2–3 days per week (wait 48 hours between resistance training sessions)	2–3 days per week (wait 48 hours between resistance training sessions)
Intensity	55%–90% of max heart rate	To the point of slight discomfort	<50% max weight 8–12 exercises	70–90% of max lift 8–12 exercises
Time	20–60 min. of continuous activity, progressive	2–4 reps, hold 10–30 seconds	15–20 reps 1–3 sets	8–12 reps 1–3 sets
Type	Large muscle groups, continual rhythmic	Static stretch, controlled dynamic stretching	Resistance training (free weights/machines), body weight, circuit training	Resistance training (free weights/machines)

Figure 12. Applying the FITT Formula to different exercise types.

to avoid injury. For example, if you want to add progress to your cardio program by adding time to your workout, you may want to add only 1–3% onto your time. You can increase the progression once your body adapts to the overload. The amount of overload required varies from person to person. Make sure to listen to your body to determine how much overload you should use. There is a difference between soreness or muscle fatigue and the sharp pains or aches that might indicate injury or overuse.

Specificity means that we choose particular activities to work particular parts of the body and challenge particular systems. With specificity, we want to train in the way that we want our bodies to change or improve. The gains that we make are directly tied to the type of workout that we do and exercises that are done. For example, if you found out with a

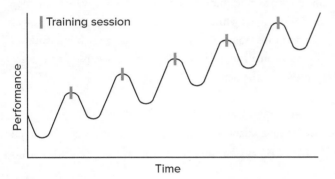

Figure 13. Progressive overload works to improve performance.

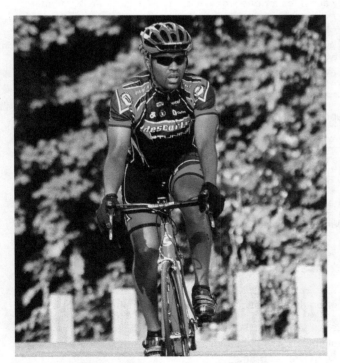

Figure 14. Different exercise can reduce painful impact on your muscles and joints.

sit-and-reach test that your flexibility is "poor," then you will want to include more stretches for the hamstrings and lower back as part of your workout (see Chapter 5). Maybe you are not happy with your push-up score after completing a push-up assessment. You will want to include push-ups and other upper body strength movements in your fitness program.

There is even specificity within types of fitness. A runner who focuses on sprints rather than distance for cardiorespiratory exercises is mostly training their anaerobic pathways and preparing their heart mostly for anaerobic movement. They are not focused on cardiorespiratory endurance. A body builder has to lift weights a certain way to get his body to look a certain way. A power lifter also lifts weights, but does it in a very different way in terms of intensity and the number of repetitions and sets.

Reversibility is essentially the "use it or lose it" principle and the opposite of progressive overload. Any improvements in fitness are reversible if the individual does not maintain his or her exercise program. A person needs to continue to be active across his or her lifespan to maintain the benefits of fitness. If you have had to take time off from your workout due to an injury, health issue, or major life event, make sure that you progress gradually with your workout.

Injuries can sometimes prevent you from continuing your normal fitness program. Try to look for other ways that you can maintain your fitness level. For example, Aunt Marge twisted her knee in a rather rambunctious game of duck-duck-goose during recess. The knee pain is temporarily keeping her away from her running plan. She needs to look for ways to exercise that don't bother her knee while it's healing. She might try using an elliptical machine, cycling, or swimming (Figure 14).

Recovery is the amount of time needed to rest and recover between exercises or workouts. Tissues experience slight damage when a body part is overloaded. It needs to rebuild—this is how muscles strengthen. Recovery is important to this rebuilding process and will be discussed in later chapters. It's important not to confuse recovery with inactivity. Unless you've sustained an injury, resting 1–2 days between the training of specific body parts (such as when lifting weights) usually gives ample time for recovery. This doesn't mean that you should stop exercising entirely during those days. That could lead to reversibility and force you to start over again at a lower intensity. Instead, alternate the days on which you exercises different parts of your body.

Overcoming Barriers to Regular Exercise

The FITT principle helps you put your best foot forward with exercising, but you should be prepared to struggle to meet goals at times, particularly if you are new to exercise. There are plenty of reasons not to exercise, and you should be ready to meet your own resistance with answers to the most common excuses to skip your workout session (Figure 15).

Injuries or accidents can happen with any form of physical activity, though most often exercise is beneficial and safe for most people. You can lessen your risk by keeping some personal considerations in mind as you structure your plan. These include injury prevention and safety (such as warm-up and cool-down times or previous injuries), adequate preparation for your environment and activity (such as clothing, weather, and air quality), as well as any previous medical conditions (e.g. high blood pressure or pregnancy).

There is no doubt that we live in a fast-paced age where we are on the move constantly and our schedules become quite busy. We've begun to rely on technology to solve this problem and have grown impatient with tasks and issues that can't be fixed with a simple Internet search. Our health and fitness is a physical practice that takes dedicated time and attention, not something we can manage with a click of a smart device

(though there are supportive applications).

It's easy to find reasons not to exercise, such as lack of time, energy, motivation, resources, money, skill, knowledge, or support from our social influences. In Chapter 1, we discussed steps toward behavior change and learning what it means to enable and reinforce behavior. Many of our reasons not to exercise come down to our ability to make those changes and put the systems in place that will help us be successful.

It's important to know that physical activity can also be built into our activities of daily living. We can mow the lawn, do heavy gardening, bike to work, walk to the store, walk or jog with the dog, and make other adjustments to our routines that help us get our heart rate pumping and squeeze in activity to contribute to our 150 minutes. Try jumping rope or doing squats while you watch television, or doing lunges as you move from room-to-room. Read your homework on your stationary bicycle or stair climber. The possibilities are endless and the benefits well worth it.

Injury Prevention and Safety

You should adapt your fitness plan to your age, personal limitations, surroundings, and previous experience with

Lack of Time	Identify available time slots. Monitor your daily activities for one week. Identify at least three 30-minute time slots you could use for physical activity.
	Add physical activity to your daily routine. For example, walk or ride your bike to work or shopping, organize school activities around physical activity, walk the dog, exercise while you watch TV, or park your farther away from your destination so you have to walk further.
	Select activities requiring minimal time, such as walking, jogging, or stairclimbing.
Social Influence	Explain your interest in physical activity to friends and family. Ask them to support your efforts.
	Invite friends and family members to exercise with you. Plan social activities involving exercise.
	Develop new friendships with physically active people. Join a group, such as the YMCA or a hiking club.
Lack of Energy	Schedule physical activity for times in the day or week when you feel energetic.
	Tell yourself that if you give it a chance, physical activity will increase your energy level. Then, try it!
Lack of Motivation	Plan ahead. Make physical activity a regular part of your daily or weekly schedule and write it on your calendar.
	Invite a friend to exercise with you on a regular basis and write it on both your calendars.
	Join an exercise group or class.
Lack of Resources	Select activities that require minimal facilities or equipment, such as walking, jogging, jumping rope, or calisthenics.
	Identify inexpensive, convenient resources available in your community like community education programs, park and recreation programs, or worksite programs.

Figure 15. Most common excuses for sedentary behavior have reasonable solutions. Some can even add more fun to your life.

an activity to help prevent injury and keep you safe during physical activities.

Know your limits — Begin slowly, especially if an exercise is new to you, and remember to keep your FITT principle SMART. Assess your fitness level first and make decisions based on your capabilities. Don't be fooled by weight loss and fitness programs that you see on television or online that show out of shape people suddenly working out at high levels and dropping lots of weight or gaining fast muscle. It isn't reasonable to expect to be able to run three miles if you haven't run even one in several years. Listen to your body and what it is telling you about your intensity level – don't compare yourself to anyone but you.

Choose the appropriate type of activity — Choose activities that are safe for you, particularly if you have a previous injury or a physical limitation. For example, if you have a chronic knee injury, then you will want to choose a form of exercise that doesn't aggravate your knee and cause pain.

Cost might also be a factor for you, but it shouldn't be a deterrent. There are many ways to exercise that don't cost a dime in membership fees, training sessions, or classes. Famous NFL running back Herschel Walker built his healthy physique using only his surroundings and his own body weight for resistance. He performed push-ups, sit-ups, ran sprints and made use of what he had available and what he could afford, which when he first started exercising was nothing. Remember the FITT principle — pick a type of exercise that you can do and that will help you progress (Figure 16).

Warm up and cool down — The primary purpose of warming up and cooling down the body is to prevent injury. Warm-ups are important for gradually increasing blood flow and building connections with the neuromuscular system. They allow the heart to prepare for increased activity and help you avoid a sudden increase in blood pressure. Exercise can be hard on cold muscles and stiff connective tissues (e.g. ligaments, tendons) and can not only limit range of motion and overall performance, but also result in sprains, strains, tears, and pulled muscles.

A typical warm-up begins with exercising at a lower speed or intensity initially, starting with light work to the

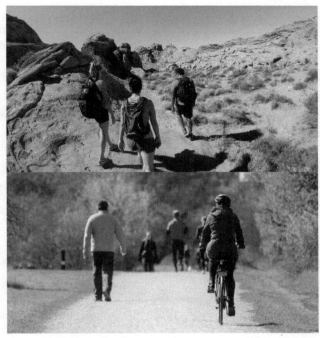

Figure 16. Pick an exercise that you enjoy doing, either alone or with friends.

cardiovascular system (e.g. walking or jogging). The particular body part being worked during that training session is then warmed up as well. For example, if you are lifting weights, start with a smaller weight initially, giving the muscle time to warm before moving to your target weight.

The cool down begins at the end of the workout as the participant slowly and progressively lowers the intensity. Cool-downs help the body gradually return to its resting state. A warm-up and cool-down should each be about 5–10 minutes, but a longer time for either may be necessary. Factors such as the fitness level of the individual, the time of day, intensity of the workout, and even the temperature may call for more time for the body to adjust. People often integrate stretching into their warm-up. This is done only after the body is warm and with dynamic stretching (controlled, repetitive stretches). Static stretching (long holds in stretched positions) should only be done when the body is thoroughly warm and is most effective and safe at the end of your workout. More information on stretching appears in Chapter 5.

Exercise Preparation: Clothing

You should always consider your surroundings and other environmental concerns before exercising. Proper preparation can help you stay safe, comfortable, and help you perform well. Take a few minutes to consider your situation before heading out the door:

- What will the climate be like where I'm exercising? Will it be hot, cold, windy, humid, smoggy, rainy, foggy, dark, sunny, and so on? What clothing will I need so I'm comfortable and protected? Do I need to layer? Do I need to wear sunscreen, bug repellant, or bring extra water?

- What type of equipment do I need to be safe? Do I need a mouthguard, shin-guards, a helmet, reflectors, a headlamp? Do I have the right shoes for the activity and terrain?

There are many things to consider, as you will see by the following sections. Not to worry. People who do a sport or activity routinely often find these considerations to be second nature. They can take stock of their situation and adapt to it quickly just by having the right equipment and knowledge.

Shoes

Most of us don't need to be told twice to go shoe shopping. It's that one item of clothing without judgment and three-way mirrors. Shoes do not care about the size of your waistline. Besides the great shopping experience, a comfortable pair of shoes can make a difference in how successful we are with our exercise routine.

Some shoes are specialized for the activity (Figure 17). Even traditional running/tennis shoes can be broken into categories based on the type of training you do (e.g. walking, distance running, CrossFit). People who do the same activity 3 or more days each week often find it worth the investment to buy a specialized shoe. But it's not just a matter of picking a nice-looking shoe in your normal size with a sign that says "cross-training" underneath it. Try using the **STRETCH test** when selecting a pair of shoes:

S—Wear the same **socks** you would use for your activities.

T—**Try** them out. Run or walk around a bit, simulating the movements you will use during exercise.

R—**Re-lace** the shoes. New shoes right out of the box are often not laced as they would be during exercise. Start at the toe and ensure that you lace the in the traditional, crisscross manner with enough pressure to make them secure and comfortable.

E—Try them on at the **end** of the day when your feet are their largest.

T—**Test** your toes. You should have three-eighths to one-half of an inch from your longest toe to the end of the shoe while standing and be able to wiggle your toes.

C—**Comfort** should be instant. Your shoes should not need to be broken in.

H—Your **heels** should be hugged by the shoe and not slipping as you move.

Replace your shoes when they start to show signs of wear and tear. A good pair of shoes can go a long way toward helping prevent discomfort and even injury during your workout. How often they last varies depending upon how often they're used and the pattern with which your feet strike the surface, usually about 3–6 months.

Sports Bras and Athletic Supporters

Ladies, your daily bra is not designed for impact, heavy movement, or significant sweat. Sports bras offer additional support and come in many styles. The larger your breasts, the more support you may need to prevent strain on your neck and back and enable you to move freely and quickly.

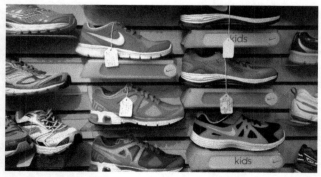

Figure 17. The right equipment can prevent injuries.

Guys, protect yourself. A lack of support can be just as uncomfortable for you as for women, but impact to the area can be more damaging and incredibly painful. Wear an athletic strap (or similar undergarment) for support during exercise and add an athletic cup for protection when playing sports, particularly those with moving objects or potential contact with other players. It only takes one unprotected blow to teach you the importance of these barriers. It's best to learn it without having to first experience it.

Exercise Preparation: Weather

It's cold, windy, and you're pretty sure that's sleet hitting the sidewalk as you're tying your shoes. You duck back into the house for a moment, grab a sweatshirt, and head out for your run. The can-do attitude is admirable and something to celebrate. However, it's important not to put yourself, and your fitness goals, at risk by subjecting yourself to an unsafe environment. Keep the elements of nature in mind when exercising, particularly outdoors. Extreme temperatures, snow, wind, rain, and humidity can present problems if you don't plan ahead.

Cold

Cold may seem like it is relative to what we are used to. When Grandpa Fred comes to visit you from Minnesota in January, he wears his short-sleeved shirts and shorts for his power-walk in 32 degree temperatures (he's a pretty active senior). To him Salem, Oregon feels quite comfortable, even warm. That doesn't mean his body can necessarily tolerate extreme temperatures any better than yours. It just means he hasn't seen such "warm" weather in a while and he has gotten a little too excited. This is why the feeling of being cold is not always the best barometer for risk. Better measurements are **temperatures** and **wind chill factors**. Temperatures measure the intensity of heat, while wind chill factors adjust that measurement by accounting for how the speed of the wind moves heat away from the skin.

On most cold days, the best approach is to dress in layers:

- **A bottom layer** made from a synthetic material, such as polypropylene, will draw sweat away from the body unlike cotton, which tends to keep the moisture next to your skin. Moisture next to the skin can make you feel colder.

- Add a **middle layer** of fleece or wool for warmth.

- Finish with a **top layer** of something breathable and, if you live where it rains a lot, waterproof.

- Be prepared to remove these layers and replace them as needed. If it's windy as well, consider adding gloves, a scarf, or head protection.

This may seem like obvious and simple advice, but we often neglect these small steps. Take a moment to shield your skin and those delicate digits from wind chafing and numbness (let's face it—it hurts like crazy when you bump numb fingers against something).

No matter how prepared you are some days are just too cold for outdoor exercise. Temperature and wind go together in the winter. The thermometer might read 30 degrees, but with the wind chill it may feel like 20 degrees. It's important to know the wind chill index (the temperature you feel) when exercising outdoors in the winter because frostbite and hypothermia can be dangerous. Your local weather channel provides this information routinely as do many online sources.

Frostbite occurs when the skin and underlying tissues begin to freeze. It primarily affects exposed areas of the skin, such as your ears, nose, and cheeks, along with your fingers and toes. Numbness, loss of feeling, and stinging are common warning signs. We often rub cold areas of the body, but this can irritate the problem even more by damaging the skin. If it's numb, you may not realize how hard you are rubbing. It's a bit like receiving a numbing injection at the dentist. While your mouth is numb, you're most at risk of biting your cheek or lip and not feeling it.

Your best approach is to go inside and warm slowly. However, if the frostbite is severe, it's possible to have irreversible damage that can lead to amputation of the affected area. The National Weather Service offers you guidelines on how quickly frostbite can occur (Figure 18).

Hypothermia can also be quite dangerous. When your body's temperature (98.6) drops well below normal (approximately 95 or lower), it begins to lose heat faster than it produces it and responds with severe shivering, slurring speech, fatigue, poor coordination, and confusion. The confusion in particular can be very dangerous. It's not uncommon for individuals with hypothermia to make poor choices, such as removing

		Temperature (F)																
		40	35	30	25	20	15	10	5	0	-5	-10	-15	-20	-25	-30	-35	-40	-45
Wind (mph)	5	36	31	25	19	13	7	1	-5	-11	-16	-22	-28	-34	-40	-46	-52	-57	-63
	10	34	27	21	15	9	3	-4	-10	-16	-22	-28	-35	-41	-47	-53	-59	-66	-72
	15	32	25	19	13	6	0	-7	-13	-19	-26	-32	-39	-45	-51	-58	-64	-71	-77
	20	30	24	17	11	4	-2	-9	-15	-22	-29	-35	-42	-48	-55	-61	-68	-74	-81
	25	29	23	16	9	3	-4	-11	-17	-24	-31	-37	-44	-51	-58	-64	-71	-78	-84
	30	28	22	15	8	1	-5	-12	-19	-26	-33	-39	-46	-53	-60	-67	-73	-80	-87
	35	28	21	14	7	0	-7	-14	-21	-27	-34	-41	-48	-55	-62	-69	-76	-82	-89
	40	27	20	13	6	-1	-8	-15	-22	-29	-36	-43	-50	-57	-64	-71	-78	-84	-91
	45	26	19	12	5	-2	-9	-16	-23	-30	-37	-44	-51	-58	-65	-72	-79	-86	-93
	50	26	19	12	4	-3	-10	-17	-24	-31	-38	-45	-52	-60	-67	-74	-81	-88	-95
	55	25	18	11	4	-3	-11	-18	-25	-32	-39	-46	-54	-61	-68	-75	-82	-89	-97
	60	25	17	10	3	-4	-11	-19	-26	-33	-40	-48	-55	-62	-69	-76	-84	-91	-98

Frostbite Times	30 Minutes	10 Minutes	5 Minutes

Wind Chill (F) = $35.74 + 0.6215T - 35.75(V^{0.16}) + 0.4275T(V^{0.16})$ Where T = Air Temperature (F) V = Wind Speed (mph)

Figure 18. Wind chill can make it feel colder than it is. Frostbite is a real danger in low temperatures, so plan accordingly.

garments and exposing themselves to greater risk. Get indoors or to shelter quickly and warm slowly. This is the key with both frostbite and hypothermia. Seek medical help if you suspect hypothermia or experience pain that doesn't resolve.

Exercising outdoors in the winter takes a bit of preparation. Look at the temperature and wind chill index (both available through your local weather channel or online), and for icy conditions that may create slipping hazards.

There may be times when it's too cold or risky to exercise outdoors. It doesn't mean that your routine has to freeze as well. It just means that you need to hit the treadmill or dust off one of those aerobics DVDs your mother gave you for your birthday. Calisthenics, weightlifting, yoga—the options are endless and present ample opportunity to keep you on track and maybe even work some muscles you haven't challenged in a while.

Heat

Heat can be relative to the person and what they are used to, at least to an extent. Last summer Grandpa Fred went to visit some retired friends in the town where he grew up in Texas. He noticed a few people running outdoors in 105 degree temperatures at 2:00 in the afternoon. The sun was blazing and the air was without the slightest breeze. He was a bit dumbfounded that people ran in this heat. However, since he used to walk to school every day in the same heat, uphill both ways (hats off to Grandpa Fred), he figured he could handle it. He went out for his walk at 3:00 only to return at 3:15, red-faced and miserable. Fortunately, he was smart enough to know early on that he wasn't adapted to the climate and relocated his

workout before he had serious problems.

Many of us would likely feel the same. In the cloudy Northwest where we rarely experience that level of heat for more than a few days each year, most of us wouldn't consider moving too far away from an air-conditioned gym—we spend so much of the year slogging through mud puddles that our bodies aren't as acclimated to the heat. But then again after months of rain the temptation for sun can be too much to resist for some of us. As with cold, planning ahead can help you avoid health risks:

Dress appropriately to keep yourself cool, as well as protect your skin. Wear a hat and light-colored, lightweight clothing that fits loosely and allows sweat to evaporate. Remember, cotton keeps the sweat next to your skin, so look for materials that will pull it away.

Wear sunscreen. Let's repeat that word—sunscreen, sunscreen, sunscreen. You almost never hear someone say that they wish they had worn less sunscreen, especially someone with a severe burn or blisters. Keep in mind that you will need to reapply often if you will be outside and active (sweating) for a long time. The more fair-skinned you are, the more often you should reapply regardless of how high your lotion's sun protection factor (SPF) is.

Exercise earlier in the morning or later in the evening when the temperatures are lower, if possible.

Temperature (F)															
80	**82**	**84**	**86**	**88**	**90**	**92**	**94**	**96**	**98**	**100**	**102**	**104**	**106**	**108**	**110**

Relative Humidity	80	82	84	86	88	90	92	94	96	98	100	102	104	106	108	110
40	80	81	83	85	88	91	94	97	101	105	109	114	119	124	130	136
45	80	82	84	87	89	93	96	100	104	109	114	119	124	131	137	
50	81	83	85	88	91	95	99	103	108	113	118	124	131	137		
55	81	84	86	89	93	97	101	106	112	117	124	129	137			
60	82	84	88	91	95	100	105	110	116	123	130	136				
65	82	85	89	93	98	103	108	114	121	128	137					
70	83	86	90	95	100	105	112	119	126	134						
75	84	88	92	97	103	109	116	124	132							
80	84	89	94	100	106	113	121	129								
85	85	90	96	102	110	117	126	135								
90	86	91	98	105	113	122	131									
95	86	93	100	108	117	127										
100	87	95	103	112	121	132										

Caution	Extreme Caution	Danger	Extreme Danger

Figure 19. It can be unsafe to exercise in extreme heat. Be aware of the temperature before going outside to exercise.

Check your local weather channel or an online source for the heat index. The National Weather Service offers guidelines for what temperatures and relative humidity (how it feels) could pose potential health problems (Figure 19).

Stay hydrated. Dehydration can cause loss of coordination, muscle cramps and fatigue, nausea and vomiting, headaches, and heat-related illness, such as heat stroke (Figure 21). It isn't as simple as aimlessly guzzling water, particularly if you're an athlete in competition. This can result in a feeling of fullness that impacts performance or even over-hydration (never drink more than 1 liter of fluid in an hour). The American College of Sports Medicine offers the following recommendations (Figure 20).

High humidity can pose a greater challenge. Heat and humidity can raise your core body temperature. Your body will try to cool itself by sending blood away from the muscles and toward the skin. This in turn increases your heart rate. Humidity can be a bit like trying to exercise in a sauna. The sweat stays trapped on your skin, which can raise the body temperature even higher.

Our bodies are designed to adapt to heat, but our natural cooling systems can only handle an overload for a certain period of time, particularly when we begin to sweat excessively or become dehydrated. Potential heat-related illnesses (degrees of hyperthermia) include:

Heat Cramps—muscles feel painful and spasms/contractions may occur, muscles may feel firm to the touch, body temp may be normal

Heat Exhaustion—profuse sweating, cramps, dizziness, fatigue, headache, cool moist skin, pulse may be slow/weak

Heat Stroke—dry/hot skin with no sweating, rapid/weak pulse, confusion, possible seizures, body temp above 105, loss of consciousness

Time	Additional Step	Time	Drinking Amount
Before	Check your urine color.	4 Hours Before 10–15 Minutes Before	16–20 fluid ounces of water or sports drink 8–10 fluid ounces of water
During	---	Every 15–20 minutes (if exercise is less than 60)	3–8 fluid ounces of water, or sports beverage
After	Weigh yourself again to determine how much fluid you've lost.	---	20–24 ounces of water or sports drink for every pound lost

Figure 20. Be aware of your hydration level before, during, and after exercise.

Signs of Danger	Treatment	
Heat		
Heat Cramps	Heat cramps are painful muscle contractions following exercise. They begin an hour or more after stopping exercise and most often involve heavily used muscles in the calves, thighs, and abdomen.	Rest and passive stretching of the muscle, supplemented by commercial rehydration solutions or water and salt, will rapidly relieve symptoms. Water with a salty snack is sufficient.
Heat Exhaustion	Most people who experience acute collapse or other symptoms associated with exercise in the heat are suffering from heat exhaustion—the inability to continue exertion in the heat.	Most cases can be treated with supine rest in the shade or other cool place and oral water or fluids containing glucose and salt; subsequently, spontaneous cooling occurs, and patients recover within hours.
Heat Stroke	Early symptoms are similar to those of heat exhaustion, with confusion or change in personality, loss of coordination, dizziness, headache, and nausea that progress to more severe symptoms.	Maintain their airway if victim is unconscious. Move to the shade or a cool place out of the sun. Use evaporative cooling: remove excess clothing to maximize skin exposure, spray tepid water on the skin, and maintain air movement over the body by fanning. Alternatively, place cool or cold wet towels over the body and fan to promote evaporation. Apply ice or cold packs to the neck, armpits, groin, and as much of the body as possible. Vigorously massage the skin to limit constriction of blood vessels and prevent shivering, which will increase body temperature.
Cold		
Frostbite	Frostbite is the term that is used to describe tissue damage from direct freezing of the skin. Frostbitten skin is numb and appears whitish or waxy.	Once the area has rewarmed, it can be examined. If blisters are present, note whether they extend to the end of the digit. Proximal blisters usually mean that the tissue distal to the blister has suffered full-thickness damage. For treatment, avoid further mechanical trauma to the area and prevent infection.
Hypothermia	When people are faced with an environment in which they cannot keep warm, they first feel chilled, then begin to shiver, and eventually stop shivering as their metabolic reserves are exhausted.	Modern clothing, gloves, and particularly footwear have greatly decreased the chances of suffering cold injury in extreme climates.

Figure 21. Watch for these dangerous symptoms of temperature-related injuries.

Move to indoor activities when the heat index is too high. If your tough, resilient, never-give-up Grandpa Fred won't exercise in a particular climate, there is no shame for you in doing a few miles on the treadmill or taking an aerobics class. Safety is about preparedness and attention to the risk factors of whatever weather conditions are happening on a given day. See Figure 21 for methods to identify and treat temperature-related illnesses.

Air Quality

Smog or other air pollutants are a significant problem in many parts of the country and can make outdoor exercise uncomfortable or hazardous to your health. Poor air quality, unlike cold and heat, is *not* relative to what you are used to, though many people become accustomed to seeing it. As much as possible, make use of parks, trails, and other green spaces where vehicle emissions are lower, avoiding busy roads where you'll breathe a lot of vehicle exhaust. Areas with tall buildings and traffic lights are a hot spot as the starting and stopping of vehicles and restricted air movement from the structures can create a higher pollutant zone.

Check your local news channel (or the Environmental Protection Agency's *AirNow* website) before you head out and heed warnings that the quality of air may not be suitable on a particular day. The **Air Quality Index** (AQI) provides a good indication of when the air is healthy, marginal, or even hazardous to your health. It is calculated based on four primary concerns: ground level ozone, particle pollution, carbon monoxide, and sulfur dioxide (Figure 22).

Ozone is normally a good thing. It's that layer high in the atmosphere that protects us from harmful rays from the sun. **Ground level ozone** is different. According to the Environmental Protection Agency (EPA), ground level or "bad" ozone is not emitted directly into the air. It is created by chemical reactions between oxides of nitrogen (NO_x) and volatile organic compounds (VOC) in the presence of sunlight. NO_x and VOC emissions come from sources like industrial and power plants and vehicle exhaust, among others.

Particle pollution can happen when the air accumulates an excess of fine or course particles, such as when a forest fire occurs. Cars, factories, wood-burning fireplaces, and other sources can also produce particles. **Carbon monoxide pollution** is very common, and its largest producers are the vehicles we drive. It develops when the carbon in our fuels does not burn completely, which happens more often in cooler months. **Sulfur dioxide** is a gas that comes from fuels that

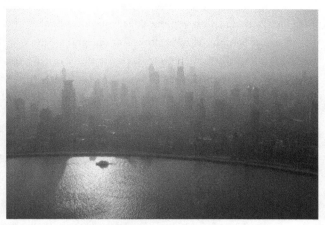

Figure 22. Poor air quality can affect your physical activity.

contain sulfur, such as coal and oil. This type of pollution is higher near industrial areas and power plants.

Poor air quality can make it difficult to breathe as deeply as necessary, can damage the cells in your lungs, make you more at risk for infection, and even cause chest pains or permanent lung damage. The EPA has established the AQI to help you determine the "health" of the air on a given day (Figure 23).

Some individuals—such as people with asthma or other respiratory conditions, heart disease, children, older adults, or people frequently exposed to poor air quality—may be more sensitive to issues with air quality. Change your outdoor run or bicycle ride to one on the treadmill or stationary bike when conditions are too risky for you.

Air quality is impacted by more than just pollution. **Seasonal allergies** can often make breathing uncomfortable.

Air Quality Index Levels	Numerical Value	Color	Meaning
Good	0 to 50	Green	Air quality is considered satisfactory, and air pollution poses little or no risk.
Moderate	51 to 100	Yellow	Air quality is acceptable; however, for some pollutants there may be a moderate health concern for a very small number of people who are unusually sensitive to air pollution.
Unhealthy for Sensitive Groups	101 to 150	Orange	Members of sensitive groups may experience health effects. The general public is not likely to be affected.
Unhealthy	151 to 200	Red	Everyone may begin to experience health effects; members of sensitive groups may experience more serious health effects.
Very Unhealthy	201 to 300	Purple	Health alert: everyone may experience more serious health effects.
Hazardous	301 to 500	Maroon	Health warnings of emergency conditions. The entire population is more likely to be affected.

Figure 23. The AQI lets you know if its safe to exercise outdoors.

Take allergy medication or move your workout indoors if the pollen count is high. Most weather stations and weather-related websites offer pollen counts, particularly during the spring and summer months.

Higher altitudes can also pose a temporary challenge. The pressure in the atmosphere is reduced, which means less oxygen. Your body has to draw on its own supply more at higher altitudes than lower. This causes the body to circulate more blood and the heart to work harder. You may experience nausea, shortness of breath, headaches, or feel lightheaded.

The good news is that this is temporary. Your body will acclimate to the higher elevation and even thrive. The heart adjusts and does less work to gain oxygen, which is good.

You may not reap the benefits if you're only vacationing in the mountains a few days but over time your body will adapt and function well. In the meantime:

- Reduce the intensity or duration of your workout.

- Give your body time to adjust.

- Increase hydration and carbohydrate intake.

In Chapter 3 you will learn about how the heart and lungs work together to circulate blood and oxygen. Until your body adapts your heart rate will be elevated and you will need the additional fuel stores.

Exercise Preparation: Safety Concerns

Many safety issues are about considering the external conditions to your workout. Be cautious of the rules designed to keep you safe, whether it is while you are biking, hiking, swimming, lifting weights at the gym, or any other activity. Adapt to your surroundings as needed. For example, if traffic is particularly heavy or the road you are on does not have a sufficient bike lane, consider changing your route to one that is more accessible or utilizing parks or trails. Follow the safety guidelines (such as particular rules in the weight room or pool) and be cautious of others who may be compromising them.

Yet safety is about more than external factors – it's about your own specific needs. Individuals with a chronic health condition or disability (Figure 24), women who are pregnant (Figure 25), or people who have a prior injury (Figure 26) should contact their health care provider for guidance with

their fitness plan. Most people with health issues are still able to work up to moderate-intensity activity, but that is a decision between you and your health care provider.

Many people with **disabilities** can benefit from physical activity, particularly since it can often help with improved

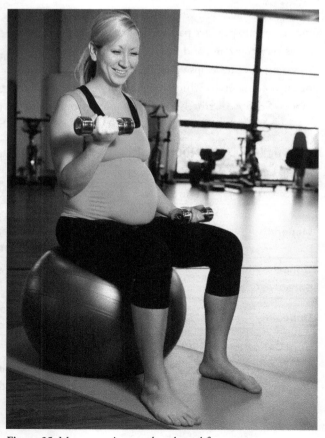

Figure 24. Design fitness plans to work with disabilities.

Figure 25. Many exercises can be adapted for pregnancy.

Injury	Symptoms	Solutions
Ankle Sprain	Tenderness, swelling, bruising, stiffness	An ankle sprain should fully heal on its own between two and twelve weeks. If it doesn't, visit a health care provider.
Groin Pull	Pain and tenderness on inner thigh, pain when bringing legs together	Ice your inner thigh and compress it using an elastic bandage or tape. Stretching also assists tissue healing, but always use caution stretching an injured muscle.
Hamstring Strain	Pain in the back of the thigh and lower buttock when walking, straightening the leg, or bending over	Compress your leg and rest it while elevated above your hip joint. Avoid putting weight on the injured leg.
Shin Splints	Ache or throb in shins after a short run or sprint	Rest your body, ice your shin, and take anti-inflammatory pain medicine.
ACL Tear	A feeling of looseness in the knee joint, inability to put weight on joint, swelling within first 24 hours	A mild to moderate knee ligament injury may heal on its own, in time. To speed the healing, you can rest the knee. Avoid putting much weight on your knee if it's painful to do so. You may need to use crutches for a time.
Patellofemoral Syndrome	Pain in the knees, especially when sitting with knees bent, squatting, jumping, or using stairs. It is also common to have a popping or grinding sensation	Tape or use a brace to stabilize the kneecap, avoid bending your knees for long periods of time, and rest them with ice.
Tennis Elbow	Pain focused on the outside of the arm, where your forearm meets your elbow	Tennis elbow can usually be treated with exercise, physical therapy, and medications such as ibuprofen, naproxen, or aspirin.

Figure 26. Most common injuries from exercise have easy home treatments.

ability to perform activities of daily living. Whether the disability is the result of an acute event, like a stroke or spinal cord injury, or something congenital, like cerebral palsy or muscular dystrophy, an exercise program can be developed to suit your individual abilities and needs. Thanks to advances in technology, science, and health care, we have many options available today to help people live their best life. This includes a wealth of both adaptive equipment and knowledge.

Moderate-intensity exercise is safe during **pregnancy** for most women, and the risks of pre-term delivery or pregnancy loss are very low. It is always best to consult with your health care provider before beginning an exercise plan. Some evidence indicates that in addition to the physical benefits already discussed in this chapter, exercise can help prevent preeclampsia (high blood pressure) and gestational diabetes and may even help reduce the length of labor (though these studies are not conclusive).

It's important to keep in mind how active you were before you became pregnant. If you were sedentary, it wouldn't be advisable to begin a high-intensity program right away. Start with light or moderate activity, listen to your body, and stop if you feel uncomfortable. Avoid exercises that are completed while lying on your back after your first trimester – the growing baby can put pressure on the main artery to your heart and make you feel dizzy. Always avoid sports that are high contact, involve swift-moving objects, or present a fall risk. For example, playing basketball, horseback riding, and skiing should be avoided.

Babies bring a lot of change and your exercise routine can help you adjust to your new life. Your body requires an initial period of rest and healing after delivery. Once you get clearance from your health care provider, exercise can help you get back to your pre-pregnancy state and improve your mood (important when your body is adjusting to changing hormone levels). It also helps you have more healthy years spent with your child and gives you the opportunity to start setting a great example for how they care for themselves as they grow.

It's important to understand your disability and your body's capabilities. Adapt the guidelines or establish a program in consultation with your health care provider. Some individuals are able to follow the federal guidelines for moderate intensity, while others have to make adjustments to ensure safety or to focus on their own specific needs. People with dementia, mental illness, or developmental disabilities may need supervision with activities.

Special Concern: Chronic Medical Conditions

Many people living with a chronic medical condition find that exercise can pose challenges. But refraining from physical activity often only compounds physical issues, leading to worsening or additional conditions. Individuals with asthma, Type 2 diabetes, or high blood pressure should be especially careful of how they exercise.

According to the CDC, 18.4 million American adults suffer from **asthma**. This is a chronic illness in which the airways of the body, responsible for carrying oxygen to and from the lungs, become irritated, swollen, and narrow. Certain irritants or allergies trigger an asthma attack, causing the person to wheeze, cough, and experience shortness of breath and tightness in the chest. Some of these triggers include cigarette smoke, pet dander, mold, dust mites, and air pollution. Changes in the weather, colds, and even exercise can trigger an attack. These are usually treated with inhaled corticosteroids (long-term use) or bronchodilators (fast-acting).

Exercise itself does not cause asthma. As we begin to breathe heavier during exercise, we often do so through our mouth, which tends to bring in colder, dryer air. It is this cool air that acts as the trigger. Activities that are more likely to bring on an attack include any in cold, dry environments, such as hockey or skiing, and exercise that needs constant activity, such as long-distance running or soccer. Activities that are less likely include those that require short bursts of energy, like gymnastics, volleyball, and baseball, as well as walking, biking leisurely, or swimming in a warm, humid environment.

You can lessen the risk of triggering an attack by wearing a scarf over your mouth and nose during cooler weather, taking your medication prior to exercise, and doing a sufficient warm-up so the body (particularly the airways) has time to adjust to the intensity. It can also help to focus on breathing in through your nose at a steady pace or even do breathing exercises (Yoga can be great for this). No matter the exercise, always keep your inhaler with you and consult your health care provider for other recommendations prior to beginning an exercise program.

Exercise is highly recommended for individuals with **Type 2 diabetes** because it can reduce weight and help control blood sugar levels. The precautions for exercising with diabetes relate to your blood sugar levels. Individuals who take insulin should discuss their exercise plans with their health care provider to determine how to monitor the amount of insulin they take. Your health care provider may recommend that you take less insulin or eat a small snack prior to exercise to avoid low blood sugar. Good hydration helps keep the kidneys functioning well and can also help reduce risk. Some individuals with Type 2 diabetes who experience weight loss as a result of a healthy diet and exercise find that they need less insulin, if any.

High blood pressure, or hypertension, occurs when the blood pushes harder than normal against the artery walls. Regular physical activity reduces blood pressure. There are a few safety measures to keep in mind for people who've been diagnosed with high blood pressure:

Take it slow at first. Don't attempt vigorous activity right away if you're just beginning an exercise program. Start with lower intensity and build up over time.

Avoid lifting weights. You can revisit this exercise if your blood pressure gets under control.

Don't consume caffeine. Caffeine is a stimulant and it raises blood pressure.

Stand slowly. Sudden changes in blood flow can cause slight dizziness, even in those without hypertension.

Monitor your breathing. Always breathe during exercise and slow down if you become out of breath. You should be breathing a little heavy but still able to speak.

Dealing with Common Injuries

Many people try to overdo it when beginning an exercise plan or increasing intensity. Grandpa Fred, for example, joined a Silver Foxes fitness program at the senior center near his home. The center offered many classes that challenged muscles he had not worked in years. He knew he was fit for his age and was sure that he could keep up with the other seniors in the aerobics class—truth be told, he was showing off a bit. He strained his hamstring the first day.

It's important to consider your current level of fitness, age, previous injuries, and increase activity gradually to avoid injuries. Typically, the most common injuries are to our bones, joints, tendons, and ligaments, often related to repetition or overuse.

Sprains and Strains

A **sprain** is a tearing or stretching of your ligaments, the tissue that connects your bones together. A **strain** is the tearing or stretching of a muscle or tendon (the tissue that joins muscles to bone). A sprain in the ankle or a strain in the back can be quite common. Use the **PRICE method** to treat a sprain or strain:

P — Protect the injured body part, such as with a splint to immobilize, and don't put further pressure on it.

R — Rest the injured body part. This is critical to heal the injury.

I — Ice the area every few hours for no more than 20 minutes at a time for the first 24–48 hours. Ice can help reduce swelling and ease pain. Be sure to put a barrier between the ice and your skin to prevent skin damage.

C — Compress the injured area, such as with an elastic bandage. This can reduce pain and limit swelling. Do not wrap so tightly as to cut off the blood flow to the area.

E — Elevate the area so that it is above the heart and the blood flows away from it. This helps keep blood and fluid from building up in the injured area and reduces swelling.

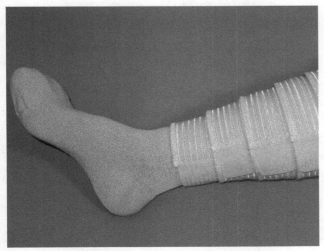

Figure 27. Compression wraps can provide temporary pain relief.

If pain does not improve in a few days, it may be more than a sprain or strain. See a health care provider right away if the pain worsens, increases when you move or apply pressure to the injured area, or won't move at all.

The inner thigh area of your leg (groin) and the back of your thigh (hamstring) are also common areas to experience pulls and strains. These typically occur with side-to-side movements or from overstretching. These can also be treated using the PRICE method.

Pain and swelling on the shin area of the leg (the inside, tibia area of your lower leg) usually results from overwork. Sudden increases to your level of activity are a common cause of **shin splints**. The muscles and tendons of the shin area simply aren't prepared. Your friend Kendal, the track star with the 6-minute warm-up mile, once broke her ankle and spent 2 months immobilized. Kendal eagerly returned to the track not long after the cast was removed. Unfortunately, she didn't build up as slowly as she should have (the state championships were getting close and she wanted to be ready). She developed a severe case of shin splints and was sidelined again for the rest of the season – no championship race for her.

Any runner or competitive athlete will tell you that shin splints can be difficult to treat. In fact, they are much easier to prevent:

Build intensity gradually, especially if you are a beginner or have had time off due to an injury. This is your first line of defense.

Strengthen the surrounding area, such as the calf muscles and ankles. Resistance bands are excellent for this.

Avoid running or jumping on concrete (such as sidewalks). Asphalt, dirt, tracks, treadmills, and wooden floors are much more forgiving and will absorb some of the shock.

Invest in a good pair of shoes. Consider using an orthotic insert for better support, particularly if you've struggled with them in the past. These can be purchased over-the-counter or customized for you at many specialty shoe stores. Use the STRETCH test in this chapter for help choosing the best shoe for you.

Treat shin splints with ice, rest, and anti-inflammatory medication. Once they are feeling better, be sure to return to your exercise program slowly and strategically, giving your shins and the muscles surrounding them time to strengthen and work up to the higher intensity.

Some athletes find that wrapping the area or using compression sleeves helps give more support and lessen pain (Figure 27). If they do not go away, see your health care provider to make sure the injury isn't more serious, such as a stress fracture, or for a referral to physical therapy.

Knee injuries can occur from overuse or from sudden stops or directional changes, as well as from impact. The most common injury is the anterior cruciate ligament (ACL) tear. These can require surgery and should be addressed by a health care provider. Sometimes the knee hurts, but you don't recall doing anything to it – it is most likely not serious and the pain will go away in a few days with ice and rest. If you experienced impact or felt (or even heard) the injury occur, watch for signs of significant swelling, redness, warmth of the area, significant tenderness or pain, and fever. See a health care provider if one of more of these occur.

Conclusion

This chapter gives you tools to understand what it means to be physically fit. We described:

- Definitions of physical activity, exercise, and fitness and what it means to be fit
- The benefits of being physically fit
- The guidelines for beneficial activity levels
- The data on how active we are as a nation
- Steps and considerations in developing your own fitness plan

Your next steps should include assessing your own activity level and using the information to create a fitness pan that includes daily physical activity. You can increase your lifespan and have a positive impact on your wellness by staying active throughout your life. This plan can help you take the first steps on that journey.

Reflection Questions

1. What is the difference between physical activity and exercise? Does your lifestyle tend to incorporate physical activity or exercise?

2. Identify three benefits of exercise that are meaningful to you. Why have you selected these benefits?

3. Are you satisfied with your current level of physical activity? Why or why not?

4. Which of the health-related components of fitness plays the largest role in your life currently?

5. Select a health-related component of fitness that you would like to improve or maintain. What are some SMART goals for this component of fitness?

6. What are some of the general considerations a person should make when creating a safe, effective fitness plan?

7. Identify a weather-related exercise challenge. Describe what it is and how it can impact a person's health. What can a person can do to reduce the likelihood that this problem will occur? How can air quality during exercise impact health?

8. Identify a health-related challenge to increasing fitness level. What should a person with this challenge do if they want to become or stay physically active? Identify an exercise-related injury. What is the typical cause and treatment for the injury you have selected?

Chapter 3
Cardiorespiratory Fitness

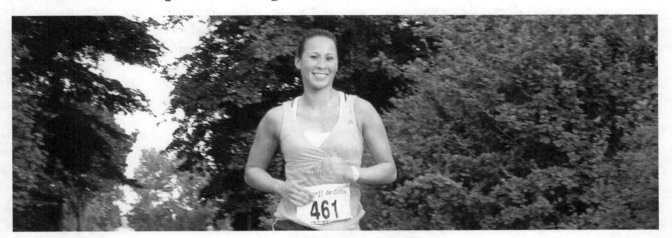

Learning Objectives

1. Describe how the body produces the energy it needs for exercise.

2. List the major health effects and benefits of cardiorespiratory exercise.

3. Explain how cardiorespiratory endurance can be assessed.

4. Describe how frequency, intensity, time (duration) and type of exercise affect the development of cardiorespiratory endurance.

5. List some of the different options that people have for cardiorespiratory training programs.

6. Apply the FITT formula to create a safe and effective cardiorespiratory training program.

You've probably heard the term "cardio" used in relation to exercise many times. Cardio is the nickname we've assigned to one of the most important health-related components of our overall fitness – cardiorespiratory fitness. Our cardiorespiratory fitness is the ability of the heart and lungs to work together to perform sustained, moderate to high levels of physical activity. People who exercise learn to love doing cardio, and we often assign nicknames to those we love. They love it because they know that cardiorespiratory fitness contributes to an improved overall quality of life, longevity, and disease prevention.

In fact, your level of cardiorespiratory fitness (CRF) is a strong predictor of your mortality. A low level of CRF endangers your heart and health as much as or more than smoking, high blood pressure, and Type 2 diabetes. Even if you have a serious health condition like high blood pressure, a higher level of CRF can lower your risk of early death from that condition.

There are so many reasons to have good CRF, as you'll soon see. Good CRF lets you perform physical activity normally, without needing to worry about becoming over tired or injured as a result. Imagine your new puppy, Larry, makes a break for it when you open the door (he'd been eyeing that squirrel through the window for some time). You certainly want to catch him before he hits the open field, but will your body be up to the task? With good CRF, even unexpected physical activity is manageable for you. You don't have to worry about losing Larry forever because you couldn't chase after him.

This chapter defines the elements of the cardiorespiratory system, describes how chemical energy is produced in your body, and explains the dimensions of wellness that are most impacted by cardiorespiratory fitness. It also describes how to assess your CRF and outlines how to implement a cardiorespiratory fitness program in your own life.

Defining Cardiorespiratory Fitness

Cardiorespiratory fitness is the ability of your circulatory and respiratory systems to supply oxygen to your skeletal muscles during sustained physical activity. These systems work together to fuel the body during exercise, pumping oxygen and blood to your muscles (Figure 1). Your heart is a muscular organ. It needs exercise to stay fit and strong, just like any other muscle. Routine exercise strengthens the heart muscle and improves its efficiency, helping it do a better job.

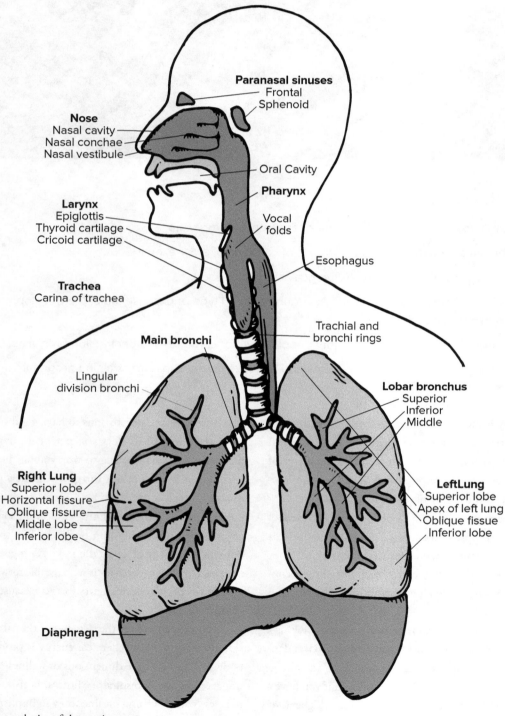

Figure 1. The complexity of the respiratory system.

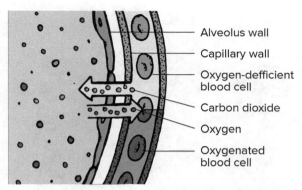

Figure 2. Oxygen and carbon dioxide exchange in the alveoli.

- Alveolus wall
- Capillary wall
- Oxygen-defficient blood cell
- Carbon dioxide
- Oxygen
- Oxygenated blood cell

A stronger heart means more blood reaches your muscles and lungs, oxygen levels in the blood rise, and your capillaries (tiny blood vessels) widen, allowing them to carry more oxygen to the body and carry away waste. A stronger heart also means more efficient oxygen distribution to the muscles and less air depleted from your lungs (Figure 2).

Oxygen is important in cardiorespiratory exercise. The body needs to be able to effectively move oxygen and other nutrients around the body quickly when the heart's pumping rate is elevated. The cardiorespiratory system is made up of the vascular system and the respiratory system, both of which are responsible for moving oxygen around the body.

Cardiovascular System

The **cardiovascular system** is the organ system responsible for transporting blood to the rest of the body. This system—sometimes called the **vascular**, **blood-vascular**, or simply **circulatory system**—consists of the **heart**, and a system of **vessels (arteries)**, **veins**, and **capillaries. These all** distribute oxygen throughout the body via the blood (Figure 3). Your blood also carries other essential nutrients to the cells in your body and carries away waste. The average adult male has between 5 and 6 liters of blood in his body, while the average adult female has between 4 and 5. Your blood, in some ways, is like the oil in a car. It must be clean, well-circulated, and at the appropriate level for your body to function well.

Like the engine in a car, the core of the human circulatory system is the heart, which is responsible for the circulatory process. A heart is usually the size of a fist and is located under the ribcage between the lungs, in the center of the chest. The heart, like an engine, has its own internal electrical system, valve and pump system, and fluid lines. Your heart, however, works harder than your car's engine. It's always turned on. This relatively small source of energy keeps working even when you are parked.

Heart Anatomy and Function

It's important to understand the heart's basic anatomy and function in order to understand the body's cardiovascular and respiratory systems. All of its parts are connected, and each is necessary to keep the system—and your entire body—going.

Your heart has four chambers, two upper (the right and left atria) and two lower (the right and left ventricles). Its

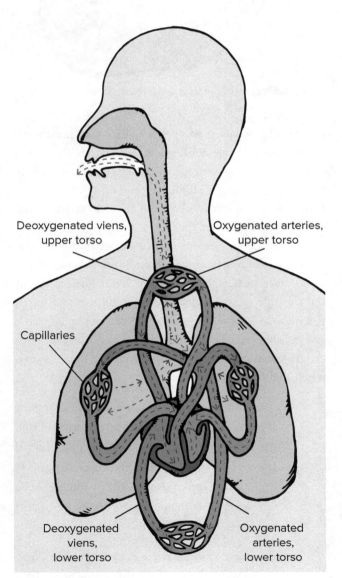

- Deoxygenated viens, upper torso
- Oxygenated arteries, upper torso
- Capillaries
- Deoxygenated viens, lower torso
- Oxygenated arteries, lower torso

Figure 3. Circulation of oxygen and carbon dioxide.

pumping action and channeling system circulates oxygen-ated blood where it needs to go and channels de-oxygenated blood to the various waste systems in the body (Figure 4). The system in charge of oxygenating your blood is the **pulmonary system**, and the system in charge of distributing that blood to the rest of your body is called the **systemic system**.

Some of the primary arteries and veins (blood vessels) in the circulatory system are directly connected to the heart. The right side of the heart has the upper and lower vena cava, the largest veins in your body. They move oxygen-poor blood from your body through the right atrium of the heart. The superior vena cava handles the oxygen-poor blood from the upper parts of your body while the inferior vena cava handles the oxygen-poor blood from the lower parts. The blood then travels through the right atrium and right ventricle, then through the pulmonary arteries (one for each lung) and into your lungs.

The blood flows through many capillaries (tiny blood vessels that supply oxygen to tissues throughout the body) inside the lungs, picking up additional oxygen, and sends the carbon dioxide waste to be released out of the lungs. This process is called gas exchange (more on this later).

The oxygenated blood then travels back into the heart through the pulmonary veins via the left atrium and ventri-cle. From here, this oxygen-rich blood is pumped through the aorta (the main artery in the heart) and to the rest of the body.

The heart, as you can see, works very hard to do its job. The amount of blood it ejects from its ventricles with each beat is referred to as the stroke volume. Your heart's stroke volume increases when you exercise to circulate more blood and oxygen – a bit like giving your car more gas to increase its revolutions. Stroke volume is an indicator of your heart's efficiency. The heart should be able to pump the amount you need based on the activity you perform.

It all may seem complex, and it is. The last time you started your car, you probably didn't think about all the moving parts it takes to keep the engine fired and running smoothly. That's probably true until your engine doesn't func-tion properly. That one broken valve or hose you usually ignore makes you realize just how important each part of the engine system is. Taking good care of your heart can keep it, and you, from breaking down too soon.

Resting Heart Rate

Your resting heart rate (RHR) is measured by the number of times your heart beats per minute (bpm) while you're at

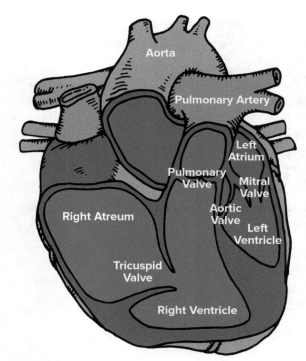

Figure 4. Diagram of the heart and its major areas.

rest. In other words, it tells you how hard your heart needs to work when you are exerting almost no effort. This can be a good indicator of your CRF. A normal RHR is between 60–100 bpm, though studies suggest that people on the higher end of this range (above 80) are often at greater risk of heart-related diseases.

A high number could mean that you are already showing signs of disease and need to see your health care provider. A low number usually means your heart is very efficient. Highly trained athletes, such as long-distance runners, may have a rate as low as 40 bpm, or even lower. A person who is inactive and has a low heart rate should also see a health care provider.

To measure your RHR, you just need a timer or stop-watch, and follow this procedure:

Place your index and middle finger on one of your pulse points. These are located on either the inside of your wrist, below the thumb-side of the hand (radial artery), or on either side of your neck adjacent to your Adam's apple (carotid artery). You should be able to feel your veins pulse with the rhythm of your heart beat.

Set a timer or use a stopwatch to clock 30 seconds. Count the number of heart beats that occur during this period and multiply it by two. That is your RHR.

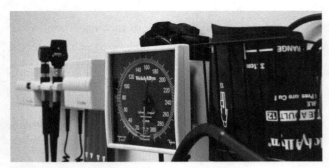

Figure 5. Blood pressure cuff.

Many factors can influence your RHR, such as blood pressure medication and activity. It's best to measure it at different times of the day, but not within a few hours of exercising. Try measuring your RHR when you first wake up in the morning to get a good baseline.

Blood Pressure

Blood pressure is the force of the blood pushing against the walls of the arteries as the heart pumps blood. Your blood pressure indicates how hard your heart is working. High blood pressure, or **hypertension**, happens when the force of your blood is too high. Hypotension happens when the force is too low. Health care workers check blood pressure using a gauge, a stethoscope or electronic sensor, and a blood pressure cuff (called a sphygmomanometer) (Figure 5). With this equipment, they measure:

- Systolic Pressure – blood pressure when the heart beats while pumping blood

- Diastolic Pressure – blood pressure when the heart is at rest between beats

Blood pressure numbers are written with the systolic number above the diastolic number. Pressure is measured in

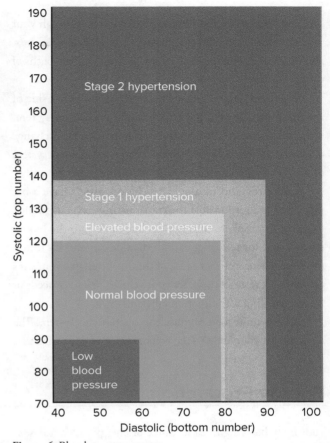

Figure 6. Blood pressure ranges.

millimeters of mercury, or mmHg. Normal blood pressure for adults is defined as a systolic pressure below 120 mmHg and a diastolic pressure below 80 mmHg. Your blood pressure changes when you sleep or wake up, when you are excited or nervous, and during activity. This is normal. However, once the activity stops, your blood pressure returns to your normal baseline range. Baseline blood pressure higher than 120/80 mmHg is considered abnormal. Chapter 9 offers more discussion on high blood pressure and what you can do to control it (Figure 6).

Respiratory System

The cardiovascular system works in tandem with the **respiratory system**. The respiratory system consists of the airways, lungs, blood vessels, and muscles that enable you to breathe. Its primary function is to exchange gas between the environment outside your body and your circulatory system.

This exchange balances oxygenation of the blood with the removal of carbon dioxide and other metabolic wastes from the blood. Gas exchange occurs in the **alveoli,** tiny air

sacs in the lungs covered with a mesh-like network of small blood vessels known as **capillaries**. Dissolved oxygen enters the **capillaries**, while carbon dioxide leaves through pulmonary circulation.

Airways are the small pipes through which air (and its oxygen) travels into the lungs. Airways also carry the gaseous waste out. The airway system includes your nose, nasal cavities, mouth, larynx (voice box), trachea (windpipe), and various bronchial tubes and their branches. Air enters through your nose or mouth as you breathe, passes through your voice box, and down your windpipe. It then separates into two paths of tubes into both your lungs.

The lungs, located near the backbone on either side of the heart, are the essential organs of the respiratory system. Once the air travels through the airway system, the exchange of gases is performed by the alveoli. These connect to a system of veins and arteries that move blood throughout the body.

Each lung and its associated blood vessels have a big job. They are responsible for transporting oxygen inhaled from the atmosphere through the body and into the bloodstream, and for releasing carbon dioxide out and back into the atmosphere. You can think of this final step like your car's exhaust—it releases the gases your vehicle no longer needs or wants, enabling it to function efficiently.

It takes quite a bit of muscle to operate this system. The muscles near your lungs—the diaphragm, intercostal muscles, abdominal muscles, and muscles in the area around your collarbone and neck—help your lungs expand and contract as you breathe. The diaphragm resides below the lungs, separating the chest cavity from the abdominal cavity, and is the primary muscle helping the lungs. The intercostal muscles between the ribs help the chest cavity expand with the lungs. The abdominal muscles are beneath the diaphragm and help a lot when breathing is fast, such as during exercise. The muscles around the collarbone and neck step in to help when other muscles aren't pulling their weight, like when a person has a lung disease.

Later in this chapter, we'll look at training adaptations in CRF that affect and are affected by your body's intake of oxygen. But first, we still need to understand more about how the body converts oxygen into energy. Like a car converting fuel to energy and then torque to move itself forward, your body uses its fuel to create chemical energy, used by your muscles each time they move.

Energy Production

Your body has a significant source of energy called **adenosine triphosphate (ATP)**, and the systems that produce that energy are the ATP-Phosphocreatine (ATP-PCr) system, the glycolytic system, and the aerobic system. These contribute to energy production in most forms of exercise.

ATP is a molecule found in every cell in your body, one that carries energy. ATP acquires its energy when food molecules (fuel) break down and then it releases this fuel as energy for other cellular processes. Scientists consider it our energy currency because it's the body's energy source for all muscle movement and fuels many of our metabolic functions as well. Later in this book you will learn about ways that fat and energy are stored. It's important to note that ATP does not store energy. Instead, it functions as the delivery driver. The body calls on other storage molecules, like fat and carbohydrates, when it needs energy. These break down into ATP which then delivers the energy where the body needs it.

The ATP-PCr, glycolytic, and aerobic systems each contribute to energy production in nearly every type of exercise, and they operate as you go about your day (Figure 7). The relative contributions of each system depend on factors like the intensity at the beginning of the exercise, your fitness level, and the availability of oxygen in the muscles.

Energy System	Type of Activity Powered	Fuels Used	Number of ATP Produced
ATP-PCr	Very high-intensity, short duration (6–10 seconds) without the use of oxygen (i.e. anaerobic); active at the onset of all activity	Creatine phosphate, Stored ATP	1
Anaerobic Glycolysis	High-intensity, short to moderate duration activities (10–90 seconds) without the use of oxygen	Blood Glucose, Muscle & Liver glycogen	2
Oxidative Phosphorylation (Aerobic)	Low- to moderate-intensity, long duration (>90 seconds)	Blood glucose, Muscle & Liver glycogen, Adipose & Intramuscular fat	From carbohydrates: 36–39 From fat: >100

Figure 7. Energy production powers different activity types, uses different fuels, and produces different amounts of ATP.

ATP-PCr Energy System

The **ATP-PCr system** fuels fast or explosive movements and only operates for a short period of time. It provides energy from the ATP stored in all of the body's cells. Creatine-phosphate (PCr), also found in all cells, is a high-energy phosphate molecule that stores energy. ATP concentrations in the cell are reduced by the breakdown of ATP to a product called adenosine diphosphate (ADP) to release energy for muscle contraction. PCr then breaks down to release both energy and a phosphate to allow reconstruction of ATP from ADP.

The body needs a continuous supply of ATP for energy—whether the energy is needed for lifting weights, walking, thinking, or even texting. It's also the unit of energy that fuels metabolism. The high-intensity bursts of activity that use ATP-PCr, such as a sprinting, standing up, throwing, jumping, or swinging a bat, don't require oxygen or build up lactic acid like prolonged activities do. The ATP-PCr system can produce energy at high rates during this type of exercise. ATP and PCr stores, which are depleted in 10–20 seconds, will last just long enough to complete the exercise.

The ATP-PCr system also replenishes itself quickly, so after a few minutes you should be able to use it again. This is good to know if you are doing a strength workout or interval training. Once this system has exhausted its fuel, the muscles still active will use a different energy system to restore the ATP and PCr.

Glycolytic System

The active muscle cell's oxygen demand exceeds its supply when exercise is of high intensity. The cell must then rely on the **glycolytic system** to produce ATP in the absence of oxygen (anaerobic). This system can only use glucose, found in the blood's plasma and stored in both muscle and the liver as glycogen. The glycolytic energy system serves as the primary energy system for all-out bouts of exercise or movements lasting from 30 seconds to 2 minutes, such as a 200-meter run. It can be accessed rather quickly, but it doesn't produce a large amount of ATP. This energy system is used at the beginning of an exercise session, or for typical movements like when you have to run a couple blocks to catch the bus, walk up several flights of stairs, or hurry to another classroom.

Lactate is the primary by-product of the anaerobic glycolytic energy system. At lower exercise intensities, when the cardiorespiratory system can meet the oxygen demands of active muscles, blood lactate levels remain close to what they are when you're resting. This is because some lactate is used aerobically by muscle and is removed as fast as it enters the blood from the muscle.

Increases in intensity change this. Lactate enters the blood from the muscle faster than it's removed from the blood, and blood lactate concentrations increase above resting levels. Lactate levels continue to increase as the rate of work increases, until the point of exhaustion. The point at which the concentration of lactate in the blood begins to increase above resting levels is referred to as the lactate threshold.

Lactate threshold provides an important marker for endurance performance. Your lactate threshold increases as your fitness level increases. Exceed your lactate threshold and you will begin to slow down. Distance runners set their race pace at, or just slightly above, their lactate threshold to avoid this. The thresholds of highly trained endurance athletes occur at a much higher percentage of their maximum aerobic capacity, and thus at higher relative workloads, than do the thresholds of untrained persons. This key difference allows endurance athletes to perform at a faster pace.

Aerobic System

The most complex energy system is the aerobic or oxygen energy system, which provides most of the body's ATP. The **aerobic system** (or oxidative system) produces ATP directly from the oxygen in the bloodstream and is the most important system to CRF. This system uses oxygen to produce ATP within the mitochondria, special cell organelles within muscle. This process cannot generate ATP at a high enough rate to sustain an all-out sprint but proves highly effective at lower rates of work (e.g., long distance running). ATP can also be produced from fat and protein metabolism through the aerobic system. Typically, carbohydrate and fat provide most of the ATP. Protein contributes only 5–10% at rest and during exercise under most circumstances.

This is the long-duration energy system. You use the aerobic system whenever you do prolonged physical activity, like a 10K run (about 6 miles), a session of Zumba, a moderate-paced walk with your dog, an indoor cycling class, or an elliptical workout. You also use this energy system throughout your day when doing something for longer than a couple of minutes.

After 2–3 minutes of exercise, the aerobic system becomes the primary to bring oxygen to the muscles. Aerobic energy pathways may take a while to use, but they are very efficient and have a significantly higher capability to produce ATP and for a much longer period. The net production of ATP for this system is 32 ATP molecules compared to 2 ATP molecules from the glycolytic system. This system is also the pathway that provides ATP to fuel most of the body's energy needs not related to physical activity, such as building and repairing body tissues, digesting food, controlling body temperature and growing hair.

The number of mitochondria (the power sources of the cell) present in the muscles' cells and the availability of oxygen are also important. Regular training increases the number of mitochondria and the body's ability to use oxygen. Your body also has to have enough carbohydrates (glucose) present to fuel this system, or you'll start to tap into protein resources, which is tough on your body.

Energy Systems Working Together

Your car has many systems that function concurrently and in different ways depending upon whether you are idling, stuck in stop-and-go traffic, cruising through town, or speeding along the interstate. All the systems are functioning at each pace, but some systems have to work more than others based on your speed. Your body's energy systems function similarly, with one system dominating the others at a given time based on your body's needs.

Remember that slippery puppy of yours, Larry, who makes a break for it to chase the squirrel he's been watching? Your first movement is a leap and failed grab in an attempt to catch the furry escape artist. At this point, your muscles use what ATP they have in them, just enough for a few seconds.

For your sprint to the tree where Larry stops to rest, about 80 meters away, your body calls upon the ATP-PCr system for help. Unfortunately, the squirrel bolts and so does Larry, heading toward an open field.

Fortunately, he stops for a moment to regain the squirrel's scent. You run after him and reach the tree in about 45 seconds. This action drew upon the glycolytic system. Apparently, you are better at running than grabbing because you miss at yet another attempt to capture the beast (it may be time to work on your agility). Now you are in for some aerobic exercise.

Larry is now running through the field, and so are you. Your aerobic system is supplying your muscles with oxygen. It takes you 7 minutes of nearly continuous running to catch up with Larry, who you only manage to apprehend because he stopped to pick up a stick.

As you can see, good CRF plays a role in both your day-to-day activities and your success when exercising. In the scenario above, you could not have caught up to Larry without a bit of aerobic training. A 7-minute run, depending on speed, could be nearly a mile – you may not be agile, but you're a decent runner. You also drew upon your fat stores by accessing your aerobic system, which helps keep your body at a healthy weight. It's a good thing that you've been working on your CRF, or chasing Larry would have been almost impossible.

Benefits of Cardiorespiratory Fitness

Good CRF has benefits associated with wellness. Improvement to your daily functioning is just one piece of the large puzzle of benefits good CRF can create. These benefits could be physical, emotional, intellectual, and even environmental.

Physical Benefits

The physical benefits of good CRF include reduced risk of disease and illness, increased life expectancy, and healthier body composition. Many factors contribute to both your wellness and your risk of disease, but CRF is a key factor because it requires aerobic exercise and a healthy diet (see Chapter 7). These lead to a whole host of physical benefits.

CRF reduces your risk of developing diseases, particularly those associated with your heart. If you are already suffering from heart disease, CRF can help make these diseases more manageable. CRF keeps blood moving through your body efficiently and widens capillaries, enabling all the parts of your body to get more oxygen and carry away waste. This, along with a healthy diet, helps keep plaque and blood clots from forming in your arteries and causing significant damage or even death. Here's what good CRF can do:

- Reduce your blood pressure and your risk of hypertension
- Reduce the triglyceride levels in your blood (these are bad fats)
- Raise your HDL (good cholesterol) levels
- Help manage your insulin and blood sugar levels, lowering your risk of Type 2 diabetes
- Reduce your risk of osteoporosis and certain forms of cancer
- Reduce your risk of becoming overweight or obese
- Help you lose weight, reducing your risk of many other chronic diseases and illnesses

At the beginning of this chapter, we mentioned that low levels of CRF often lead to increased mortality rates. In other words, a lack of aerobic exercise can lead to an earlier death, likely due to the development or poor management of disease. In general, people with good cardiorespiratory fitness live longer lives.

They also enjoy a better **body composition**. We discussed this briefly in Chapter 2 and will provide even more detail in Chapter 6. A healthy body composition essentially means that you are not carrying excess fat and have enough muscle to succeed in your activities. Excess fat is a health risk to your organs, joints, and metabolic systems. Too much fat and not enough muscle strength can also impact your ability to perform day-to-day activities because of increased fatigue.

Emotional Benefits

Your brain contains chemicals called neurotransmitters. These are chemical messengers that transmit signals throughout the body, affecting both physical and psychological functions. Low levels of neurotransmitters can lead to feelings of sadness, anxiety, and a general loss of interest in your life. These chemicals include dopamine, a chemical that triggers your reward centers in your brain. Exercise boosts dopamine levels, making you feel happier. It also gives you a sense of control over your life that can increase your confidence level. In fact, studies on neurotransmitter health and chemical triggers indicate that we can manage symptoms of depression and anxiety through exercise.

We also do a better job managing stress when we are healthy and exercising. The complications that arise from illness or disease can seriously interfere with your life. Lower risk for stress-inducing disease means less interference and less stress. Regular exercise also means you're successfully scheduling this activity into your life by taking the time to exercise. This downtime away from daily stressors gives you a few moments to focus on yourself. It might distract you from those worries that can have a negative impact. Exercise can be a powerful outlet for managing stress, especially if you find a form of exercise that you enjoy or that gives you satisfaction. We'll look at stress management in more detail in Chapter 8.

Improved cardiorespiratory fitness also contributes to your emotional health. Feeling healthy, comfortable, and confident is not superficial. It's tangible.

Your friend Jane, for example, has struggled to maintain a healthy fitness level for years. Last fall, a mutual friend ran in a 10k fun run, and that inspired Jane to try it too. But a

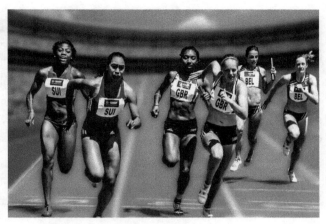

Figure 8. Competitive sports can motivate fitness.

few months later, when Jane signed up for a similar event, she found she couldn't finish the race, and didn't really find the "fun run" to be fun at all. She set a goal for her fitness—she would finish the race at the 5k fun run this coming fall. She started jogging each morning, increasing her cardiorespiratory fitness over time. In the fall, she not only finished the race but completed it without stopping to walk (Figure 8)! The tangible accomplishment of finishing the race made Jane realize that she could use her body in ways she didn't think were possible, improving her confidence.

Additional Benefits

Good CRF can also stimulate you on an intellectual level. Your muscles release certain proteins when you exercise that have a regenerative effect on the brain. The National Institute of Health supported research on a particular protein released during exercise called cathespin B. This protein is thought to directly impact the memory centers of the brain. Participants in the study found that after two weeks of regular exercise, their memories tested better than before they began the exercise routine. In this way, exercise is like a smart pill. You retain more information and generate new neurons in your brain to help you think critically and see improvement in your cognition.

Even the environment benefits from your good CRF. How? Walking, running, biking—all these types of physical activity transport you without polluting the environment. You read in Chapter 1 that motor vehicles cause a lot of pollution and poor air quality. A person cycling or walking to the store or work pollutes very little. Not only are they more active and less sedentary (great for their health) but they also lower their carbon footprint on the planet and improve the air they breathe.

Improving Cardiorespiratory Fitness

This chapter has shown you what CRF is and why you should improve it—now let's focus on how. You can improve your cardiorespiratory fitness through training, beginning with self-assessments, goal setting, and creating a training plan. This section will show you how to assess your current level of CRF, determine what kind of goals you should set, and suggest some different training methods and exercises to help meet your goals.

Assessing Your Cardiorespiratory Fitness

Your current CRF can be assessed through the Rockport Walking Test and other VO_2 max tests, resting heart rates, and blood pressure.

The Rockport Walking Test and VO_2 Max

Experts at the University of Massachusetts at Amherst's Department of Exercise Science developed this one-mile test to measure a person's aerobic capacity (or VO_2 max) based on the participant's age, weight, and gender. All you need to complete the test is a level, one-mile track, a stopwatch, a scale, and comfortable clothes and shoes. Follow this procedure:

- Weigh yourself.

- Take about 5–10 minutes to lightly warm up and stretch.

- Start the timer and walk one mile as quickly as you can (do not run or speed walk).

- As soon as you complete the mile, take your pulse while walking slowly to cool down, count the number of beats for 30 seconds, then double the number.

- Calculate your VO_2 max using the formula:

  132.853 – (0.0769 x weight) – (0.3877 x age) + (6.315 x 1 if male, 0 if female) – (3.2649 x time) – (0.1565 x heart rate)

A 30-year-old man weighing 180 pounds finished the mile in 10.55 minutes (or 10 minutes 33 seconds) and had a heart rate of 160 beats per minute (bpm). His estimated VO_2 max would be as follows:

132.853 – (0.0769 x 180) – (0.3877 x 30) + (6.315 x 1) – (3.2649 x 10.55) – (0.1565 x 160) = 54.21

Note: This manual calculation requires you to convert time to minutes by dividing the seconds by 60 and adding that number to the whole number. For example, 10 min. 33 sec. = 10 + (33/60) = 10.55 minutes.

Use the table (Figure 9) to determine where you are, then set your goals at a level you'd like to be.

The Rockport Walking Test is generally considered a safe and effective way to measure your aerobic capacity for most individuals. With level terrain, no running, low impact to the body, and no set time or pace established for completion, even inactive individuals can make use of this method to determine their cardiovascular fitness level.

The 1.5 Mile Test

This test is a lot like the Rockport test. A level track or road that enables you to complete 1.5 miles, comfortable clothes and shoes, and a stopwatch are all that are needed. For this test, however, the participant will run, walk, or a combination of the two, as quickly as possible for the entire distance. Cardiovascular endurance is measured based on how long it takes the individual to complete the run (Figure 10). Law enforcement and other government agencies often use this test to determine a potential employee's ability to meet the physical demands of the profession.

3-Minute Step Test

The 3-minute step test requires stepping up and down on a 16.25-inch step for 3 minutes at a constant rate. At the completion of the activity, heart rate is measured for 15 seconds. The lower the heart rate, the better the ability to recover from an aerobic task, a good indication of CRF.

Maximal Oxygen Uptake Norms for Men (ml/kg/min)						
Age	18–25	26–35	36–45	46–55	56–65	65+
Excellent	>60	>56	>51	>45	>41	>37
Good	52–60	49–56	43–51	39–45	36–41	33–37
Average	47–51	43–48	39–42	35–38	32–35	29–32
Average	42–46	40–42	35–38	32–35	30–31	26–28
Average	37–41	35–39	31–34	29–31	26–29	22–25
Poor	30–36	30–34	26–30	25–28	22–25	20–21
Very Poor	<30	<30	<26	<25	<22	<20
Maximal Oxygen Uptake Norms for Women (ml/kg/min)						
Age	18–25	26–35	36–45	46–55	56–65	65+
Excellent	>56	>52	>45	>40	>37	>32
Good	47–56	45–52	38–45	34–40	32–37	28–32
Average	42–46	39–44	34–37	31–33	28–31	25–27
Average	38–41	35–38	31–33	28–30	25–27	22–24
Average	33–37	31–34	27–30	25–27	22–24	19–22
Poor	28–32	26–30	22–26	20–24	18–21	17–18
Very Poor	<28	<26	<22	<20	<18	<17

Figure 9. VO_2 max ranges.

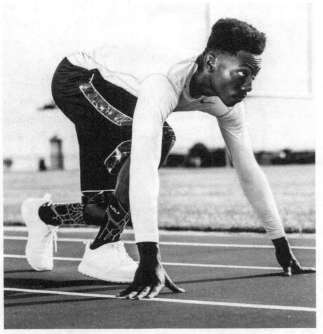

Figure 10. The 1.5 mile test is widely used to test physical ability.

Resting Heart Rate and Blood Pressure

Your resting heart rate and blood pressure can be good indicators of CRF. Earlier in this chapter you learned how to determine your RHR and whether you are in a healthy range or not. Your health care provider can check your blood pressure as described earlier. It is best not to drink coffee or smoke cigarettes for 30 minutes prior to the test. You should also use the restroom before the test and sit down for at least 5 minutes before starting. Refer to Chapter 9 for more information on blood pressure, such as healthy ranges.

Setting Goals for Cardiorespiratory Fitness

Now you know some ways to establish your baseline. You can set goals to achieve improvements in your problem areas based on what you learn from these assessments. Each should follow the SMART goal principles of being specific, measurable, achievable, relevant, and time-based. For example, if your assessment reveals that you have high blood pressure, here is a SMART goal you could set for yourself:

Specific—I want to lower my blood pressure

Measurable—From 140/90 to 130/80 mmHg

Achievable—This is a small improvement

Relevant—I will feel healthier and reduce risk

Time-based—3 months

You should also set smaller goals on the way to your large goals. The example above is a smaller goal on the way to healthy blood pressure. The long term goal might be a blood pressure 120/70 mmHg. The goal of 130/80 mmHg is closer to the healthy rate, but it isn't all the way there. This lets you celebrate the progress without feeling discouraged by the time it might take to reach your larger goal of a healthy blood pressure. Taking things in stages is wise, and small goals help you do that.

Training for Cardiorespiratory Fitness

Do you like to run? Walk? Ride a bicycle? Hike? Swim? Surf? Anything that elevates your heart rate works your CRF and the options seem endless. No matter what type of cardio you enjoy, training for CRF should follow the guidelines from the American College of Sports Medicine (ACSM) and the US Department of Health and Human Services' 2008 Physical Activity Guidelines for Americans. Fortunately, there are many ways to meet these guidelines safely while achieving variety in your training. This will keep you focused and interested in enhancing your CRF. This section offers a few examples of healthy ways to meet the guidelines.

Cross-Training

Cross-training is when a person takes advantage of different methods of training to develop a specific aspect of their fitness. Varying the type of aerobic activity you perform gives you many options. It can also help you work a variety of muscles and reduce your risk of injury. It is a good method of balancing a healthy training frequency while correctly resting other areas of your body when needed. You can vary not only your aerobic activities, but also your other types of activity, like those that work your muscles and improve flexibility. You can play soccer one day and lift weights and do yoga the next. What you choose depends on your goals and interests (Figure 11).

Your friend Kendal, the track enthusiast, does not actually run every time she works out. She has had issues with shin splints over the years and finds that she can work in her CRF in other ways and still be ready to run during competition. She runs three days, and on the other two she bicycles, takes a low-impact aerobics class, does kickboxing, and occasionally swims laps at the pool. This helps her do cardio and work a variety of muscles, keeping her from getting bored and reducing the risk of overusing her sensitive shins.

High Intensity Interval Training (HIIT)

According to the American College of Sports Medicine, High Intensity Interval Training (HIIT) involves repeated episodes of high-intensity activity followed by varied recovery times. These intense segments can range from 5 seconds to 8 minutes and are performed at 80% to 95% of a person's estimated maximal heart rate. The recovery periods (lower intensity) may last for as much time as the workout periods and are usually performed at 40–50% of a person's estimated maximum heart rate. The workout continues with alternating work and relief periods totaling 20–60 minutes.

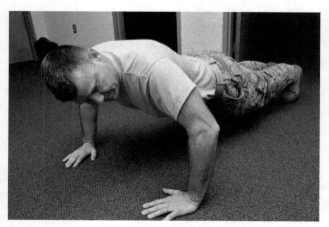

Figure 11. Cross-training improves multiple areas of fitness.

Benefit	Description
Helps build endurance	High Intensity Interval Training (HIIT) adapts to the cellular structure of muscles which enables you to increase your endurance while doing any type of exercise.
Burns calories and fat in a shorter period of time	Studies show that 15 minutes of HIIT burns more calories than jogging on a treadmill for an hour.
Effective energy use	Through HIIT, your body learns how to efficiently use the energy that comes from your body's energy system.
Boosts metabolism	HIIT helps you consume more oxygen than a non-interval workout routine. The excess amount of oxygen consumed helps increase your rate of metabolism from about 90–144 minutes after a session of HIIT.
Burn calories and fat for hours after training	When participating in such HIIT workouts, your body's repair cycle goes into overdrive.
No equipment necessary	HIIT workouts are extremely cost efficient because you need zero equipment! All you need is a little open space.
Lose fat and not muscle	Steady cardio is often associated with losing muscle. HIIT workouts, however, combine weight training (the weight being your body) and effectively allows dieters to preserve their muscle gain while still shedding weight.
Choose your own workouts	HIIT doesn't limit you to just running or biking. In fact, you can pick any cardio workout and make it an interval workout.
Good for heart health	With HIIT it's easier to push yourself to that level because of the rest interval that comes right after you reach that point.
Challenging	HIIT workouts offer a new challenge to experts and a quicker way to see results for beginners.

Figure 12. HITT training has many distinct benefits for beginners and advanced trainees.

These workouts can be performed with nearly any type of activity, including cycling, walking, swimming, elliptical cross-training, and group exercise activities. They provide similar fitness benefits as continuous endurance workouts, but in shorter periods of time (Figure 12). This is because HIIT workouts tend to burn more calories than traditional workouts, especially after the workout. The post-exercise period is called the excess post-exercise oxygen consumption (EPOC). This is generally about a 2-hour period after a workout where the body is restoring itself to pre-exercise levels, using more energy.

HIIT training has been shown to improve:

- Aerobic and anaerobic fitness

- Blood pressure

- Cardiovascular health

- Insulin sensitivity (which helps the exercising muscles more readily use glucose for fuel to make energy)

- Cholesterol profiles

- Abdominal fat and body weight while maintaining muscle mass

The ACSM states that when developing a HIIT program, you should consider the duration, intensity, and frequency of the work intervals and the length of the recovery intervals. Intensity during the high-intensity work interval should range ≥80% of your estimated maximum heart rate (Figure 13). Using the Borg Rating or Talk Test, the work interval should feel like you are

Age	Steady State Heart Rate	Interval Heart Rate
20	60–80 Beats Per Minute	100–170 Beats Per Minute
30	60–80 Beats Per Minute	95–162 Beats Per Minute
40	60–80 Beats Per Minute	93–157 Beats Per Minute
50	60–80 Beats Per Minute	90–153 Beats Per Minute

Figure 13. Target steady state and interval heart rates by age.

exercising "hard" to "very hard" or that carrying on a conversation would be difficult. The intensity of the recovery interval should be 40–50% of your estimate maximal heart rate. This would be physical activity that feels very comfortable in order to help you recover and prepare for your next work interval. The talk test isn't much help here because you will be in EPOC, and breathing may still be heightened.

The relationship of the work and recovery interval is important. Many studies use a specific ratio of exercise to recovery to improve the different energy systems of the body. For example, a ratio of 1:1 might be a 3-minute hard work (or high-intensity) bout followed by a 3-minute recovery (or low-intensity) bout. These 1:1 interval workouts often range about 3, 4, or 5 minutes followed by an equal time in recovery.

The "spring interval training method" is another popular HIIT training protocol. The exerciser does about 30 seconds of a sprint or other activity with a near full-out effort, followed by 4–5 minutes of recovery. This combination of exercise can be repeated 3–5 times (Figure 14). These higher-intensity work efforts are typically shorter bouts (e.g. 30 second sprint intervals).

HIIT training can easily be modified for people of all fitness levels and special conditions, such as people who are overweight or have diabetes. However, people who are inactive or who may have an increased coronary disease risk should get medical clearance from a health care provider before starting HIIT or any exercise training. These risks could include a family history, cigarette smoking, hypertension, diabetes (or pre-diabetes), abnormal cholesterol levels, and obesity.

You should establish a foundational level of fitness, or "base fitness level," prior to beginning HIIT training. This usually requires consistent aerobic training, such as 3–5 times

Time	Interval	Exertion Level (0–10)
5 min.	Warm-up	3–4
1 min.	Speed	7–9
2 min.	Recovery	5–6
1 min.	Speed	7–9
2 min.	Recovery	5–6
1 min.	Speed	7–9
2 min.	Recovery	5–6
1 min.	Speed	7–9
2 min.	Recovery	5–6
5 min.	Cool-down	3–4

Figure 14. Sample HITT training program with exertion levels.

per week for 20–60 minutes per session at a somewhat vigorous intensity for several weeks. Establishing appropriate exercise form and muscle strength are important before engaging in regular HIIT to reduce the risk of injury (Figure 15).

Regardless of your age, gender, and fitness level, one of the keys to safe participation in HIIT training is to modify the intensity of the work interval to your preferred level of challenge. Safety should always be your first priority. Focus more on finding your own optimal training intensities rather than on keeping up with other people.

HIIT workouts can be more exhaustive than traditional endurance workouts. A longer recovery period is often needed. Perhaps start with one HIIT training workout a week, with your other workouts being your normal workouts. As you feel ready for more challenge, add a second HIIT workout a week, making sure you spread the HIIT workouts throughout the week.

Stages	Description
Stage I	People new to cardiorespiratory exercise need to develop a baseline level of aerobic fitness to avoid over-training and exhaustion. Generally, exercising at an estimated maximal heart rate (MHR) of 65 to 75% is a safe intensity for apparently healthy adults; or 12–13 on the Rating of Perceived Exertion Scale (RPE). During this training period you should strive to gradually increase the duration and intensity of exercise bouts.
Stage II	Stage II is the introduction to interval training in which intensities are varied throughout the workout. You should use intervals ranging from 65 to 85% of MHR; or 14 to 16 RPE. Stage II differs from high-intensity anaerobic interval training in that it uses more moderate to challenging work intervals (i.e., running, not sprinting) with varying lower-intensity recovery periods (i.e. light jogging). This format also tends to be more engaging and less boring than steady state aerobic exercise.
Stage III	Stage III is a form of high-intensity interval training involving short, intense bouts of exercise (i.e. sprinting), interspersed with active bouts of recovery (i.e., light jogging). People training in stage III should use intervals ranging from 65 to 95% of MHR; or 17 to 19 RPE. The time needed to transition to stage III training is variable, perhaps requiring 2 to 3 months or longer.

Figure 15. Cardiorespiratory training should be based on experience. Rushing could result in injuries that might delay improvements.

Applying the Principles to Cardiorespiratory Fitness

You learned about the FITT principle in Chapter 2. Your cardiorespiratory fitness should involve this principle, following a plan that can strengthen your heart and lung capacity to function well.

Frequency—Adults should do 3–5 days per week of aerobic activity depending upon intensity. Moderate-intensity walking is usually safe to do every day, but the body needs time to rebuild, repair, and restore energy between high-intensity workouts. Exercising more than 5 days per week may not yield additional benefits for everyone and could lead to overuse injuries, but this varies with the individual. Incorporating different types of cardio can help avoid overuse injuries, especially if a person wants to train more than 3 days per week. Training less than 3 days per week makes it challenging to improve fitness level. Some, however, is always better than none.

Intensity—The more intense your exercise, the faster your heart will beat. You can calculate your target heart rate based on your age, and then exercise with an intensity that raises your heart rate to the target. Target heart rate is measured as a percentage of your maximum heart rate (MHR) which is the fastest your heart can beat, also based on your age (Figure 16).

A person who has been inactive may want to begin targeting the lower end of their target heart rate zone, while an active person may want their heart rate closer to 90% of MHR. You can check your heart rate during exercise. To do so, take a short break at your peak performance (or at intervals throughout) but keep walking to stay warm. Take your pulse. Use the chart to see if you are in your target zone.

For example, Claudia is 40 years old and has been measuring her resting heart rate each morning when she wakes up (a good way to get a baseline). Her average is 64 bpm. She goes on her 5k jog on Mondays, Wednesdays, and Fridays. During her jog, she turns around at the crosswalk at Dearborn and River Road—right at the halfway point—and checks her heart rate. She does this by walking back toward home at first to keep her heart rate elevated. Her fitness band that takes her pulse measures her heart rate as 145 bpm. This is right at 80% of MHR, perfect for her routine and experience level. She then resumes her jog home.

Claudia used to think that you could only burn fat by exercising at a low intensity. This is a myth. Advanced equipment in physiology labs does show that fat stores contribute a greater percentage of fuel used to power lower-intensity exercises, but that is offset by the total caloric expenditure in high intensity exercises. For example, you chose a low-intensity exercise for your one-hour session. 60% of your burned calories came from fat stores, but you only burned 100 calories. In a high-intensity one-hour session, only 40% of your burned calories came from fat stores, but you burned 500 calories. So, at low-intensity you burned 60 fat calories, while

Calculate your Maximum Heart Rate (MHR): Subtract your age from 220 Calculate your Target Heart Rate: Multiply your MHR by 0.55–0.90 based on experience level		
Age	**Previously Sedentary** Target Heart Rate Zone: 55–65%	**History of Regular Exercise to Athlete** Target Heart Rate Zone: 65–90%	**Maximum Heart Rate: 100%**
20	110–130 beats per minute (bpm)	130–180 beats per minute (bpm)	200 beats per minute (bpm)
25	107–126 bpm	126–175 bpm	195 bpm
30	104–123 bpm	123–171 bpm	190 bpm
35	102–120 bpm	120–166 bpm	185 bpm
40	99–117 bpm	117–162 bpm	180 bpm
45	96–113 bpm	113–158 bpm	175 bpm
50	93–110 bpm	110–153 bpm	170 bpm
55	90–107 bpm	107–149 bpm	165 bpm
60	88–104 bpm	104–144 bpm	160 bpm
65	85–101 bpm	101–140 bpm	155 bpm
70	82–98 bpm	98–135 bpm	150 bpm

Figure 16. Target and maximum heart rate by activity level.

at high intensity, you burned 200 fat calories (Figure 17). See the difference?

You can also determine your optimal heart rate by using the **Heart Rate Reserve** (HRR) method. Start by determining your MHR. Subtract your heart's resting rate from your maximum (RHR – MHR). Test during performance as above. For Claudia, her HRR is 116 bpm (220 – 40 = 180 – 64 = 116).

You may not always be able to measure your heart rate, but you can still get an idea of how hard your heart is working by using some simple alternative methods. One way is to measure your intensity by using the **talk-test,** which tests relative intensity. In general, if you're doing moderate-intensity activity you can talk, but not sing, during the activity. During vigorous-intensity activity, you will not be able to say more than a few words without pausing for a breath.

Another alternate method to measure intensity is to determine an activity's **Rate of Perceived Exertion** (Figure 18) using the Borg Rating of Perceived Exertion (RPE). Perceived exertion is how hard you feel like your body is working. It's based on the physical sensations a person experiences during physical activity, including increased heart rate, increased respiration or breathing, increased sweating, and muscle fatigue.

During activity, use the scale to assign numbers to how you feel (focus only on your level of exertion, not any injuries you may have). Health care providers generally agree that perceived exertion ratings between 12–14 on the Borg Scale suggest that physical activity is at a moderate level of intensity. This process is subjective, but a person's exertion rating may provide a good estimate of the actual heart rate during physical activity.

Monitoring how hard your body is working can help you adjust the intensity of the activity by speeding up or slowing down your movements. It will become easier to know when to adjust your intensity as you become more experienced. For example, a walker who wants to engage in moderate-intensity activity would aim for a level of "somewhat hard" (12–14). If he describes his muscle fatigue and breathing as "very light"

Moderate Activity 3.0–6.0 METs (3.5–7 kcal/min)	Vigorous Activity Greater than 6.0 METs (more than 7 kcal/min)
Walking, hiking, roller skating	Walking at 5 mph or faster, jogging or running, walking and climbing up a hill, mountain climbing
Bicycling 5–9 mph on level terrain	Bicycling more than 10 mph on uphill terrain
Aerobic dancing, water aerobics	Aerobic dancing step aerobics, water jogging
Calisthenics: yoga, general home exercises	Calisthenics: pushups, pull ups, karate, jump rope, jumping jacks
Weight training and bodybuilding with free weights	Circuit weight training
Boxing with punching bag	Boxing in ring, sparring, wrestling—competitive
Ballroom dancing, line dancing, square dancing, folk dancing, modern dancing, disco, ballet	Professional ballroom dancing, square dancing, folk dancing, clogging
Table tennis—competitive, tennis—doubles	Tennis—singles
Softball, basketball—shooting baskets	Football game, basketball game, soccer game, rugby
Volleyball	Beach volleyball
Frisbee, juggling, curling, cricket	Handball, racquetball, squash
Downhill skiing, ice skating	Downhill skiing—racing, ice skating, cross-country skiing, sledding, ice hockey
Swimming—recreational	Swimming—steady paced laps, water jogging, water polo water basketball
Canoeing or rowing a boat, rafting, sailing, paddle boating	Canoeing or rowing—4 mph or more
Fishing, hunting	
Horseback riding	Horseback riding—competitive, polo

Figure 17. Activities by activity level.

(9 on the scale) he would want to increase his intensity. On the other hand, if he felt his exertion was "extremely hard" (19) he would need to slow down his movements to achieve the moderate-intensity range.

Time—The federal guidelines for physical activity recommend 150 minutes of moderate-intensity activity per week or 75 minutes of vigorous-intensity. More is recommended for weight management or loss. For more extensive health benefits, adults should increase their aerobic physical activity to 300 minutes (5 hours) per week of moderate-intensity, or 150 minutes per week of vigorous-intensity aerobic physical activity, or an equivalent combination. Additional health benefits are gained by engaging in physical activity beyond this amount.

Here is an example of how you might structure your exercise plan:

Moderate intensity—30–60 minutes of continuous activity, five times per week

Vigorous intensity—20–60 minutes of continuous activity, three times per week

Time, intensity, and frequency are closely tied together. Vigorous-intensity workouts require less time to achieve similar benefits to moderate-intensity workouts. Vigorous-intensity workouts are not recommended until a person has established a solid cardiorespiratory foundation. Cardiorespiratory sessions can also be broken up into multiple ten-minute sessions if needed. Remember, a person can benefit from some activity even if they are not able to meet the time guidelines identified here.

Type—Cardiorespiratory endurance activities include rhythmic movements of large muscle groups. With that in mind, there are many options for cardio training. People often ask, "What is the best type of exercise?" The answer is simple—one that you will actually do. It should be accessible, affordable, and something that you can enjoy. Try different activities to see which ones you enjoy the most. It can be helpful to choose a variety of exercises to avoid overuse injuries and stay motivated. This could be running, aerobics class, bicycling, swimming, walking, rowing, cross-country skiing, hiking, basketball, volleyball, dancing, or any activity that elevates your heart rate to the target zone and utilizes your large muscles (Figure 19).

Cardiorespiratory exercise can be done indoors, outdoors, on a team, solo, or in a group. You might find that you enjoy a competitive form of exercise where you are playing a game or sport, or you may find a run outdoors satisfying. It may be worth taking a Physical Education course to explore an exercise mode more in-depth and gain hands-on experience.

Training Principles

You also learned about the training principles of overload, progression, specificity, reversibility, and recovery in Chapter 2. These can be easily applied to CRF training. The specificity aspect is simple—you're working your cardiorespiratory system. The recovery principle, as well, is simple for CRF. Unlike your muscles (Chapter 4), your cardiorespiratory system doesn't need a lot of time off between workouts—just follow the frequency and time guidelines. Your main concerns with these principles should be with overload, progression, and reversibility.

Your plan should account for progress toward your goal and to do that you will need to overload at times. For example, say that you started by running one mile in 15 minutes,

#	Level	Activity
6	None	Lying in bed or sitting in a chair, relaxed—Little or no effort
7, 8	Very, very light	
9, 10	Very light	
11	Fairly light	
12, 13, 14	Somewhat hard	Target range: Cardiorespiratory exercise or moderate activity—Moderate effort
15, 16	Hard	
17, 18	Very hard	Vigorous exercise or high intensity interval training—Maximal effort
19	Very, very hard	
20	Maximum exertion	

Figure 18. The Borg Rating of Perceived Exertion scale.

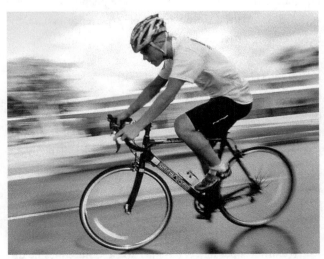

Figure 19. Cycling can be moderate or vigorous activity.

and now your body can do this comfortably. You set a goal for yourself to score above 52 on the Rockport Test and aren't quite there yet. You also have a goal of running a 5k race with a friend. Try increasing your speed to do the mile in less time or add distance to your run. Overload again when this becomes comfortable or easy for you. Remember that if you take too much time off from your cardio workouts, you may encounter reversibility and will need to work back up to your prior level.

Keep in mind that wellness takes time. Nothing happens overnight, no matter what you've seen on social media or which celebrity promotes it. Research suggests that at least 6 weeks is required to see noticeable improvement, and as much as a year or more of regular exercise is needed before a peak in fitness is reached.

Choosing a Fitness Program

Each person should carefully determine their exercise intensity based on their SMART goals and the safety of their chosen intensity. The type of cardiorespiratory exercise you choose should suit your fitness goals and your preference for activity type. If you don't like competitive sports, don't do them! Hate aerobics classes? No need to go! There are plenty of options to choose from, so pick something you enjoy. You'll have more fun and be more consistent if you develop an exercise plan that works with your personality and interests. If you're trying to get started, try several different kinds of activities to see what you like and don't like.

Also, the amount of time you spend in each cardiorespiratory fitness activity should reflect a consideration of the guidelines and safety for you. Someone who is already athletic might comfortably jump into a HIIT program, but a low-activity person exercising for the first time might want to try something easier, like starting a Couch-to-5k program, or joining a walking group. Increases to activity should be made in stages.

Scenarios: Fitness Training Plans

Here are two examples that show how people at different ages, levels of fitness, and levels of experience can safely become more active over time.

Scenario #1 – Bill: Inactive

Bill is a man who has been inactive for many years. He wants to work his way up to the equivalent of 180 to 210 minutes (3 – 3 ½ hours) of walking per week. On weekdays, he has time for up to 45 minutes of walking, and he plans to do something physically active each weekend. He decides to start with walking because it is moderate intensity and has a low risk of injury.

- Weeks 1 through 2: Bill starts at a low level. He walks 10 minutes per day, 3 days per week. Sometimes he divides the 10 minutes per day into 2 sessions. He prefers to alternate rest days and active days. (Total = 30 minutes per week)

- Weeks 3 through 8: Bill increases duration by adding 5 minutes per day and continues walking on 3 non-consecutive days each week. The weekly increase is 15 minutes. (Week 3 total = 45 minutes / Week 8 total = 120 minutes or 2 hours)

- Weeks 9 through 12: Bill adds another day of moderate-intensity activity on the weekend, and starts doing a variety of activities, including biking, hiking, and an aerobics class, gradually increasing the minutes of activity. By week 12, he is doing 60 minutes or more of moderate-intensity activity on the weekend.

Reaching his goal: Bill increased to a total of 180 moderate-intensity minutes a week over a 3-month period.

Scenario—Kim: Active

Kim is an active woman who currently does 150 minutes (2 ½ hours) per week of moderate-intensity activity. She wants to work up to at least the equivalent of 300 minutes (5 hours) of moderate-intensity activity per week. She also wants to shift some of that moderate-intensity activity to vigorous-intensity activity. Her current 150 minutes a week includes:

- 30 minutes of mowing the grass one day a week

- 30 minutes of brisk walking 4 days a week

- 15 minutes of Zumba 2 days a week

Over a month, Kim adds walking on another weekday, and she gradually adds 15 minutes of moderate-intensity activity on each of the 5 walking days each week. This provides an additional 105 minutes (one hour and 45 minutes) of moderate-intensity activity.

Over the next month, Kim decides to replace some walking with jogging. Instead of walking 45 minutes, she walks for 30 minutes and jogs for 15 minutes on each weekday, providing the equivalent of 300 minutes a week of moderate-intensity physical activity from her walking and jogging.

Reaching her goal: Kim now does a total of 180 minutes of moderate-intensity activity each week (walking and mowing the grass) and does 75 minutes (one hour and 15 minutes) of vigorous-intensity jogging. One minute of vigorous-intensity activity is about the same as 2 minutes of moderate-intensity activity, so she is now doing the equivalent of 330 moderate-intensity minutes (5 ½ hours) a week. She has more than met her goal.

Considerations for Safety and Success

There may be certain challenges along the way, particularly during times of illness or if a chronic disease is present. Chapter 2 discussed some of the methods for exercising with asthma (Figure 20), during pregnancy, with a previous injury, during extreme temperatures, and with poor air quality. Individuals who suffer from heart or lung diseases, common colds, or who are older in age may have particular challenges for practicing cardiorespiratory fitness. There are, however, strategies for developing or maintaining CRF for people with certain health conditions.

General Considerations

Several general considerations apply for any person during aerobic exercise:

- Check with your health care provider prior to exercise if you have an injury, chronic disease, or chronic pain.

- Warm up before and cool down after your workout. Begin and end your cardio workout at a lower intensity to give the body time to adjust.

- Listen to your body. If you experience chest pains, nausea, dizziness, become lightheaded, or feel significant pain in any part of your body, take a break. Stop if the pain persists. Call 911 if you suspect you are having a heart attack.

Specific Considerations

Some individuals have special circumstances to consider both as they develop an exercise program and as they perform exercise. The following information can offer some general assistance for certain conditions.

Bronchitis is a condition in which the bronchial tubes, one of the airways that carry air to your lungs, become inflamed (Figure 21). Individuals with bronchitis often have a cough that produces mucus, wheezing, shortness of breath, a low fever, and discomfort or pain in their chest. Bronchitis can be acute—the result of an infection, virus, or pollutant—or chronic, meaning long-term. Chronic bronchitis, like emphysema and chronic obstructive pulmonary disease (COPD), is an ongoing, serious condition. It occurs if the lining of the bronchial tubes is constantly irritated and inflamed, causing a long-term cough with mucus. People with chronic bronchitis become more susceptible to viruses and bacteria. Smoking is the main cause of chronic bronchitis.

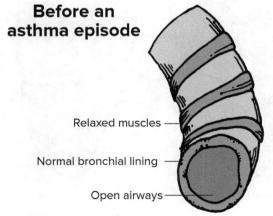
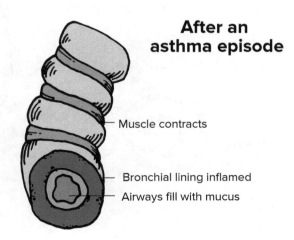

Before an asthma episode

Relaxed muscles —

Normal bronchial lining —

Open airways —

After an asthma episode

— Muscle contracts

— Bronchial lining inflamed
— Airways fill with mucus

Figure 20. How asthma affects the lungs.

Exercise can improve chronic bronchitis symptoms. Yes, you may be out of breath, but you are also working your respiratory muscles and circulating blood, with its valuable oxygen, throughout your body. Activities that boost cardiorespiratory fitness will help lessen shortness of breath, improving the body's use of oxygen, energy levels, and overall cardiovascular health. Stretching, aerobic exercise, resistance training, and even swimming are good activities for people with forms of chronic bronchitis. Always remember to build intensity gradually and listen to your body.

Controlled breathing can help lessen discomfort during exercise. Some general breathing techniques are:

- Inhaling when you begin an exercise and exhaling during the most difficult part

- Taking slow breaths and pacing your breathing

- Pursing your lips when breathing out

People who wear oxygen should be sure to consult their health care provider about when to use it during exercise.

Heart disease comes in many forms, such as congestive heart failure, coronary artery disease, and atrial fibrillation. **High blood pressure** is also associated with heart risk. CRF can bring improvements in many cases of heart disease,

though it may not reverse the disease itself. It can help manage symptoms by increasing blood and oxygen flow (and making your heart more efficient at its job), strengthening the heart and body, and lowering blood pressure and cholesterol levels that add insult to injury when it comes to the disease. It can help you be more active with fewer incidents of chest pain and other related symptoms.

As with any disease, it is important to first check with your health care provider to make sure your heart is healthy enough for exercise and what, if any, restrictions you may have. The following tips offer a basic guide to improving CRF for people with heart disease:

- Do aerobic exercises for maximum benefit to your cardiorespiratory system. Make your heart work a little harder each time but not too hard.

- Start slowly. Choose an aerobic activity such as walking or light jogging and do it at least 3 to 4 times a week.

- Always do at least a 5-minute warm-up and cool-down (See Chapter 2).

- Take rest periods before you get too tired.

- Know your resting heart rate and an acceptable rate during exercise.

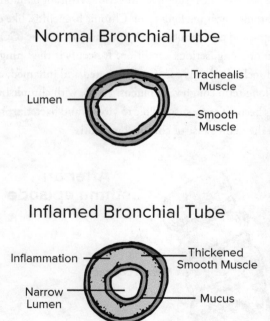

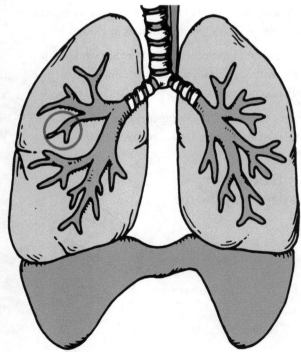

Figure 21. Progress of bronchitis in the airways.

- Know your limits. Stop and rest if you experience symptoms, such as chest pain, nausea, dizziness or lightheadedness, irregular heartbeat or pulse, or shortness of breath. Write down your symptoms, what you were doing when they occurred, and their duration so that you can share them with your health care provider.

- Stand slowly when moving from a lying, sitting, or bending position to reduce the chance of dizziness.

- Keep any medications you take for chest pain with you. Consult your health care provider about potential side effects of blood pressure medication, or any other medications, prior to exercise.

Aging can sometimes seem like a barrier to cardiorespiratory exercises. Senior citizens often have a chronic illness, lower muscle strength, weakened joints and bones, problems with balance, reduced flexibility, and even dementia. An older person who has maintained a good level of CRF throughout their life is likely to have fewer limitations and be in much better physical condition. Cardiorespiratory training will offer many of the health benefits this chapter has addressed, even for someone who has limitations from aging.

Even adults with walkers or wheelchairs can get aerobic exercise. Wheeling is active and can be done around a track. Walking is still walking, regardless of whether or not you're using a walker. Treadmills, set on a safe speed, can be a good option. The important thing is to know your capabilities and limits, follow the safety precautions and principles mentioned in Chapters 1 and 2, and gain assistance when you need it.

Sometimes small things, like fighting a **cold or flu,** can have a negative impact on your day and may make exercise difficult. Consider the following tips for how and when to continue with your program:

- It is usually safe to exercise if your symptoms are all above the neck, such as a runny nose or nasal congestion, or a slight sore throat. Consider reducing your intensity until you feel better, and be sure to hydrate well.

- Do not exercise if you have symptoms below the neck, such as chest congestion, a hacking cough, or an upset stomach.

- Do not exercise with a fever or if you are achy and fatigued.

Women often find it a challenge to exercise during their **menstrual cycle**. Hormonal changes and blood loss can sometimes cause mild dizziness and fatigue. The pain of cramps and discomfort of bloating tend to make you want to stay on the couch. Exercise during this time, however, does more to relieve the symptoms than aggravate them. The endorphins released during exercise serve as a temporary pain blocker and can also help relieve moodiness. Sweating can provide some slight relief for bloating as well. Take acetaminophen or another pain reliever, wear comfortable clothing, and use your workout to improve your condition.

If the pain is too much, take the day off. Most women do not have periods that debilitate them, so if yours is sidelining you, see your health care provider.

Regardless of your particular challenges, remember that inactivity will likely make it worse, not better. Good cardiorespiratory fitness will help you avoid additional problems and complications and can improve your quality of life by making symptoms more manageable. Your health care provider will let you know what's safe and what isn't.

Conclusion

Your next steps should include assessing your own CRF and using your results to create a CRF plan that includes raising your activity level and monitoring your intensity for safety. Try different cardiorespiratory activities so that you can find something that you enjoy, and try to work moderate activity into your life on most days of the week. You might find that if you take brief activity breaks or walks between classes, it's not that difficult to work this into your day.

Even if you're not be ready to commit to an exercise program, consider ways that you can increase your activity throughout the day, such as walking to school or walking your dog. You may already be incorporating cardiorespiratory exercise into your routine. If so, you might think about how you can take your workout to the next level and stay consistent throughout the years. Staying active with cardiorespiratory exercise can help your heart stay healthy and functioning longer. You will also likely find that you have increased energy to enjoy a good quality of life for many more years.

Reflection Questions

1. What is cardiorspiratory fitness? How can cardiorespiratory exercise affect the functioning of the cardiorespiratory system?

2. What are the major components of the cardiorespiratory system?

3. What are the different energy systems of the body? What types of activities are each used for?

4. How is energy produced for cardiorespiratory exercise?

5. In what ways might having improved cardiorespiratory fitness affect your wellness? Please consider different dimensions of wellness in your answer.

6. How is cardiorespiratory endurance assessed?

7. Create a sample plan for cardiorespiratory fitness using the FITT formula.

8. What is high intensity interval training? What are possible benefits and risks?

Chapter 4
Muscular Strength and Endurance

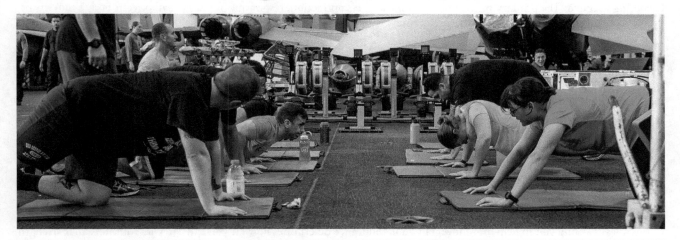

Learning Objectives

1. Describe the basic physiology of muscles and how strength training affects muscles.

2. Define muscular strength and endurance, and describe how they relate to wellness.

3. Explain how muscular strength and endurance can be assessed.

4. Apply the FITT formula to create a safe and effective strength training program.

5. Describe the effects and risks of supplements and substances that are marketed for improving strength or performance.

One component of fitness relates to the strength of our muscles and their capability to sustain that strength for as long as it is needed. We often depend on our muscles to perform without considering whether or not they are up to the challenge. We expect to be able to carry our 60-pound backpack all the way to class, even on days when we parked several extra blocks away from campus. Most of us just expect that we will be able to use our core muscles to go stand-up paddle boarding with some friends—it looks easy (Figure 1). On the other hand, many of us understand the concept of lifting weights at the gym and know that we can't lift just any weight. But in our day-to-day lives we don't think about our muscles having any limitations until we call upon them to complete a task and suddenly don't have the strength or muscle endurance to get the job done.

Your lifestyle dictates just how much strength and energy you need to get through your day. Training for strength and endurance can have a significant impact. Each of the important muscle groups can be improved using targeted training techniques, and an understanding of the muscle and its functional components can help you along the way. This chapter will define muscular strength and endurance, describe muscle structure and function, and show why muscular fitness is so important. It will then provide methods for you to assess your muscular fitness, set goals to improve it, and plan your own muscle strength and endurance training program.

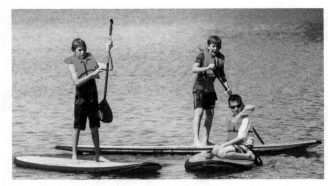

Figure 1. Paddle boarding uses core muscles.

Defining Muscular Fitness

Muscular fitness is measured by how often, for how long, and under how much resistance your muscles can contract without becoming fatigued. The primary function of your muscles is contraction, responsible for almost all of your body's movement. They control not only your obvious movements, like walking, bending, grasping objects, and running but also contract to maintain your posture, stabilize your joints, and even produce as much as 85 percent of the heat your body needs (Figure 2). Muscles are a complex system with many parts to consider. The body contains various types of muscles in addition to an array of fibers, tendons, ligaments, and other connective tissues that enable them to work on your body's behalf. Many pieces work together in each and every contraction, voluntary and involuntary.

Muscular strength is the maximal amount of force a person can exert for a short period of time. The concept is simple—lifting something involves strength. Lifting something heavy requires more strength. Your muscle's strength enables you to hold up your end of that heavy sofa your friend wants you to help him move. It helps you lift that bag of trash you really should have taken out to the dumpster 2 days and 10 pounds ago.

Muscular endurance is the ability of a muscle or group of muscles to repeatedly exert force against resistance. This enables you to do something several times without getting tired. Your strength enables you to pick up the end of that sofa for the friend who is always asking you to help him move, but your endurance determines how far you can carry it. Your muscular strength helps you lift the bag of trash, but your endurance will tell you if you will make it to the dumpster without having to set it down on the way.

Muscular power is the maximum amount of "work" that can be completed in a unit of time. "Work" is a concept from physics that specifically relates to energy transfer between the energy source and an object. Strength doesn't necessarily equal power. For example, good upper-body strength might allow you to lift a lot of weight, but it doesn't necessarily mean you can throw a ball very far—that relies on speed in addition to strength. Power is thE combination of forces that lets you transfer energy into something else.

Muscular force is the measurable output of your muscles. To use another physics example, the downward force of gravity must be matched by the upward force of your muscles if you are going to lift a weight off the ground. Your muscles have to be able to generate an equal amount of force, or more.

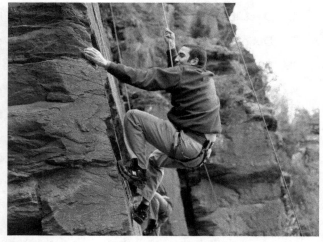

Figure 2. Rock climbing uses several muscle systems at once.

Muscle Structure

Now that the physics lesson is over, let's get to the anatomy lesson. Basic muscular structure comes in three type: skeletal, cardiac, and smooth.

Skeletal muscles are striated—they have transverse streaks, appearing striped or grooved. They usually attach to bones (Figure 3). You control skeletal muscles voluntarily through your central nervous system, which is responsible for moving your bones and supporting your skeleton. They make up 42% of the average adult male's body mass and 36% of the

average adult female's body mass. Skeletal muscles control your arms (biceps and triceps), legs (quadriceps and hamstrings), abdomen, fingers, toes, eyes, nose, and any other part of the body with bone involvement that you move deliberately. They attach to bones via **tendons**—strong, collagen-based cords. Bones attach to one another via **ligaments** and **cartilage**—other strong, collagen-based connective tissues.

Smooth muscles are non-striated muscles that operate bodily functions that aren't controlled with intentional

Skeletal Muscle Fiber

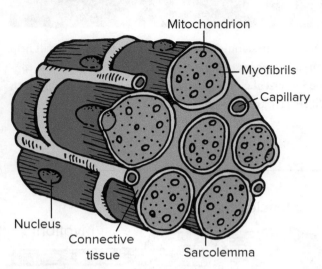

Figure 3. Skeletal muscle fiber structure.

movements. These are *involuntary*, controlled by your autonomic nervous system. These muscles are found in the walls of hollow internal areas such as the iris of the eye, veins, trachea, and urinary and digestive tracts. These muscles make a slow, rhythmic contraction.

Cardiac muscles are striated muscles found in the walls of the heart, controlled by the autonomic nervous system (Figure 4). The heart is your muscular pump responsible for circulating blood (with its oxygen and nutrients) to all other parts of the body. The muscles contract in a strong, rhythmic manner, moving approximately five liters of blood per minute.

Strength Training on Skeletal Muscles

Strength training has specific effects on skeletal muscles, including hypertrophy (an increase in the size of the muscle) and atrophy (the shrinking or wasting away of the muscle). A little knowledge of how muscles function can help you plan your training to maximize results.

As you age, in particular, your muscle mass becomes very important in helping you maintain your independence and health. A decrease in muscle mass in an older adult can lead to poor mobility, balance problems, illness, and even vision problems. A decrease in muscle strength can begin as early as age 30. By age 80, the average older adult has lost 30% of his or her muscle mass. Muscle strength declines even more rapidly than bone or muscle mass. The less active a person is, the earlier they will experience the issues that come with muscle loss.

To complicate this matter, the retirement age in the US has been increasing over the years, often due to economic reasons.

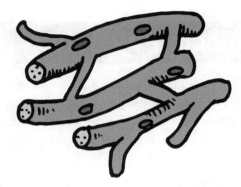

Cardiac muscle

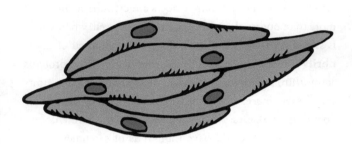

Smooth muscle

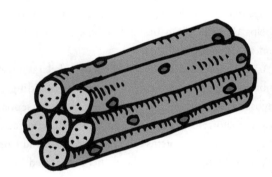

Skeletal muscle

Figure 4. Structure patterns in different muscle types.

People often work beyond age 65. In fact, the Social Security Administration doesn't pay full benefits until age 66 for current retirees and people born after 1960 can expect to work until at least 67 for these benefits. Many people often choose to work even longer to save more for their retirement. The need to stay active and healthy as long as possible may be crucial to avoid being forced to retire from muscle loss-related injuries. Strength training may mean more to you than just your health by the time you are in your sixties—it could mean your livelihood.

Muscle Physiology

Skeletal muscles can be trained for greater strength and endurance, so understanding more about their physiology will help you know why training yields improvements. So, let's get back to the anatomy lesson for a moment. Each skeletal muscle contains different types of tissue—muscle, connective, nerve, and blood or vascular. The muscles can vary in size from tiny, such as those in the eye or ear, to large, such as those in the leg. Their fibers play an important role in their function.

Muscle Fibers

Skeletal muscles consist of multiple bundles of cells called muscle fibers. Skeletal muscle fibers are cylindrical and have more than one **nucleus** (the "brain" of your cell, where DNA is stored) in their cells. These fibers are composed of **myofibrils**—myofibrils contain filaments made of the proteins actin (thin) and **myosin (thick)**. These are repeated in units called **sarcomeres**, the basic functional units of the muscle fiber (Figure 5). One sarcomere contains many filaments and each muscle cell could have thousands of sarcomeres. The sarcomere creates the striated appearance of skeletal muscle and forms the basic machinery necessary for muscle contraction. These bundles of fibers, like many other cells in the body, are delicate. A layer of connective tissue covers them and helps them hold up under frequent or even constant movement (Figure 6).

According to **sliding filament theory**, skeletal muscles function by the actin filaments of muscle fibers sliding past the myosin filaments during muscle contraction. Essentially, the friction shortens the muscle and causes the contraction (Figure 7). Additional proteins called **tropomyosin** and **troponin** bind to the filaments and keep them separated. **Motor units** are the groups of fibers controlled by a particular neuron terminal from your brain. When a motor unit is activated, all of its fibers contract. The energy needed to make this movement possible, called ATP (see Chapter 3) is produced by **mitochondria** in the muscle cells.

Types of Muscle Fibers

Your muscles have two main types of fibers: **slow-twitch muscle fibers**, or type I, and **fast-twitch muscle fibers**, which come in two varieties—type IIa and IIx. Most of your muscles contain both types of fibers, though not in the same quantity.

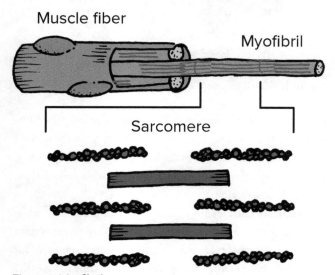

Figure 5. Myofibril structure.

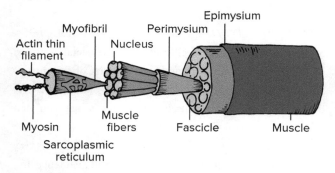

Figure 6. Muscle structure.

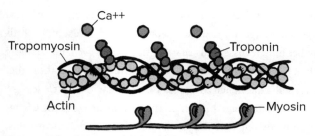

Figure 7. The elements of sliding filament theory.

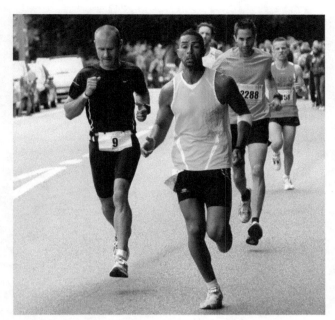

Figure 8. Long-distance running requires strong slow-twitch muscles fibers.

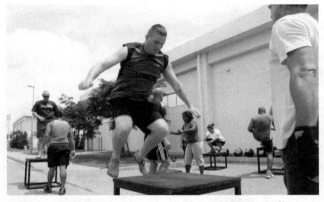

Figure 9. Bursts of movement require fast-twitch muscle fibers.

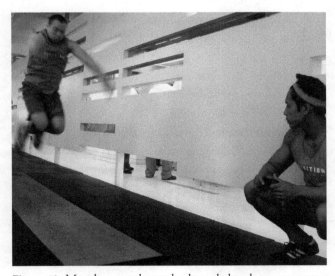

Figure 10. Muscles propel your body and absorb momentum.

Slow-twitch fibers appear darker or redder because they contain a high number of capillaries. They also have a good amount of **myoglobin** (a red protein) that allows the muscle fiber to store oxygen. They resist fatigue relatively well. The body uses them for activities such as long-distance running and bicycling (Figure 8). Certain parts of the body may have more slow-twitch fibers than fast-twitch. The muscles responsible for your posture, for example, may contain more because they must be frequently in a state of endurance.

Because slow-twitch muscle fibers enable endurance, cardiovascular training and activities that focus on prolonged endurance are important to their enhancement. Activities like long runs, swimming laps, and long bicycle rides are all good for your slow-twitch fibers.

Fast-twitch muscle fibers handle short-term bursts of movement (Figure 9). These fibers typically generate energy through an anaerobic process, meaning they utilize carbohydrate combustion rather than oxygen to create fuel. Fast-twitch muscle fibers have fewer capillaries and aerobic enzymes. They contract quickly but fatigue faster than slow-twitch fibers because they use more energy. The body recruits them for activities that require shorter spurts of energy such as sprinting, jumping, and catching objects (Figure 10). Muscles that are naturally responsible for quick movement on a regular basis, such as those in the eye, may have more fast-twitch fibers, but like slow-twitch, we can perform exercises that activate these particular fibers in all of our muscles.

Type IIa fast-twitch muscle fibers (also called intermediate fast-twitch) can use either aerobic or anaerobic metabolism to generate energy. Type IIa also resist fatigue fairly well. Essentially, they are a combination of slow-twitch (type I) and fast-twitch (type II). **Type IIx** fibers, the typical fast-twitch fibers, use anaerobic metabolism and excel at rapid movement. These fibers fatigue quickly. While training, using force and resistance against the muscles helps the body's readiness to recruit these fibers when needed. Lifting heavy or moderately heavy weights with shorter repetitions, for example, will activate these fibers, as will doing sprints or agility drills.

No definitive evidence exists to suggest that we can convert certain types of fibers from slow to fast or fast to slow, but exercising both will enable your body to be ready for different forms of activity.

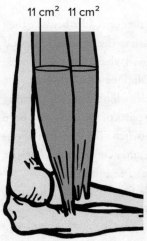
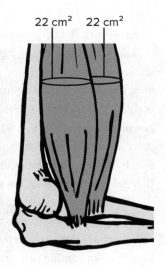
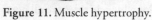
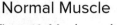

11 cm² 11 cm²   22 cm² 22 cm²

Figure 11. Muscle hypertrophy.

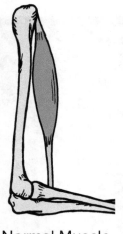
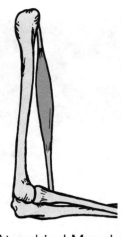

Normal Muscle   Atrophied Muscle

Figure 12. Muscle atrophy.

Hypertrophy is the growth in the size of the organ or tissue by increasing its cells—an increase in mass—in this case the muscles (Figure 11). Hypertrophy generally refers to increases in two areas—sarcoplasmic and myofibril. **Sarcoplasmic** refers to the fluid in the muscle. **Myofibril** refers to the fibers. Both can increase during training, though it is the growth in the size (not quantity) of the myofibril that we generally see when muscles gain strength. Fast-twitch muscle fibers are more likely than slow-twitch to undergo hypertrophy.

Atrophy occurs when proteins in the muscle fibers begin to break down and muscle mass decreases (Figure 12). Your body naturally experiences protein loss, to a certain extent, for cellular health, replacing unwanted proteins with new proteins. Shrinkage of the muscles, however, is rarely a positive thing. This can occur as a result of poor nutrition, disease, or a lack of use. Your muscles are vital to the production of energy for your body. Extensive muscle loss puts you at risk for metabolic disorders, such as diabetes, and your body may be ill-prepared to handle any serious illnesses that may come your way, like cancer.

Genetics

Research suggests that your genes play a significant factor in the amount of each type of muscle fibers a person has. We all know people who seem naturally predisposed to developing muscle or have the lean makeup of a distance runner. Your friend Jake, a power-lifter, seems like he's been buff since kindergarten (with Jake around, you never had to worry about bullies). He may have more fast-twitch muscle fibers and may have gravitated to this sport out of a natural ability to excel. Likewise, when your friend Kendal was in school, she always found stamina tests in P.E. to be child's play. She now runs 3 miles in under 16 minutes on her college's track

team. Endurance activities may have come a bit more easily to her because her muscles contain more slow-twitch fibers.

Regardless of an individual's makeup, exercising for both strength and endurance will still improve overall performance. Someone who works to strengthen their fast-twitch muscle fibers, for example, may still be able to lift a heavier weight than someone who is genetically predisposed to muscular makeup but doesn't exercise. If Jake ever slacks on his weight-lifting routine and you really step yours up, who knows? Maybe you'll finally be able to arm-wrestle him and win.

Muscle Roles

Your muscles play different roles depending on how they are used. They typically work as a team. A muscle providing the main force in a movement is considered the **agonist**, while the muscle that opposes it is the **antagonist**. For example, during a bicep curl, the bicep does most of the work and serves as the agonist, while the tricep muscle (the antagonist) relaxes. In an arm extension, their roles reverse. The tricep becomes the agonist and the bicep is the antagonist. The antagonist doesn't always relax. Sometimes it works to slow down a motion to help maintain control. Lift a heavy weight during a bicep curl and the tricep will contribute a certain amount of tension for support.

You also have muscles called **stabilizers** that help keep your joints safe. These function as either a **synergist** or a **fixator.** A synergist helps movement by stabilizing the joint where the movement occurs. A fixator stabilizes at the origin of the agonist and the joint it moves over. Your hip and shoulder joints, for example, have fixators for stability. In a bicep curl, the rotator cuff muscles serve to stabilize the movement and protect the shoulder—they serve as fixators. The muscles around the elbow (brachioradialis and brachialis) are the synergists.

Benefits of Muscular Strength and Endurance

We've been discussing how your muscles work and how they support you. Every time you pitch in to help move a couch or take out the trash, your muscles bear the burden. It may seem like all these poor organs do is help you labor, and what fun is that? But think of all the good times you and your muscles have shared — the hikes, surfs, ballgames, dances — the fun has been endless. There are a million reasons to keep them fit and happy. We all can benefit from good muscle fitness in more ways than we might imagine. Activities focused on muscle strength and endurance can yield many emotional and psychological benefits in addition to the physical benefits you might expect.

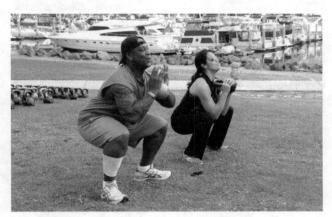

Figure 13. Muscle fitness leads to increased mobility.

Type	Benefits
Walking	Maintain a healthy weight
	Prevent or manage various conditions, including heart disease, high blood pressure, and Type 2 diabetes
	Strengthen bones and muscles
	Improve mood
	Improve balance and coordination
Running	Lose weight
	Boost confidence
	Relieve stress
	Eliminate depression
Strength Training	Help keep weight off
	Help protect bone health and muscle mass
	Be stronger and fitter
	Help develop better body mechanics
	Play a role in disease prevention
	Boost energy levels and improve mood
	Burn more calories
Weight Training	Increase physical work capacity
	Improve ability to perform activities of daily living
	Improve bone density
	Promote fat-free body mass and decrease natural mass loss
	Increase strength of connective tissue, muscles, and tendons
	Improve quality of life

Figure 14. Benefits of different training types.

Physical Benefits

As mentioned in Chapter 2, the benefits of exercise are extensive. Working on the strength and endurance of your muscles in addition to cardiovascular exercise contributes even more to your overall health and fitness than aerobic activity alone. The federal Physical Activity Guidelines recommend at least 2 days per week of muscle strengthening activity.

Recent studies indicate that only 29.3% of adult Americans meet these guidelines — 34.4% of men and 24.5% of women. Young adults aged 18–24 meet these guidelines most often at just over 44%. This number drops nearly 10% for people aged 25–34 and the percentage continues to decline with the age of the population. Only 21.7% of adults over 65 meet them. Overweight individuals are even less likely to meet the guidelines at any age. It would seem that many Americans do not realize their importance in maintaining physical functioning and avoiding physical limitations throughout their lives (Figure 13).

Improved Performance

Strength and endurance training enable you to complete your activities of daily living with greater ease. With our fast-paced lives, it can be difficult to find the time, and squeezing 2–3 days of this type of training can take a back seat to work, school, and household responsibilities.

Yet creating a plan to physically improve your body can make all the difference in the fulfillment of your responsibilities. Healthy muscle mass and muscle stamina enable you to get through your day-to-day tasks more quickly without fatiguing, whereas a decreased muscle mass will inhibit your functional ability. Climbing stairs, carrying boxes or loads of laundry, and just meeting the demands of your workload becomes easier with increased strength, energy, and stamina (Figure 14).

Have you ever had a broken bone, sprained ankle, or simply taken a bad fall? Then you understand how quickly life becomes complicated by injuries. Simple things like climbing stairs and taking a shower become anything but simple. No one is immune to accidents, but the risk of certain injuries can be reduced with good muscle strength.

Even just increased reaction time, certainly important in athletics and certain types of recreation, is invaluable in helping us avoid accidents in our daily lives. How many accidents have you, or could you have, avoided with quick reaction? Muscular strength and endurance lead to faster reaction times and can help you catch yourself before a serious injury occurs.

Your skeletal muscles connect to bone, tendons, and ligaments, all of which benefit from exercise and all of which help keep your body balanced and in proper alignment. Athletes in particular know the importance of training these muscles for injury prevention (Figure 15). When a muscle area and its connective tissue weakens, it isn't ready when called on during sudden physical movements. This increases risks for more damage.

Reduced Risk of Diseases

Research indicates that one of the leading causes of chronic disease and premature death is a lack of physical activity. As we age, we begin to lose muscle and bone mass along with strength. Some of this loss can be avoided with regular strength and endurance exercises. In fact, maintaining skeletal muscle mass has been shown to produce positive health outcomes by providing energy reserves in the event of stress or illness.

Your muscles impact more than you may realize. The loss of density in bone minerals becomes one of the largest risk factors for fractures. For most of us, bone mass peaks during our thirties. After that time, we can begin to lose bone. Like muscle, bone is living tissue that responds to exercise by becoming stronger. Young people who exercise regularly generally achieve greater peak bone mass (maximum bone density and strength) than those who do not. Strong muscles that can maintain stamina not only help reduce the risk of falls, they strengthen bone mass to lower the risk of fracture, too (Figure 16). This is especially important for older adults and people who have been diagnosed with osteoporosis (Figure 17).

Osteoporosis is a disease that thins and weakens the bones. They become fragile and break easily, especially the bones in the hip, spine, and wrist. Women average 2–3% bone loss each year for the first 5–8 years after menopause, and men average 1% loss per year after age 50. For every 10% of

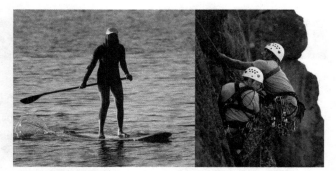

Figure 15. Athletic activities that require balance emphasize muscle strength.

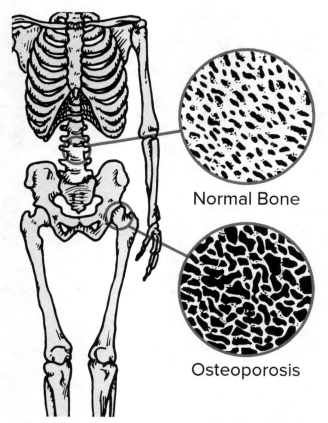

Normal Bone

Osteoporosis

Figure 16. Osteoporosis bone damage.

bone mass lost, the risk of fracture nearly doubles. Women, because they lose bone mass so quickly after menopause, are at a higher risk of osteoporosis. Strong muscles can lessen the risk of injury and reduce your chances of developing osteoporosis.

You likely hear a lot about body fat, maybe even on a daily basis. Products that promote weight loss, products that remove belly fat, and about a million different diet plans – they're all over the television and social media. The fads and gimmicks may not be the best idea, but the people behind them do have one thing in common. They know the health risks of excess body fat.

Symptoms	Causes	Risk Factors
Back pain	Your bones are in a constant state of renewal. New bone is made and old bone is broken down. The higher your peak bone mass, the more bone you have "in the bank" and the less likely you are to develop osteoporosis as you age.	Sex, age, race, family history, body frame size, hormone levels, thyroid problems, dietary factors, steroids and other medications, seizures, gastric reflux, cancer, transplant rejection, medical conditions, lifestyle choices
Loss of height		
A stooped posture		
A bone fracture that occurs much more easily than expected		

Figure 17. Osteoporosis can have a severe impact on your body.

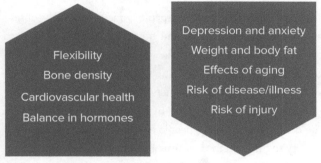

Figure 18. Strength training has benefits beyond strength.

Your body composition matters. According to the National Institute on Aging, an increase in body fat along with a decrease in lean muscle mass, often lead to common diseases and even disability, particularly as a person ages. Strength training can increase or maintain your lean body mass and reduce fat in the body – without the gimmicks. People with more muscle burn more calories than people with less, even when at rest. Healthy percentages of body fat lower your risk of developing chronic diseases, such as Type 2 diabetes, high blood pressure, and heart disease (see Chapter 6 on Body Composition and Chapter 9 on Chronic Diseases).

Improved Athletic Performance

Improved muscular fitness can have benefits for recreational or serious athletes, in addition to making them less at risk for injury. Ever watch an outfielder make a diving catch during a baseball game, skid on his stomach across the turf, roll, and come up with the ball still in his glove? Or a soccer player jump high in the air, kick a ball into the goal, hit the ground in a roll and jump up to celebrate? Impressive, right?

Many sports involve strength or endurance training (or a combination of both) as a regular part of their fitness regimen. Studies indicate that improved strength and improved athletic performance go hand-in-hand. More strength means achieving greater power, faster. This means more explosiveness off the blocks for sprinters, more vertical jumping power for basketball players, more punch off the spring floor for gymnasts, and so on. It also means balance and body alignment that helps them prevent or control their falls and reduce the risk for many types of injuries.

Muscular endurance training can be just as beneficial as strength. Even those athletes that seem as though muscle size and strength would be most important need endurance. Have you ever considered how much time football players spend in full gear, running up and down the field? They need the strength to carry the load, block, and tackle but need the stamina to do it safely and successfully.

Additional Physical Benefits

Improved muscle and bone health with age, improved body composition, a higher metabolism (even when resting), and the avoidance of injury and physical limitations—the list of benefits to strength and endurance training is long. And yet, the list goes on. It helps many other parts of our body that are less noticeable (Figure 18). Your posture, for example, can be improved. A strong core (torso) makes significant contributions in the way we manage nearly every activity—sitting, standing, walking, doing chores, all of these become easier and less painful, particularly in the lower back, when you maintain good muscle fitness. Even your digestion and sleep are improved through this type of physical training. This leads to an overall improvement in your quality of life and happiness.

Emotional and Psychological Benefits

Your confidence in your ability to handle your daily routine, the feeling of good health, and how comfortable you are with the appearance of your body can all impact your emotional and psychological wellness. It might sound odd, but the strength and endurance of your muscles can play an important role in helping you manage day-to-day difficulties with a positive attitude.

Strong muscles can help improve your overall psychological state. There have been many studies evaluating the effect of exercise on feelings of distress and personal well-being. On average, active Americans had significantly lower odds of feeling distressed and higher odds of having a more positive sense of their well-being than people who were inactive. Your physical health directly impacts your emotional and psychological health – something you shouldn't undervalue.

Improved Self-Esteem and Energy

Strong muscles that perform when you need and want them to, healthy body composition, feeling comfortable in your clothes and with your abilities – these impact your self-esteem. These benefits shouldn't be thought of as non-physical, because they are caused by altered brain chemistry. This happens through changes with neurotransmitters and the increased release of the endorphins mentioned earlier. Improved body image, contentment with health, and a general ability to manage your day with less stress boosts your confidence level physically and emotionally. For more information on body composition, see Chapter 6. These same endorphins

that make you happy also hinder your body's ability to signal pain and give you a euphoric feeling. You push your muscles physically beyond the limits they're used to when you train them. Your body registers this as stress or pain and releases endorphins to compensate. This is why runners experience what we call "runner's high." These endorphins, along with a higher metabolism, give you added energy.

Reduced Anxiety and Depression

Anxiety disorders, such as panic attacks, phobias, obsessive-compulsive disorders, and post-traumatic stress, impact over 16 million people in the US alone. According to the American Psychiatric Association, approximately 8 percent of women and 4% of men experience depression, costing the US around $83 billion annually in treatment. These issues can be debilitating, causing people to lose interest and a general ability to function in their lives and can even lead to suicide.

Physical activity, including strength training, in more than 100 population-based studies, has been shown to offer protection against symptoms related to these mental health concerns. Studies estimate that the odds of depression lower by as much as 30–45% with regular activity. Moderate intensity resistance training, in particular, has been shown in clinical studies to reduce anxiety both immediately following a training session and long-term if the program persists. Even one session of weight training can reduce anxiety for approximately 2 hours after your workout, so imagine the results with a regular training plan in place.

Improving Muscular Strength and Endurance

To improve your muscular strength and endurance, you must first assess your current levels. Then you will be able to set goals, plan your improvements, and choose training exercises that target your improvement areas effectively and safely.

Imagine this for a moment. The stage is set. The Olympic rings hover in the background and a barbell with a seemingly undefeatable amount of weight on either end sits menacingly in the center of the floor. A large, burly man with impressive arms and legs the size of tree trunks approaches the set of weights and breathes deeply. With his body perfectly positioned, the veins bulging from his neck, and a series of grunts he jerks the massive weight to his chest, then over his head, before dropping it to the floor with a resounding clang. This is a 1-RM, often used as a way to measure one person's strength against another.

The one-repetition maximum (1-RM) refers to the heaviest weight you can lift with your maximum effort in a single repetition for any specific exercise. This could be a bench press, bicep curl, squat, or any other activity. Professional bodybuilders and weightlifters use this measurement competitively, but for the rest of us this serves as a good indicator to determine our current strength and track our progress. There are two methods for assessing your 1-RM.

Actual 1-RM

The procedure is fairly simple:

- Decide which muscle groups to test and which exercises you will perform to complete the test. The bench press and leg press are commonly done, but the test can be used to measure any muscle group.

- Complete a set of the exercise using a weight with which you can perform 15 repetitions.

- Add a small amount of weight and complete another set of up to 15 repetitions. Keep adding weight and completing sets until you reach a weight that you cannot lift for even one repetition. The weight prior to that is your 1-RM.

- Re-test at designated intervals (usually once per month) using the same methods and exercises.

It is important to note that the warm-up process for this should not be skipped. To choose a heavy weight and attempt to lift it without properly warming up can result in injury.

Estimated 1-RM

Estimating your 1-RM is a safer way to establish your current baseline, but if you do not lift weights routinely it may not be an option. If you know that you can routinely bench 150 pounds for 10 repetitions, you can use these numbers to estimate your 1-RM using the following formula:

$$1\text{RM} = w\left(1 + \frac{r}{30}\right), \text{ assuming } r > 1$$

This is the Epley formula. There are several different formulas used and some deliver slightly different results, which is why the actual 1-RM test is more accurate. For this formula, if you could lift 150 pounds for 10 repetitions your 1-RM would be 200 pounds. A different formula, such as the Brzycki, might yield a slightly different number, but you will still get a reasonable baseline for measurement.

Muscle Mass (Bodybuilding)

Before you set and measure specific goals in muscle mass, it can help to determine your Lean Body Mass (LBM), or the amount of weight you carry on your body that isn't fat. You can also calculate your percent body fat. A trainer or dietician can help you do this with calipers or with the use of various machines.

Once you've learned your current maximum capabilities, set a date to re-evaluate and measure your progress. This assessment of your muscular strength and endurance will be an ongoing process of any training.

Setting Goals for Muscular Strength and Endurance

You may have very specific types of improvements you want to make based on your lifestyle or profession. You may just want to see overall improvements to your strength and endurance. Do you have to carry a 70-pound firehose up a ladder? Do you work in an office? Play football? Identify the kind and amount of improvements you want to see in your strength and endurance based on your needs and wants. This is important to setting goals. Remember to use SMART goals to help you achieve improvements and avoid discouragement.

For example, imagine your 1-RM baseline for a squat-press is 75 pounds. You're training to be a firefighter and know that you will need to carry your own weight, plus the hose or even a person, up or down a ladder. Here is a SMART goal you could set for yourself:

Specific – I want to increase my 1-RM

Measurable – From 75 pounds to 90 pounds

Achievable – This is a small improvement

Relevant – I will be more successful at my job

Time-based – in 2 months

Your goals can be based on how you function throughout your day or more specific to the activity you perform. Specific goals are easier to measure, track, and adjust. Your long-term goal in this scenario might be to increase your 1-RM in your squat-press to 200 pounds. You know that you need to hit this mark but understand that progress takes time and benchmarks along the way are important.

The same applies to building endurance. Say you currently run one mile before your muscles fatigue. You may have a short-term goal of 2 miles as a way to build toward better muscle endurance. Maybe your long-term goal is 3 miles.

Goals for building muscle mass and power can be fairly easy to set and measure, depending on why you want to improve in this area. Maybe you are a sprinter and want to get faster out of the blocks—this is based on reaction time and easy to track. Maybe you assessed your lean body mass and were at the high end of normal (see Chapter 6). Set a SMART goal that includes an easy measuring system, like your home scale for weight or your pants size, until you get closer to your long-term goal. Then have your lean body mass reassessed.

Goals with activities of daily living may not be as easy to notice, at least until you are called upon to perform something out of the ordinary. It could be that once each month your office receives a large box of copy paper, and you always have to call for help to have it carried in. Your goal may be to perform this task without assistance.

Consider your needs, daily activities, and current health. If you have an illness, such as Type 2 diabetes, you may have a goal of reducing or eliminating your insulin intake. If your blood pressure is high, you may be hoping to lower it. If your body composition may be affecting your health, determine a reasonable, healthy weight or percentage of body fat and set short-term goals for improved numbers. Remember that most of these changes take time to achieve. Everyone benefits from muscle fitness. Not everyone has the same capabilities, limitations, or capacity for muscle, and our physical make-up dictates, to some extent, how we will train. Some considerations people must face when improving muscular fitness are their biological sex, age, and other genetic factors. Be consistent, let your SMART goals keep you on track, and be proud of the accomplishments along the way.

Gender

Women who want to maintain their health and lifelong independence should incorporate strength training into their fitness plan (Figure 19). They benefit from improving their muscular fitness in similar ways that men do. Women in particular may consider benefits related to improving bone density and reducing their risk of osteoporosis.

Some women may be hesitant about strength training for fear of developing a bulky appearance, but they needn't worry. Hormonal differences between biological males and females mean that women are generally unable to develop large muscles. Some women may be genetically predisposed to gaining larger muscles than others, but most will not be able to achieve the same muscle size as a man. Consider some

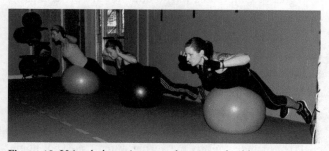

Figure 19. Using balance in strength training build core muscles.

of the fittest, most muscular female athletes—swimmers and gymnasts. Compared to the average woman, they are quite muscular. Yet given the number of hours they train, anywhere from 20 to 30 per week or more, their muscles still to do not achieve the same size of their male counterparts, in general.

For women who do want to improve their muscle mass, they would want to follow guidelines for increasing strength that are similar to the guidelines for men—moderate to heavy load, high volume with short rest periods.

Age

Your ability to build muscle size declines as you age, starting around 25–30. But that doesn't mean that an older person doesn't feel the benefits to their health and functional level. People can improve their strength and endurance at any age. Studies show that strength and endurance training help people develop and maintain independence, prevent illness and injury, maintain a healthy weight, and improve motor skills.

A major consequence of muscle wasting is an increased risk of falling. The Centers for Disease Control reports that falls are the leading cause of unintentional injury-related death for elderly adults. The statistics about falls and risk of fracture are striking. The lifetime risk of a fracture for men and women is about 40%. In addition, one in four women will sustain a low-trauma fracture (i.e., a fracture caused by a fall from standing height or less) after age 50.

For this reason, elderly individuals need to be proactive with strength training to both strengthen muscle and improve balance but also cautious and, if inexperienced or showing signs of cognitive decline, supervised during exercise.

Genetics

Individuals respond to strength training in different ways. Studies indicate that no specific gene can be consistently linked to athletic performance or success. They suggest that genetics likely factor into a person's success with training, but it is still unclear which parts of our genetic code impact that success. As mentioned earlier in this chapter, scientists believe that the amount of fast-twitch vs. slow-twitch muscles a person has plays a significant role in the types of activities at which we excel.

Body size, body composition, and muscle fiber development also have a genetic component, and each plays a role in the physical strength training success. Hand grip strength, for example, has been linked to genetic factors by scientists as recently as July 2017.

Training for Muscular Strength and Endurance

Your plan for muscular strength and endurance should include identifying what types of training exercises will best target your improvement goals and what types of equipment you will need to use. There are three main types of training—static exercise, isokinetic training, and dynamic exercise.

Static exercise, also known as isometric exercise, utilizes resistance rather than motion of the joints. It involves tension or contraction of the muscles as they push against an object or hold the object (or body position) steady (time under tension). Put your hands together in front of your chest with your fingers pointing upward and push your palms together until you feel your biceps contract. This is an example of static exercise. Essentially, it involves placing your body in a position where you are squeezing or flexing your muscle and holding that position for a predetermined amount of time, such as when you do a plank to work your abdominals (Figure 20). Other examples of static exercises include a spine extension, glut bridge, wall sit, boat pose, and side plank.

Static training improves muscle endurance as well as strength. This type of exercise can also be done with weights in a variety of ways. For example, you may do three bicep curls (3 reps) and be unable to complete another, but you can hold the weight so that your bicep is in the flexed position for another 10 seconds. The muscles might shake but that's normal. Static training forces your muscles to fatigue faster.

Isokinetic exercises are those where a special machine applies variable resistance to your limbs while in constant motion. One example of this is a stationary bike with increasing resistance to simulate inclines. It is more difficult for an athlete to overdo it or lose pace because the speed and resistance can be set where users can't exceed the limit.

Unlike static exercise, **dynamic training** involves the full range of motion of the muscle and movement of the joint. The muscle contracts through movement. The speed of contraction varies because muscle is weaker at its longest and shortest, and stronger in the middle of the range of motion. The muscle is able to increase strength more effectively than with static training because you are using the muscle's entire range of motion.

Dynamic training is the most common type and what we do during movement-based exercises, such as bicep curls, tricep dips, bench presses, squats, or crunches. This type of training offers a lot of variety and can be done almost anywhere. Dynamic exercises can be performed with free weights, machines, resistance bands, stability balls, kettle bells, and medicine balls.

Static exercise holds the tension for a certain period of time, while dynamic utilizes rhythmic repetition. When a muscle is shortened during a contraction it is considered **concentric.** When it is lengthened during a contraction, it is considered **eccentric**. In a bicep curl, the raising would be concentric and the lowering would be eccentric, working the entirety of the muscle. There is usually greater potential for a muscle to produce

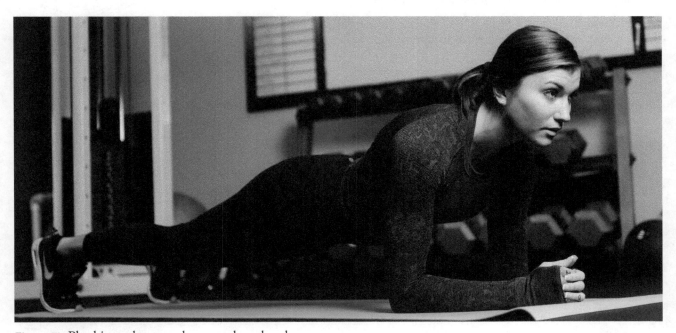

Figure 20. Planking takes muscle strength and endurance.

force during the eccentric contraction—a person can usually lower more weight than they can lift (Figure 21).

Both types of contractions have training benefits. Dynamic training works well for most individuals and can be more effective for increasing strength. For those with joint issues who struggle with full range of motion, static may be preferred for safety. A person could also incorporate static exercises into their dynamic strength routine to help increase muscular endurance and facilitate muscular fatigue as mentioned earlier.

You will train based on what you want to achieve. Do you need more power or strength? Is your endurance important? Do you want to see a greater mass or less body fat? See (Figure 22) as a guide.

Training Options

Many training options are available for each type of improvement, including weight training options, functional training options, plyometrics, and more. Your choices depend largely on your preferences, lifestyle, goals, and what is available to you. You can improve your strength with all of these training options.

Weight machines are available at nearly every gym and for home purchase (Figure 23). They isolate the muscle group and allow you to complete the movement without a spotter because the machine's cables and pulleys hold the weight for you. You can work most muscle groups using various machines, such as the lat pull down, leg press, rowing machine, and many others.

They can be great for beginners and people rehabilitating from an injury because they make it safe and easy to isolate the muscle groups. People lifting on their own often prefer machines because they don't need a partner and are less likely to sustain an injury. People doing strength circuits, in which they cycle through several exercises targeting different muscles, also may prefer the machines to save time in set-up.

Machines do have some drawbacks. They don't mimic normal human movement (which helps us with our day-to-day activities) or work smaller, stabilizing muscles. They can also be expensive for home use or require a gym membership.

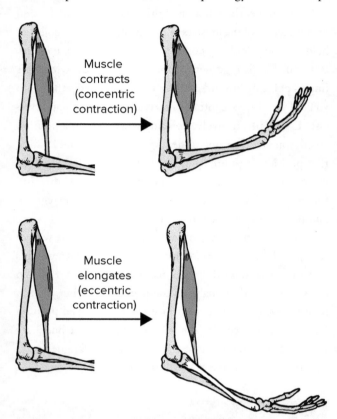

Figure 21. Concentric and eccentric muscle contraction.

Type	Description
Muscle Power	Improving a muscle's explosive power, meaning its ability to perform a powerful movement in minimal time. Examples include launching into a fast sprint or jumping. Training for muscle power is generally used to help people improve their sporting performance. It involves doing one to six repetitions of each exercise at maximum speed.
Muscle Strength	All types of weight training will improve your strength. But this technique aims to improve absolute strength—meaning the ability to lift or push heavy weights. It involves one to six repetitions of each exercise performed relatively slowly.
Muscle Hypertrophy	This type of training aims to increase the amount of lean muscle in the body. It's especially useful for weight loss. It can also help with achieving a lean, toned look. For older adults, it can help counteract or reverse the age-related muscle loss that can lead to frailty.
Muscular Endurance	This kind of training helps muscles to be able to keep performing a movement for a prolonged period of time such as in rowing. Training for muscular endurance involves doing 20 repetitions or more at a controlled speed, generally for one to three sets.

Figure 22. Different types of strength training help accomplish different things.

Free weights require more assistance (Figure 24). You may need a spotter for many types of exercises. They do, however, allow you to use the full range of motion of the muscle, something that benefits you with your daily activities. They also tend to work those smaller, stabilizing muscles more and can promote greater strength gains. They offer more variety and allow you to combine muscle groups. Functional training, discussed next, usually incorporates free weights, along with other strength equipment. The ability to slightly change body position with free weights can help you develop strength, balance, and coordination.

The drawback to free weights is that you really need a proper knowledge of good technique. Weight machines are easy because they usually have instructions on them and your exposure to injury comes primarily from not knowing how much weight to attempt. You can work the same muscle groups with free weights as with weight machines, but free weights put more responsibility on the individual to know and maintain correct form in the activity. If you want to get the most out of your weight training, and you have available assistance and the knowledge to complete the task, free weights can be an excellent choice.

Functional training involves exercises that prepare the body for daily life. Have you ever heard the phrase "practice the way you perform?" These exercises tend to focus on activities that build the muscles you use daily. For example, throughout the day, you might climb stairs, squat to pick up dropped objects, bend, turn, sit, stand, and so on. Many of these movements involve use of your core muscles, those that stabilize you. Exercises such as squats, lunges, abdominal work, and movements with medicine balls or stability balls force you to activate your core and improve your daily functioning. They work the muscles you use to perform.

Neuromotor exercise is a type of functional training that also takes a very practical approach to muscle training, recommended for 2–3 days per week. Exercises should involve motor skills, such as balance, agility, coordination, and gait. This includes proprioceptive exercises, those that help build body awareness, like tai chi and yoga. This helps you improve physical function, flexibility, and prevent falls, especially as you age.

Core training is related to functional training but focuses specifically on core muscles. Like functional training, core training tends to encourage the core muscles to work as stabilizers, which is how they normally function, but core training may not include the entire body. Core muscles are hidden beneath the exterior musculature people typically train. These deeper muscles include the transverse abdominals, multifidus, diaphragm, pelvic floor, and many other deeper muscles.

These muscles support the upper and lower body through their daily movement. A weak core often leads to problems. Your body may be unable to support your movements effectively and you are more likely to sustain an injury or have lower back pain. Core exercises can include planks and side planks, deadlifts, bar exercises including toe-to-pull-up-bar leg lifts, and medicine ball chest passes. Pilates and yoga can also do a great job of working your core muscles.

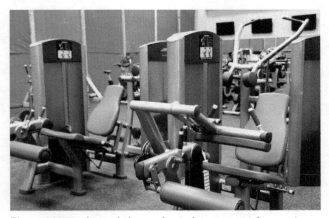

Figure 23. Weight machines mechanical connect weight to actions.

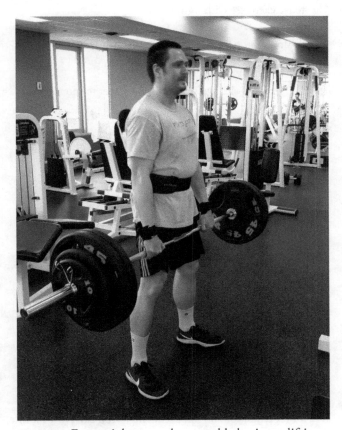

Figure 24. Free weights must be assembled prior to lifting.

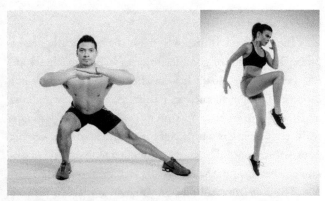

Figure 25. Strength movements can build muscle.

Plyometrics focuses on speed, strength, power, and agility, often utilizing a series of jumps and leaps to build athletic performance. Jumping onto and off of boxes from different directions (box jumps and lateral box jumps), vertical leaps, broad jumps, and skater jumps (side to side movements that mimic ice or roller skating) are typical examples. These exercises train you to be quicker on your feet and more agile.

Many exercises can be completed at home with little to no assistance from anyone. Resistance bands, medicine and stability balls, Pilates, calisthenics—the options seem endless. You don't have to pay for a gym membership. You can still train at little cost and with little space. Buy a Pilates DVD and some resistance bands, use your body for resistance, and put your knowledge to work (Figure 25).

Applying the Principles to Muscular Strength and Endurance

So, how often should you work your muscles and how do you go about it? Sample training programs are widely available online for all ability levels. Here we cover the FITT Principle (see also Chapter 2) and the American College of Sports Medicine guidelines for implementing an effective training program.

Frequency—Adults should train each major muscle group 2 to 3 days each week using a variety of exercises and equipment. Wait at least 48 hours between resistance training sessions.

Intensity—In muscular strength and endurance training, intensity refers to the amount of weight or resistance used. This is often calculated as a percentage of the 1-RM you are capable of.

For strength training, a load equal to 60–70% of your 1-RM is recommended for beginners and a load of 80–100% of your 1-RM for advanced training. Lighter intensity works better for older adults or people who are just getting started.

Intensity should be higher for people who have been exercising for some time or who want to build muscle mass.

For hypertrophy (muscle mass), a load equal to 70–85% of your 1-RM is recommended for beginning and intermediate training. A load of 70–100% of your 1-RM is recommended for advanced training.

For endurance, a different approach is needed. You need to overload to build endurance – the muscle needs to be stressed beyond its normal ability. Intensity in endurance training relates to time instead of weight. Loads should therefore be lower, always less than 70% of your 1-RM. If you can easily do 8–12 reps, increase the weight on the next set. You want to choose a weight that you can do 8–12 reps (with proper form) that feels challenging. Increase the weight if it feels easy. Reduce the weight if your form isn't good.

Time—Training programs for muscular strength include the following exercises:

- 1–3 sets of 8–12 repetitions for beginner to intermediate training
- 2–6 sets of 1–8 repetitions for advanced training
- Rest period: 2–3 min for higher intense exercises that use heavier loads; 1–2 minutes between the lower intense exercises with light loads

Training programs for muscular hypertrophy include the following exercises:

- 1–3 sets of 8–12 repetitions for beginner to intermediate
- 3–6 sets of 1–12 repetitions for advanced
- Rest period: 2–3 min for higher intense exercises that use heavier loads; 1–2 minutes between the lower intense exercises with light loads

Training programs for muscular endurance include the following exercises:

- 2–4 sets of 10–25 repetitions
- Rest period: 30 seconds to 1-minute between each set

Type—The type of exercise you choose will depend upon your fitness goals. Muscle movement exercises are possible for all muscle groups, and your chosen groups should be the focus of the exercises (Figure 26).

A common myth exists that you can target train a specific area for fat reduction, or "spot reducing." You can't lose fat in a particular area by exercising that area only. You can alter the

Muscle Group	Free-Weight	Machine-Based	Body Weight
Chest	Supine Bench Press	Seated Chest Press	Push-ups
Back	Bent-over Barbell Rows	Lat Pulldown	Pull-ups
Shoulders	Dumbbell Lateral Raise	Shoulder Press	Arm Circles
Biceps	Barbell/Dumbbell Curls	Cable Curls	Reverse Grip Pull-ups
Triceps	Dumbbell Kickbacks	Pressdowns	Dips
Abdomen	Weighted Crunches	Seated "Abs" Machine	Crunches, Prone Planks
Quadriceps	Back Squats	Leg Extension	Body Weight Lunges
Hamstrings	Stiff-leg Deadlifts	Leg Curls	Hip-ups

Figure 26. Example resistance excercise for different training options.

muscle in that area, and you can lose fat from your body, but the fat doesn't have an awareness that the muscle underneath it is working. You can't control which parts of your body lose fat.

Comprehensive strength programs need a balance between muscle groups. You should be exercising a variety of groups across the different days of your training. Some exercises move just one joint, while others require multi-joint movement. A good training program will include both (Figure 27). Keep in mind as you plan that some types of training, such as Cross-Fit, HIIT, and even some aerobics classes work many muscles and joints during a session.

Training Principles

Safe, noticeable progress with your muscles, as with CRF, involves the training principles of overload, progression, specificity, reversibility, and recovery. The principle of **specificity** suggests that to improve something, you need to train it. This is why we target specific muscle groups in our exercise plan and **progressively overload** these targets, adding intensity to our workouts slowly and incrementally to achieve our goals (see also Chapter 2). The more you do a specific exercise, the better you will become at it. What you choose to train depends on your goals.

Training Goal	Frequency	Intensity	Time
Muscle Strength (beginner)	2–3 days/week per muscle group	60–70% 1-RM	1–3 sets of 8–12 repetitions Rest: 1–3 minutes
Muscle Hypertrophy (beginnger)	2–3 days/week per muscle group	70–85% 1-RM	1–3 sets of 8–12 repetitions Rest: 1–3 minutes
Muscle Endurance (beginner)	2–3 days/week per muscle group	>70% 1-RM	2–4 sets of 10–25 repetitions Rest: 30 seconds to 1 minute
Muscle Strength (intermediate)	2–3 days/week per muscle group	60–70% 1-RM	Rest: 1–3 minutes
Muscle Hypertrophy (intermediate)	2–3 days/week per muscle group	70–85% 1-RM	1–3 sets of 8–12 repetitions Rest: 1–3 minutes
Muscle Endurance (intermediate)	2–3 days/week per muscle group	>70% 1-RM	2–4 sets of 10–25 repetitions Rest: 30 seconds to 1 minute
Muscle Strength (advanced)	2–3 days/week per muscle group	80–100% 1-RM	2–6 sets of 1–8 repetitions Rest: 1–3 minutes
Muscle Hypertrophy (advanced)	2–3 days/week per muscle group	70–100% 1-RM	3–6 sets of 1–12 repetitions Rest: 1–3 minutes
Muscle Endurance (advanced)	2–3 days/week per muscle group	>70% 1-RM	2–4 sets of 10–25 repetitions Rest: 30 seconds to 1 minute

Figure 27. Sample strength training program.

If you want to strengthen your core muscles for stand-up paddle boarding, you need to include core movements regularly in your training. You will want to incorporate exercises for your abdominals, lower back, and hips. You will want to include functional movements that challenge the core muscles to hold your body in different positions.

Regardless of the type of activity, if you do not repeat it, improve at it, and gradually overload, you will see limited results. You are not likely to experience a significant improvement in your arm strength, for example, if you lift weights only once every 3 weeks. If you want to build strength in your arms but do only running, you may see some muscle definition, but since you have not specifically targeted the arms, you will not see the increase in strength you had hoped. (See Chapter 6 "When You Are Trying to Gain Weight" for more information on safe ways to build muscle).

Adequate rest and **recovery** prevents muscle atrophy and contributes to hypertrophy. Give the worked muscles 2–3 days rest between workouts. Be aware of which muscle groups you work each time you train. If you work your upper body on Monday, for example, you shouldn't work it again until Wednesday or Thursday. The fibers experience microscopic tears during training and they need time to rest and rebuild, which is what increases strength. You should not be idle too long, however, or you may experience shrinkage of the muscle.

The amount of rest depends on your level of soreness.

Resting for 2 days is a general guideline, but 3 may be necessary for a particular muscle group if you are still sore.

Within 24 to 72 hours following exercise, it is common to feel **Delayed Onset Muscle Soreness** (DOMS), particularly after eccentric muscle contraction or increasing overload. The minute tears the fibers experience are likely what causes the pain, although this is not entirely understood. Swelling, stiffness, and loss of strength often occurs when you increase a particular activity and challenge your muscles beyond what they are used to — this is a sign of progress. You can limit soreness by adding intensity more gradually to your workouts, warm-up, and cool-down. You can also try a few of the following techniques to help keep soreness manageable and keep you on target with your exercise program:

- Stretching gently
- Staying hydrated
- Taking anti-inflammatory medications, such as ibuprofen
- Using massage, foam rollers, or heat and cold treatments

Ultimately, taking it easy, but not stopping your exercise can be the best way to combat soreness. You may not be able to go full force with your activity level some days, but light exercise will help keep the blood circulating to your muscles and heal them more quickly than complete rest. It also prevents **reversibility**.

Considerations for Safety and Success

Your friend Jake once had the idea that he would train for a World's Strongest Man competition, but he didn't go about it quite the right way. He tends to gain muscle mass easily and was already in great shape, so he thought he could make quick progress. He began working both his upper and lower body 6 days per week. It only took him a few weeks to realize that he was mostly just getting overly sore. His muscles grew so fatigued that he injured his hamstring and had to take time off. He could not properly prepare for the competition and had to put off his goal.

You've learned in this chapter about the structure of your muscles, the benefits of training them, setting SMART goals, and ways to plan a program. But there is a science behind these strategies and ways to use this science to your advantage.

Exercise guidelines for any training program must consider the amount of rest and recovery time between sessions, the specificity and progressive overload of any exercises you perform, and the prevention of injuries during and after workouts.

Safety

Safety and injury prevention should be taken seriously, not only because they protect your health, but also because temporary lapses in your training program resulting from injury can cause reversibility, or the loss of your progress (Figure 28). Be sure to warm-up before and cool-down after every workout, follow proper form and technique, use a spotter when lifting weights, breathe correctly, ensure the safety of your equipment, and use the right fuel for your developing muscles.

Warm-Up and Cool-Down

These activities are an important part of your exercise plan to reduce the risk of injury and lessen soreness. A strength warm-up may include a few minutes of light aerobic activity at a slower speed or lower intensity. This allows your heart rate to elevate gradually and the blood to begin flowing to your muscles.

Spend a few minutes walking after you train to allow your heart rate time to return gradually to its normal resting rate if it is elevated. Stretching the muscles you targeted while you are cooling down can be ideal because the blood is still flowing and the joints are still warm from the activity. This can also help reduce soreness and keep your training on schedule in addition to improving your flexibility.

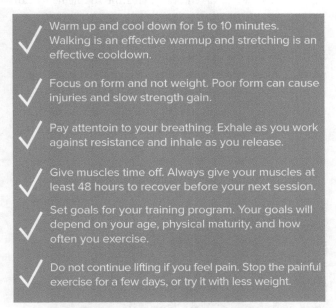

✓ Warm up and cool down for 5 to 10 minutes. Walking is an effective warmup and stretching is an effective cooldown.

✓ Focus on form and not weight. Poor form can cause injuries and slow strength gain.

✓ Pay attentoin to your breathing. Exhale as you work against resistance and inhale as you release.

✓ Give muscles time off. Always give your muscles at least 48 hours to recover before your next session.

✓ Set goals for your training program. Your goals will depend on your age, physical maturity, and how often you exercise.

✓ Do not continue lifting if you feel pain. Stop the painful exercise for a few days, or try it with less weight.

Figure 28. Safety is important in strength training.

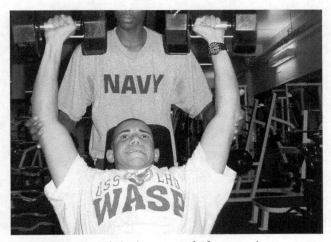

Figure 29. A spotter helps keep you safe if you overshoot your strength goals.

Form and Technique

Strength and endurance training work well to improve your health, but the risk of injury increases when you aren't properly educated on the correct way to complete the activity. If you are just beginning a weight-training routine at the gym, it may seem like a good idea to watch the guy next to you and see how he uses a particular piece of equipment, or to listen to your friend who had that one weight-lifting class in high school. A better approach is to spend some time educating yourself.

Most gyms have staff and trainers available to show you how to use equipment, not to mention detailed instructions hanging next to each apparatus. If you are training outside the gym, do your homework. Read the instruction manual that came with your medicine ball or spend some time on the Internet to find instructions from an expert in your chosen activity. Here are some general guidelines for weight training:

Lift only the amount of weight that you can while still having correct form. You should be able to complete your set raise and lower it without discomfort. The better your form, the better your results.

Go slow. Speed is not always an asset. Form is more important. Slow, controlled movements will yield better results and lower your risk of injury.

Listen to your body and work within your limits. Doing more sets after you can no longer maintain your form will not lead to better results. Some individuals can do only one set, while others can do more. It depends on the activity, the body part you're training, and how many sets you complete. Doing more than you can handle may lead to injury.

Listen to pain. If an activity hurts, try the movement in a different way to see if it feels differently. If not, stop. Try again in a few days with a smaller weight. Talk to your health care provider if the pain persists.

Be safe. If you have an injury, focus on the muscle groups you are able to work.

Use a Spotter

You should always have someone with you when using heavy free-weights to strength train. A bit of fatigue, pulled muscle, or incorrect form could result in a lot of weight on your body unexpectedly. You may need help to place the weight in the starting or finishing position, if the weight tilts, or if you can't complete a lift (Figure 29).

Breathe

Breathing is important when exercising. It may sound obvious, but some people have a tendency to hold their breath when they exert force. Your muscles need oxygen to do their job. How you breathe can be important as well. Try exhaling as you lift and inhaling as you lower – if you reverse the order, you may find it harder to do that next repetition without ready oxygen. Your heart also dislikes it when you hold breath for too long. It lowers your heart rate at a time when it should be elevated and less oxygen circulates where it needs to go.

It is the same principle if the weight is your body. While doing crunches or push-ups, for example, exhale as you raise your upper body and inhale as you lower. For endurance activities, like running, athletes often find that a controlled, rhythmic pattern, breathing in through your nose and out through your mouth, often helps stamina and can prevent those nagging side cramps.

Equipment Safety

Your equipment should be in good working order. Most equipment requires regular maintenance. If something is loose, broken, or making a strange noise, don't use it until it is repaired properly. You always want to check that bands are not cracked, stability balls are adequately inflated, weights are clear of cables or stacked to the right size, machines are locked into place, and weights are secured with collars (devices that secure weight to a barbell or dumbbell). Even experienced people often take shortcuts or skip safety steps in their eagerness to train. This can result in injury and lost time from your training program.

Dietary Supplements

Spend just a few hours watching television or surfing the Internet and you'll likely come across at least a few advertisements for products claiming to help you build muscle or burn fat. Even some flawed training programs recommend the use of dietary supplements to help you achieve your goals, but they should be taken with great care because of the inherent risk and dangers associated with their misuse. We do not recommend using dietary supplements for any reason (Figure 30).

The US Food and Drug Administration regulates these products but they are classified differently than drugs. The FDA does not require manufacturers to prove the safety of these products prior to distribution, though they can have products removed from the shelves if they later prove harmful. The FDA also do not evaluate whether or not these supplements prove effective in achieving what they claim to achieve. Illegal supplements have other consequences, such as health implications and legal risks.

Supplements range from those designed to boost energy, increase protein levels, or add amino acids to the body, to those designed to increase testosterone levels (see "Substances"). All should be considered closely before being incorporated into your nutritional or training plan.

Creatine is an amino acid that occurs naturally in the body and is stored mostly in our muscle cells. You get creatine from your diet by eating red meat and seafood. Creatine can also be made in a laboratory and taken in the form of creatine supplements. When taken orally, creatine supplements can increase the creatine levels in the muscles, which help transport energy to the part of the body that needs it during contraction. It works well for activities requiring short bursts of energy, which is likely why trainers often recommend it for bodybuilders. It does not work well when combined with caffeine and could even have adverse effects if taken with other stimulants. The body can only store a certain amount of creatine,

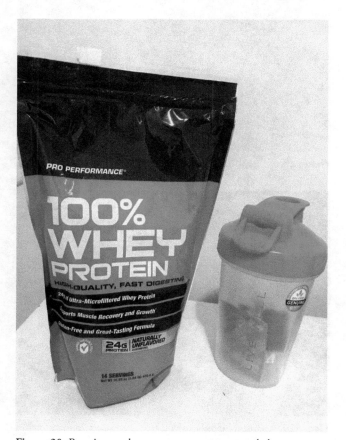

Figure 30. Protein supplements are not recommended.

and taking in too much is not beneficial. We don't yet know the long-term risks of creatine use.

Protein powders are usually made from whey, soy, or casein (a milk protein), though whey is the most common. Whey protein is considered complete because it contains all 9 amino acids needed by the human body. Your body needs protein to help it convert food into energy and process toxins. You need approximately .36 grams per pound of body weight each day.

People doing increased strength training often need more protein and will add a protein powder to compensate. A good guide is 0.68–1.0 gram per kilogram of protein daily when trying to build muscle. Protein supplements are generally considered safe, but they are an expensive way to consume protein. We recommend protein from real food sources, a healthier way to consume more protein. Keep in mind that you may not need to add additional protein if you already consume an ample amount for training, as most Americans do.

Substances

Substances like **testosterone boosters** and **steroids** are sometimes used by athletes to increase their performance and muscular appearance, which may work in the short term. They can increase muscle size and help people recover faster. They are also illegal and dangerous. Anabolic steroids are a man-made version of testosterone, a male hormone. It seems ironic that these man-made, man-enhanc-

ing materials should actually (after long-term use) shrink testicles, enlarge male breasts, and lower sperm count, but they do. This is in addition to an increased risk of prostate cancer; kidney, liver, and heart damage; mood swings ("roid rage"), and irritability.

In women we see a potential for male-pattern baldness, a deepened voice, facial hair, and an interrupted menstrual cycle. After long-term use, women become more "manly" and men lose certain aspects of their masculinity. Both are at risk for serious health problems. When steroids are used alongside other supplements, such as creatine and protein powders, there is an increased potential for kidney injury.

Various herbal supplements also allege to naturally boost the testosterone levels men lose as they age and, in theory, help improve or maintain muscle mass. The jury is still out on many of these supplements, but most seem to do little if anything to contribute to muscle growth. More information on supplements is available online:

- National Center for Complementary and Alternative Medicine: nccih.nih.gov/

- National Institutes of Health Office of Dietary Supplements: ods.od.nih.gov/

- Federal Trade Commission: www.consumer.ftc.gov/articles/0261-dietary-supplements

- Food & Drug Administration Supplements: www.fda.gov/Food/DietarySupplements

Conclusion

Your next steps should be assessing your muscular strength and endurance and using what you find to create a muscle fitness plan that includes targeting areas of improvement and identifying training exercises. You may not be asked to assess your own fitness during this course, but you might consider activities that you do each day that may be easier or more enjoyable if you had greater muscular strength and endurance. Consider some ways you can adapt or change your other fitness programs to include muscle strength and endurance to stay challenged and motivated to improve your overall health and wellness.

Reflection Questions

1. What are the different types of muscle fibers that are in the human body? Please describe.

2. For each type of muscle fiber, can you give an example of an activity or exercise that predominantly uses the muscle fiber type?

3. What is the process of muscle hypertrophy? Why and how does muscle atrophy occur?

4. How satisfied are you with your current level of muscular strength and endurance? Please explain.

5. Consider the different benefits of muscular strength and endurance. In what ways might your quality of life be different if you made improvements in your muscular strength and endurance or were able to maintain a high level of muscular strength and endurance long-term?

6. What are some of the different options that people have with strength training programs?

7. Create a sample program for muscular strength and endurance using the FITT formula.

8. What are important safety considerations a person should keep in mind with regards to muscular strength and endurance?

9. Identify some of the health concerns associated with testosterone boosters and steroids. Why do you think some people use these substances despite the possible risks?

Chapter 5
Flexibility

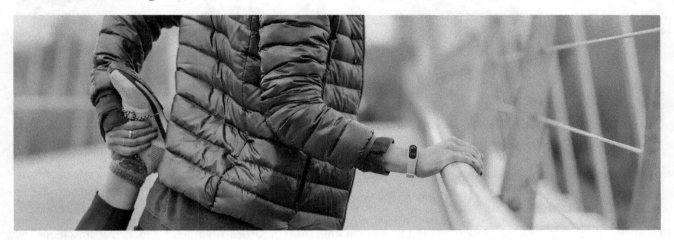

You're out for a run a few weeks before your vacation. You've always wanted to hike the Pacific Crest Trail, and you decide that some initial trail running would be a good way to prepare for the terrain and build your cardiorespiratory stamina. It sounds like a good plan until one morning, you take a longer than normal stride to avoid a puddle and tear your Achilles tendon. The good news is that your arms are about to get a major workout. The bad news is that you're about to be on crutches for at least the next four weeks. Crutches don't hike the PCT. Your vacation will be a bit delayed.

With better flexibility, you might have avoided this scenario. Your body's flexibility is linked to your ability to move and remain pain-free. You can achieve sufficient flexibility through training, and every other kind of fitness training (including runs and hikes) will be less likely to cause injury or pain.

This chapter defines and compares static and dynamic flexibility, shows why flexibility is so important, describes how to assess your flexibility, and details how to achieve better flexibility resulting in safer and more satisfying exercises.

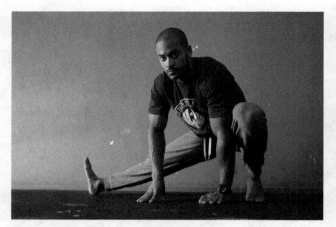

Figure 1. Static flexibility is improved by static stretching.

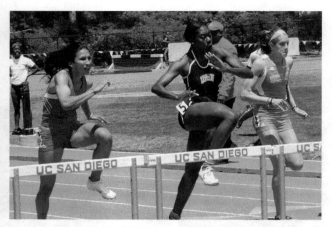

Figure 2. Dynamic flexibility is improved by dynamic stretching.

Defining Flexibility

Flexibility is your body's ability to execute its full **range of motion** (ROM), particularly around muscles that cross joints and induce bending movements. Each specific joint has its own degree of flexibility. You could be flexible in your legs, for example, but find that turning your head to check your blind spot in traffic is difficult because the range of motion in your neck seems limited. For this reason, flexibility exercises that target specific muscle groups or parts of the body are important in helping us function comfortably and safely. Each joint depends on variables such as the rigidity of surrounding tendons and ligaments. These are the strong connective tissues between muscles and bones.

You can lose your flexibility with inactivity, but regular stretching can improve it. You don't have to be extremely flexible to notice health benefits and improvements in your abilities, yet flexibility is an often-overlooked aspect of fitness that is important to maintaining overall wellness.

Flexibility has two types, static and dynamic. Static stretches impact your **static flexibility**—muscle movement conducted while staying relatively still with the rest of your body. An example of this is bending to touch your toes. How far you can reach and hold the stretch? A slow, steady stretch like this one involves no other motion than the bend—no bouncing, pulsing, or quick repetitions (Figure 1).

Dynamic stretches impact your **dynamic flexibility**, or the absolute range of motion you can achieve through movement, such as swinging your arms across your body to see how far they can reach. In your toe touch, rather than holding the position, you would do slow, controlled repetitions of the movement (Figure 2).

In your day-to-day life, you often challenge your body in ways that involve both dynamic and static flexibility. When you run, jump, hop off a curb, or suddenly reach out to catch something, your dynamic flexibility impacts whether you can do it. It enables you to use the full range of motion of the joint. Really stretching to reach something, bending in any direction to pick something up, or even tying your shoes draws on your static flexibility to complete the task comfortably. It sounds simple enough, but it actually has a great deal of value.

Factors that Determine Flexibility

A variety of factors affect your flexibility, some that you can control and others you can't. Some factors, such as joint structure and function, can't be changed. Other factors, such as muscle length at rest, can be changed. The goal in flexibility training is to have a full normal range of motion, not to create extreme flexibility. It's possible to have too much flexibility, just as it's possible to have too little.

Some factors that affect flexibility are joint structure and function, connective tissue, nervous system regulation, injury and disease, genetics, biological sex, and age.

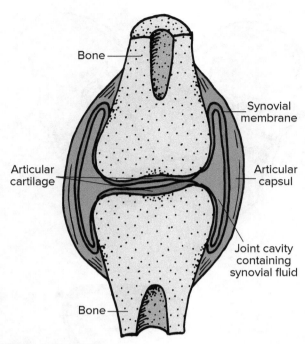

Figure 3. Basic joint structure.

Joint Structure and Function

Everywhere that two or more bones join together in your body is a joint. Joints can either be rigid, like the joints in your skull, or movable, like in your elbows and knees (Figure 3). Some joints have greater range of motion than others due to their design. Some move a lot, some move a little, and others don't move at all. Joints are classified functionally by how they move, and structurally by how they are composed.

There are three main types of joints—fibrous (synarthrodial), cartilaginous (synchondroses and sympheses), and synovial (diarthrosis).

Fibrous joints do not move. Fibrous connective tissues, like ligaments, hold them together (Figure 4). The roots of your teeth, for example, anchor into your jaw with fibrous joints, just like the parts of your skull and other areas where the bones join but are not intended to move.

Cartilaginous joints are partially moveable. These bones connect to each other with **cartilage**, a hard connective tissue. The vertebrae in your spine or where your ribs anchor to your

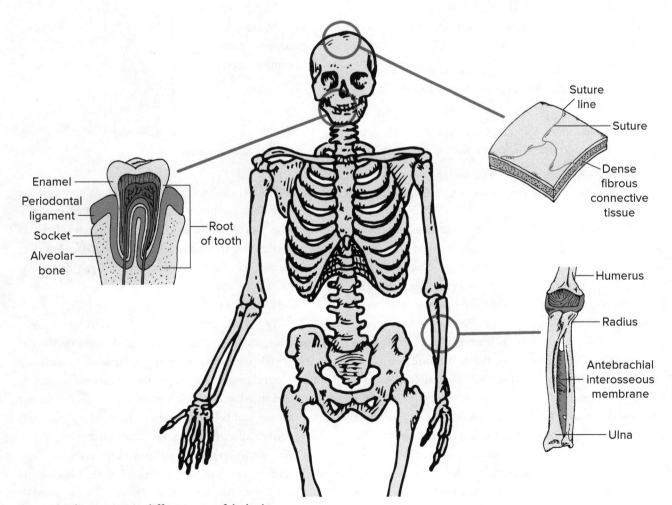

Figure 4. Fibrous joints in different parts of the body.

breastbone are examples of cartilaginous joints (Figure 5). Children have many temporary cartilaginous joints called growth plates. As they grow, bone replaces these plates and become permanent.

Synovial joints are very moveable and are what we often think of when we imagine a joint. Your knees, elbows, fingers, shoulders, and neck are all examples of synovial joints. They contain cartilage, membranes, and a joint cavity filled with lubricating fluid. The entire joint is surrounded by a collagenous type of capsule and a membrane that secretes the fluid into the joint to keep it moving efficiently. You have six different types of synovial joints:

- **Hinge**—Flexes and extends, such as your elbow and knee

- **Pivot**—Rotates one bone around another on its own axis, such as the first few vertebrae of your neck that enable your head to move

- **Ball and socket**—Flexes, extends, rotates, abducts (movement away from the body), and adducts (movement toward the midline of the body), such as your shoulder and hip (Figure 6)

- **Saddle**—Flexes, extends, rotates, abducts, adducts, and circumducts (360 degrees of movement), such as your thumb

- **Condyloid**—Flexes, extends, rotates, abducts, adducts, and circumducts, such as your wrist

- **Gliding**—Gliding movements, such as those that occur with the bones of your hand (intercarpal joints)

The shape of synovial joints determines in what way and degree a joint can move (Figure 7). Some synovial joints, such as the elbow and knee, allow movement in one direction. Other synovial joints, such as the hip and shoulder, allow movement in all directions. Joints that allow for a greater amount of movement have a higher risk of injury, as they tend to be more flexible. Flexibility varies by joint because the structure varies between joints. There is no single test to measure flexibility.

Joint structure and function can limit flexibility because not all of your joints have a great range of motion. Many joints can move in almost any direction, while others, like your knees and elbows, only bend one way. When we see athletes like gymnasts on television, we are shocked by the ways they can tumble and bend. We assume that their backs are quite flexible. In reality, many of their movements are possible through

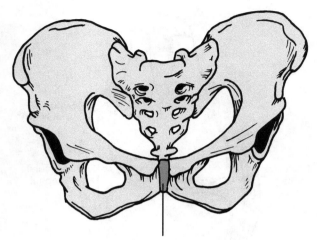

Pubic symphysis

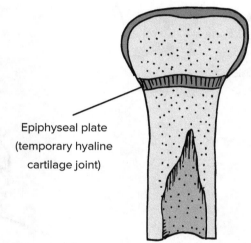

Epiphyseal plate
(temporary hyaline
cartilage joint)

Figure 5. Cartilageonous joints.

the flexibility of their shoulders and hips, which have a greater range of motion. You may want to be able to bend your back or any other part of your body in a certain way, but your joints will only allow you to bend so far before its unsafe. Any time you move a joint beyond its natural capacity, you risk injury.

Connective Tissue and Nervous System Regulation

Connective tissues are vital to the range of motion you experience in your joints and muscles. Collagen and elastin are proteins found in your connective tissues that allow them to stretch and then bounce back. Over time, connective tissues can lose water and collagen, or they can build up too much collagen. Both affect the way your body stretches.

Different tissues vary in the way they can maintain a new length or return to their original length. **Ligaments**, for example, are a tough connective tissue. They respond to

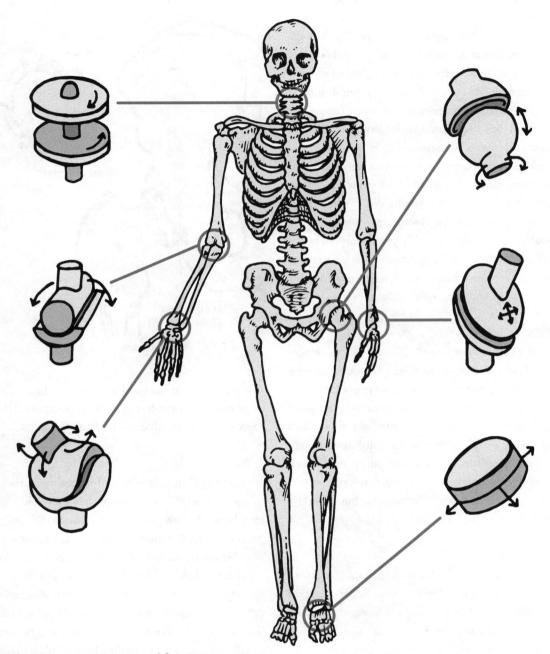

Figure 6. Different joint types structure and function.

stretching but do not have a fixed memory of their original shape — they don't spring back like a rubber band after being stretched too far. Some injuries result from ligaments stretching to a length that becomes unsafe or painful.

Deep connective tissue, such as **fascia** and **tendons**, provide stability for the joint and prevent too much movement. A layer of fascia wraps around all of your muscles, organs, nerves, and nearly every part of your body — it really holds us together. It's elastic but tough, and is designed to maintain tension — a bit like lycra clothing. Tendons are tough

tissues that connect muscles to bones, primarily. They work a bit like bungee cords, keeping your bones, joints, and muscles in place but moveable. You can run, jump, and do whatever your body needs to do because fascia and tendons are naturally pliable and stretch to your movements. They also limit your range of motion to prevent injury.

These connective tissues need care just like your muscles. Sometimes in a person's efforts to increase muscle mass, they neglect to work on their flexibility. This can cause the connective tissues around the joint to be too tight, limiting movement.

In the same way, if a person's normal way of moving throughout the day emphasizes or de-emphasizes one particular muscle group or body part, those areas may have a limited range of motion. For example, if you have a job where you sit most of the day, your hamstrings can become shortened from a lack of stretching and even cause lower back pain. Flexibility can help rebalance this potential harm.

Connective tissues have other important features as well. Your muscles, tendons, and ligaments have **stretch receptors** that activate when your muscle is lengthened or compressed. They send a message—called **proprioceptors**—to your brain or spine through your nervous system. They facilitate your body's awareness of your limbs and other body parts. The last time you put on your shirt, you didn't have to watch your arm go through the sleeve to know it happened, thanks to your proprioceptors.

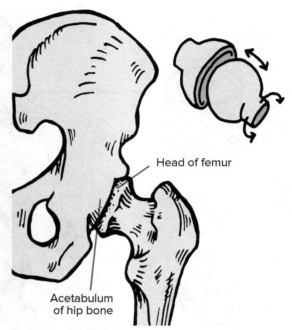

Head of femur

Acetabulum
of hip bone

Figure 7. Ball and socket joint.

Genetics

Genetics play a role in how flexible you can be. Some people have more flexible connective tissues than others., such as people with **hypermobility**, or what we might call being "double-jointed." They can move their joints into positions that would injure the rest of us. This may not always be a good thing. Many people with hypermobility never experience any physical problems, but others become prone to pain, stiffness, joint dislocation, and have a higher risk of injury.

Everyone benefits from flexibility training, but not everyone will easily be able to do a back-bend or the splits.

Biological Sex

Females are generally more flexible than males, likely due to the amount of the hormone relaxin in their bodies. Relaxin encourages muscle lengthening and joint looseness. In fact, women's joints, ligaments, and muscles are usually looser during pregnancy due to increased relaxin. This is especially true for pelvic joints. Joints may remain looser for several months after childbirth. Testosterone, the primary male sex hormone, makes muscles larger and has the opposite effect, which is why men may have more challenges in flexibility

training. This can be good for strength, but it limits range of motion. As a result, men may need additional flexibility exercises just as much or more than women do.

Use and Age

It's easy to think that joint and flexibility issues only relate to age because of how common they are in older adults. But even in youth, how you use your body has the largest impact on your range of motion. Flexibility issues often happen to younger adults because of changes in their lifestyle.

For example, a sedentary job can lead to decreased energy for physical activities. Long periods without activities that utilize your range of motion can cause your muscle fibers to degrade and connective tissue to undergo a type of scarring usually associated with a healing injury. This is called **fibrosis**. The excessive tissue limits mobility and impedes the muscle's ability to regenerate. There isn't much you can do to prevent age-related fibrosis. However, staying flexible to prevent injury-related fibrosis can help keep joints movable.

Injury and Your Joints

For a joint injury, treatment usually includes avoiding movements that cause pain, but it doesn't mean resting completely. If an injury is serious, resting the area might be recommended. If you've had a joint injury, you're well aware that

after immobilizing one of your joints, even for a short time, it can be very difficult to move that part of your body again. Imagine that you break your ankle. You spend four weeks or more in a cast keeping the bone, its joint, and the surround-

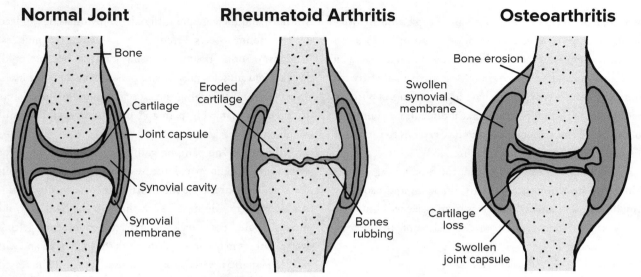

Figure 8. A normal joint compared to joints affected by rheumatoid arthritis and osteoarthritis.

ing tissues in a fixed position. This means that your ankle is not exercised, and the rest of your body isn't doing as much moving either while you're on crutches—except for maybe your upper body and abdominals. When you finally remove the cast, things don't just go back to normal. It can take a long time for the ankle to be ready for strenuous exercise and even longer before it stops swelling the minute you even look at your running shoes. Naturally, your flexibility will be impacted. You find that you have to actively work to regain that range of motion.

Injuries can challenge your flexibility, and repeated injuries to a particular joint can lead to arthritis in the area, even at a young age. Athletes often play through their pain because of their desire to compete, but this can lead to long-term complications. It's important to know how to manage and heal from an injury to safely get back in action quickly. Your health care provider should be able to advise you on what activities are safe and effective and tell you when you can perform them.

Disease and Your Joints

Certain diseases that affect the joints, such as **arthritis**, can impact flexibility, creating a complicated situation for exercising. People with arthritis often find moving their joints difficult and uncomfortable, yet movement is one of the things that help reduce the pain and swelling (Figure 8).

Osteoarthritis is one of the most common forms of arthritis. It occurs most often in older adults or in people who are either inactive or over-active with certain joints. Cartilage can begin to wear down, causing bones begin to rub together during movement. This is why some people need a knee or hip replacement. The pain can become unbearable and the movement so difficult that an artificial version of the joint becomes necessary. This can happen as a result of aging, joint disease, or an injury that damages the cartilage.

Rheumatoid arthritis is an autoimmune disease where the body's immune system confuses healthy tissue with bacteria, and attacks the tissues surrounding a joint. This can be very painful, resulting in not only the pain, swelling, and limited range of motion associated with osteoarthritis, but also fatigue, fevers, and damage to other organs. Health scientists don't yet understand what triggers the autoimmune conditions of rheumatoid arthritis.

Gout is another form of arthritis. It occurs most often in men and frequently will begin in their big toe, though it can affect other joints as well. The attacks can be sudden. A man might go to sleep feeling fine but wake up with a big toe

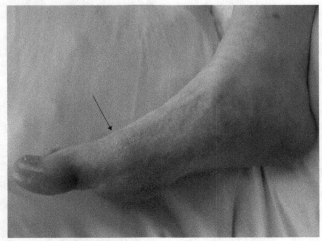

Figure 9. Affected foot of a gout patient.

swollen, red, and throbbing with pain. People who are overweight or those who eat a lot of foods high in purines—a chemical compound that gets broken down into uric acid by the body—are more prone to gout. Meat (particularly fatty red meat) and certain types of fish have high amounts of purines. Eating a lot of these foods can make it difficult for your body to process all the uric acid, causing uric crystals to form that the body stores around joints (Figure 9).

Other diseases that can impact the functioning of your joints include fibromyalgia, lupus, diabetes, and psoriasis. Any disease that affects the joints or muscles will limit the joint's range of motion and complicate attempts to exercise.

Exercising with Joint Pain

It's important to keep moving if you have joint pain or limited flexibility. Inactivity can reduce range of motion, increase stiffness, and increase pain. In older individuals, it can lead to contractures—a shortening or hardening of muscles, tendons, or other tissues—causing joints to become rigid. Weak, rigid muscles mean more pressure on the joint itself. Exercising and stretching the muscles around painful joints is crucial in managing pain and preventing further loss of mobility.

The motto "no pain, no gain" doesn't exactly apply for some types of joint-related diseases. Some people's joints will certainly feel better once they learn to exercise through pain. A better motto might be "work through the pain to avoid increased pain." Focus on keeping the discomfort from getting worse. Others may not be able to work the joint at all and will have to plan their exercise routine around it to avoid increased pain. Talk with your health care provider if you have a joint disease or joint injury to find out how you can safely stay active.

Benefits of Flexibility

The importance of good flexibility can often be overlooked when we think of our overall health. Most of us wouldn't put flexibility on the list of things they picture when they imagine getting healthier. When you envision the healthiest version of yourself, what comes to mind? A healthy weight? Larger muscles? Increased athletic performance? Maybe you imagine life with fewer trips to your health care provider. The fact is that improving your flexibility contributes to all of these and more. It isn't just about being able to impress others in a yoga class or do a cartwheel. Improved flexibility can support improvements in many aspects of your overall wellness.

Physical Benefits

Think of all the times during your physical education classes in school or classes at the gym that someone has asked you to bend forward and touch your toes. If you couldn't do it, likely you laughed and made a comment about not being very flexible. You may not have given it much thought after that. It's not uncommon for people to underestimate the power of flexibility. There are many benefits to flexibility that can keep you active and independent throughout your lifespan.

Joint Health

According to the US Department of Health and Human Services, joint pain can be one of the most common barriers to an active life, particularly as we get older. Joint health is improved by maintaining flexibility and can help you avoid bigger problems that stem from poor joint health (Figure 10).

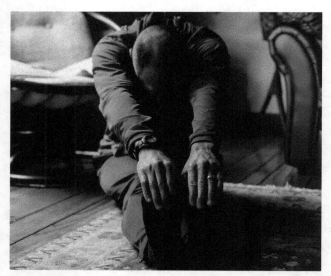

Figure 10. Stretching is important to maintaining mobility.

If your flexibility declines, your body must compensate in other ways. You might stop doing activities that are uncomfortable, which speeds the problem by further reducing your flexibility and activity level even more. Your posture, agility, and balance can be impacted from limitations in range of motion. Worst of all, poor joint health can lead to chronic pain that is difficult, if not impossible, to improve.

The end result of poor joint health is often irreversible. Research suggests that once contractures occur, stretching does very little to help because of the shortening of the ligaments and tissues. Someone with arthritis in their hands and wrists might be permanently bent in a certain direction. This is very painful. Flexible muscles and tissues at the joint enable it to move efficiently and keep it healthier longer.

Performance

Flexibility can improve performance, particularly when you focus on flexibility training that addresses the type of movement necessary for your activities such as your favorite sports and hobbies, or for your job. To efficiently perform the movements you need, whether it's throughout your nor-

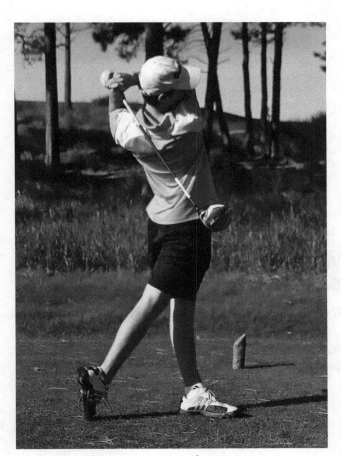

Figure 11. Flexibility impacts range of motion.

mal day or during exercise, you need flexible joints to maintain your balance and remain pain-free. In a competition, this impacts how much power you can exert. In your normal day, this impacts your ability to make the movements you need to do your job well (Figure 11).

Imagine watching a runner sprint during a race. Now imagine yourself trying to sprint to catch the bus. Now imagine a horror movie hero, running from the chainsaw-wielding monster. Did any of these runners fall down in your imagination? Maybe the horror movie victim gets caught or trips as they try to look back at their pursuer, but it's hard for most of us to imagine an athlete falling during an event. Sure, it happens, and true, it's a movie, but you never see someone with high athletic training fall victim in these scenarios. Nope—they're flexible, agile, and ready to move at a moment's notice.

Everyone's performance benefits from flexibility training. Runners need increased flexibility in their legs and hips. Swimmers need a full range of motion in their shoulders. For those of us who don't compete, we need good flexibility to keep our workouts consistent, comfortable, and efficient (and to keep us on our toes if we ever do need to make a run for it).

Reduced Pain

Flexibility can reduce your risk of lower back pain, especially with the right kinds of stretches. Flexibility in your joints and muscles enables you to maintain good posture and balance. This helps you avoid other aches and pains, too, particularly in the back, shoulders, and neck.

How many times have you been told to stand up straight? This is a well-known instruction for a good reason. Take a moment to fully extend your back and abdomen upright, keeping your shoulders back. You'll feel the stretch, and if you tend to slouch, you'll feel the muscle exertion as well. You can make things easier on your body by keeping these muscles and joints flexible. Poor posture can lead to poor balance, which can lead to injury. It can also cause your body to compensate in other ways, adapting to the poor position. This can cause further discomfort in other areas of your body.

Your back is not the only part of your body susceptible to injury and pain. Your joints and connective tissues, as mentioned, can cause a great deal of chronic discomfort if not tended to properly. Your muscles, as well, need that range of motion in order to be ready to protect you from injury. Flexibility won't prevent every injury, but it can lower the risk of injuries, and it's an important part of any rehabilitation from a previous injury.

Overall Health

Flexibility improves overall health by reducing muscle tension, lowering blood pressure, and relieving muscle cramps. Muscle tension relates to a muscle's length. A longer muscle will be less tense, and stretching focuses on lengthening the muscle. It may seem strange, but when your body is stretched and flexible, your arteries are as well. Regularly working on flexibility helps you avoid arterial stiffness. Stiff arteries can lead to high blood pressure and cardiovascular disease. Muscle cramps happen when muscles gets tight and contract involuntarily. Stretching, which lengthens the muscle, can help relieve a cramp, making it easier to keep exercising and improve your overall health.

Emotional and Psychological Benefits

The benefits already mentioned may not have surprised you, but there are many more that may be less obvious. Whether it's that run from the chainsaw monster, a long night of studying, or just a busy day, good flexibility can help. Think of your typical day, or even the craziest day you've had recently, and imagine how much better you'd feel with some of the following benefits of good flexibility:

Reduced stress and increased relaxation — Stretching forces you to relax your muscles. Routinely relaxing your muscles teaches your body to release tension. Stress is a form of tension. Flexibility training, in a sense, hard-wires your body to relax and relieve any form of tension it encounters. Additionally, illness and injury can create significant stress in your life. The reduced risk of illness and injury that flexibility provides limits these as potential added stressors.

Relief from regular aches and pains — Stress can also cause psychosomatic responses in the body, causing physical symptoms of distress. Its reduction can make you feel better both emotionally and physically.

Flexibility training stretches your muscles and connective tissues that cause pain when tense. This helps generate relief except when there is an injury (such as a fracture or torn ligament) present.

Lowered breathing rate — If you've ever taken a yoga class, you know the importance of regulated breathing. Part of stretching is knowing how to breathe as you stretch. This patterned breathing can be relaxing and, when done routinely, can lower your breathing rate, which is great for cardiorespiratory health as well.

Improved mood — What happens when you reduce stress, relieve pain, limit your illnesses, and feel confident in your abilities? It stands to reason that you see an overall improvement in your mood.

It sounds good, right? The benefits of flexibility connect with wellness in more ways than physical. When you take care of your body's flexibility, you're focusing on your whole body and its functioning as well as feeling good.

Improving Your Flexibility

Your first step before setting your SMART goals is assessment — you need to know where you are before you can decide where you want to be. Flexibility can be assessed using several joint-specific measurements and simple ability tests that can help you target your less-flexible joints for training. Here you'll find several tests to help you assess the flexibility of different joints. Be sure to warm up for 5 to 10 minutes before completing any assessment.

Age (years)	15–19	20–29	30–39	40–49	50–59	60–69
Men						
Excellent	≥39 cm	≥40 cm	≥38 cm	≥35 cm	≥35 cm	≥33 cm
Very good	34–38 cm	34–39 cm	33–37 cm	29–34 cm	28–34 cm	25–32 cm
Good	29–33 cm	30–33 cm	28–32 cm	24–28 cm	24–27 cm	20–24 cm
Fair	24–28 cm	25–29 cm	23–27 cm	18–23 cm	16–23 cm	15–19 cm
Needs Improvement	≤23 cm	≤24 cm	≤22 cm	≤17 cm	≤15 cm	≤14 cm
Women						
Excellent	≥43 cm	≥41 cm	≥41 cm	≥38 cm	≥39 cm	≥35 cm
Very Good	38–42 cm	37–40 cm	36–40 cm	34–37 cm	33–38 cm	31–34 cm
Good	34–37 cm	33–36 cm	32–35 cm	30–33 cm	30–32 cm	27–30 cm
Fair	29–33 cm	28–32 cm	27–31 cm	25–29 cm	25–29 cm	23–26 cm
Needs Improvement	≤28 cm	≤27 cm	≤26 cm	≤24 cm	≤24 cm	≤22 cm

Figure 12. Sit-and-reach results by age and gender.

Sit-and-Reach

The sit and reach test measures the flexibility of your lower back and hamstrings. You will need a sit-and-reach box—with the footline set at 26 cm—and a partner.

1. Sit with your bare feet flat against the box.

2. With your hands parallel to the box, lean forward toward the ruler portion of the box as far as possible. Keep your hands side by side. Your legs should be straight, but do not lock your knees.

3. Exhale and drop your head between your arms as you reach to extend the stretch as far as you are able.

4. Hold for 2 seconds.

5. Have your partner measure your reach distance.

6. Repeat until you have an average.

On the following chart, find the rating that corresponds with your score (Figure 12).

Shoulder Flexibility

You will need a partner and either a ruler or tape measure for this test.

1. Raise your right arm over your head.

2. Bend at the elbow and reach between your shoulders as far as you can with your palm against your back.

3. Extend your left arm toward the ground.

4. Bend at the left elbow and raise your hand between your shoulders as far as you can with your palm against your back.

5. Your partner should measure the distance between the fingers of your right and left hand, or the amount of overlap, to the nearest quarter of an inch. If your fingers meet or overlap, the number is positive. If your fingers do not meet, the score is a negative number.

6. Repeat with your other arm.

Your score is the average of the two measurements. Find your rating in the table that corresponds with your measurement.

Hamstring Flexibility

For this assessment, you need a goniometer or other joint measurement tool (optional) and a partner.

1. Lie on your back with your arms at your sides.

2. Bend one knee, keeping the foot flat on the floor and extend the other leg straight.

3. Raise the extended leg so it is at least at a 90-degree angle, perpendicular to the floor.

4. Compare the range of motion in the raised straight leg relative to a 90-degree position. If a partner and a measuring instrument are available, you can obtain a more precise measurement of the joint angle.

5. Repeat with your other leg.

If you can't raise your leg so that it is vertical to your hips, your hamstring flexibility is below average. Beyond perpendicular would be above average.

Setting Goals for Flexibility

What areas of your body lack flexibility? How do you use your body on a daily basis? What would you like to be able to do that you can't right now? Do you have a family history of joint disease you'd like to actively avoid or a previous injury to keep in mind? Consider your situation and think about what goals are appropriate for you. Remember to keep them SMART. For example, say that in your shoulder flexibility assessment your fingers were 4 inches apart. You want to be able to climb the rock wall at the gym with your friends and know that you need flexible shoulders for this. Here is a SMART goal you could set for yourself:

Specific—I want to decrease the separation between my fingers in my shoulder flexibility test
Measurable—From 4 inches to 2 inches
Achievable—This is a small improvement
Relevant—It will help me climb the rock wall
Time-based—2 months
Your ultimate goal might be to have your fingers touch, but you wisely set a smaller goal along the way. You also may find that you reach a level of flexibility that works for you or that you reach your maximum flexibility before your fingers touch. Each person is different, and you should listen to your body.

Training for Flexibility

Stretching has been considered an effective tool to boost performance levels, improve range of motion, and lower the risk of injury for many years. Unsurprisingly, there are many ways to stretch. Flexibility training techniques include static, ballistic, and dynamic stretching, as well as proprioceptive neuromuscular facilitation (PNF) and myofascial release.

Static stretching involves only the bend of the joint you are stretching. You should stretch until you feel a slight tension, or just beyond, and hold it until you feel a slight discomfort. The benefits occur during the hold (usually about 20–60 seconds), which allows the muscle group time to relax and lengthen. Repeat the stretch and hold 2–4 times for ideal improvement to your flexibility. Normally, the length of the stretch can be improved a little with each repetition. This improves muscle elasticity and joint mobility.

People who are new to stretching often prefer static stretching because of the low risk of injury, provided they aren't attempting to place their body into an unnatural position. Listen to your body telling you "enough!" with that slight discomfort. We've all seen those people that can sit on the floor and pull their foot behind their head, but nothing is gained for them but attention and, potentially, pain. Static stretching is not just for beginners. It's effective for everyone and not as time consuming as some of the other methods.

Static-active stretching is achieved through the strength of the agonist muscle. The individual assumes a position and holds it in place with no other assistance. For example, from a standing position, bend your knee, bringing your leg behind your body. This actively engages the force of your hamstrings (the agonists). Hold it there, engaging no other power than the strength of the hamstring. Don't use your hands to hold your foot back! This means that your quadriceps (antagonists)—now lengthened—are being stretched while the hamstring is being strengthened. The hold time for this stretch should be approximately 20 seconds. This can be a bit demanding. Many of the movements in yoga and Pilates are static-active.

Static-passive stretching utilizes some form of assistance with the stretch, either an object, a partner, gravity, or your own body (Figure 13). You can do the stretch described above,

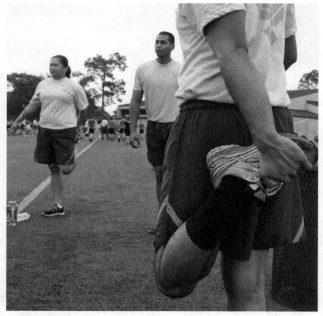

Figure 13. Static-passive stretching.

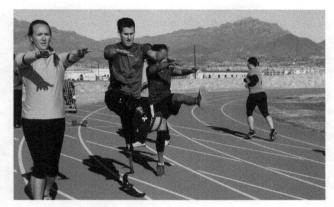

Figure 14. Ballistic stretching.

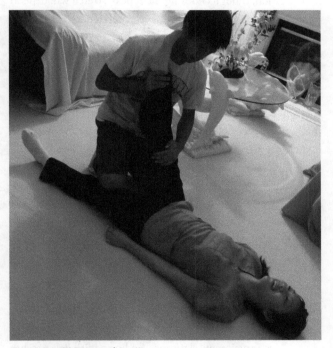

Figure 15. PNF stretching.

but if you use your hands to hold your foot behind your back, it's a static-passive stretch instead. This type of relaxed stretching is more common than static-active. For another example, place your foot on top of a bar, bench, or chair with your leg extended at a 90-degree angle and slowly bend toward your knee as far as you can, holding the stretch for 10–30 seconds.

Whether active or passive, static stretching works well on warm muscles for cooling-down *after* a workout and for stretching tired or sore muscles. Studies suggest that static stretching *before* intense activity or athletic competition can *limit* performance in most age groups. In adults over 65, static stretching is good at any point during exercise.

Ballistic stretching requires momentum, and quick, bouncy movements. Repeatedly kicking or swinging your

leg up to touch your toes to your hand extended high in the air would be an example (Figure 14). By propelling your legs forward, you use the speed of the limb to push its joint past its normal range of motion.This type of stretching can improve flexibility, but it is riskier. It does not allow the muscle time to relax and adjust to the stretched position. It is often used with certain athletic activities to prepare the body for specific movements, especially in sports where there is kicking, throwing, running, batting, or other ballistic movements.

Dynamic stretching involves controlled repetitions of movement through a joint or muscle's range of motion. For example, a slow lunge down and up would stretch the quadriceps. Standing while slowly extending one leg out in front at a time is a dynamic hamstring stretch. The movements in dynamic stretches are never extended past the normal range of motion of the joint. Unless you work for the circus, it isn't necessary for most of us to be able to pull our ankles past our ears.

Dynamic stretching works great as a warm-up to aerobic activity or competition because it engages the joint in a range of motion similar to what we experience in our active lives. Keeping your movements controlled and intentional can improve performance. Recent studies have suggested that dynamic stretching before athletic events may improve performance.

Proprioceptive neuromuscular facilitation (PNF) is a more advanced form of stretching that requires both the stretching and the contraction of the muscle. In a PNF stretch, stretch the muscles like you would in a static stretch, then contract the muscle group while under some form of resistance to prevent movement, such as against an object or with the help of a partner (Figure 15). The contraction would be held for a certain amount of time (6 seconds, for example). Then release the contraction, staying in a static stretch for 20 or 30 seconds, then rest and repeat. PNF not only stretches the muscle group but also serves as a form of strength training. Studies have shown that doing PNF before jogging or other moderate or low-intensity exercises actually increases performance. It also serves as an excellent post-workout activity to improve range of motion and strength.

Myofascial release uses stretching, compression, direct pressure, and other techniques to release restricted areas of fascia, ideally creating a biochemical and mechanical change that allows for more efficient movement. Foam rollers and other special products can assist in targeting and releasing the tissue. Because of the amount of stretch that it provides, don't do this prior to high-intensity exercise.

F	Frequency of Exercise	How Often	Minimum 2 to 3 times a week. Best to do some stretching daily.
I	Intensity of Exercise	How Hard	You should stretch to the point where you feel tension, not pain.
T	Time of Exercise	How Long	15–30 minutes total. Static stretches of warm muscles; 15–60 seconds, 3 sets
T	Type of Exercise	Which Exercises	After warm up: dynamic stretch, prepares body for exercise. After cool down: static stretch, most improvement gains for flexibility.

Figure 16. The FITT Formula in flexibility training.

Applying Training Principles to Flexibility

The FITT Formula can be applied to a flexibility training program in the same manner we apply it to other aspects of fitness (Figure 16). This will enable you to create a plan that will be effective and safe. The following guidelines from the American College of Sports Medicine can be helpful:

Frequency—Stretching should be done at least 2 or 3 days per week, though more often is safe. People new to stretching should start with 2 days per week and gradually increase the frequency. Building it into your exercise program can make the process simpler and increase the benefits of your workout. For example, if you perform a cardiovascular activity 4 days per week, dynamic stretching as part of your warm-up will help prepare your body and improve performance, and static stretching afterwards can be part of your cool-down to improve flexibility.

Intensity—Each joint in your body has a different capacity for range of motion. How far you stretch depends on what you feel. You should experience slight tension but not pain. Once you feel tension, slowly move just past the tension to challenge the body part. The tension helps you establish your threshold and set goals with your stretching. You have to use your own perceptions to determine the appropriate intensity level for stretching. As you hold a stretch, try to relax and breathe comfortably. If you can't, you might be attempting to stretch too far.

Time—The amount of time for each stretch will depend on the type of movement performed, whether static, dynamic, or PNF. A static stretch should be held for 15–60 seconds on average, for 2 to 4 repetitions. Beginners may need to hold it for a shorter time period. Rest between stretches for 30 seconds. A PNF stretch would also be held for the length of time of the contraction (5 to 6 seconds or more) and stretched approximately 30 seconds afterwards, for 2 to 5 repetitions. It should take you approximately 10–15 minutes to complete a flexibility training routine.

Type—You should establish a routine to work each major muscle group, though choosing the type of stretch will depend upon your specific needs, skill level, preferences, and goals. Make sure to include stretching exercises for the neck, shoulders, upper and lower back, pelvis, hips, and legs. If your range of motion is limited in a particular area, say your shoulders, you may choose to put more focus there. It can be helpful to assess flexibility in different joints to help set up a program that will be beneficial. Beginners may want to choose static stretching over PNF or dynamic stretching. Some people prefer group activities, like a yoga class, instead of a 10 to 15-minute training program (Figure 17). Stretching exercises can be static, dynamic, PNF or a combination, just so long as you are stretching with your progress and safety in mind.

Like applying the FITT Formula, training principles like specificity, progressive overload, adaptation, and reversibility can be used to enhance your flexibility training program.

Specificity—Determine the flexibility of a certain muscle/tendon group, then choose stretches that will focus on your major muscle groups, adding additional stretches for those that have a lower range of motion.

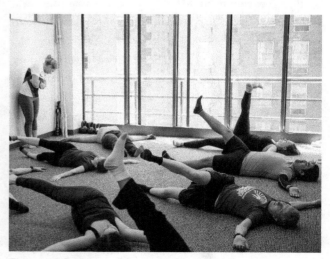

Figure 17. Group stretching activity.

Progressive Overload—Each time you push your body past that point of tension a bit more, you are overloading. You may notice that when you initially assessed your hamstrings, your fingers only reached your ankles but now they reach the top of your shoe. Rather than trying to reach your shoe, you focused on the point of tension and going beyond it. Eventually, you may reach your heels.

Adaptation—As your flexibility improves, your muscle/tendon groups should see increased range of motion, resting muscle length, and greater force during muscle contractions. This will enable you to establish new target areas or set new goals if you choose.

Reversibility—It may take time to notice, but if you stop training your flexibility will eventually decrease. This also happens gradually with age, which is why maintaining a program is so important.

Considerations for Safety and Success

Flexibility training requires attention to your current level of fitness, personal abilities, and limitations. Any form of exercise can pose risks if you have a lack of knowledge or fail to listen to your body. As discussed, certain joints only move certain ways, so body awareness is important.

As with any physical activity, stretching has safety concerns that everyone should consider before attempting. Stick to a routine like any other kind of training (Figure 18). The following safety tips can help you avoid injury:

- Always breathe smoothly and at a normal rate while stretching.

STRETCH REPETITIONS, SETS, AND SESSIONS			
Flexibility Exercise/ Stretch	**# of repetitions per set**	**# of sets per session**	**# of sessions per week**
Hamstrings	4 per side	1	After every aerobic or strength session
Alternative Hamstrings	4 per side	1	After every aerobic or strength session
Calves	4 per side	1	After every aerobic or strength session
Ankles	4 per side	1	After every aerobic or strength session
Triceps	4 per side	1	After every aerobic or strength session
Wrists	4 per side	1	After every aerobic or strength session
Quadriceps	4 per side	1	After every aerobic or strength session
Double Hip Rotation	4 per side	1	After every aerobic or strength session
Single Hip Rotation	4 per side	1	After every aerobic or strength session
Shoulder Rotation	4 per side	1	After every aerobic or strength session
Neck Rotation	4 per side	1	After every aerobic or strength session
Side Leg Raise	4 per side	1	After every aerobic or strength session

If you are not currently doing aerobic or strength activities, do flexibility and stretching at least 3 times per week for at least 20 minutes per session.

Figure 18. Sample flexibility training program.

- Check with your health care provider before beginning if you've had an injury, particularly to your knee or hip.

- Stretch to the point of tension, not pain. Stretching should never hurt.

- Use controlled movements. Avoid bouncing or jerking while static stretching.

- Keep your joints soft. Your arms and legs can be straight, but your joints should have a slight bend to avoid locking them in place.

- Modify stretches as needed. If you cannot perform a stretch in the recommended position, on the floor for example, try using a chair. Make a slight adjustment if you feel pain or feel unsafe.

Warm-Up and Cool-Down

Stretching should never be performed on cold muscles. Static stretches in particular can lead to injury if done before the body is warm. This is why stretching after cardiovascular exercise or weight training makes sense. The purpose of warming up is to prepare the muscles for activity, raising the temperature of the muscles, and circulating the blood.

To prepare for cardiovascular exercise, begin at a lower intensity for a few minutes to warm up your muscles, then proceed to your chosen pace. A good time for static or PNF stretching is at the completion of your cardio. For dynamic stretching, start at a lower intensity, perform the dynamic stretches, then resume your cardio. There may be times you choose to focus only on flexibility training. Even then, warm up your muscles by walking or jogging first. If you are unable

to, dynamic stretching can be a good warm-up. If the stretching session was intense and involved movement (power yoga, for example), then it would be a good idea to end with gentler movements to slow down your breathing. Otherwise, stretching can be a great way to cool-down from more intense exercise.

Stretches to Avoid

Our knowledge of the body has come a long way even in the last 20 years. Some stretches are no longer considered safe because they don't follow with the intended rotation of the joint. The following should be avoided:

- Stretches that extend your neck backward. Years ago, it was considered good to put your neck through a 360-degree rotation, but now we know better. You can put your chin to your chest and raise it or put either ear toward your shoulder, but do not roll your head in a circle or stretch your head toward your back.

- Stretches that flex or extend your back in an unsupported way, such as standing straight leg toe touches (standing hamstring stretches), plows, donkey kicks, or seated hamstring stretches where both legs are extended. The range of motion of your back is only partial (it has cartilaginous joints) and these can put a strain on your lower back. They can also cause you to hyperextend your knee joint.

- Stretches that take your knee out of alignment with your ankle, such as deep knee bends or hurdler's stretches. Your form in exercises involving your knee is important in lunges, squats, and any other leg movements.

Posture and Lower Back Health

No discussion of flexibility would be complete without addressing one of the most commonly cranky parts of your body—your back. It seems like one little move can lead to a lot of discomfort. Your posture is the position of your body when your torso is erect, such as when you are standing or sitting. Your back muscles can be injured by bad posture.

Your spine is divided into three sections, the **cervical spine** (the uppermost part of the spine in your neck), the **thoracic spine** in your chest, and the **lumbar spine** in your lower back. The spine is made up of bones called **vertebrae,** with cushiony **discs** between them. These all stack on top of

one another, forming a column that stands vertically when you stand.

You have 7 vertebrae within your cervical spine (numbered C1 to C7 from top to bottom), 12 vertebrae in the thoracic spine (T1 to T12), and 5 vertebrae in the lumbar spine (L1 to L5). Some people have 6 lumbar vertebrae. The lumbar spine, which connects the thoracic spine and the pelvis, bears the bulk of the body's weight and has the largest vertebrae.

Nearly 80% of people experience back pain at some point in their life, particularly in the lower back. This can range in intensity from a dull, constant ache to a sudden, sharp sensation that leaves the person incapacitated. Pain can begin abruptly as a result of an accident or by lifting something heavy, or it can develop over time due to age-related changes of the spine. Sedentary lifestyles also set the stage for low back pain, especially when a weekday routine of getting too little exercise is punctuated by a strenuous weekend workout. Basically, if you spend your week sitting on the couch, don't be surprised if you get hurt trying to move it by yourself.

Most back injuries occur with little knowledge of how they happened, but some typical causes of back pain include having poor posture, lifting a heavy object incorrectly, being in poor physical shape and/or overweight, having poor flexibility, having weak core muscles (abdomen/torso), twisting beyond the back's tolerated range of motion, or making sudden movements that stress the back muscles. You are at greater risk for back injury during times of stress or fatigue.

You can prevent most back injuries by developing good habits before you're in a higher risk situation, like when lifting a heavy object. Some good habits include:

- Practicing good posture when standing or sitting. Keep your head up, shoulders back, pelvis straight, and stomach in (not sucked in). Keep your feet on the floor when sitting.

- Using good body mechanics. This will vary with the movement, but in general, knees (and all joints) should be slightly bent, pelvis in neutral position—not tipped either way. It can take practice and work to learn what neutral is and then getting the body to adjust to neutral, especially if a person has picked up poor posture habits over time.

- Lifting a heavy object only what you can handle it from a position that enables you to use good body mechanics. Ask for help or use a hand truck.

- Exercising your core muscles. Weak abdominals force your back to work harder to move your torso.

- Taking breaks when sitting or standing for long periods.

Exercises to Prevent and Manage Back Pain

Since most people will suffer from back pain, it's important to be aware of the healing techniques we can use during those times. Many exercises can help improve your core and flexibility safely and reduce pain, particularly for chronic sufferers.

Partial crunches—Lie on the floor on your back with your knees bent, with feet flat on the floor and your hands behind your head (sit-up position). Tighten your stomach muscles and raise your head and shoulders off the floor without bending your neck or pulling your elbows in. Keep your elbows back. Make the abdominals do the work, not your head or back. At no point should your feet or lower back leave the ground. Breathe out as you raise your head and shoulders, hold for one second, lower back to the floor, then repeat. Beginners should do approximately 3 sets of 12 crunches and work up from there as you gain strength (Figure 19).

Hamstring stretches—Lie on the floor on your back with one knee bent. With the other leg, wrap a towel around the ball of your foot and extend it up as straight as you can, pushing your heel toward the ceiling. Hold it for approximately 20 seconds, then repeat 2 to 4 more times per leg.

Back extensions—Lie on the floor on your stomach. Push with your hands so that your shoulders lift off the floor. You can rest on your elbows if it is more comfortable. Hold the stretch for a few seconds, then lower your shoulders back to the floor.

Pelvic tilts—Lie on the floor on your back with your legs bent and feet flat. Keeping your upper back on the floor, contract your pelvic and raise your hips and pelvis, keeping the muscles tight. Hold for around 10 seconds, then slowly lower. Repeat 8 to 12 times.

Bird dog—Begin on the floor on your hands and knees. Your hands should be directly below your shoulders

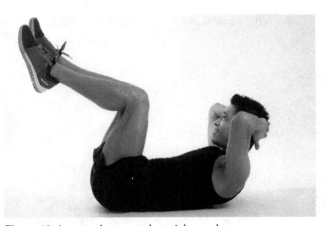

Figure 19. A correctly executed partial crunch.

and knees below your hips. Keep your head looking down. Extend your right arm straight in front of you as you extend your left leg straight behind. Hold for 7 or 8 seconds. Repeat with the opposite side.

Wall sits—Stand in front of a wall and lean your back against it. Walk your feet out until you can slide down the wall into a squat, similar to sitting in an imaginary chair. The muscles in your thighs, abdomen, and buttocks should contract. Hold for 10 to 15 seconds. Gradually increase the time until you can stay in a hold for one minute.

Conclusion

Your next steps should be to assess your flexibility and set SMART goals for improving flexibility. Then design a training program that ideally targets those joints that are most affected by the other training plans you have put in place so far.

Consider the impact that a regular flexibility program might have on your health. Think about improving your flexibility by incorporating different stretches into your fitness routine, making sure to incorporate stretching into your cool-down routines. If you find yourself sitting for long periods of time, stand up and stretch. Practice the recommended postures for sitting and standing that are described in this chapter. Adjust your workspace so that you have good alignment when doing schoolwork. For 80% of people, your back will thank you.

Reflection Questions

1. What is the basic structure of a synovial joint?

2. How satisfied are you with your current level of flexibility?

3. Consider the different benefits of flexibility training. In what ways might your quality of life be different if you made improvements in your level of flexibility or were able to maintain a high level of flexibility long-term?

4. What are some of the different options that people have with flexibility training programs?

5. Create a sample program for flexibility using the FITT formula.

6. What are important safety considerations a person should keep in mind with regards to flexibility training?

7. Why is low-back health important?

8. What exercises can be done to help prevent and manage back pain?

Chapter 6
Body Composition Basics

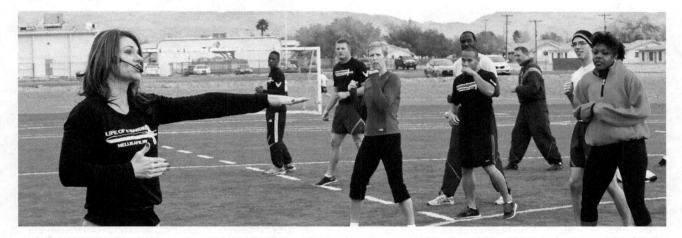

Learning Objectives

1. Define fat-free mass, essential fat, and nonessential fat, and describe their functions in the body.

2. Describe the scope of obesity as a public health concern in the US.

3. Explain how body composition affects overall health and wellness.

4. Describe how body mass index, body composition, and body fat distribution are assessed.

5. Explain the factors that contribute to body composition, including genetics, biological sex, age, ethnicity, lifestyle, and environmental factors.

6. Identify and describe the symptoms of eating disorders and the health risks associated with them.

7. Design a personal plan for achieving and maintaining a healthy body composition that includes nutrition and physical activity.

Your body may be composed of many parts that keep it running smoothly—blood, organs, water, bone, muscle, and other complex systems that work together—but this chapter's description of body composition is different. **Body composition** relates specifically to two components—lean mass and fat mass. This may sound simple, but it's not. Every person is made up of the same basic components but not every person has the same body composition, nor should they.

We often look at different ranges in the proportion of fat to lean mass on a person's body to measure their health. There are established ranges that correspond to the lowest risk of disease and death in the general population, and other ranges that focus on what is healthy for specific groups. Different types of athletes have their own optimal level of body fat or weight-related standards that makes them successful at their sport. You wouldn't expect a football player to have the same body composition as a gymnast, nor a basketball player to have the same as a body builder. In fact, athletes in the same sport but in different positions will often have different body compositions. In football, the typical body fat percentage of a wide receiver is quite different than the typical body fat percentage of an offensive lineman.

Your cousin Ann has been a gymnast since she was three years old. When you watch her compete, it's hard to imagine how she can fly around the uneven bars the way she does. She seems like a natural. In fact, it takes years of training, proper body mechanics, and some serious muscle tone, especially in her core, to reach this ability. An excess of body fat could impact her ability to perform skills that require strength and precision. Most of us, however, do not need to maintain the low level of body fat required of elite athletes. What we need is to stay healthy and limit our risk of disease. We can all work to achieve a body composition that will help us maximize our quality of life.

The notion of an "ideal" body composition can sometimes be complicated by misinformation. In this age of instant information and viral circulation of knowledge, we frequently find ourselves overwhelmed with "facts"—testimonials of success stories, images of current notions of a healthy appearance, and the latest diet trend. We may find it difficult to know what is best for us. First, let's look at why our society talks so much about body composition.

Obesity continues to be a major public health problem in the US, with nearly 70% of people registering over a normal weight and over half of those registering as obese (Figure 1). Obesity contributes to 3 of the top 4 causes of death (heart disease, cancer, and stroke), and still the number of obese individuals continues to rise. Even 10 extra pounds of fat can have adverse health effects, so understanding body composition basics is more important than many of us realize.

Throughout this chapter, we want to challenge the idea

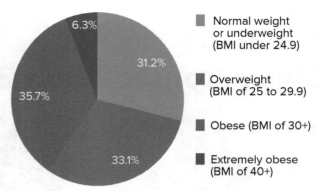

Figure 1. Average BMI of US adults age 20 and older.

of an "ideal body." Weight, though it can be a good measuring tool at times, is not the only number to focus on. As you will learn in this chapter, body composition has other factors that go beyond the scale or your physical appearance.

This chapter defines body composition and the way fats are stored in the human body, describes the benefits of a healthy body composition and weight management, and illuminates the challenges many people face when attempting to change or maintain their body composition and weight. It also recommends methods for assessing, improving, or maintaining your body composition through physical activity and healthy eating—the most effective long-term strategies for managing weight.

Defining Body Composition

Your body composition is the make-up of fat, muscle, bone, water, and other lean tissue in your body. Your body composition is usually defined simply as the percent of your body that is fat. For example, if you weigh 160 pounds and you learn that your body fat percentage is 20%, then you have 32 pounds of fat in your body and 128 pounds of lean tissue.

Not all fat is bad. In fact, your body needs between 3–5% (in males) and 8–12% (in females) of what we call **essential fat** just to survive (Figure 2). This fat helps your body regulate energy, cushions and protects your organs, and stores some of the essential nutrients your body needs.

Fat and Metabolism Basics

It likely comes as no surprise that food plays a significant role in the formation of body fat. Your body immediately uses some of the food you eat for energy. We measure this food in calories. Any calories not needed for use right away are stored as fat or sugar for later energy use. Excess fats are stored primarily as **triglycerides**. Your body breaks these down when it needs extra energy, such as when you exercise.

Until it's ready to be used, your body stores fat as **adipose**

tissue, which is considered an organ of the endocrine system. This system is responsible for the balance and release of many hormones and for helping regulate metabolism and appetite, in addition to maintaining your body temperature. Humans have two types of adipose tissue, white and brown. Most adipose tissue is white. Brown tissue is most common in newborns. It forms under the skin, around muscles, and vital organs. It generates heat by consuming energy, something infant humans

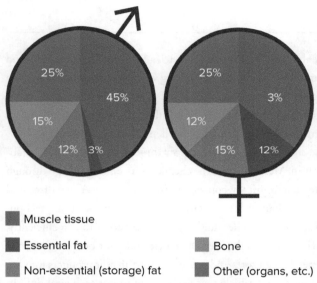

Muscle tissue

Essential fat

Non-essential (storage) fat

Bone

Other (organs, etc.)

Figure 2. Healthy body composition differs for males and females.

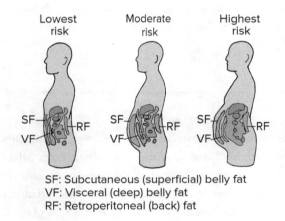

SF: Subcutaneous (superficial) belly fat
VF: Visceral (deep) belly fat
RF: Retroperitoneal (back) fat

Figure 3. Some fats are more dangerous than others.

and other mammals, particularly those that hibernate, need during times of inactivity. This tissue decreases as we age and is nearly non-existent by the time we reach adulthood.

Visceral fat is adipose tissue stored in the abdominal cavity. It surrounds the organs there, such as the intestines, liver, and pancreas. This fat is different than what you can see or feel directly under your skin, which is considered **subcutaneous fat**. Your body needs a certain amount of subcutaneous fat to store energy, regulate body temperature, and protect the skin and organs. It can be found all over the body, but the largest amounts of it generally occur on the abdomen, hips, thighs, and buttocks.

Any amount of excess fat, regardless of type, can have a negative impact on your health. Many people think of subcutaneous fat when they think about excess fat because they can see it, but visceral fat can actually be more dangerous because of the way it can impact vital organs (Figure 3). People with an excess of visceral fat (abdominal obesity) are more prone to cardiovascular damage, colon cancer, diabetes, and several other chronic diseases.

Visceral fat releases different bioactive molecules and hormones, such as adiponectin, leptin, tumor necrosis factor, resistin, and interleutin-6 (IL-6). These hormones play a role in risks for Type 2 diabetes, elevated glucose levels, hypertension, cardiovascular disease, and certain cancer-related issues.

It is a safe assumption that if you have a large amount of subcutaneous fat in your abdominal area, then you likely have too much visceral fat, too. It is possible, however, to have visceral fat without significant abdominal fat—you may not even know it is there.

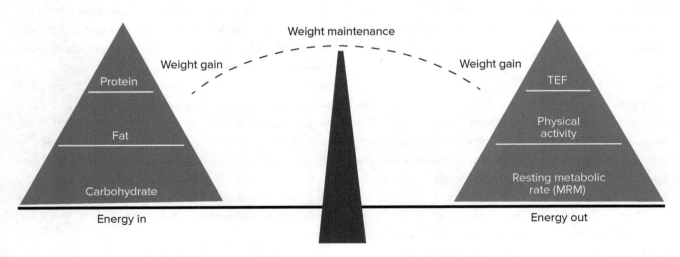

Figure 4. The energy balance equation helps define the balance between energy in and energy out and its impact on weight gain or loss.

The Energy Balance Equation

Energy imbalances lead to fat storage. According to the National Institutes of Health, the simple concept of balancing our energy in and energy out, can keep you healthy. We call this the **energy balance equation** (Figure 4). The body takes in calories (energy in) through food and drink. It then uses this energy (energy out) to function while performing activities ranging from digesting food and breathing, to moving and exercising. When you take in more energy than you can use right away, your body stores it either as sugar in your liver and muscles, or as fat (triglycerides) in your adipose tissue. It stays put until you use it. If the energy out never increases to the point where this stored fat becomes needed, it'll remain there. The longer this energy imbalance occurs (taking in more energy than the body can use), the more fat tissue accumulates.

This tissue develops in two ways: by multiplying and by enlarging. By the time you reach adolescence, your fat cells stop multiplying and begin swelling when you consume more than your body can use. This leads to an increase in your overall size and the formation of cellulite, the dimpling that occurs just under the skin from swollen cells in subcutaneous fat.

Your body converts energy through a process called metabolism. **Metabolism** is the chemical process that cells go through to sustain life by converting fuel to energy. As we discussed in previous chapters, your body runs a bit like a car. You put fuel, oil, and other fluids into your car for it to run efficiently. The difference between a vehicle and your body is that your metabolism sorts and processes the different products for you, unlike your vehicle that expects you to put each vital fluid in the correct place. Your metabolism is much smarter. It converts food/fuel into energy, proteins, fats, acids, and carbohydrates. It even eliminates waste (no oil change necessary).

Factors that Affect Body Composition

Not everyone's body metabolizes food at the same rate, but you do have control over many aspects of your body's composition. A healthy diet and physical activity can help you live your healthiest life and reduce your risk of disease, but not everything is within your control like diet and exercise. Your body composition can be affected by multiple factors. Your biological sex, ethnicity, age, environment, and even your genes play a role in how your body looks, develops, and functions. You can't control these factors. You can control other factors such as lifestyle choices and how you manage stress.

Genetics

Your genetic makeup can affect your body composition. According to the Centers for Disease Control (CDC), lifestyle choices tend to play the largest role, but research suggests that our genes—which are responsible for giving our body cues for how to handle environmental changes—can have an impact.

Past studies of family members, twins, and adopted children offered indirect scientific evidence that some of the variation in weight among adults is due to genetic factors. For example, a key study that compared the body mass of twins—raised together or apart—found that inherited factors had more influence than childhood environment. In rare cases, obesity occurs in families according to a clear inheritance pattern caused by changes in a single gene. Affected children feel extremely hungry and become obese because of consistent overeating (hyperphagia). So far, rare variants in at least nine genes have been implicated in this type of obesity.

In most people who are obese, no one genetic cause can be identified. Studies have found more than 50 genes associated with obesity, but most with very slight impact. Research continues in this area, but the CDC now suggests that most obesity seems to result from complex interactions among many genes and environmental factors.

For most of us, the factors affecting our body composition are more multi-dimensional than just our genetic history. Even in cases where suspect genes may be present, they are only expressed under certain circumstances. You may not be able to control many aspects of what you inherit, such as bone structure or the number of fast-twitch muscles in your body, but genetic tendencies related to the development of fat tissue can largely be managed with health choices.

The Set-Point Theory

Research in body composition is being done to better understand metabolism and the different mechanisms that can help with weight control, and there continue to be new insights. One theory is that each person's body is genetically predisposed or programmed to maintain a certain weight, it's natural weight. For example, if you're at this natural weight and you eat too much, your body will increase temperature and speed up metabolism to burn the extra calories. If you don't eat enough, you lose energy as your body slows down in an attempt to maintain this predetermined weight. This is why, according to this theory, it can be challenging to lose weight. Your body will send you signals by increasing your hunger, telling you to eat, essentially fighting against you.

This theory can get a bit cloudy. In reality, you may have various "settling points" at which your body will become comfortable again. We often call them "plateaus" influenced by energy and macronutrient intake. It can be difficult to get past them. But, your body's fight to maintain a set weight may be weaker than you imagine. Consider how easy it is for your body to go the direction you *don't* want it to, even if it is unlike the weight you've traditionally maintained most of your life. Much of this is because of the nature of typical diets in the US and constant exposure to enticing, high-calorie foods. You can get past the body's desire to maintain this set weight—and get past the different settling points—by paying close attention to your energy balance equation and doing a fair assessment of your needs vs. wants. That's not to say it's always easy. Let's face it, people often want an easier approach.

Biological Sex

Women generally have a higher percentage of body fat than men, and they tend to store it around their hips and thighs, giving them more of a pear shape. Hormones likely play the largest role in this. Estrogen and testosterone respond differently in the body, with testosterone leading to more muscle mass. Men, though they may gain weight all over, tend to have a larger accumulation of fat around their abdomen. More weight around the mid-section means more visceral fat, which is more dangerous to your health than the subcutaneous fat around your thighs.

Males are generally born larger, but most of the biological differences in body composition begin in puberty. As their hormone levels begin to change, males will see an increase in muscle mass, whereas females will gain fat. Hormones play a role again for women during and after menopause. This usually occurs between the ages of 45 and 55. The body's production of estrogen and progesterone, two hormones made by the ovaries, varies greatly during this transitional period that

eventually leads to the ending of a woman's menstrual cycle. The body begins to use energy differently at this time, fat cells change, and women may gain weight more easily. They may also begin to see more of the visceral fat that men experience.

As testosterone declines with age, men see an even higher risk of visceral fat. In general, adult men tend to be overweight more often than women, approximately 38% in comparison to 28%. However, when they are overweight, women are more likely to be obese. Men have a naturally higher resting metabolic rate (RMR) than women, most likely due to the difference in muscle between the average man and woman. A higher RMR means that a man will have a higher metabolism and burn more calories than a woman, even at rest.

Age

Many of the hormonal changes listed above change over time, but changing hormone levels are only one of the factors that affect your body composition as you age. Your muscle mass and bones also play an important role. As mentioned in previous chapters, these begin to deteriorate over time, particularly over age 60.

In general, for every ten years that a person is not involved in strengthening activities, they will lose 4–6 pounds of muscle. A 30-year-old person will have a greater quantity of bone and muscle than a 70-year-old with the same weight and height. A person's ability to gain new muscle or strengthen their bones declines with age, so later efforts to improve body composition should relate to weight control and maintenance. Obesity tends to be highest among middle-aged adults at around 40%, followed by older adults at 37%, and younger (age 20–39) at 32% (Figure 5).

Ethnicity

Your race and ethnicity can also play a role in body composition, though it is difficult to determine how much of this is related to sociocultural or socioeconomic differences as compared to inherited ones. These factors, which take malnutrition and life-

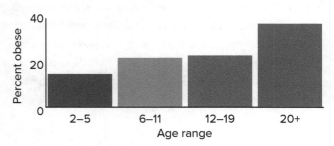

Figure 5. Obesity percentage in the US by age.

style issues into account, impact the physical development of an individual. There are, however, some tendencies among different groups. Blacks, for example, tend to have a larger musculoskeletal mass than whites, Hispanics, and Asians. Asians tend to have a smaller bone density than whites, Hispanics, or blacks. More research is needed to fully understand the dynamics and how this truly impacts body composition.

Lifestyle

Your lifestyle choices are the largest factors contributing to your body composition. Regardless of your biological sex, family history, race, or ethnicity, your health and those aspects of it that you can control often come down to this. You make lifestyle choices every day that impact how you feel and how your body functions, including your food intake, physical activity, sleep, and other habits. You control the energy balance equation for your body. The food choices you make and your decision to be physically active (or not) has the largest impact on body composition.

Along with proper diet and exercise comes the need for enough rest to allow your body to regenerate. In fact, your body grows muscle during your deepest sleep periods, and muscle leads to a higher metabolism. It stands to reason that sleep deprivation can also lead to lower metabolism. But not getting enough sleep can also lead to unhealthy eating habits. Research suggests that when you do not get enough sleep, your endocannabinoid (eCB) system is activated, similar to activation caused by smoking marijuana. Essentially, it triggers the reward center of your brain, causing you to crave foods that make you feel better. Over time, this leads to gains in fat tissue. Imagine a person who both smokes marijuana and suffers from sleep deprivation. That could be a serious increase in caloric intake.

Habits such as smoking, excessive consumption of alcohol, and drug use can also contribute to your body composition. According to the US Surgeon General, people who smoke tobacco tend to store higher amounts of visceral adipose tissue than people who don't, putting them at greater risk for Type 2 diabetes and other chronic illnesses in addition to a higher percentage of body fat. Alcohol, like any other sugary drink with empty calories, contributes to body fat as well. In addition to adding excess calories, too much alcohol can slow your metabolism, making the energy out process of the energy balance equation even more difficult.

Stress

When you have a final exam tomorrow, an essay due soon that you haven't even started, or your boss just called you in to work on your one day off, it can start to feel like you just can't seem to get ahead of things. Stress seems to be a recurrent theme when we talk about health, so it might not surprise you to learn that increased body fat is a side effect of stress.

Some people quickly gain weight when they're stressed. A National Institutes of Health study has uncovered a potential molecular connection between stress and weight gain. A molecule called **neuropeptide Y** (NPY) is involved in the growth of the blood vessels necessary to support new tissue formation. This is released from certain nerve cells during stress. Other research has suggested that NPY and its receptors play a role in appetite and obesity. Putting these results together, researchers think that NPY may be involved in new fat growth during stressful situations. In high-fat, high-sugar diets, researchers found that fat cells produced more NPY and more fat tissue.

Additionally, when your body experiences stress it releases a hormone called **cortisol**. This triggers a release of insulin that lowers your blood sugar and causes you to look for sugar to put in your body. A study done among healthy female university students showed that as stress levels increased during the semester, their levels of cortisol, binge eating, anxiety, and depression increased among many of them. At the same time, their concern over their weight and shape decreased, and they showed less concern with their eating habits. Over half the participants gained an average of 5 pounds. The increase in cortisol seems to have a direct connection to the other behaviors. Researchers consider this information critical in helping people understand the relationship between stress and eating behaviors and the importance of stress management (Figure 6). For more information on stress management, see Chapter 8.

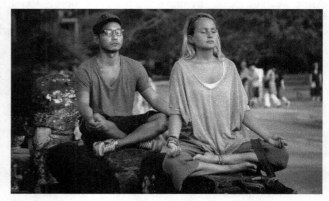

Figure 6. Stress management can lower cortisol levels.

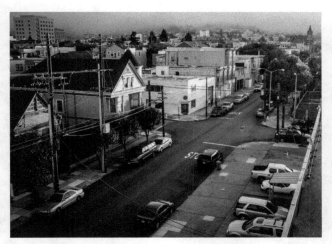

Figure 7. Neighborhoods influence physical activity.

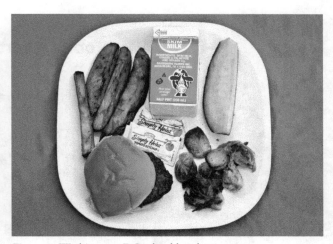

Figure 8. Washington, DC school lunch.

Environment

Your environment can play a role in your body composition as well. The CDC suggests that obesity is epidemic in populations of Americans that lead sedentary lives and consume high calorie foods. This is not always deliberate. It can be the result of a lack of infrastructure and resources that provide access to healthy foods.

In other chapters, we discuss how some areas have poor access to health care. But think about how many neighborhoods don't have sidewalks, safe trails, or parks (Figure 7). This discourages physical activity. Consider how the place you spend your time impacts your diet. Do your workplace or school have nearby food resources that provide healthy options? Access to easily available, healthy food is crucial. If your neighborhood has greater access to fast food than to a grocery store, you will have to plan around your environment (Figure 8). This is difficult for many people who face challenges with transportation, money for whole foods, and time.

A **food desert** is an area with low access to healthy food. To qualify as a "low-access community," at least 500 people and/or at least 33% of the census tract's population must reside more than one mile from a supermarket or large grocery store (for rural census tracts, the distance is more than 10 miles). Food deserts are typically low on whole food sources, but they could also be high on local quickie marts that provide a wealth of processed, sugar, and fat-laden foods that are known contributors to our nation's obesity epidemic (Figure 9).

Your physical location is not the only factor. Your family environment has likely made or still makes a difference in how you treat and view your body. The examples set by the people around you help to form your habits. If you grew up eating doughnuts for breakfast rather than oatmeal, and burgers and fries at the drive-thru for lunch rather than a salad bar, you may not have learned the value of healthy meals. If you were raised to spend most of your leisure time watching television rather than getting active, you may not realize the impact your environment has had on your health. It's not too late, but these habits have a big impact.

Even the **region of the country** you live in can impact your body. A lack of health education or an established community ideology that revolves around negative habits is common in some parts of the country. If fried foods are common in your community, or if frequent, large gatherings with food at the center are part of your culture, you may find it difficult to see foods like this as a choice. It's more of a way of life. This is what we call an **obesogenic environment** or **obesogenic society**, one that encourages or contributes to obesity and makes weight management difficult. If many people in your home or community are overweight or obese and are content to be so, they may not understand or support the merits of a healthy body composition.

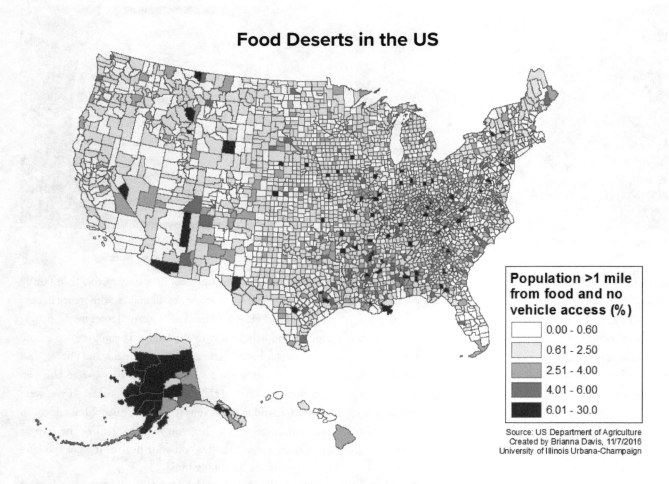

Food Deserts in the US

Population >1 mile from food and no vehicle access (%)

☐	0.00 - 0.60
☐	0.61 - 2.50
☐	2.51 - 4.00
☐	4.01 - 6.00
■	6.01 - 30.0

Source: US Department of Agriculture
Created by Brianna Davis, 11/7/2016
University of Illinois Urbana-Champaign

Figure 9. A food desert is where there are predominantly unhealthy food choices available.

Healthy Body Composition

Weight can be an important factor in determining if you have a healthy body composition, but it's not the only factor. For example, it doesn't tell us anything about a person's level of visceral fat. The misconception that weight is the primary determiner of someone's health is very common, but using weight to determine if you're overweight or obese doesn't take into account what's happening with your body's muscle mass, water, and fat levels. Someone could be reasonably thin through most of their body, but have a substantial amount of visceral fat. Someone who lifts weights may weigh more overall than someone of comparable height but be in better health due to the way their body is composed of a lower quantity of fat tissue.

How much body fat is the right amount? The American College of Sports Medicine suggests ranges for men and women by age (Figure 10). The human body has an essential fat threshold that never changes, even as you age. For men, this is 2–5%, and 10–13% for women. Acceptable limits cover a wide range that varies by age.

Weight-Related Issues

The CDC defines overweight or obese as having weight that is higher than what is considered a healthy weight for a given height, as measured by the body mass index (BMI). BMI is a person's weight divided by their height. You'll learn how

Age (years)	20–29	30–39	40–49	50–59	60+
Male					
Essential Fat	2–5%	2–5%	2–5%	2–5%	2–5%
Excellent	7.1–9.3%	11.3–13.8%	13.6–16.2%	15.3–17.8%	15.3–18.3%
Average	14.1–17.5%	17.5–20.4%	19.6–22.4%	21.3–24%	22–25%
Poor	>22.4%	>24.2%	>26.1%	>27.5%	>28.5%
Female					
Essential Fat	10–13%	10–13%	10–13%	10–13%	10–13%
Excellent	14.5–17%	15.5–17.9%	18.5–21.2%	21.6–24.9%	21.1–25%
Average	20.6–23.6%	21.6–24.8%	24.9–28%	28.5–31.5%	29.3–32.4%
Poor	>27.7%	>29.3%	>32.1%	>35.6%	>36.6%

Figure 10. The ACSM's recommended body composition changes over the lifespan.

to calculate your own BMI later in this chapter (See section on "Assessing Your Body Composition"). There are different ways to measure and define the categories overweight and obese, and these are detailed later in this chapter.

Based on BMI data, more than one third of people in the US are **overweight** (BMI of 25–29.9) (Figure 11). From 2011–2014 **obesity** rates (BMI of 30 or more) were a little over 36% in adults, an increase from 1999 rates, and 17% in children, which has held stable. Among women, the rates were higher at 38.3% than men at 34.3%. Obesity rates were lowest among Asian adults (11.7%), followed by white (34.5%), Hispanic (42.5%), and black (48.1%) (Figure 12).

Disparities in weight also exist by geographic region (Figure 13). The southern US has the highest prevalence of obesity at 31.5%, with Alabama, Louisiana, Mississippi, and West Virginia at 35% or more. The Midwest follows at 30.7%, the Northeast at 26.4%, and the West at 25.2%. Nationwide, the combined number of adults either overweight or obese is approximately 70%. The US is at a point where the prevalence of overweight and obesity is considered an epidemic that costs billions of health care dollars annually and many lives. Average life expectancy, though it has increased over the century, may soon start decreasing due to rising obesity-related health problems.

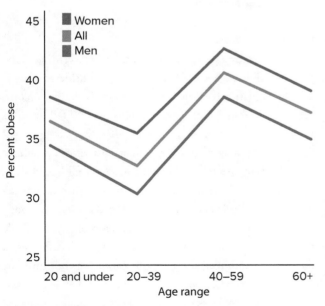

Figure 11. Percentage of obesity in the US by age and gender.

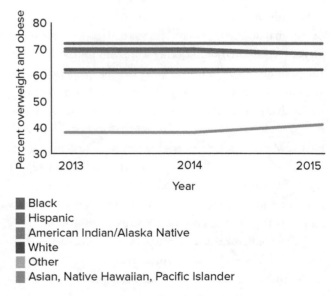

Figure 12. Percentage of overweight people in the US people by race.

Prevalence of Self-Reported Obesity Among U.S. Adults by State.

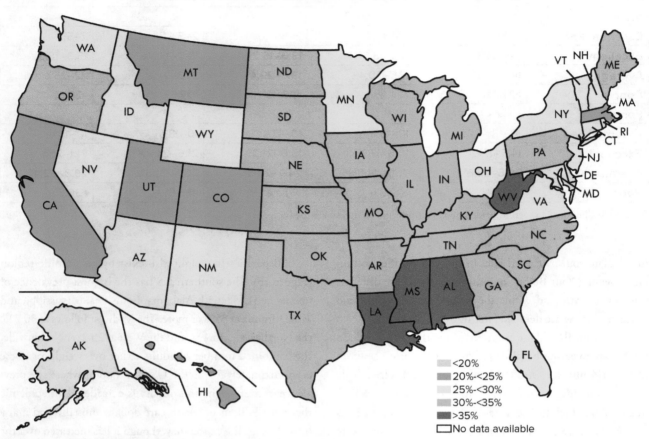

Legend:
- <20%
- 20%-<25%
- 25%-<30%
- 30%-<35%
- >35%
- No data available

Figure 13. Obesity is most common the midwest and south.

Health Effects

Excess fat tissue leads to a decline in physical capabilities. Your daily activities may cause fatigue you more quickly, or you may find yourself avoiding situations that involve a higher level of exertion. In other words, an unhealthy body composition places limits on you. This happens slowly, so you don't realize it right away. It may be months before you notice that you've been choosing the elevator over the stairs due to avoiding physical strain rather than just for convenience. Many of us simply aren't honest with ourselves about the shape we are in. We adjust to our bodies, then adjust again if we gain more fat, and tell ourselves that we are doing just fine and are happy. If you wait until you aren't fine, returning to health can get more and more difficult.

Excess adipose tissue increases your risk of experiencing a multitude of health-related issues, such as Type II diabetes, cardiovascular disease, cancer, stroke, depression, anxiety, high cholesterol, high blood pressure, gallbladder disease, sleep apnea, osteoarthritis, and others. All of these issues lead to fewer healthy years in your life, a higher potential of living with an obesity-related disability, and an increased risk of

premature death. When you neglect maintaining a healthy body composition, you aren't fine.

Underweight

It is possible for a person to have a body fat level that is too low. An adult with a BMI below 18.5 is considered **underweight**. A National Health and Nutrition Examination Survey in 2006 found that 1.8% of adults over 20 fall into this range. In a nation of 235 million adults, that's roughly 4.2 million underweight adults, representing a serious problem.

This is often a result of malnutrition or health issues, but it could also be the result of an eating disorder such as anorexia nervosa or bulimia nervosa. As mentioned earlier, your body needs a certain amount of fat to function properly. Too little fat can cause many problems. The resulting deficiencies in fat-soluble vitamins A, D, E, and K can make your immune system less effective. For example, vitamin deficiencies can cause an increased risk of illness, weakened bones, damaged vision, and even lessen your blood's ability to clot properly. Body fat helps regulate insulin and hormones, and an inadequate fat percentage can lead to diabetes and problems with

Eating Disorders	Characteristics
Anorexia Nervosa	Emaciation, relentless pursuit of thinness, and unwillingness to maintain a normal, healthy weight Distorted body image (seeing oneself as overweight even when dangerously thin). Intense fear of gaining weight Extremely disturbed eating behavior Weight loss through excessive diet and exercise, use of self-induced vomiting, or misuse of laxatives, diuretics, or enemas Lack of menstruation
Bulimia Nervosa	Recurrent, frequent binge-purge cycles: eating an unusually large amount of food followed by compensatory purging (vomiting or use of laxatives or diuretics), fasting, or excessive exercise Feeling a lack of control over eating Fear of gaining weight Unhappiness with body size and shape Disgust or shame about eating behavior Normal weight or slightly underweight
Binge Eating Disorder	Recurrent, frequent episodes of binge eating; no compensatory purging Feeling a lack of control over eating Disgust or shame about eating behavior Overweight or obesity

Figure 14. Characteristics, symptoms, and dangers of eating disorders.

reproduction or fertility. Low body fat can lead to kidney problems and the loss of your menstrual cycle in women. It can also impact your skin, causing it to sag or appear wrinkled. In serious cases, the body begins to break down muscle instead of fats to get the energy it needs to function.

Body Image and Eating Disorders

You've been working to create the perfect profile picture for your social media account. You've tried multiple filters, taken your selfie from various angles and in different lighting levels, and finally come up with an image that you think might be worthy. And yet, you're still uncertain. After an hour of tweaking your picture to be the best version of you, you still can't bring yourself to post it. Could it be that this cultivated version you spent so much time on really isn't an improvement upon the original? Are you trying to live up to an unrealistic expectation of what your body should look like? Are you comparing yourself to someone else who also spent hours crafting an image that barely resembles them in real life?

No discussion of body composition would be complete without addressing body image. The overwhelming discussion of the gap between expectations and reality is an important part of learning what it means to be healthy. This issue is enormous. Most middle and high schools in the US devote time to educating young individuals about positive body image and warning them about eating disorders. Despite this knowledge during their formative years, people often still struggle to see their body for what it is—an amazing and complex vessel with an important job. They focus instead on criticizing their own appearance for not meeting the unrealistic expectations they are surrounded by. So many of us, old and young, focus more on our body's appearance than its power. Our own view of our body is often subjective rather than objective, as we are generally our own worst critics. How do we shift the focus from an "ideal" body to a healthy body? Let's first take a look at the different aspects of body image.

Body image is an individual's perception of their physical body and their thoughts and feelings related to it, whether positive or negative. There are four aspects to body image:

1. **Perceptual**—How you see or perceive your body. You may perceive yourself as under or overweight, though it may not be accurate.

2. **Affective**—How you feel (satisfied or dissatisfied) about your body (weight, shape, or individual parts). Many people have an emotional reaction to changes in their body.

3. **Cognitive**—How you think about your body. This could be a preoccupation with your weight or body shape or a belief that you would be happier with yourself if you were thinner or had more muscle.

4. **Behavioral**—How you behave as a result of your body image. Some people self-isolate or engage in destructive behaviors (excessive exercising, vomiting, or not eating enough) in an attempt to change their body.

A **positive body image** exists when a person accepts and appreciates their body and treats it with respect. This has an impact on a person's overall self-esteem and leads to a more positive outlook and healthier behaviors. A **negative body image** is a sense of dissatisfaction with the body. This can result in habits that can negatively affect your physical, emotional, and social health. Problems can arise when a person has a negative body image, including stress, anxiety, depression, disordered eating, and other negative health habits. People with a negative body image are also more likely to attempt to change it with expensive and potentially risky surgeries.

This negative image can also contribute to an eating disorder. Do you ever feel out of control around food, avoid gatherings with food involved, lie about having eaten, or throw away food that you should have consumed? Are you afraid to miss a day of exercise, afraid that you'll gain wait if you eat normally, or do you force yourself to vomit after you eat? Do you worry that you may be fat but no one is telling you? These feelings, fears, and actions can indicate a problem with how you relate to your body.

You may notice these types of unusual behaviors in a friend. Are they withdrawing from social activities? Adopting an overly restrictive diet? Leaving meals to visit the bathroom? Exercising excessively? Repeatedly talking about losing weight? Maybe they frequently eat a large amount of high sugar or high fat foods in a sitting or express shame or disgust about what they've eaten.

Eating disorders, such as anorexia nervosa, bulimia nervosa, binge-eating, disordered eating, or eating disorders not specified are mental illnesses often associated with a poor body image. They occur most often in teens and young adults but can affect people at any age. Individuals with this type of illness will go to extremes with food, severely limiting intake or severely overeating, depending on the disorder (Figure 14).

Among US children ages 13–18, 2.7% of them have eating disorders. Girls make up more than half of this percentage. In adults, the numbers are slightly lower at 0.6% for anorexia, and 0.6% for bulimia, though a bit higher for binge-eating at 2.8%. Research suggests that these disorders develop for many potential reasons, such as genetic, biological, psychological, and social factors. The risk factors can be complex but most relate to a negative body image.

Body image issues can stem from a "thin ideal" perpetuated by social and peer pressure to be thin (Figure 15). Friends, family, teachers, and even simple acquaintances can all have an impact on how we view ourselves. A lack of family support, a history of being overweight, or frequent comments on an individual's weight can contribute to this negativity. Probably the worst catalyst is media representations of human bodies. Photos of thin, "perfect" models and magazine covers with airbrushed, muscular abdominals and large biceps constantly stare at us. Worse yet, the people in these photos may not even look the way they appear, since digitally altering photographs of models is so common. Social media and "reality" television have added yet another level to unrealistic images and expectations. Teens and young adults in particular spend a great deal of their time with

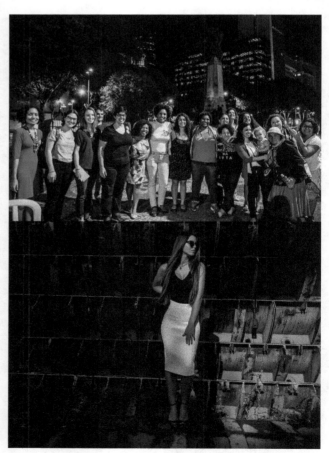

Figure 15. Body image often relies on an unrealistic standard.

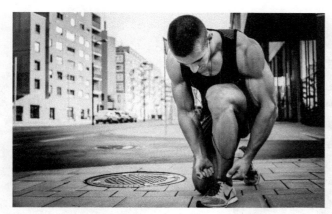

Figure 16. Men also experience body image insecurity.

Effects of Anorexia

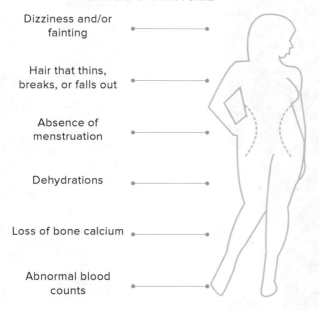

Dizziness and/or fainting

Hair that thins, breaks, or falls out

Absence of menstruation

Dehydrations

Loss of bone calcium

Abnormal blood counts

Figure 17. Anorexia negatively affects the body in many ways.

media outlets like these, adding more pressure for them to fit in with what is often a false reality.

All eating disorders are 2.5 times more common in women than in men, but lower numbers in men does not mean that men don't experience eating disorders. Men, on average, are less likely to develop eating disorders, but they do report being dissatisfied with their appearance and bodies in similar ways, such as feeling pressured to appear muscular. A recent has study showed that men and women respond in nearly identical ways to questions regarding self-confidence "when [they are] with attractive persons of the other sex," or "when the topic of conversation pertains to physical appearance," and "during certain recreational activities." Both men and women reported experiencing negative emotions at least "sometimes"

and "moderately often." This shows that men and women are equally insecure about their bodies when the idea of "the body" is directly or indirectly confronted in social situations (Figure 16).

Anorexia Nervosa

Individuals with **anorexia nervosa** have a strong fear of gaining weight, which leads to them restricting their food intake and exercising excessively. Sometimes they may assign rigid rules about food, such as low-calorie limits or only eating food of one color. They see themselves as overweight even though they may be normal or underweight, and in an attempt to lose more weight, they don't eat enough food to maintain their bodily functions (Figure 17). If left unresolved, this can lead to them becoming dangerously thin, which has physical risks associated with it. Cardiovascular issues are a significant and potentially fatal risk, since anorexia can lead to low blood pressure, an irregular heartbeat, or even heart attack. They are also at risk for thinning bones, cessation of their menstrual cycle in women, anemia, and kidney stones or kidney failure.

Symptoms of anorexia include weight loss, moodiness, missed periods, brittle hair and nails, yellow skin, weakness, dizziness, confusion, and a lack of desire to socialize. People with anorexia nervosa often spend more time alone and avoid eating around others, or say they've eaten when they haven't. They often restrict their food or weight as a means of gaining control over one part of their life when they feel other parts of their life are out of control.

Anorexia nervosa is more common among women, but recent studies show that many men are also being diagnosed. In women, it may be a concern over weight, while in men they may over-diet and over-exercise to gain more muscle. Both are the result of an unrealistic image of what the body should look like.

This can be a very difficult illness to treat and generally involves psychological and behavioral therapy. In extreme cases, the person will need to be hospitalized to manage their physical decline, treat their underlying mental illness, or both, before it becomes fatal.

Bulimia Nervosa

Unlike anorexia, people with **bulimia nervosa** may be at a healthy weight because they do typically eat. They will sometimes eat a large amount of food and then attempt to get rid of it or thwart the weight gain by vomiting, taking

Blood
Anemia

Heart
Irregular heart beat,
heart muscle weakened,
heart failure, low pulse
and blood pressure

Body Fluids
dehydration, low
potassium, magnesium,
and sodium

Kidneys
Problems from diuretic abuse

Intestines
Constipation, irregular bowel
movements (BMs), bloating, diarrhea,
abdominal cramping

Hormones
Irregular or absent period

Brain
Depression, fear of gaining weight,
anxiety, dizziness, shame,
low self-esteem

Cheeks
Swelling, soreness

Mouth
Cavities, tooth enamel erosion,
gum disease, teeth sensitive to
hot and cold foods

Throat & Esophagus
Sore, irritated, can tear and
rupture, blood and vomit

Muscles
Fatigue

Stomach
Ulcers, pain, can rupture,
delayed emptying

Skin
Abrasion of knuckles,
dry skin

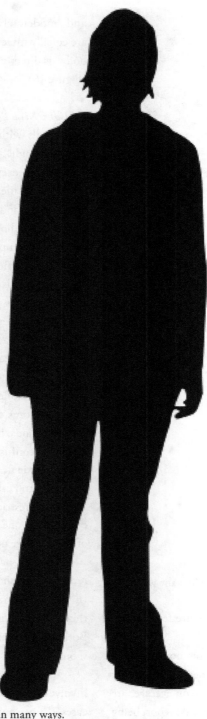

Figure 18. Bulimia negatively affects the body in many ways.

laxatives, exercising a great deal, or fasting. This doesn't necessarily occur on a daily basis. Someone with bulimia may binge eat as a result of stress or anxiety or in response to hunger if they've been cutting back on their food intake. This would be followed by a purge, such as deliberately vomiting what they consumed. The purge often, but not always, follows a large binge.

As with anorexia nervosa, this occurs more often in women and is linked to a strong concern with body image. Over time, this can lead to stomach or intestinal damage from overeating and laxative use, ulcers and throat damage from vomiting, tooth decay, dehydration, and electrolyte imbalance which can lead to heart failure (Figure 18). Because people with bulimia often have a normal weight or are merely

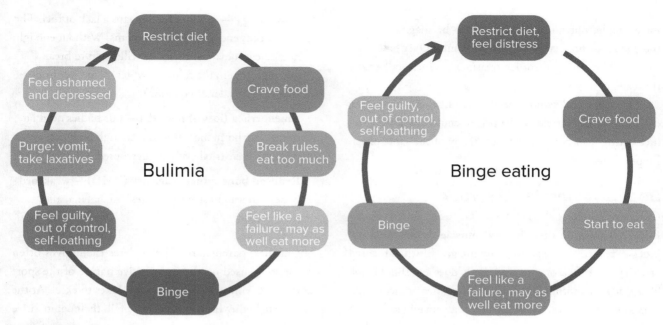

Figure 19. Bulimia and binge eating cycles.

overweight, it can be difficult to identify the problem. Symptoms include trips to the bathroom following eating, broken blood vessels in the eyes, damaged knuckles (from inducing vomiting), and acid reflux.

Binge Eating Disorder

People with a **binge eating disorder** are often overweight or obese. They don't limit food or attempt to purge it. Rather, they engage in episodes during which they eat large amounts of food within a short period of time (two hours, for example). They will eat until they are uncomfortable, even if they weren't originally hungry, often reporting a sense of feeling out of control (Figure 19). After a binge, they often experience feelings of disgust and embarrassment.

Not everyone who is overweight or obese has a binge eating disorder, nor is every person with a binge eating disorder overweight. This can be a difficult illness to diagnose as people who binge eat often engage in the activity when no one is around. It is also difficult because many of us have engaged in the activity at one time or another (though maybe not to the same extent) and may not see it as a problem if we are not around the person often. It is considered a disorder when a person binge eats at least once per week for approximately three months.

These individuals may also have problems with substance abuse, depression, or other mental illnesses. People with a binge eating disorder are at higher risks of osteoarthritis, chronic

kidney problems, Type 2 diabetes, or high blood pressure and high cholesterol, both of which can lead to stroke and heart disease.

Disordered Eating

It is possible to have more than one eating disorder in a person's lifetime, particularly when we recognize it as a mental illness that is difficult to overcome. For some, particularly people who train heavily for a sport, their eating can become disordered in an attempt to control their weight and manage their performance, or even to keep their coaches happy. Crash diets, irregular eating patterns, and binge eating can often occur during this process in an attempt to find what works. However, disordered eating can occur in any part of a population.

Extreme dieting can be one form of disordered eating. Someone with this illness may become preoccupied with sticking to their diet, upset if they break the rules, and may avoid social situations where they may be expected to eat what is available. This can also lead to other, specified eating disorders.

Eating Disorders Not Specified (EDNOS)

Eating disorders not specified (EDNOS), or other specified feeding and eating disorders (OSFED), are those that don't fit neatly into one category. The person may have some symptoms of anorexia nervosa or bulimia nervosa, for example, but not often enough to be diagnosed with the disease or not yet having weight issues. Over half of all cases seen at eating disorder treatment centers fall under this category.

The signs and symptoms are the same as other eating disorders. If left untreated, the person could develop a specified eating disorder or experience many of the same physical problems.

Body Dysmorphic Disorder and Muscle Dysmorphia

Body dysmorphic disorder and **muscle dysmorphia** are illnesses related to a negative body image, this time focused on a distorted sense of what their body does and should look like. Body dysmorphic disorder occurs when someone has a fixation on a perceived defect (even an imagined one) in their appearance, or a certain part or characteristic of their body. For someone with this disorder, the flaw seems all-important and can consume their daily thoughts. The person will often seek plastic surgery or surgeries to correct their perceived flaw.

Muscle dysmorphia is more common among men and results in a fixation with becoming more muscular, no matter how much muscle they already have. It is generally grouped with disordered eating like a reverse anorexia because food and exercise play a significant role in the formation of muscle. A person with this disorder may see their body as healthy even if they are so muscular they experience discomfort and deformation. Like any other disorder related to poor body image, body dysmorphic disorder and muscle dysmorphia can be treated with therapy and medical intervention.

Female Athlete Triad Syndrome

For women who train competitively for a sport, developing **female athlete triad syndrome** is a real risk (Figure 20). Participants in sports like gymnastics, figure skating, cross-country running, rowing, or any other sport where having a low body fat is important to performance are at higher risk. These athletes may think that any excess body fat impacts their training and performance, whereas a lean body and good muscle tone will put an athlete at their peak. Rather than being at their best skill level, the athlete will over-train, resulting in:

1. **Disordered eating**—the push for a performance-ready body can lead to overly rigid or restrictive eating patterns and other eating disorders.

2. **Low energy**—a lack of food means a lack of fuel. The body needs energy to run its systems. Without enough fat and carbohydrate the body will begin to break down protein in the muscles, which is counterproductive (energy balance equation).

3. **Amenorrhea (loss of periods)**—our bodies need fat to regulate hormones. Without enough body fat, a woman's menstrual cycle is interrupted.

4. **Reduced bone mineral density (BMD)**—weakened bones can lead to stress fractures, osteopenia, and osteoporosis.

Coaches, parents, and the athletes themselves often become so focused on the competitive nature of the sport that they are willing to do whatever it takes to excel. At the point where bodily functions begin to fail, their competitive nature has worked against them and caused a loss of their health in exchange for a perceived competitive edge.

The warning signs for female athlete triad syndrome are similar to other eating disorders—decreased food intake, excessive exercise, and vomiting, with the added symptoms of fatigue and stress fractures. Health care providers must work in conjunction with the athlete's family and coaches to reverse these issues. Increased caloric intake and reasonable exercise are usually the first steps. Some athletes will be placed on oral contraceptives or other hormonal supplementation to resume their menstrual cycle, along with calcium, vitamin D, and other vitamins and minerals to enhance BMD.

Like other eating disorders, this can be challenging to

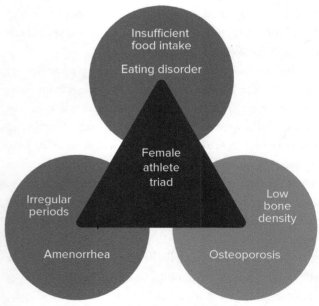

Figure 20. Components of the female athlete triad.

treat. Ironically, these highly competitive individuals are often unwilling to risk being what they would consider unhealthy, so getting them to recognize the harm their excessive training is doing can be difficult. As a result, one effective treatment approach is to make counseling and treatment a condition of their continued participation in their sport.

Treatment of Eating Disorders

Most people with these illnesses get better with treatment and go on to have a healthy, practical relationship with food and exercise. Health care providers usually take an interdisciplinary approach that involves psychotherapy, nutrition therapy, support groups, and medicine such as antidepressants. Some people who have eating disorders will need to be hospitalized to monitor their weight, ensure they are taking in enough food, and monitor their heart rate to ensure they are physically safe. Many geographic areas have designated treatment facilities or special programs within hospitals for people with eating disorders.

If you think you may have a problem with an eating disorder, the most important step is to speak to your health care provider. They will ask you questions about your eating and exercise habits and run laboratory tests to rule out any other possible health problems. Honesty is the key. Since many people with eating disorders are isolated and secretive, they can go undiagnosed for a dangerously long time. It's important to be truthful with your health care provider about your behaviors and feelings, even if it's uncomfortable.

So much of the problem with eating disorders stems from a negative perception of your body. But we can change the ideal of a perfect body to an ideal of good health. The National Eating Disorders Association offers the following tips for keeping a positive image:

- Wear comfortable clothes that you feel good in and that work for your body (not against it)
- Make a list of things you like about yourself that aren't related to your weight or body
- Consider yourself as a whole person, not just at your physical appearance
- Surround yourself with positive, supportive people

- Be a critical viewer of social media and other outlets—don't take things at face value
- Avoid negative or berating self-talk
- Set positive goals focused on health rather than a specific weight or size
- Avoid comparing yourself to others
- Say positive things to yourself every day
- Every morning when you wake up, thank your body for resting and rejuvenating itself so you can enjoy the day
- Every evening when you go to bed, tell your body how much you appreciate what it has allowed you to do throughout the day

You may find this list a little simplistic or even humorous. Talk to yourself? Say "thank you" to your body? But think about how many times you've spoken negatively to or about yourself and felt down afterwards. Imagine if you spoke in a positive way to yourself on a regular basis instead. Imagine if you saw your body as something to be cared for and respected, not punished. That's really what a healthy body composition is all about. Remember what your body is meant to do. Realistic goals and ideals can help you embrace your body and take care of it in a reasonable way.

Resources

There are a wealth of local, regional, and national resources to help people who have or may have eating disorders find treatment options and support for their condition. Help is available, and it should never be difficult to find it. Here are a few national resources available on the web:

1. **Something-Fishy.org**—an online site raising awareness about eating disorders and collecting resources for treatment, recovery, and ongoing support

2. **NationalEatingDisorders.org**—the National Eating Disorders Association's online resource hub, including resource collections at the state and local level

3. **APA.org/helpcenter/eating.aspx**—the American Psychological Association's page on eating disorders, offering information and explanations of disordered eating from a clinical psychological perspective

Benefits of a Healthy Body Composition

Think of a time when you feel your healthiest and all you're able to do and accomplish. How did you feel about yourself?. That feeling of comfort and confidence in your body highlights the many benefits of a healthy body composition. It can have positive impacts on many factors related to your overall wellness, from the physical to the emotional and even economical.

By maintaining a healthy body composition, you have more energy and stamina, and you're ready to participate in whatever comes your way. You become a more functional member of your family and society.

You substantially reduce the risks of disease and premature death and avoid placing limitations on your activities. Excess body weight also increases your risk of cardiovascular disease, Type 2 diabetes, joint problems, sleep apnea, digestive problems, gallbladder and liver disease, asthma and other respiratory problems, and certain forms of cancer (breast, prostate, esophageal, endometrial, kidney, and others). Obesity can also reduce your years of healthy life.

You may not be happy just because you are physically fit. Having a healthy amount of body fat does not in itself reduce stress, but the exercise and healthy eating needed to achieve and maintain a healthy body does. As discussed in previous chapters, the body releases hormones during exercise that help your mood and energy levels. In addition, reducing your risk of illness and disease reduces those events as stressors in your life.

A healthy body composition can also help you maintain a positive body image. Individuals with a poor body image often struggle with anxiety, depression, or eating disorders. Obese individuals can also experience social anxiety related to their weight that can disrupt their lives, such as an unwillingness to participate in social functions and self-seclusion. A healthy body composition won't solve all your problems, but it can reduce those within your control.

The health care costs related to body composition are too big to ignore. National estimates of health care costs related to obesity in 2018 were $344 billion. In addition to this, the CDC estimates that the productivity costs related to obesity-related absenteeism due to health issues is $3.38 billion nationwide. Obese workers also experience "presenteeism," or a loss of productivity even while at work. This has the potential to cost a person their job and livelihood.

Assessing, Improving, and Maintaining Your Body Composition

Understanding the amount of energy your body needs can be a great starting point for assessing your body composition, so let's return to the body energy equation. We've established that your body, like your car, needs fuel to run efficiently, but we also know that overflowing your tank serves no good purpose. So how do you determine the size of your tank?

The energy balance equation directly affects the way we process and store fat in our bodies. It is the concept of energy in and energy out. If you take in the exact amount of energy you need, burn as many calories as you consume, you have a *neutral* balance. If you consume more than your body can use, you have a *positive* balance, meaning you will gain fat. Using more than you consume during the day, your body utilizes stored fat, and you have a *negative* balance, meaning you will lose fat.

This section will help you determine the size of your tank, provide strategies for filling it the right way, and help you know when your energy in and energy out need rebalancing.

Measuring RMR, TEE, and BMR

Just as your car's engine idles at a certain number of revolutions per minute, your body has a **resting metabolic rate** (RMR). This is the amount of energy the body needs to complete its basic physical processes, like breathing, brain function, and blood circulation. Essentially, this is the energy it needs to expend to keep you alive or keep your motor running. This doesn't include calories burned during movement (Figure 21). There are factors that can affect your RMR, such as how active you are (fitness level) and your age, biological sex, and weight loss efforts. Knowing your RMR can help you determine how much energy you need to consume and how much exercise you need during the day. This isn't a perfect measuring tool. It doesn't explain why some people gain or lose weight easier, and it doesn't account for the different factors that influence RMR (Figure 22). However, it's a good starting point to help you measure progress with weight loss or weight management.

There are several different methods for measuring RMR. The following is the Mifflin-St. Joer equation:

- **Males:** (9.99 x weight in kilograms) + (6.25 x height in centimeters) – 4.92 x age) + 5

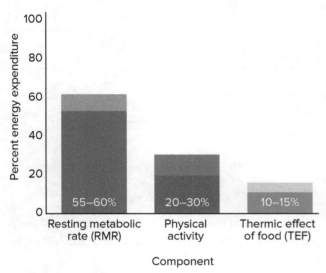

Figure 21. Energy expenditure in percent ranges.

Factor	Description
Body Mass	A person with greater body weight will have a higher resting metabolism than a smaller person.
Body Composition	Muscle burns more calories than fat, even at rest.
Age	Metabolism declines naturally in adults at a rate of about 2-3% per decade because of loss of lean muscle.
Gender	Men normally have a higher metabolism than woman due to body mass and body composition.
Hormones	Certain hormones can increase or decrease metabolism.
Nutritional Supplements	Certain supplements can increase or decrease metabolism.
Nicotine	Tobacco products can increase resting metabolism from 3–7%.
Pharmaceuticals	Prescription and over the counter drugs can increase or decrease metabolism.
Fever and/or Infection	An increase in body temperature will increase metabolism.
Stress/Emotional Excitement	Good and bad stress could cause an increase in metabolism due to an increased utilization of stress hormones epinephrine and norepinephrine (catecholamines).
Exercise	Strength training can lead to a chronic increase in metabolism because of the increase in lean muscle mass.
Weight Loss	The two main reasons for a decrease in resting metabolism are that 1) a smaller body requires fewer calories and 2) during weight loss the body may try to conserve energy in response to a lower calorie intake.
Caloric Restriction	Restrictive diets consisting of less than 1000 calories per day can result in an acute decrease in resting metabolic rate.

Figure 22. Factors that affect metabolism.

Level of Activity	Description	Activity Factor	
		Male	Female
Sedentary	Little to no activity	0.3	0.3
Lightly Active	You move a bit for work, stand and walk around a little with short bursts of moderate activity	0.6	0.5
Moderately Active	Same as lightly active with added 1.5–2 hours of moderate activity (e.g., jogging)	0.7	0.6
Very Active	You're active all day, comparable to 9–13 miles of running (army recruits, full-time athletes, laborers)	1.1	0.9
Extremely Active	You run the equivalent of 14–16 miles/day (lumberjacks, coal miners-heavy labor and exercise)	1.4	1.2

Figure 23. Determining your activity level helps you calculate your resting metabolic rate.

- **Females:** (9.99 x weight in kilograms) + (6.25 x height in centimeters) – (4.92 x age) – 161

For example: a male who weighs 150 pounds (68.03 kg), is 72 inches (182.88 cm) tall, and 25 years-old would have an RMR of 1705 calories per day.

(9.99 x 68.03) + (6.25 x 182.88) – (4.92 x 25) + 5 = 1705

For another example: a female who weighs 180 pounds, is 65 inches tall, and 44 years-old would have an RMR of 1472 calories per day.

(9.99 x 81.82) + (6.25 x 165.1) – (4.92 x 44) – 161 = 1472

(Note on the metric system: 1 pounds = .4536 kilograms and 1 inch=2.54 centimeters)

Let's take into account how active these people are to get a more realistic number by estimating their Thermic Effective of Exercise (TEE):

To calculate your TEE, multiply your RMR times the appropriate activity factor from the table (Figure 23). For example, if the man in the previous example is lightly active, the activity factor to use is 0.6. His calculated RMR is 1705 calories per day, so his TEE is calculated as follows:

TEE = RMR x activity factor

TEE = 1705 x 0.6 = 1023 calories/day

Add those calories to his daily total from RMR and you'll find he needs 2,728 calories each day to maintain his weight at his current activity level.

If the woman in the example is moderately active, the activity factor it the same at 0.6. Her calculated RMR is 1472 calories per day, so her TEE is calculated as follows:

TEE = 1472 x 0.6 = 883 calories/day

Add those calories to her daily total from RMR and you'll find she needs 2,355 calories each day to maintain her weight at her current activity level.

Basal metabolic rate (BMR) is often used interchangeably with RMR, but it is slightly different. Both are an estimate of the energy required by the body at rest, including breathing, circulation, maintaining body temperature, and building and repairing cells. BMR is more precise, but RMR is a more practical way of finding your metabolic rate because BMR can only be determined in a lab or clinical setting, and you can calculate your own RMR at home.

Assessing Your Body Composition

How do you know if you have a healthy ratio of lean mass to fat mass? Body composition can be assessed in several different ways, including the Body Mass Index, percent body fat measurements, and body fat distribution tests.

Body Mass Index

The **Body Mass Index** (BMI) is a simple method used by many health care providers to estimate body fat. BMI is calculated by taking a person's weight (in kilograms) and dividing it by their height (in meters) squared (Figure 24). If the metric system is too much for you, you can also divide your weight (in pounds) by your height (in inches) squared, and then multiplying the result by 703. According to the CDC, weight that is higher than recommended based on a person's height can be considered either overweight or obese (Figure 25).

For example: If your weight is 150 pounds and you are 5'5" (65"), your BMI would be 24.96, just inside the normal or healthy weight range.

$$150 \div (65^2) \times 703 = 24.96$$

This method makes it easy for the average person to determine their approximate body composition. It does have some limitations. BMI does not take muscle into account nor does it directly measure fat, so it may not be accurate for someone who does strength training. Studies show that it can be a bit less accurate for men, who tend to have more lean mass, and for the elderly, who tend to have higher fat percentages. However, it offers a general, good idea of how your body is composed. You can use it to set initial goals and as an easy way to track your progress. It has also been used as a basic method of assessing disease risks.

Many other methods can be used to assess your **body fat percentage** and **lean mass percentage**—the amount of fat you have in your body compared to the amount of lean mass. Knowing your percentage of body fat can be more useful because it takes fat into consideration, rather than simply weight and height like BMI. This eliminates discrepancies over the amount of bone, muscle, and water versus the amount of fat in your body.

There are several methods for assessing percent body fat, including underwater weighing, skinfold measurements, bioelectrical impedance analysis, air displacement plethysmography, and different waist measurements.

Underwater Weighing

Underwater weighing, also known as hydrostatic weighing, uses Archimedes' principle of displacement to determine how much fat a person has (Figure 26). Archimedes' principle tells us that a buoyant force will be exerted on a submerged object equal to the weight of the water that the object displaces. Muscle and bone weigh more than fat, so when the person is submerged and weighed, professionals can compare their normal weight to their submerged weight. Someone with a lower percentage of body fat and more muscle will weigh more in the water. Someone with a higher percentage of body fat will weigh less. This test is considered to be very accurate. The drawback is that the equipment is specialized and expensive, so it requires a trained professional.

Formula and Calculation
Kilograms and meters
Formula: weight (kg) / [height (m)]2 Example: Weight = 68 kg, Height = 165 cm (1.65 m) Calculation: $68 \div (1.65)^2 = 24.98$
Pounds and inches
Formula: weight (lb) / [height (in)]2 x 703 Example: Weight = 150 lbs, Height = 5'5" (65") Calculation: $[150 \div (65)^2] \times 703 = 24.96$

Figure 24. How to calculate BMI.

≤18.5	18.6–24.9	25.0–29.9	≥30.0
Underweight	Healthy	Overweight	Obese

Figure 25. BMI ranges.

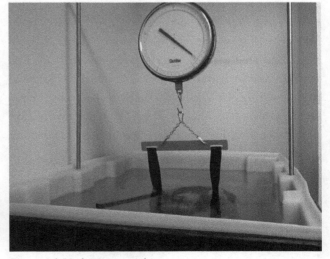

Figure 26. Underwater weighing.

Skinfold Measurements

In a **skinfold thickness test** a professional uses a special caliper to measure the amount of subcutaneous tissue a person has in seven sites on their body (abdominals, thigh, biceps, triceps, calf, scapula, and waist). The process is simple for a trained person and can be done anywhere. It may not work well for people who are quite obese or very lean due to the caliper's inability to grasp the tissue. It is fairly reliable when done correctly, though it does focus only on subcutaneous fat and cannot measure visceral fat (Figure 27).

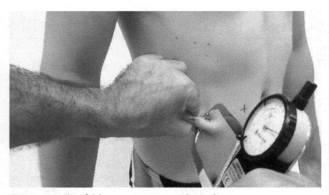

Figure 27. Skinfold measurement with a caliper.

Bioelectrical Impedance Analysis

Bioelectrical Impedance Analysis (BIA) measures resistance within the body to a small, electrical current (Figure 28). This provides an estimate of the person's total body water, with which it is able to estimate their body fat. This can be done in several ways. One involves electrodes placed on the wrist and ankle. Another uses a machine. The participant stands on a special scale that sends the current through the body. Fat does not conduct electricity well and will make the flow of the current difficult. This resistance enables the machine to determine body fat. It is fairly accurate if done correctly, but there are many variables that come into play, such as the amount of fluid in the body.

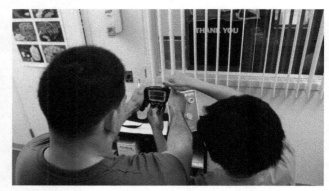

Figure 28. BIA test interface.

Bod Pod

The **Bod Pod** is an air displacement plethysmograph (ADP). Instead of using water, like in underwater weighing, the Bod Pod uses air (Figure 29). The participant is enclosed in a cocoon-like machine that measures the volume of air displaced by the body in order to measure the person's body volume. It is very accurate, though not quite as accurate as underwater weighing. The results can be affected by the person's hydration level and breathing patterns. This could be problematic for someone who cannot tolerate enclosed spaces and finds breathing in them difficult. It works well for most ages and sizes and does not require a substantial amount of time. It's a better option than underwater weighing for people who cannot be submerged in water safely. Like underwater weighing, however, the equipment is expensive and not everyone has access to it.

Waist Measurement Methods

Many of the above options require access to professionals and equipment. But there are other methods as easy as the BMI calculation that can help you establish a good baseline

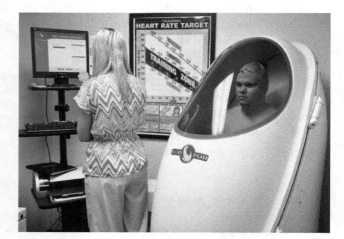

Figure 29. Bod Pod in use.

by looking at your **body fat distribution.** This is the pattern in which fat is stored over the body. For example, some people carry a lot of weight around their abdomen, while others carry it around their hips and thighs. By measuring certain areas of the body, you can obtain ratios that help determine your risk for certain diseases.

You can estimate the way your fat is distributed by measuring your waist circumference. In women, a measurement over 35 inches is considered high risk, and in men a measurement over

40. A high circumference shows an elevated risk of cardiovascular disease, Type 2 diabetes, and hypertension. In participants who are obese and will exceed the numbers, there is no way to measure incremental risk of disease (for example, there is no guide that says each inch equals a certain percentage of increased risk), but it offers a good guideline and a tool by which to measure progress.

This doesn't mean that you can do crunches and try to focus on simply toning up your abdominals. It doesn't work that way. It means that you likely have more body fat overall (including visceral fat) than is healthy—not just what is around your waist—and need to work toward a healthier body composition to protect your health.

Measuring your **waist-to-hip ratio** is another method for determining abdominal fat and can be particularly helpful with identifying possible danger associated with visceral fat. Measure your waist at its most narrow point and your hips at their widest, then divide your waist measurement by your hip measurement. Women with ratios over 0.71 and men with over 0.83 are at risk for health issues.

Another way to determine abdominal obesity is to compare your waist to your height. Measure your waist and height using the same units (inches, for example). A healthy number is below 0.5.

Setting Goals for a Healthy Body Composition

Setting goals for changing body composition and creating a plan for weight management should involve measurable goals based on improving overall health or avoiding individual health risks. These will likely require a range of physical activity and nutrition changes to see results.

Set SMART Goals

Set some short-term goals and reward your efforts along the way. If your long-term goal is to lose 30 pounds of fat and to control your high blood pressure, some short-term eating and physical activity goals might be a good start. For example:

Specific: I will eat more vegetables

Measurable: By replacing a starch or carbohydrate with a vegetable at dinner 5 days each week

Achievable: This is a small change

Relevant: It will help me lose weight and feel healthier

Time-based: I will do this for two weeks and then make additional changes

Remember to keep them specific and measurable. For example, "Exercise More" is not a specific goal. But if you say, "I will walk 15 minutes, 3 days a week for the first week," you are setting a specific and realistic goal for the first week. Remember, small changes every day can lead to big results in the long run.

Remember that reasonable goals are *achievable* goals. By achieving your short-term goals day-by-day, you'll feel good about your progress and be motivated to continue. Unrealistic goals, such as losing 20 pounds in two weeks, can leave you feeling defeated and frustrated. Losing 5 or 8 pounds in one month would be more realistic and achievable.

You should also expect occasional setbacks. These can happen when you get away from your plan for whatever reason—maybe the holidays, longer work hours, final exams, or another life change. Get back on track as quickly as possible. Also, take some time to think about what you would do differently if a similar situation happens.

Keep in mind that everyone is different. What works for someone else might not be right for you. Just because your neighbor lost weight by taking up running, doesn't mean running is the best option for you. Try a variety of activities—walking, swimming, tennis, or group exercise classes to see what you enjoy most and can fit into your life. These activities will be easier to stick with over the long term.

Make a Commitment

You have many good reasons to improve or maintain your body composition. This book has given you many related to your health, but you likely have others that are more personal to you. Start simply by making a commitment to yourself. Many people find it helpful to sign a written contract committing to the process. This contract may include things like the amount of weight or fat you want to lose, the date you'd like to lose it by, the dietary changes you'll make to establish healthy eating habits, and a plan for getting regular physical activity.

It can help to write down the reasons why you want to work on this aspect of wellness. It might be because you have a family history of heart disease or simply because you want to feel better in your clothes. Post these reasons in a place where they can serve as a daily reminder of why you want to make this change in your lifestyle.

Take Stock of Where You Are

Consider talking to your health care provider. He or she can evaluate your height, weight, and explore other weight-related risk factors you may have. Ask for a follow-up appointment to monitor changes in your weight or any related health conditions.

Keep a "food diary" for a few days, in which you write down everything you eat. By doing this, you become more aware of what you are eating and when you are eating. This can help you determine if you are eating mindlessly, as many of us do, and help you set goals and create a plan to avoid this (See "Reflect, Replace, Reinforce").

Next, examine your current lifestyle. Identify things that might pose challenges to your weight loss efforts. For example, does your work, school, or travel schedule make it difficult to get enough physical activity? Do you often find yourself surrounded by sugary foods? Think through things you can do to help overcome these challenges.

Finally, think about aspects of your lifestyle that can help you stay focused. For example, is there an area near your school or workplace where you and some friends can take a walk at lunchtime? Is there a place in your community with exercise facilities for you and child care for your kids?

Healthier Eating Habits

You learned earlier in this section how to determine your RMR or BMR. These numbers can help you understand your body's metabolism and consider the strategies that will help you manage your energy balance. The food you consume on a daily basis can help or harm you in this process.

It is often difficult to know how to approach your nutritional plan given the sheer abundance of possibilities available on television, through books, and online. There is a constant change and flow of information in popular culture today. Many of the trendy diets may result in initial weight loss but are frequently unsustainable, resulting in people regaining any pounds lost and sometimes gaining even more. There are, however, some healthy nutrition strategies that focus on the basic concept of reducing energy in. By simply reducing the portion size of a beverage, or substituting a sugary drink with something unsweetened, you can reduce the amount of energy you consume (Figure 30).

Type of Beverage	Calories in 12 ozs	Calories in 20 ozs	Difference
Fruit punch	192	320	128
100% apple juice	192	300	108
100% orange juice	168	280	112
Lemonade	168	280	112
Regular lemon/lime soda	148	247	99
Regular Cola	136	227	91
Sweetened lemon iced tea (bottled)	135	225	90
Tonic water	124	207	83
Regular ginger ale	124	207	83
Sports drink	99	165	66
Fitness water	18	36	18
Unsweetened iced tea	2	3	1
Diet soda (with aspartame)	0*	0*	0
Carbonated water (unsweetened)	0	0	0
Water	0	0	0
*Some diet soft drinks can contain a small number of calories that are not listed on the nutrition facts label.			

Figure 30. Calorie amounts in drinks.

The energy balance equation is important knowledge in managing your body composition. But the food you consume can help or harm you in ways beyond your waistline. Foods high in saturated fat, sugar, and even artificial ingredients can impact your body. Consider the quality of the energy you consume to get the most value from it. According to the *Dietary Guidelines for Americans 2015–2020*, a healthy eating plan:

- Emphasizes fruits, vegetables, whole grains, and fat-free or low-fat milk and milk products

- Includes lean meats, poultry, fish, beans, eggs, and nuts

- Is low in saturated fats, trans fats, cholesterol, salt (sodium), and added sugars

- Stays within your daily calorie needs

You don't have to give up your favorite comfort foods entirely. Healthy eating is all about balance. You can enjoy your favorite foods even if they are high in calories, fat or added sugars. The key is balancing them out with healthier foods and more physical activity.

Here are some general tips for consuming your favorite comfort foods:

1. **Eat them less often.** If you normally eat these foods every day, cut back to once a week or once a month. You'll be cutting your calories because you're not having the food as often.

2. **Eat smaller amounts.** If your favorite higher-calorie food is a chocolate bar, have a smaller size or only half a bar.

3. **Try a lower-calorie version.** Use lower-calorie ingredients or prepare food differently. For example, if your macaroni and cheese recipe uses whole milk, butter, and full-fat cheese, try remaking it with non-fat milk, less butter, light cream cheese, fresh spinach and tomatoes. Just remember to not increase your portion size.

The point is, you can figure out how to include almost any food in your healthy eating plan in a way that still helps you lose weight or maintain a healthy weight (Figure 31). For more information on nutrition, see Chapter 7.

Portion Sizes

The amount of each thing you eat matters, too. It helps to have an idea what one serving of a particular food looks like in order to know how much to eat. Dieticians and other nutrition experts often recommend that you use familiar objects to gauge portion sizes. A portion of fruit, for example, is the size of your fist. A serving of meat should be about the size of a deck of cards. The best way is to read the label of what you are eating, not only to determine whether the food is healthy but also to find the measurement of one serving. The size and number of portions of a particular food will

Meal	Food Substitute Ideas
Breakfast	Substitute some spinach, onions, or mushrooms for one of the eggs or half of the cheese in your morning omelet. The vegetables will add volume and flavor to the dish with fewer calories than the egg or cheese. Cut back on the amount of cereal in your bowl to make room for some cut-up bananas, peaches, or strawberries. You can still eat a full bowl, but with fewer calories.
Lunch	Substitute vegetables such as lettuce, tomatoes, cucumbers, or onions for 2 ounces of the cheese and 2 ounces of the meat in your sandwich, wrap, or burrito. The new version will fill you up with fewer calories than the original. Add a cup of chopped vegetables, such as broccoli, carrots, beans, or red peppers, in place of 2 ounces of the meat or 1 cup of noodles in your favorite broth-based soup. The vegetables will help fill you up, so you won't miss those extra calories.
Dinner	Add in 1 cup of chopped vegetables such as broccoli, tomatoes, squash, onions, or peppers, while removing 1 cup of the rice or pasta in your favorite dish. The dish with the vegetables will be just as filling but have fewer calories than the same amount of the original version. Take a good look at your dinner plate. Vegetables, fruit, and whole grains should take up the largest portion of your plate. If they do not, replace some of the meat, cheese, white pasta, or rice with legumes, steamed broccoli, asparagus, greens, or another favorite vegetable. This will reduce the total calories in your meal without reducing the amount of food you eat. But remember to use a normal- or small-size plate—not a platter. The total number of calories that you eat counts, even if a good proportion of them come from fruits and vegetables.
Snacks	Most healthy eating plans allow for one or two small snacks a day. Choosing most fruits and vegetables will allow you to eat a snack with only 100 calories.

Figure 31. Healthy food substitution ideas.

depend on how much energy (calories) you need to take in and how much you expect to expend. Remember the energy balance equation.

You should also be trying to balance your food groups and eat foods low in saturated fats and sugars. One combo meal at a fast food restaurant may be 1500 calories. Choosing to eat only this during the day rather than three balanced meals plus healthy snacks would be the wrong approach to both energy intake and portion control.

Reflect, Replace, Reinforce

What do you eat each day that helps your body? What foods don't help or maybe even harm it? What do you consume that adds empty calories? Sometimes it just takes thought and maybe a little honesty with yourself. On your way to school this morning you bought a 20-ounce café mocha. How many of those calories provided nutrients vs. fat or sugar? You could have swapped it for a regular latte with 2 percent or non-fat milk, but you told yourself that it was okay because it served as your breakfast. True, the overall calories may have been the equivalent of a cup of coffee and a bowl of oatmeal, but you aren't likely to be as full. In fact, by lunch you may be quite hungry, feeling foggy, and lacking in willpower.

The CDC's recommendations for good nutrition are based on a systematic approach to each habit. They recommend you **reflect** on all of your specific eating habits, both bad and good, and your common triggers for unhealthy eating; **replace** your unhealthy eating habits with healthier ones; and **reinforce** your new, healthier eating habits.

Reflect

Create a list of your eating habits. Keep a food diary for a few days in which you write down everything you eat, your location, what you were doing, and the time of day you ate it. Keep track of how you were feeling emotionally and physically when you ate. Were you hungry? Bored? This knowledge will help you uncover your habits. For example, you might discover that you always seek a sweet snack to get you through the mid-afternoon energy slump.

Highlight the habits on your list that may be leading you to overeat. Many common eating habits can lead to weight gain. These include:

- Eating too fast
- Always cleaning your plate

- Eating when not hungry
- Eating while standing up (maybe mindlessly or too quickly)
- Always eating dessert
- Skipping meals (even just breakfast)

Look at the unhealthy eating habits you've highlighted. Look at your notes on how you typically feel at those times. What triggered you? Were you tired? Stressed out? Be sure you've identified all the triggers that cause you to engage in those habits. Identify a few habits you'd like to work on improving first. Don't forget to pat yourself on the back for the things you're doing right. Maybe you almost always eat fruit for dessert, or you drink low-fat or fat-free milk. These are good habits. Recognizing your successes will help encourage you to make more changes.

Create a list of "cues" or "triggers" by reviewing your food diary to become more aware of when and where you're "triggered" to eat for reasons other than hunger. Often an environmental "cue" or a particular emotional state is what encourages eating for non-hunger reasons. Maybe you always eat when you sit down in front of the television or when your friend comes over.

Circle the cues on your list that you face on a daily or weekly basis. Going home for the Thanksgiving holiday may be a trigger for you to overeat, and eventually, you want to have a plan for as many these eating cues as you can. But for now, focus on the ones you face more often.

Ask yourself these questions for each cue/trigger you've circled:

1. **Is there anything I can do to avoid the cue or situation?** This option works best for cues that don't involve others. For example, could you choose a different route to work to avoid stopping at a fast food restaurant on the way? Is there another place in the break room where you can sit so you're not next to the vending machine?

2. **For things I can't avoid, can I do something differently that would be healthier?** Obviously, you can't avoid all situations that trigger your unhealthy eating habits, like your friend's birthday party. In these situations, evaluate your options. Could you bring a healthier snack or beverage to the party? Could you sit farther away from the food so it won't be as easy to grab something? Could you plan ahead and eat a healthy snack before going?

Replace

Replace unhealthy habits with new, healthy ones. For example, you may realize that you eat too fast when you eat alone. Make a commitment to share a lunch each week with a friend, or have a neighbor over for dinner one night a week. Other strategies might include putting your fork down between bites or minimizing other distractions (i.e. watching the news during dinner) that might keep you from paying attention to how quickly—and how much—you're eating.

Here are more ideas to help you replace unhealthy habits:

1. **Eat more slowly.** If you eat too quickly, you may "clean your plate" instead of paying attention to whether your hunger is satisfied.

2. **Eat only when you're truly hungry.** Don't eat only because you're tired or anxious, or feeling an emotion besides hunger. If you find yourself eating when you are experiencing an emotion besides hunger, such as boredom or anxiety, try to find a non-eating activity to do instead. You may find a quick walk or phone call with a friend helps you feel better.

3. **Plan meals ahead of time.** This ensures that you eat a healthy well-balanced meal.

Reinforce

Finally, make sure to reinforce your new, healthy habits with positive, healthy rewards. Maybe this is small reward like a visual reminder that only you know about (like a gold star for every good day), or maybe it's a bigger thing like a night at the movies when you reach a month of good behavior. Be patient with yourself, especially at first. Habits take time to develop. It doesn't happen overnight. Be proud of the positive choices you make. When you do find yourself engaging in an unhealthy habit, stop as quickly as possible and ask yourself: Why do I do this? When did I start doing this? What changes do I need to make? Be careful not to berate yourself or think that one mistake "blows" a whole day's worth of healthy habits.

Physical Activity

A healthy diet has to go with physical activity. Training to lower your body fat percentage (the most common option for improving body composition) should be based on reaching a negative energy balance. That is don by reducing the energy you take in from nutrition *and* by increasing your energy out through physical activity. One pound of fat = 3,500 calories, and health professionals typically recommend a weight loss rate of 0.5–2 pounds of fat loss per week. To create a loss of one pound of fat per week, a person should have a deficit of 500 calories per day, ideally from a combination of increasing activity level and making changes to your nutrition. Sometimes it's not possible to do both, depending on individual circumstances. Some people, for example, aren't eating enough calories, or they might already have a high level of physical activity.

Most of the time, you can create that deficit from both activity changes and eating habit changes—gradual, sustainable changes. For example, most people can find 250 calories per day that they can reduce—changing your café mocha to a non-fat latte can save a good number of calories. Try going all the way down to black coffee to really cut calories out of your morning coffee drink. Adding 30 minutes of physical activity each day will usually burn at least a few hundred calories. This could yield one pound of fat lost in the week. If there is a day during the week that a person isn't burning the extra calories through physical activity, which is often the case, they would need to create a larger energy deficit through nutrition changes. And that can become more challenging, depending on their current habits (Figure 32).

Losing one-half to 2 pounds per week can be challenging for some people. It's a good idea to track progress regularly so that you can see if what you are doing is effective, and if you find that you aren't making gradual, steady progress, it's time to reassess and troubleshoot.

There are many healthy, simple ways to boost physical activity and increase your energy out. It is important to remember the FITT principle when planning your physical fitness program and adjust based on your goals. More information on healthy physical activities is available in Chapters 2–5.

General Strategies

To lose weight, try increasing your activity level to 50 minutes of moderate or 25 minutes of high-intensity activity per day for modest gains. For more significant gains, increase to

Gender	Age (years)	Activity Level		
		Sedentary	Moderately Active	Active
Female	2–3	1,000	1,000–1,400	1,000–1,400
Female	4–8	1,200	1,400–1,600	1,400–1,800
Female	9–13	1,600	1,600–2,000	1,800–2,000
Female	14–18	1,800	2,000	2,400
Female	19–30	2,000	2,000–2,200	2,400
Female	31–50	1,800	2,000	2,200
Female	51+	1,600	1,800	2,000–2,200
Male	2–3	1,000	1,000–1,400	1,000–1,400
Male	4–8	1,400	1,400–1,600	1,600–2,000
Male	9–13	1,800	1,800–2,200	2,000–2,600
Male	14–18	2,200	2,400–2,800	2,800–3,200
Male	19–30	2,400	2,600–2,800	3,000
Male	31–50	2,200	2,400–2,600	2,800–3,000
Male	51+	2,000	2,200–2,400	2,400–2,800

Figure 32. Caloric needs by age and gender.

300 minutes of moderate or 150 minutes of high-intensity aerobic activity per week (Figure 33).

Adding strength training to your routine can also help improve weight loss. Muscle helps boost your metabolism and improve your overall strength and stamina for your workout routines.

Add a sport or new exercise to your routine. If you enjoy soccer or basketball, join a club and become more active in that way. Take up cycling, kickboxing, yoga, or some other new activity that you haven't tried. The variety can keep you from getting bored and help you stay on track with your goals.

If you've not been physically active in a while, you may be wondering how to get started again. The CDC offers some good tips to help you begin:

1. **Look for opportunities to reduce sedentary time and to increase active time.** For example, instead of watching TV, try taking a walk after dinner.

2. **Set aside specific times for physical activity.** Schedule sessions to make it part of your daily or weekly routine.

3. **Start with activities, locations, and times you enjoy.** For example, some people might like walking in their neighborhood in the mornings; others might prefer an exercise class at a health club after work.

4. **Try activities with friends or family members.** Being in a group can help with motivation and mutual encouragement.

5. **Start slowly.** Then, work your way up to more physically challenging activities. For many people, walking is a particularly good place to begin.

6. **Break up your daily activity goal into smaller amounts of time.** For example, you could break the 30-minute a day recommendation into three 10-minute sessions or two 15-minute sessions. Just make sure the shorter sessions are at least 10 minutes long.

Considerations for Safety and Success

Diet plans, programs, books, and TV shows will often claim you can achieve a faster weight loss—even as much as 10 pounds per week. If you consider that one pound of fat contains about 3,500 calories, you will realize that it's just not physiologically possible to lose 10 pounds of fat in one week. That would mean that you had an energy deficit of 5,000 calories each day, which is not possible unless you spend the entire day doing vigorous exercise. That wouldn't be safe, of course, and would be challenging even for a professional athlete.

Moderate Physical Activity	Approximate Calories/30 Minutes for a 154 lb Person	Approximate Calories/Hr for a 154 lb Person
Hiking	185	370
Light gardening/yard work	165	330
Dancing	165	330
Golf	165	330
Bicycling (<10 mph)	145	290
Walking (3.5 mph)	140	280
Weight lifting	110	220
Stretching	90	180
Vigorous Physical Activity	Approximate Calories/30 Minutes for a 154 lb Person	Approximate Calories/Hr for a 154 lb Person
Running/jogging (5 mph)	295	590
Bicycling (>10 mph)	295	590
Swimming	255	510
Aerobics	240	480
Walking (4.5 mph)	230	460
Heavy yard work	220	440
Weight lifting (vigorous effort)	220	440
Basketball (vigorous)	220	440

[1]Calories burned per hour will be higher for persons who weigh more than 154 lbs (70 kg) and lower for persons who weigh less. Source: Adapted from Dietary Guidelines for Americans 2005, page 16, Table 4

Figure 33. Calories used by common physical activities.

It's important to also remember that we need to eat enough, too, so that we consume enough calories and essential nutrients for the body to do its many jobs. People often try to restrict their calorie intake too much, and their body will slow down metabolism in an effort to hold onto the required calories your body needs. Finding the right energy balance can be tricky. Health experts usually suggest finding out how many calories a person needs to maintain their body weight (using an energy expenditure formula like TEE), and then reducing calories by 200-300 per day.

There are more aggressive approaches to weight loss or weight management than those described here, including diet programs, supplements, medications, and even surgery. These aren't all necessarily recommended by health professionals. Some of these may have significant science behind them and others have never truly been tested or proven to be effective long-term. If you are considering a particular approach, speak to your health care provider or nutritionist before proceeding.

Fads, Diet Books, and Programs

As a general rule, be cautious of programs that offer rapid weight loss and quick fixes. There is no one food, no matter how super, that will magically remove fat any more than there is one food alone that will cause you to gain it. Plans with extreme restrictions on particular food groups, limits on food combinations, rigid and boring menus, and promises of fat loss without exercise are a dime a dozen and most likely not going to work. You may even end up missing out on vital nutrients in your diet. Consider whether you could really eat that way for the rest of your life. If you can't, it isn't for you.

If you want to participate in a structured program, look for a plan that promotes reasonable weight loss, such as one or two pounds per week. It should also discuss ways to keep weight off long-term, manage stress, change eating habits, deal with challenges, and get support. Losing body fat isn't a simple process—it requires knowledge and behavioral changes aimed at gaining or maintaining health.

Supplements

Many advertised supplements claim to reduce your weight or build muscle. These often contain ingredients that are untested or under-tested and possibly unsafe. The names of the ingredients can be so unfamiliar that without research, you may be ingesting multiple forms of caffeine or other stimulants that could be hazardous. There simply isn't a quick fix for weight loss or muscle growth. Claims about rapid weight loss should be viewed with extreme skepticism. Even some vitamins and minerals are dangerous when taken in high doses.

Supplements are not regulated in the same way as medications or food. The manufacturers are given responsibility for testing their products and ensuring safety, not the Food and Drug Administration. If a product is found to be dangerous, it is removed from the market, which means it could be on the shelves for a while before the negative issues are reported. These companies are also under no obligation to prove whether their products work as advertised.

The substances comfrey, chaparral, lobelia, germander, aristolochia, ephedra (ma huang), L-tryptophan, germanium, magnolia-stephania, and stimulant laxative ingredients, all have noted safety concerns. You should definitely avoid these substances. Check the labels of any supplement you are considering for these ingredients.

Medications

There are some over-the-counter medications on the market intended to help with weight loss, such as orlistat (xenical and Alli), lorcaserin (Belviq), phentermine, benzphetamine, diethylpropion, naltrexone combined with bupropion (Contrave), and others. These medications, depending upon the product, are designed to either slow the absorption of fat or suppress your appetite. They may help you lose 5 or 10 pounds, on average, but unless combined with a healthy diet and fitness plan, consumers usually regain the weight once they stop taking the medication. Sometimes health care providers will recommend these in patients with BMI's over 30 and serious health issues in an effort to kick-start the weight loss process.

These should not be taken without first seeking the advice of a health care provider. Their side effects can be serious, ranging from diarrhea, constipation, dry mouth, insomnia, and headaches to increased blood pressure, heart palpitations, depression, and even liver failure. Even if approved by your provider, typical use is limited to only short terms like a few weeks.

Surgery

In extreme situations, health care providers will perform bariatric surgery to help a patient lose weight. Gastric bypass, gastric sleeves, and adjustable gastric bands are just a few but all are designed to limit the amount of food that gets to the stomach or the size of the stomach in general.

Gastric bypass, for example, involves the surgeon stapling the stomach into two sections, creating a small, upper pouch about the size of a walnut (Figure 34). The food goes directly into this pouch. It is so small that people can only eat about one ounce of food at a time. Your health care provider also connects a part of your small intestine directly to this pouch. This enables the food to pass through the body more quickly and the person to absorb fewer calories.

A gastric band is similar. Your health care provider places a band around the top of your stomach to create a small pouch. Your health care provider can adjust the band by injecting or removing a salt-water solution inside of it. A gastric sleeve, on the other hand, is permanent — surgeons remove most of your stomach. Again, the goal of these is to make you feel fuller, faster and eat less.

Most people can expect to lose 10–20 pounds the first month after surgery. Within a year, they may be able to lose half of the weight the need to as long as they continue to take in small portions. Bariatric surgery does not replace healthy habits, but may make it easier for someone to consume fewer calories and be more physically active. Most people regain some weight over time, but weight regain is usually small compared to their initial weight loss. The individual may need counseling in addition to surgery to help them manage any emotional issues that lead to overeating. The surgical approach is aggressive and can lessen your desire to eat but cannot stop you from reverting to old habits.

Health care providers use surgery only when someone's health is seriously at risk due to excess fat, such as a BMI over 40 and/or serious weight-related illness, such as heart disease or Type 2 diabetes. These surgeries are major and

Roux-en-Y Gastric Bypass

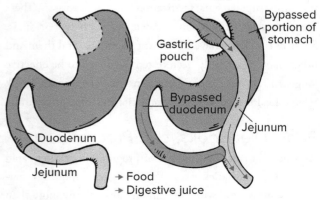

Figure 34. Gastric bypass divides the stomach into sections.

involve a significant recovery time. A patient can expect to experience initial pain, temporary drains and catheters, and a liquid diet until they are able to keep food down. They can also expect to pay a lot of money. On average, bariatric surgery costs between $15,000 and $25,000, depending on what type of surgery you have and whether you have surgery-related problems.

Liposuction

Liposuction removes isolated areas of subcutaneous fat deposits. In this procedure, health care providers will insert a tube (cannula) and a suctioning device through the patient's skin and into the area chosen for fat removal. This procedure will permanently remove fat cells from the targeted spots on the body. If a person gains a small amount of weight after liposuction, the remaining fat cells will grow. More than a 10% weight gain will result in new fat cell growth. The patient will see it in other parts of the body first, those that did not have the procedure. For example, if a person has fat removal on their abdomen, hips, and thighs they may see fat develop more in their face, arms, or chest. The liposuctioned areas will not grow as rapidly, but with continued weight gain they can still accumulate fat.

Liposuction comes with risks. Swelling and bruising is a given after treatment, but some people can also experience infections, skin sagging, and edema and seromas (fluid build-up). In some cases, patients may have an over-correction or under-correction. This means that too much or too little fat was removed from a spot, leaving the shape of the body part no longer contoured as it should be.

Usually only about 5 or 6 pounds can be removed safely in one treatment, so it isn't intended for someone with obesity. Like most surgeries, it is not a substitute for healthy eating and exercise. Someone who eats well, exercises, and maintains their weight will see better results than someone who is looking for a quick fix to an unresolved issue.

When You Are Trying to Gain Weight

Some people are interested in gaining weight and must consider healthy strategies. This means you may need to increase your caloric intake (positive energy balance) by consuming more healthy foods. You also may need to incorporate strength training into your exercise program to build muscle mass. There are some simple tips that can help you add calories and gain weight in a healthy way:

- If you have a small appetite, try eating several small meals each day and drink fluids after meals.

- Add concentrated calories to your food such as shredded cheese on your baked potato or almond butter on your toast.

- Prepare oatmeal and other hot cereals with milk instead of water and top them with fruits, nuts, or honey.

- Add healthy oils to salads, like olive oil, whole olives, avocados, nuts, and seeds.

- Add 1–2 tablespoons of dry milk powder to soups, casseroles, liquid milk, and mashed potatoes.

- Choose nutrient-rich foods like whole grains, fruits, vegetables, lean protein, nuts, seeds, and healthy fats are important to your diet.

- Try adding smoothies and shakes with fresh fruit and milk and adding some flaxseed.

The important thing is to remember quality over quantity. Adding calories with candy bars may increase your weight, but they won't be beneficial to your health and body composition. It's also important to be realistic about your body type. Remember to focus on your health, not on looking a certain way that may not be realistic for you.

If you've tried to gain weight in a healthy way and are still struggling, there may be an underlying problem. Visit your health care provider if you are under weight and suspect you may have an illness or eating disorder causing the weight loss that needs to be addressed.

Conclusion

Your next steps should include assessing your body composition, setting goals for improving your health based on body composition or BMI, and planning a healthy energy balance for achieving your goals. It's important to keep weight management in perspective and focus on health. Do an honest appraisal of your body image. Is it accurate and fair, or is it negative and unhealthy? If you feel that you might have disordered eating or a disturbance in body image, you should get help from the sources listed in this chapter.

Reflection Questions

1. Explain the difference between visceral fat and subcutaneous fat. Which is more likely to be harmful for health? Why?

2. Briefly describe the scope of obesity as a public health concern in the US.

3. What does it mean to be underweight? What are possible health effects associated with being underweight?

4. What is the energy balance equation? What are the different components?

5. What is body image? How does it develop?

6. Identify three strategies that you would recommend to someone for improving their body image.

7. Explain the difference between anorexia nervosa, bulimia nervosa, binge eating disorder, and disordered eating. How are they similar?

8. How is body composition assessed?

9. Create a sample plan for achieving or maintaining a healthy body composition that includes strategies for nutrition and physical activity.

Chapter 7
Nutrition

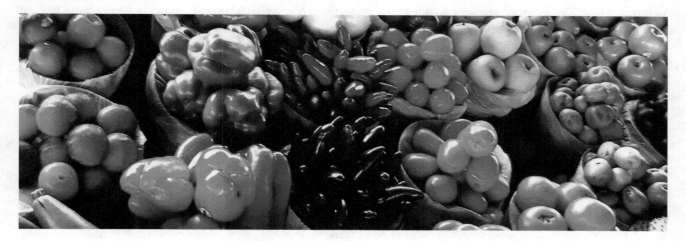

Learning Objectives

1. Discuss the connection between nutrition habits and health.
2. Describe the functions and healthful food sources of the essential nutrients.
3. Describe the components of MyPlate and the US dietary guidelines.
4. Explain how to use food labels and other consumer tools to make informed choices about foods.
5. Discuss nutritional guidelines for vegetarians and for special population groups.
6. Create a personal nutrition plan that promotes wellness.

When kids play sports, it's common for them to get a snack at halftime or at the end of their game. Most soccer players can instantly remember the feeling of eating orange slices at halftime, or getting rewarded with a juice box and granola bar after a game. It's comforting to be fed after playing hard.

How many times have you had chicken soup when you had a cold or heard the phrase "an apple a day keeps the doctor away?" These sayings and experiences are common because nutritious food is an essential part of a healthy life and contributes to several areas of wellness. The positive effects can be immediate, such as resolving hunger and replenishing energy, or long-lasting since healthy eating fuels the healing of injuries and prevents illness or disease. Eating a healthy snack or a healthy meal does a lot of good for your body.

What you eat affects your health on many levels, which is why you need to understand nutrition and make educated choices. Proper nutrition has the amazing power to keep you healthy and happy, and improper nutrition can also wreak havoc on your body. Your nutritional intake should be aligned with health guidelines and other health and fitness goals you have. Each of us is a little different, so you'll probably discover that you can take some general guidelines and experiment until you find the nutrition plan that works for you.

This chapter first defines nutrition and essential nutrients. It then presents guidelines for healthy nutrition and potential plans for meeting those guidelines. The chapter includes a discussion of several common dietary concerns and how they affect individuals.

Defining Nutrition

Nutrition is the process of gaining essential nutrients and energy from the foods you consume, those you need for your body to function properly. It connects to wellness due to the long-term effects both healthy and unhealthy nutrition can have on your quality of life. Combined with physical activity, your diet can help you to reach and maintain a healthy weight, reduce your risk of chronic diseases (like heart disease and cancer), and promote your overall health.

Deficiencies, excesses, and imbalances in diet can produce negative impacts on health. About half of all American adults—117 million individuals—have one or more preventable chronic diseases, many of which may lead to various health problems such as obesity, osteoporosis, and diabetes. Many are related in large part to poor quality eating patterns. Cardiovascular disease, high blood pressure, Type 2 diabetes, some cancers, and poor bone health often occur as a result of inattention to nutrition. More than two-thirds of adults and nearly one-third of children and youth are overweight or obese. These high rates of overweight and obesity and chronic disease have persisted for more than two decades and come not only with increased health risks, but also at high cost. For more information on chronic disease, see Chapter 9.

Many Americans do not meet the recommended guidelines for essential foods and nutrients and exceed what is recommended on foods that in large quantities can be detrimental to their health, such as saturated fats, sugars, and sodium. Before you plan your nutrition, it is important to be aware of nutritional requirements and the essential nutrients that are used by the body to meet those needs.

Nutrition and Energy

Your body needs energy to operate all of your vital organs and systems. We measure this energy as **calories**, units of energy taken in through food. Scientifically, it is defined as the energy required to heat 1 kilogram of water by one degree Celsius. The total number of calories a person needs each day varies depending on a number of factors, including the person's age, biological sex, height, weight, and level of physical activity.

If you want to lose, maintain, or gain weight, the number of calories you should consume may need to change. Remember the energy balance equation from Chapter 6? A positive balance (more in, less out) means you gain weight, neutral balance (equal in and out) means you maintain your weight, and negative balance (less in, more out) means you lose. You need to understand how many calories your body needs to power its systems and then determine what you need to take in to reach your goal.

Your body needs a certain amount of energy to manage basic functions, such as breathing, digestion, and the function of your vital organs. This is the resting metabolic rate (RMR) you learned about in Chapter 6. Beyond this, it needs additional energy to move based on your body composition, size, and activity level. If you are physically smaller or less active, for example, you might need fewer calories, whereas a

professional athlete might need a few thousand calories in a day. Estimates range from 1,600 to 2,400 calories per day for

Calories Per Day*			
Height	**Activity Level****	**Men**	**Women**
5 ft. (60 in.)	Sedentary	1,950–2,200	1,700–1,850
	Low active	2,150–2,400	1,900–2,100
	Active	2,400–2,700	2,150–2,300
	Very active	2,650–3,000	2,400–2,600
5 ft, 6 in. (66 in.)	Sedentary	2,200–2,500	1,900–2,100
	Low active	2,400–2,750	2,150–2,300
	Active	2,700–3,050	2,400–2,600
	Very active	3,000–3,400	2,700–2,950
6 ft. (72 in.)	Sedentary	2,450–2,800	2,150–2,350
	Low active	2,700–3,050	2,350–2,600
	Active	3,000–3,400	2,650–2,900
	Very active	3,350–3,850	3,000–3,300

Figure 1. Estimated calorie needs per day by height, activity level, and sex.

adult women and 2,000–3,000 calories per day for adult men.

In the table on calories per day ranges (Figure 1), you can see average caloric intake needs based on height. Further information is available when categories are separated by age (Figure 2). Within each age and sex category, the low end of the range is for sedentary individuals. The high end of the range is for active individuals. Due to the reductions in basal metabolic rate that occur with aging, calorie needs generally decrease for adults as they age. Data is based on a male of 5'10" and 154 pounds and a woman of 5'4" and 126 pounds.

Keep in mind that these are just guidelines and would need to be adapted based on your height and weight. They would also need to be adjusted based on your weight gain or loss goals. In Chapter 6, we discussed identifying your RMR or BMR and estimating your Thermic Effective of Exercise (TEE) to calculate your energy needs based on your activity level.

It's important to note that you don't need to count calories every day, but tracking your diet periodically can give you a sense of how close you are to meeting the nutrient recommendations and help to identify patterns of eating and overall caloric intake. Tracking your food intake during the week and during the weekend may tell you if your food habits vary, which is true for most people. Counting calories alone isn't enough, however. Your body needs essential nutrients to survive, too. Most people get plenty of calories but not enough essential nutrients.

Energy Density vs. Nutrient Density

Not all calories are created equal. Some foods have a lot of calories but little nutritional value, while some are packed with nutrients but not with calories. **Energy density** is the amount of energy or calories in a particular weight of food and is generally presented as the number of calories in a gram (kcal/g). Foods with a lower energy density provide fewer calories per gram than foods with a higher energy density. For the same number of calories, a person can consume a larger portion of food lower in energy density than food higher in energy density.

Energy density values are influenced by the composition of foods. Water lowers the energy density of foods, because it has an energy density of 0 kcal/g and contributes weight but not energy to foods. Fiber also has a relatively low energy density (1.5–2.5 kcal/g). On the opposite end of the energy density spectrum, fat (9 kcal/g) is the most energy dense component of food, providing more than twice as many calories per gram as carbohydrates or protein (4 kcal/g). In general, foods with a lower energy density (i.e., fruits, vegetables, and broth-based soups) tend to be foods with high water content, lots of fiber, or little fat.

We can also consider a food's **nutrient density** (the amount of nutrients per calorie). Foods with a high nutrient density offer valuable calories because the energy comes from their essential nutrients without empty (not valuable)

Calories Per Day for Males					Calories Per Day for Females			
Age	Sedentary	Moderately Active	Active		Age	Sedentary	Moderately Active	Active
18	2,400	2,800	3,200		18	1,800	2,000	2,400
19–20	2,600	2,800	3,000		19–20	2,000	2,200	2,400
21–25	2,400	2,800	3,000		21–25	2,000	2,200	2,400
26–30	2,400	2,600	3,000		26–30	1,800	2,000	2,400
31–35	2,400	2,600	3,000		31–35	1,800	2,000	2,200
36–40	2,400	2,600	2,800		36–40	1,800	2,000	2,200
41–45	2,200	2,600	2,800		41–45	1,800	2,000	2,200
46–50	2,200	2,400	2,800		46–50	1,800	2,000	2,200
51–55	2,200	2,400	2,800		51–55	1,600	1,800	2,200
56–60	2,200	2,400	2,600		56–60	1,600	1,800	2,200
61–65	2,000	2,400	2,600		61–65	1,600	1,800	2,000
66–70	2,000	2,200	2,600		66–70	1,600	1,800	2,000
71–75	2,000	2,200	2,600		71–75	1,600	1,800	2,000
≥76	2,000	2,200	2,400		≥76	1,600	1,800	2,000

Figure 2. Calorie needs per day by sex, age, and activity level.

Higher Energy Density	Lower Energy Density
Regular hamburger patty (4 oz) =235 calories	Lean hamburger patty (4 oz) =167 calories
Medium croissant (2 oz) = 231 calories	Two slices of whole wheat bread =138 calories
Slice of apple pie = 356 calories	Large apple (8oz) = 110 calories
Fried chicken w/skin and batter (3 oz) = 479 cal.	Roasted chicken breast, skinless (3 oz) = 141 cal.

Figure 3. Calorie comparisons of common foods.

calories. The most nutrient-dense foods include vegetables, fruits, whole grains, seafood, eggs, beans and peas, unsalted nuts and seeds, fat-free and low-fat dairy products, and lean meats and poultry—all with little or no saturated fat, sodium, and added sugars.

Research indicates that a diet that focuses on foods with low energy density and high nutrient density—one that is rich in fruits, vegetables, whole grains, lean meats, and low-fat dairy products—helps people lower their calorie intake. At the same time, eating low-energy-dense foods helps people control their hunger and maintain feelings of satisfaction and fullness. This is important when trying to stick to an eating plan. Making nutrient dense and low energy (low calorie) choices can be fairly simple. Just look at a few comparable foods side by side (Figure 3).

Because the foods on the right have less fat, sugar, and added fillers, they contribute fewer calories at the same portion size. The basic nutrients may be comparable in the meats, but one is lean rather than fatty. The apple contains 3g of fiber and is rich in vitamins A and C compared to the slice of pie filled with sugar and fat. The whole wheat bread contains fiber, calcium, and potassium, while the croissant packs in nearly 6g of fat and lots of sodium.

It's simple to choose better versions of the foods you eat regularly. You can also seek out foods that pack a large nutrient punch. A large serving of kale, for example, has 2g of fiber, 3g of protein, and only 50 calories. Other foods that are standouts in the nutrient-rich class include salmon, liver, potatoes, berries, broccoli, almonds, and sweet potatoes.

Essential Nutrients

We've discussed nutrient density, but what exactly is a nutrient? A **nutrient** is a chemical compound in food that the body uses to function and maintain health. An **essential nutrient** refers to nutritional requirements that a person must meet through dietary intake because their body can't produce them in sufficient quantities on its own. There are six classes of essential nutrients—carbohydrates, fat, protein, vitamins, minerals, and water.

Nutrients come in two types—macronutrients and micronutrients. **Macronutrients** (carbohydrates, fat, and protein) are the powerhouses, fueling your body to keep things running. Your body can't produce these nutrients on its own, so you must take them in through your diet. **Micronutrients** are called that because your body needs them in smaller amounts like milligrams and micrograms rather than full grams. As these enter your digestive system, they break down in the stomach and then are absorbed into the blood stream through the walls of your intestines (passive diffusion). Compared to macronutrients, your body absorbs micronutrients very quickly.

Carbohydrates

Carbohydrates are one of the main types of nutrients, the body's primary source of energy, and generally the largest source of calories in your diet. Common sources of carbohydrates include bread, pasta, cereal, grains, dairy products, fruits, vegetables, rice, and beans. There are 4 calories in 1 gram of carbohydrates. Carbohydrates offer a pretty efficient source of calories, which your body needs to create energy. Carbohydrates consist of sugars, starches, and fibers.

Carbohydrates play a role in the functioning of the nervous system, metabolism, and muscles. Your digestive system changes carbohydrates into glucose (blood sugar) then your body uses this sugar for energy for your cells, tissues, and organs and to fuel your muscles, which is particularly important when during exercise. It stores any extra sugar in your liver and muscles for when it is needed. Without this nutrient, your body resorts to breaking down protein from your muscles to get energy.

Carbohydrates are considered either simple or complex, depending on their chemical structure. **Simple carbohydrates** include sugars found naturally in foods such as fruits, vegetables, milk, and milk products. They also include sugars added during food processing and refining. The sugars and starches in carbohydrates provide glucose, the main energy source for the brain, central nervous system, and red blood cells. Glucose also can be stored as glycogen (animal starch) in liver and muscle, or, like all excess calories in the body, converted to body fat. Simple carbohydrates break down very quickly into glucose and energy.

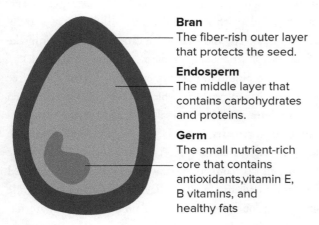

Bran
The fiber-rish outer layer that protects the seed.

Endosperm
The middle layer that contains carbohydrates and proteins.

Germ
The small nutrient-rich core that contains antioxidants,vitamin E, B vitamins, and healthy fats

Figure 4. Parts of a whole grain.

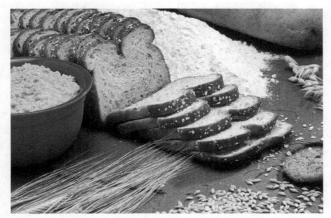

Figure 5. Whole grains can be found in many breads.

Complex carbohydrates include whole grain breads and cereals, starchy vegetables, and legumes. These take longer to break down in your body, which means they don't elevate your blood sugar as quickly. This is particularly important for someone who is diabetic. Many of the complex carbohydrates also contain fiber. Dietary fibers are non-digestible forms of carbohydrates, such as those found naturally in plants. This is why fruits, vegetables, and beans help provide a feeling of fullness and promote healthy laxation. The complexity of fruits and vegetables varies. The sugars in fruits, for example, make them simple yet their vitamin and fiber content make them more complex than something like cane sugar or white flour. Fiber has a lot to do with whether a carbohydrate is simple or complex. Diets high in fiber also have been linked to reduced risk of diabetes, colon cancer, obesity, and other chronic diseases. This is where the old "apple a day keeps the doctor away" adage comes from.

Whole Grains

Whole grains are products made from the entire grain seed, usually called the kernel, which consists of the bran, germ, and endosperm (Figure 4). The bran is the outer shell of the grain that protects the seed—for us, it provides fiber, B vitamins, and trace minerals. The germ, which nourishes the seed, contributes antioxidants, vitamin E, and B vitamins to our diet. The endosperm provides energy in the form of carbohydrates and protein. If the kernel has been cracked, crushed, or flaked, it must retain the same relative proportions of bran, germ, and endosperm as the original grain in order to be called whole grain. Many, but not all, whole grains are also sources of dietary fiber (Figure 5).

You've heard on television, online, and now here in this chapter that whole grains provide a valuable form of carbohydrate. The tricky part is actually making sure that the grains you eat are in fact "*whole*" grains. You may buy something brown or that looks grainy and think it must be healthy—the box says so! However, a lot happens to a grain during the milling (refining) process. This is when your pristine-looking white bread and white flour achieves its appearance. But even those that look whole may not be. Often many of the components mentioned above are removed and other starches and flours added in that wouldn't be considered whole. In fact, unless the word "whole" is in front of the ingredient listed on the food label, you may need to do a bit of investigation.

Flour can be one of the trickiest to determine. The US Food and Drug Administration (USDA) recommends looking for those labeled as: cracked wheat, whole-wheat flour, crushed wheat, graham flour, entire-wheat flour, bromated whole-wheat flour, or whole durum wheat flour.

That covers the flour, but what about all of the other products that contain grains? Savvy consumers know that nowadays labels are designed to sell and can be deliberately misleading. Manufacturers want you to consider their cereal or their bread as healthy, especially with the push toward whole grains. But honesty is not always their policy. The USDA has some tips for this as well. Look for some common and usual names for whole grains:

- The word "whole" listed before a grain: "whole wheat"
- The words "berries" and "groats" designate whole grains: "wheat berries" or "oat groats"
- Rolled oats and oatmeal: old-fashioned, quick-cooking, and instant oatmeal

Other whole-grain products that do not use the word "whole" in their description, but are a whole grain: brown rice, brown rice flour, wild rice, popcorn, bulgar, rye, quinoa, millet, triticale, teff, amaranth, buckwheat, or sorghum.

If you're wondering why whole grain is better than many refined grain, it comes down to nutritional content. Many refined grains lack the fiber and many other nutrients that are lost during the refining process. Some are "enriched," meaning a few nutrients will be added back in but rarely do they have the same health benefits. Whole grains contribute to lower body weight and lower incidences of heart disease, Type 2 diabetes, and cancer. But many refined grains lack the nutrients that aid your body. The *2015 Dietary Guidelines for Americans* recommend that at least half of your grain consumption be whole grains.

Gluten

Some grains—such as wheat, barley, rye, and spelt—contain a naturally occurring protein called **gluten**. This protein acts as a binder to keep the food together. It's what gives that stretchy consistency to dough when we make pizza, bread, and pastries. Yet this innocent little protein has been getting a bad reputation the last few years, getting blamed for any number of issues ranging from weight gain, headaches, and intestinal issues to poor cognition and attention deficit disorder.

Studies indicate, however, that gluten is a healthy protein for most individuals. Not only is evidence lacking to support many of the pop culture theories on gluten-free diets, gluten

may actually serve as a pre-biotic, promoting the growth of good bacteria in your gut and helping out your gastrointestinal system. Remember those diseases whole grains help prevent? People often avoid many healthy grains in an attempt to avoid gluten, which results in an absence of beneficial whole grains in their diet. This increases the risk of heart disease, Type 2 diabetes, and stroke.

For some individuals, gluten can be a serious health risk. **Celiac disease** is an autoimmune disorder that causes the body to sense gluten as a toxin. This leads to many side effects, including fatigue, bloating, constipation, diarrhea, weight loss, malnutrition, and intestinal damage. It is estimated that approximately 1% of the population has celiac disease, though it is commonly undiagnosed or misdiagnosed. There are other individuals that have milder reactions to gluten (gluten sensitivity) or allergies that involve skin reactions. For people with celiac disease or any form of gluten allergy, the only treatment is to avoid gluten. Most people, however, eat gluten their entire lives with no issues.

People with gluten sensitivity or Celiac disease must be careful to avoid gluten, but it's important not to replace gluten-containing foods with more red meat, full-fat dairy, starchy vegetables, sweets, and fats, which can lead to a higher intake of cholesterol, saturated fat, sodium, and unwanted calories.

It's also best to limit commercially prepared gluten-free snacks and bakery products, which are typically high in refined carbohydrate, fat, sugar, and salt—just like their gluten-containing counterparts. In the US, gluten-free foods tend to be lower in folate, thiamin, riboflavin and niacin. This may be because in this country most wheat products are enriched with folic acid, thiamin, riboflavin, niacin and iron, while gluten-free flours, cereals and bread products typically are not.

However, gluten-free whole grains, such as amaranth, quinoa, buckwheat, teff, millet, corn and rice, are good natural sources of folate, thiamin, riboflavin, niacin and iron—as well as protein and fiber.

Fiber

Dietary fiber, or what we simply call fiber, is sometimes referred to as "roughage." It is a type of carbohydrate found in plant foods and made up of many sugar molecules linked together. But unlike other carbohydrates (such as starch), fiber binds together in such a way that it cannot be readily digested in the small intestine. There are two types of dietary fiber, soluble and insoluble, and most plant foods contain some of each kind.

Soluble fiber dissolves in water to form a thick gel-like substance in the stomach and is broken down by bacteria in the large intestines. This type of fiber, because it breaks down in the body, has calories. Soluble fiber can interfere with the absorption of dietary fat and cholesterol. This, in turn, can help lower low-density lipoprotein (LDL or "bad") cholesterol levels in the blood, reducing your risk of cardiovascular disease. It also slows digestion and the rate at which carbohydrates and other nutrients absorbed into the bloodstream. This can help control your level of blood glucose (blood sugar) by preventing rapid rises in blood glucose following a meal. Soluble fiber is found in a variety of foods, including: beans, fruits, oats (such as oat bran and oatmeal), nuts, seeds, and vegetables.

Insoluble fiber does not dissolve in water and passes through the gastrointestinal tract relatively intact and, therefore, is not a source of calories. Insoluble fiber provides "bulk" for stool formation and speeds up the movement of food and waste through the digestive system, which can help prevent constipation. Both soluble and insoluble fiber make you feel full, which may help you eat less and stay satisfied longer. Insoluble fiber is found in a variety of foods, including: fruits, nuts, seeds, vegetables, wheat bran, and whole grain foods such as brown rice, whole grain breads, cereals, and pasta.

The *2015 Dietary Guidelines for Americans* recommends consuming a variety of nutrient-dense foods and beverages containing dietary fiber. The recommended healthy amount of fiber intake is 38g for men and 25g for women. Most Americans, however, do not get the recommended amount of dietary fiber. This is considered a "nutrient of public health concern" because low intakes lead to potential health risks.

The FDA suggests using the Nutrition Facts Label as your tool for increasing consumption of dietary fiber. The label on food and beverage packages shows the amount in grams (g) and the Percent Daily Value (%DV) of dietary fiber in one serving of the food. Food manufacturers may voluntarily list the amount in grams per serving of soluble and insoluble fiber on the label (under Dietary Fiber). They are only required to list soluble fiber and/or insoluble fiber if the package labeling states something about fiber health effects or the amount contained in the food (for example, "high in insoluble fiber").

The Daily Value for fiber is 25g per day. This is based on a 2,000-calorie diet—your Daily Value may be higher or lower depending on your calorie needs. When comparing foods, choose foods with a higher %DV of dietary fiber. The goal is to get 100% of the Daily Value for dietary fiber on most days. Keep in mind that 5% DV or less of dietary fiber

per serving is low, and 20% DV or more of dietary fiber per serving is high.

To bring more fiber into your diet, the FDA recommends that you look for whole grains on the ingredient list on a food package. Ingredients are listed in descending order by weight—the closer they are to the beginning of the list, the more of that ingredient is in the food. They also recommend trying some of the following options:

Switch from refined to whole grain. Most commonly consumed foods (such as breads, cereals, pasta, and rice) have whole grain versions available.

Limit refined grains and products made with refined grains. Many of these products (such as cakes, chips, cookies, and crackers) can be high in added sugars, saturated fat, and/or sodium and are common sources of excess calories.

Add beans to your diet. Beans (such as garbanzo, kidney, or pinto), lentils, or peas can be great in salads, soups, and side dishes—or serve them as a main dish!

Start your day with a bowl of whole grain breakfast cereal. High fiber cereals (such as bran or oatmeal) that are low in added sugars can be topped with fruit for sweetness and even more fiber!

Choose fruit. Any fruit, whether fresh, frozen, dried, or canned in 100% juice, can be a good as snack, salad, or dessert.

Keep raw, cut-up vegetables handy for quick snacks. Choose colorful dark green, orange, and red vegetables, such as broccoli florets, carrots, and red peppers.

Try unsalted nuts and seeds. Replace some of the meat and poultry in your diet with unsalted nuts and seeds.

It's important to note that fiber should be increased gradually in your diet. Sudden, large increases can result in gas, bloating, and cramping. Take it one step at a time and drink plenty of water along with higher fiber foods.

Added Sugars

The role of carbohydrates in the diet has been the source of much public and scientific interest. These include the relationship of carbohydrates with health outcomes, including coronary heart disease, Type 2 diabetes, body weight, and tooth decay. In most studies, however, little evidence has surfaced to support these theories or those related to poor cognition or behavior. Very few studies link carbohydrates to obesity, and some even suggest that their fiber content helps promote weight loss.

What *does* contribute to these diseases and works against weight loss—and your health in general—is **added sugar**. These are the "carbs" that give carbohydrates a bad name. Added sugars are sugar carbohydrates (caloric sweeteners) added to food and beverages during their production. This type of sugar is chemically indistinguishable from naturally occurring sugars, but the term "added sugar" has become increasingly used in nutrition and medicine to help identify foods characterized by added energy. They have no nutritional value, only adding "empty calories." Despite this, the average American consumes 22 teaspoons of added sugar each day!

Added sugars negatively impact your health in a few different ways. First, the consumption of these empty calories often leaves your diet unbalanced. In a nutritional comparison between an apple and a piece of pie, the whole apple contains only the sugars naturally occurring in the food while the slice of pie contains a great deal of added sugars. A person who eats the slice of pie fills up on a lot of empty calories compared to the person eating the apple. Your stomach can only hold so much food. Each meal is a choice. If you choose the empty calories, and fill yourself, you aren't likely to eat as many nutritionally dense foods (Figure 6).

If you ate a healthy diet *and* added sugar, would you be fine? Studies are pointing to a solid "no." How exactly excess sugar impacts the heart isn't yet clear, but individuals who consumed a healthy diet in addition to an excess amount of added sugar still had higher rates of heart disease.

It's easy to consume more sugar than you mean to. You and your brother recently decided to eat "clean," removing most processed food and added sugar from your diet. You both did really well for the first few weeks because you focused only on whole foods, nothing out of a package or wrapper. But then you decided to take a road trip. You chose to plan ahead to avoid too many stops at fast food restaurants—great idea. But you needed to find foods that didn't take up so much cooler space—there's only so much room in your car and the Grand Canyon is a long way. While trolling the aisles, he begins picking out boxes of fruit and nut bars, and whole grain cereal. A little fruit, a little protein, some whole grains—no problem. Until you looked at the label. The bars contained

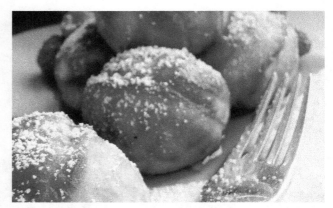

Figure 6. Added sugars can affect heart health.

high fructose corn syrup and cane sugar. The box of whole grain cereal, though whole-wheat flour was the main ingredient, contained malt syrup and fruit juice concentrate. Are these the same as table sugar? In short: yes!

Added sugar goes by many different names. It doesn't matter how natural and unprocessed it sounds. The body doesn't differentiate between naturally occurring sugar and those that are added to the food. Looking at the total grams of sugar on the label is your best approach. Getting to know some of the names of different forms of sugar can also help when it comes to reading the labels and making choices. Some, like cane sugar, molasses, corn syrup, honey, and most things that say "syrup," "crystals," or "sweetener" behind another word are almost always forms of sugar. Others can be harder to identify, like dextrose, fructose, and maltose.

Recommended Carbohydrate Intake

Current dietary guidelines recommend consumption of carbohydrate-containing foods, including vegetables, fruits, grains (at least 50% of them whole), nuts and seeds, and milk products as part of a healthy diet. The recommended intake of carbohydrates is measured as grams or as a percentage of your total calories, called the **Acceptable Macronutrient Distribution Ranges** (**AMDR**). These ranges take into account disease risk reduction and the intake of essential nutrients. The US Dietary Guidelines suggest that 45–65% of your calories come in the form of carbohydrates.

How about that worrisome carbohydrate, added sugar? The American Heart Association recommends consuming no more than 6 (women) to 9 (men) teaspoons of added sugar each day. That's 100–150 calories or 24–36g at most. Just to give you an idea, that is the number of calories in one can of cola. The US Dietary Guidelines (2015–2020) have for the first time recommended that added sugar be limited to 10% of your diet.

Recommended Intake During Fitness Training

A person participating in a fitness training program, particularly when it involves endurance at a high level, may need additional energy for their muscles. This comes in large part from carbohydrates, the primary fuel sources for the body. Endurance athletes often have less body fat to draw from for energy during competition. This is ideal for health on a day-to-day basis, but when exercising it means your carbohydrate intake must be adequate to keep your body from robbing protein from your muscles to use as energy. Regardless of body fat, you need carbohydrates while training to maintain energy levels and performance (Figure 7). Great sources of quick energy include fruits (bananas and berries), brown rice, and yogurt.

The Academy of Nutrition and Dietetics recommends the following levels of intake:

Type of Training	Daily Carb Needs per Kilogram	Daily Carb Needs per Pound
Moderate duration and low intensity	5 to 7 grams per kilogram	2.3 to 3.2 grams per pound
Moderate- to heavy-training load and high intensity	6 to 10 grams per kilogram	3 to 4.5 grams per pound
Extreme training and high-intensity races (longer than 4 to 5 hours)	> 8 to 12 grams per kilogram	> 3.6 to 5.5 grams per pound

Figure 7. Additional carbohydrates are needed for fitness training.

Fats

These days you can find a fat-free version of almost everything, from chips and desserts to salad dressing and margarine. Fat-free this and fat-free that. Some are good (some foods don't really need fat to taste good), some have added sugar to mask taste and texture, and some are totally inedible. When people try to reduce their fat intake, they can choke down foods that their dog wouldn't even steal a bite of. Would it surprise you to learn that it's okay to eat fat, and that you *need it* in your diet?

Fats are another of the three macronutrients, the essential nutrients that contain energy. You need a certain amount in your diet to stay healthy. Fats provide needed energy in the form of calories. In fact, they are the most concentrated source of energy in your diet. Fat has 9 calories per gram, more than twice the number of calories in carbohydrates and protein, which each have 4 calories per gram. During cardiorespiratory exercise, your body uses primarily calories from carbohydrates you have eaten. After 20 minutes of steady-state training, the body depends more on calories from fat to keep you going.

Fats do more than just provide energy. They help your body absorb important vitamins—called fat-soluble vitamins—including vitamins A, D and E. The fats you consume also give your body essential fatty acids called linoleic and linolenic acid—"essential" because your body cannot make them itself or function without them. You need them for brain development, control over inflammation, and blood clotting. You also need fat to keep your skin and hair healthy and to fill your fat cells, which insulate your body and help keep you warm.

Fats also make foods more flavorful and help you feel full. Eating some fats as part of a healthy and satisfying diet is essential, though it is also harmful to eat too many. The tastiness of fatty food is paid for with a load of calories. This is why all fats, including healthy fats, can contribute to weight gain when eaten in large amounts. Fats may be vital to your health, but a fat-rich diet will give you way more calories than you need. Fats that aren't used for energy get stored in your body as (you guessed it!) fat.

Like carbohydrates, not all fats are equal. The term "healthy fats" probably sounds like an oxymoron, but some types of fat are healthier than others. Choosing a small amount of healthy fats from plant sources—including nuts and seeds, good sources of omega-3 fats—more often, and choosing less healthy fats from animal products can help lower your risk for heart attack, stroke, and other major health problems. Unhealthy fats increase your risk for these diseases and others, such as Type 2 diabetes. Not only might you be tipping the scale on energy balance when you consume too much fat, but you could be affecting the inside of your body, even if you have a healthy body composition.

	Butter (1 Tbsp)	Stick Margarine (1 Tbsp)	Soft/Tub Margarine (1 Tbsp)	Canola Oil (1 Tbsp)
Calories	100	100	60	120
Total Fat	11g	11g	7g	14g
Saturated Fat	7g	2g	1g	1g
Trans Fat	0g	3g	0.5g	0g
Cholesterol	30mg	0mg	0mg	0mg

Figure 8. Calorie, fat, and cholesterol comparisons in commonly used fats.

Saturated Fat

All fats are made up of saturated and unsaturated fatty acids. Fats are called **saturated** or **unsaturated** depending on how much of each type of fatty acid they contain.

Imagine a building made of solid bricks. This building's bricks are similar to the tightly packed bonds that make **saturated fat**. The bonds are often solid at room temperature, like butter or the fat inside or around meat. Animal products such as beef, pork, and chicken contain saturated fat. Leaner animal products, such as chicken breast or pork loin, often have less saturated fat. We also typically find it in stick margarine, shortening, and coconut and palm oil, as well as in snack foods, chocolates, baked goods and other desserts, and deep-fried and processed foods (Figure 8).

Saturated fats raise your LDL (bad) cholesterol level. A high ratio of LDL to HDL cholesterol increases your risk for heart attack, stroke, and other major health problems. You'll learn more about cholesterol and its dangers in Chapter 9, but the most important thing to remember about it is that this soft, waxy substance can clog your arteries. When you light a candle for a few minutes and then blow it out, the wax is in between hard and liquid, sort of soft and glue-like—it still runs a bit if you tip the candle but can't easily be washed away by other liquids. This is similar to what happens in your arteries when blood tries to pass build-ups of cholesterol. It gets in the way, interfering with blood flow and adding potentially life-threatening risk.

Saturated fats store well and take a long time to spoil, which is pretty important if you don't own a refrigerator, but a dubious claim-to-fame once it enters your body. Any food that takes an unusually long time to spoil likely contains more gifts from man than from nature. Unfortunately, saturated fats make up too high a percentage in the average American diet, which leads to numerous negative effects on overall health, especially cardiovascular health because of its impact on your arteries. This data from the National Health and Nutrition Examination Survey (NHANES) tells us just how much saturated fat the average person consumes compared to how much is recommended (Figure 9).

You can't avoid saturated fat completely (Figure 10). It would be almost impossible to remove every ounce of fat from your meat, and if you could, it would be more like jerky.

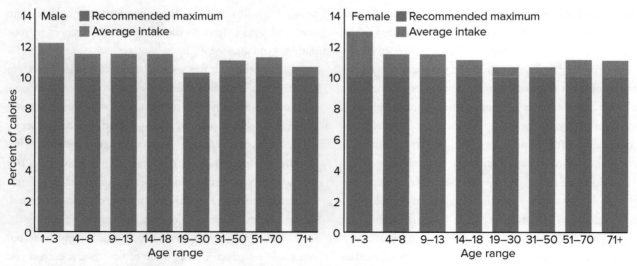

Figure 9. Saturated fat intake (orange) compared with recommended amount (blue), by age, gender, and percentage of total calories.

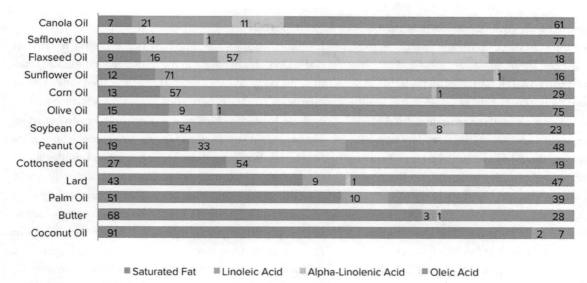

Figure 10. Cooking oils each have a different composition of dietary fats.

Saturated fats, however, are not essential for life, so reducing them as much as possible is both safe and healthy.

Unsaturated Fat

Imagine the links in a chain that bend, move, and flow. The chain links are similar to the loose bonds that make **unsaturated fat** fluid or liquid at room temperature, like the oil on top of a salad dressing or in a can of tuna. Unsaturated fat typically comes from plant sources such as olives, nuts, corn, or seeds but is also present in fish. There are two types of unsaturated fats—monounsaturated and polyunsaturated.

Monounsaturated fats are healthier forms of fat. Monounsaturated oils include olive, avocado, sunflower, safflower, canola, peanut, and most nuts. You may have heard people praise the merits of olive oil. There is a good reason for that. Eaten in moderate amounts and in place of saturated fats, monounsaturated fats can lower your LDL (bad cholesterol) levels, help your body regulate blood sugar, promote healthy cell regeneration, and improve your immune system. They also contain Vitamin E, which is great for your vision.

Polyunsaturated fats are also considered healthier and found in plants, salmon, vegetable oils, and some nuts and seeds. These contain **omega-3** and **omega-6 fatty acids**, essential fatty acids that the body needs for brain function and cell growth. Your body does not make these acids, so you can only get them from food. Good sources of omega-3 acids include fatty fish—such as salmon, mackerel, and sardines—walnuts, flaxseeds, canola oil, and unhydrogenated soybean oil. **Omega-3 fatty acids** are good for your heart in several ways. They help reduce triglycerides, a type

of fat in your blood; reduce the risk of an irregular heartbeat (arrhythmia), slow the build-up of plaque in your arteries, and slightly lower your blood pressure.

Good sources of omega-6 acids include vegetable oils, such as sunflower, safflower, corn, soybean, and walnut oils. **Omega-6 fatty acids** may help control your blood sugar, reduce your risk of diabetes, and lower your blood pressure.

It's great to get more omega-3 acids into your diet like the ones in many kinds of fish, but some fish can be tainted with mercury and other chemicals. Eating tainted fish can pose health risks for young children and pregnant women. You can reduce your risk of exposure by eating a variety of fish. Pregnant women and children in particular should avoid fish with high levels of mercury. These include swordfish, shark, king mackerel, and tilefish. However, if you are middle-aged or older, the benefits of eating fish outweigh any risks.

Most health experts agree that the best way to reap the benefits of omega-3 is from food. Whole foods contain many nutrients besides omega-3s. These all work together to keep your heart healthy. If you already have heart disease or high triglycerides, you may benefit from consuming higher amounts of omega-3 fatty acids. It may be hard to get enough omega-3s through food. Ask your health care provider if taking fish oil supplements might be a good idea.

Recommended Fat Intake

The American Heart Association recommends reducing saturated fat intake to less than 7% of your total calories. This concurs with similar recommendations made by the US Department of Health and Human Services, which suggest that limiting saturated fat consumption to less than 10% each day would positively affect health and reduce the prevalence of heart disease (Figure 11).

The recommended AMDR for fat for adults is 20–35%. There are no specific guidelines on the exact amount of healthy fat people should consume, but of the recommended AMDR, we know that no more than 10% of that should be saturated. That means that you should work toward a range between 10% and 25% of your diet as unsaturated fats. The American Heart Association suggests that people try to consume between 5–10% of their daily calories from omega-6 fatty acids, which most people already do. They also recommend eating at least 2 servings a week of fish rich in omega-3s. For reference, a serving is 3.5 ounces (100g), which is slightly bigger than a checkbook.

If you're using more saturated fats than recommended, replacing the fats you regularly use with healthier options can be done with simple changes (Figure 12). Swap your partially hydrogenated oil with olive or canola oil. Try frying your morning eggs (if you just can't master poaching) in a small amount of olive oil rather than butter or bacon fat. Buy low fat dairy products (be careful to check the label for added sugar). Add some nuts and seeds to your salad instead of processed croutons and bacon bits. You may be surprised at how easy and satisfying a few simple changes can be.

Trans-Fat

It's difficult to describe just how bad **trans-fat** is for your body. Don't bother looking for recommended intake guidelines for trans-fat—it's zero! Trans-fat is the Frankenstein's monster of fat. Trans-fatty acids form when oils (even healthy oils) are hardened through a process called hydrogenation. Hydrogenated fats, or trans-fats, are often used to keep some foods fresh for a long time. Trans-fats are to fats like plastic is to garbage—it just doesn't biodegrade in any natural way.

This process began in the early-twentieth century with margarine and shortening. Once food manufacturers learned how to partially hydrogenate oils, it began turning up in many processed foods to extend their shelf life (Figure 13). Many restaurants (particularly fast food) used trans-fat for years, enabling them to replace the oil in their fryers less often. Trans-fats have since come under scrutiny for their health effects and many companies and food chains have begun to remove the fat from their products. Much of this came in response to measures by city and county governments to restrict trans-fat usage within their communities. The USDA put its own efforts to work by requiring trans-fat to be separated from other fats on food labels to fully inform consumers what they put in their bodies. In other words, it's a serious problem.

Trans-fats can raise LDL cholesterol levels in your blood. They can also lower your HDL (good) cholesterol levels. In

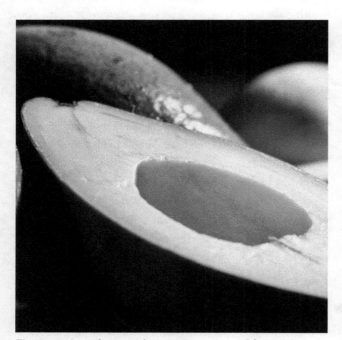

Figure 11. Avacados are rich in monounsaturated fat.

Higher Fat Foods	Lower Fat Alternative
Whole milk	Low-fat, reduced-fat, or fat-free milk
Sour cream	Plain low-fat yogurt
Cheese	Fat-free cheese, reduced calorie cheese
Ramen noodles	Rice or noodles
Pasta with white sauce	Pasta with red sauce
Regular ground beef	Extra-lean ground beef such as ground turkey
Pork	Pork tenderloin or trimmed, lean smoked ham
Whole eggs	Egg whites or egg substitutes
Regular margarine or butter	Light spread margarines, whipped butter

Figure 12. High fat foods can be substituted with healthier options.

Saturated Fat	Trans-Fat
High-fat cuts of meat (beef, lamb, pork)	Commercially baked pastries (cookies, muffins, cakes, pizza dough, pie crusts)
Chicken with the skin	Packaged snack foods (crackers, microwave popcorn, chips)
Whole-fat dairy products (cream/milk)	Stick margarine
Butter	Vegetable shortening
Palm and coconut oil (snack foods, non-dairy creamers, whipped topping)	Fried foods (french fries, fried chicken, chicken nuggets, breaded fish)
Ice Cream	Candy Bars
Cheese	Pre-mixed products (cake mix, pancake mix, chocolate drink mix)
Lard	Doughnuts, especially frosted or cream-filled

Figure 13. Where to find saturated and trans fats in common foods.

addition to high cholesterol levels, they cause inflammation that also can lead to heart disease, and stroke, and contribute to insulin resistance increasing your risk of Type 2 diabetes. Research conducted at the Harvard School of Public Health suggests that even a small amount of trans-fat, such as 2%, can increase your risk of heart disease by 23%. And those numbers are incremental. Every 2% increase adds an additional 23% risk!

How to Spot Trans-Fat on Labels

According to the Food and Drug Administration, tran-fat content must be expressed as grams per serving to the nearest 0.5g increment. If a serving contains less than 0.5g, the content, when declared, must be expressed as "0g." This means that even though the label indicates no trans-fat, you could still be eating it and, as discussed, even small amounts can be detrimental to your health. Look at the ingredients on the label. Any substance listed as hydrogenated or partially hydrogenated is trans-fat.

Proteins

Proteins are one of the three classes of macronutrients and the building blocks of life. Every cell in the human body contains them. Proteins are large, complex molecules that play many critical roles in the body. They do most of the work in your cells, and your body requires them for the structure, function, and regulation of its tissues and organs. You need protein in your diet for growth and development at every stage of life, from the womb to adulthood.

Function	Description	Example
Antibody	Antibodies bind to specific foreign particles, such as viruses and bacteria, to help protect the body.	Immunoglobulin G (IgG)
Enzyme	Enzymes carry out almost all of the thousands of chemical reactions that take place in cells. They also assist with the formation of new molecules by reading the genetic information stored in DNA.	Phenylalanine hydroxylase
Messenger	Messenger proteins, such as some types of hormones, transmit signals to coordinate biological processes between different cells, tissues, and organs.	Growth hormone
Structural component	These proteins provide structure and support for cells. On a larger scale, they also allow the body to move.	Actin
Transport/ storage	These proteins bind and carry atoms and small molecules within cells and throughout the body.	Ferritin

Figure 14. Proteins serve many purposes in the body.

Proteins consist of hundreds or thousands of smaller units called **amino acids**, which attach to one another in long chains. These acids are the organic compounds that build together to form protein. Up to 20 different types of amino acids can be combined to make a protein. Your body makes 11 amino acids on its own but 9 of them are essential, they must come from food.

The sequence of amino acids determines each protein's unique 3-dimensional structure and its specific function. Proteins can be described according to their large range of functions in the body (Figure 14). As you can see, amino acids from proteins have many jobs from building muscle and connective tissue fibers to making hormones and antibodies.

Their lowest priority is energy production. Proteins have 4 calories per gram, just like carbohydrates. Your body doesn't use this nutrient in the same way it uses carbohydrates. It constantly breaks proteins down into acids, reassembles or rearranges them, and uses them again. Your muscles are the only part of your body that really stores any protein. Your body only accesses muscle protein for energy when other sources, such as carbohydrates or fat, are depleted. This is why you need to maintain a healthy amount of body fat and carbohydrate intake, particularly when you exercise regularly. However, any excess protein that the body can't use for its daily functions converts to fat, just like everything else.

The human body needs amino acids in large enough amounts to maintain good health. Amino acids are found in animal sources such as meats, milk, fish, and eggs, but you don't need to eat animal products to get all the protein you need in your diet. They are also found in plant sources such as soy, beans, legumes, nut butters, and some grains (such as wheat germ and quinoa).

Complete, Incomplete, and Complementary Proteins

Dietary proteins aren't all the same. They consist of different combinations of amino acids and are characterized according to how many of the essential amino acids they provide.

Complete proteins contain all of the essential amino acids in adequate amounts. Animal foods (such as dairy products, eggs, meats, poultry, and seafood) and soy are complete protein sources, but they don't have the same nutritional value. The type of fat (saturated or unsaturated) and other nutrients they provide, for example, will vary depending upon the animal or soy source.

Incomplete proteins don't have enough, or any, of one or more of the essential amino acids, making the protein imbalanced. Most plant foods (such as beans and peas, grains, nuts and seeds, and vegetables) are incomplete protein sources. They are still high-quality foods both for protein and other nutrients. You just need to have a balance of various protein sources throughout the day to ensure you consume all of the essential amino acids.

Complementary proteins are two or more incomplete protein sources that, when eaten in combination (at the same meal or during the same day), compensate for each other's lack of amino acids. For example, grains are low in the amino acid lysine, while beans and nuts (legumes) are low in the amino acid methionine. When you eat grains and legumes together (such as rice and beans, or peanut butter on whole wheat bread), they form a complete protein.

Good Sources of Protein

One ounce (30 grams) of most protein-rich foods contains 7 grams of protein. One ounce equals, for example:

- 1 oz of meat fish or poultry
- 1 large egg
- ¼ cup of tofu
- ½ cup of cooked beans or lentils
- 1 Tbsp peanut butter

Healthy sources of protein include:

- Turkey or chicken with the skin removed, or bison
- Lean cuts of beef or pork, such as round, top sirloin, or tenderloin (trim away any visible fat)
- Fish or shellfish
- Pinto beans, black beans, kidney beans, lentils, split peas, or garbanzo beans
- Nuts and seeds, including almonds, hazelnuts, mixed nuts, peanuts, peanut butter, sunflower seeds, or walnuts (just watch how much you eat, because nuts are high in fat)
- Tofu, tempeh, and other soy protein products
- Low-fat dairy products
- Whole grains—these contain more protein than refined or "white" products

Food	Serving	Calories	Protein (g)
Black Beans	.5 cup	114	8
Quinoa	1 cup	222	8
Tofu	.5 cup	94	10
Soy Milk	1 cup	132	8
Peas	.5 cup	67	5
Spinach, cooked	.5 cup	41	3
Oatmeal	.5 cup	79	3
Pumpkin Seeds	1 oz	159	9
Sunflower Seeds	1 oz	140	6
Peanut Butter	2 tbsp	188	7
Almonds	1 oz	163	6
Pistachios	1 oz	185	4

Figure 15. Foods with high protein content.

You'll notice that the meat selections above are all "lean" meats. The USDA recommends that most of your protein sources be lean selections to cut down on saturated fat. Trimming away fat, removing skin, and buying lean cuts of your favorite meats can help you do this. They recommend choosing seafood at least twice a week as the main protein food, particularly those rich in omega-3 fatty acids, such as: salmon steak or filet, salmon loaf, or grilled or baked trout. They also suggest choosing beans, peas, or soy products as a main dish or part of a meal often. Some choices are:

- Chili with kidney or pinto beans
- Stir-fried tofu
- Split pea, lentil, minestrone, or white bean soups
- Baked beans
- Black bean enchiladas
- Garbanzo or kidney beans on a chef's salad
- Rice and beans
- Veggie burgers
- Hummus (chickpeas spread) on pita bread

Choosing unsalted nuts as a snack, on salads, or in main dishes can also help you integrate healthy proteins in your diet. Here are some ways to use nuts to *replace* meat or poultry:

- Use pine nuts in pesto sauce for pasta
- Add slivered almonds to steamed vegetables
- Add toasted peanuts or cashews to a vegetable stir-fry
- Sprinkle a few nuts on top of low-fat ice cream or frozen yogurt
- Add walnuts or pecans to a green salad instead of cheese or meat

Meatless or Meat-Restricted Diets

You probably know at least one or two people who have chosen **vegetarian** or **vegan** diets to avoid animal proteins, either for health, personal, political, or environmental reasons. You may even have that one vegan friend (or maybe it's you) that doesn't seem to be able to eat anything when you go out for burgers with friends. You've watched them eat a pile of lettuce so many times that you worry they will waste away. Your vegetarian friends fill up on so many processed carbohydrates, even French fries, that they seem to be defeating the purpose of their "healthy" diet.

Because they don't consume animal protein, this means that many of the forms of protein they consume are considered incomplete. This doesn't mean, however, that they can't maintain adequate nutrition levels. It just means that they need to seek out a variety of proteins. Some proteins, like quinoa and soy, have all the essential amino acids. It also helps to eat whole foods as much as possible, avoiding processed products that easily fill your stomach and leave no room for good sources of nutrition. This chart can give you an idea of the types of plant sources that are rich in protein (Figure 15).

Recommended Protein Intake

The amount of protein you need in your diet depends on your size. The recommended daily intake of protein for healthy adults is 0.8g per kilogram (0.36g per pound) of body weight. A man weighing 200 pounds should be eating about 72g. The recommended AMDR for protein is 10–35% of your daily calories. Studies suggest that the average American man consumes approximately 100g each day and the average woman 70g, more protein than they really need for good health.

Individuals looking to increase muscle mass through strength training may need to increase their protein intake. But they may be getting enough from food without any additional effort. You probably know proteins as the major component of muscle. Some people may think the way to build body muscle is to eat high-protein diets and use protein powders, supplements and shakes. However, most Americans already eat about 12–18% or more of their calories as protein. Before adding protein to your diet, and saturated fat along with it, keep track of the amount of protein you already consume to determine if the addition is really necessary.

Women who are pregnant or breastfeeding also need more protein (up to 0.59 grams per pound of body weight). The daily recommended intake for pregnant women is 71g a day, but this may change based on weight.

Health Risks

The medical community has raised many concerns about high-protein diets. There's no solid scientific evidence that most Americans need more protein. These diets operate on varying ideas about the consumption of carbohydrates, particularly grains and sugars. The general theory is that carbs create sugar, which creates fat, which creates problems. Less carbs means less fat (again, in theory). The exact approaches vary. These diets often (though not always) boost protein intake at the expense of some fruits and vegetables, and particularly grains, so dieters can miss out on healthy nutrients. This could possibly increase their risk of cancer.

Many high-protein diets are high in saturated fat and low in fiber. Research shows this combination can increase cholesterol levels and increase the risk of heart disease and stroke. These diets generally recommend dieters receive 30% to 50% of their total calories from protein. Depending upon the type of protein consumed, this could lead to an amount of saturated fat far above and beyond the American Heart Association's recommendation of 7% and the recommended AMDR of no more than 10%.

In addition to an increased risk of heart disease, too much protein can impact other parts of your body. People on high-protein diets excrete more calcium through their urine than do those not on a high-protein diet. If a person sticks to a high-protein diet long term, the loss of calcium could increase their risk of developing osteoporosis. Additionally, people with kidney disease should consult their health care provider before starting a high-protein diet. Research suggests people with impaired kidneys may lose kidney function more rapidly if they eat excessive amounts of protein—especially animal protein.

The jury is still out on the merits of low carbohydrate, high protein intake. Just as with the controversies over saturated fat, it's important to remember balance. As with anything in life, too much of a good thing is usually no longer good, with few exceptions.

Vitamins

When you were a child, your parents probably gave you a sweet, crunchy, animal-shaped treat every morning—but only one. Unlike your other snacks of fruit, cheese, or crackers, you only got a tiny bite of this snack. You were told it was good for you, so why couldn't you have more? Well, you may not have even needed that one you got. The truth is that most healthy people don't need a vitamin supplement if their diet is adequate.

Vitamins are a group of substances that the body needs for normal cell function, growth, development, and to maintain life and health. How they are stored depends upon the type of vitamin (more later on this). Vitamins have many different jobs—helping you resist infections, keeping your nerves healthy, and helping your body get energy from food or your blood to clot properly. By following the Dietary Guidelines,

Sources of Fat-Soluble Vitamins	
Vitamin A	Dark-colored fruit, dark leafy vegetables, egg yolk, fortified milk and dairy products (cheese, yogurt, butter, and cream), liver, beef, and fish
Vitamin E	Avocado, dark green vegetables (spinach, broccoli, asparagus, and turnip greens), margarine (made from safflower, corn, and sunflower oil), oils (safflower, corn, and sunflower), papaya and mango, seeds and nuts, wheat germ and wheat germ oil
Vitamin D	Fish (fatty fish such as salmon, mackerel, herring, and orange roughy), fish liver oils (cod's liver oil), fortified cereals, fortified milk and dairy products (cheese, yogurt, butter, and cream)
Vitamin K	Cabbage, cauliflower, cereals, dark green vegetables (broccoli, brussels sprouts, and asparagus), dark leafy vegetables (spinach, kale, collards, and turnip greens), fish, liver, beef, and eggs

Figure 16. Some foods provide several different vitamins.

Sources of Water-Soluble Vitamins	
Biotin	Chocolate, cereal, egg yolk, legumes, milk, nuts, organ meats (liver, kidney), pork, yeast
Niacin (vitamin B3)	Avocado, eggs, enriched breads and fortified cereals, fish (tuna and salt-water fish), lean meats, legumes, nuts, potato, poultry
Thiamine (vitamin B1)	Dried milk, egg, enriched bread and flour, lean meats, legumes (dried beans), nuts and seeds, organ meats, peas, whole grains
Vitamin B12	Meat, eggs, fortified foods such as soymilk, milk and milk products, organ meats (liver and kidney), poultry, shellfish
Folate	Asparagus and broccoli, beets, brewer's yeast, dried beans (cooked pinto, navy, kidney, and lima), fortified cereals, green, leafy vegetables (spinach and romaine lettuce), lentils, oranges and orange juice, peanut butter, wheat germ
Pantothenic acid	Avocado, broccoli, kale, and other vegetables in the cabbage family, eggs, legumes and lentils, milk, mushroom, organ meats, poultry, white and sweet potatoes, whole-grain cereals
Pyroxidine (vitamin B6)	Avocado, banana, legumes (dried beans), meat, nuts, poultry, whole grains (milling and processing removes a lot of this vitamin)
Vitamin C (ascorbic acid)	Broccoli, brussels sprouts, cabbage, cauliflower, citrus fruits, potatoes, spinach, strawberries, tomato juice, tomatoes
NOTE: Animal sources of vitamin B12 are absorbed much better by the body than plant sources.	

Figure 17. Vitamins are available naturally across many food groups.

you will get enough of most of these vitamins from food.

There are 13 essential vitamins the body needs to work properly. They are: vitamins A, B1, B2, B3, B6, B12, C, D, E, and K; pantothenic acid, biotin (B7), and folate (folic acid and B9).

Types of Vitamins

Vitamins are grouped into two categories: fat-soluble and water-soluble. **Fat-soluble** vitamins remain stored in the body for long periods of time in the liver and fat tissues. Your body does not need these every day, and they absorb more slowly than water-soluble. They do need to be replaced in the body regularly. The four fat-soluble vitamins are vitamins A, D, E, and K. These vitamins absorb more easily in the body in the presence of dietary fat (Figure 16).

There are nine **water-soluble** vitamins. The body must use water-soluble vitamins right away. Any leftover water-soluble vitamins leave the body through the urine. Vitamin B12 is the only water-soluble vitamin that can be stored in the liver for many years (Figure 17).

Function and Sources

Each of the vitamins listed below has an important job in the body (Figure 18). A vitamin deficiency occurs when you do not get enough of a certain vitamin, which can cause health problems. For example, if you don't get enough vitamin C, you could become anemic. Vitamin A prevents night blindness. Not eating enough vitamin-rich foods—such as fruits, vegetables, beans, lentils, whole grains and fortified dairy—may increase your risk for health problems, including heart disease, cancer, and poor bone health (see section on "Deficiencies in Vitamins and Minerals").

Antioxidants

Antioxidants are man-made or natural substances that may prevent or delay some types of cell damage, and counteract the damage of free radicals. **Free radicals** are highly unstable molecules that are naturally formed when you exercise and when your body converts food into energy. Your body can also be exposed to free radicals from a variety of environmental sources, such as cigarette smoke, air pollution, and sunlight. Free radicals can cause "oxidative stress," a process that can trigger cell damage. Oxidative stress is thought to play a role in a variety of diseases including cancer, cardiovascular diseases, diabetes, Alzheimer's disease, Parkinson's disease, and eye diseases such as cataracts and age-related macular degeneration.

Diets high in vegetables and fruits, which are good

Vitamin	Job
Vitamin A	Helps form and maintain healthy teeth, bones, soft tissue, mucus membranes, and skin
Vitamin B6 (pyridoxine)	Helps form red blood cells and maintain brain function
Vitamin B12	Important for metabolism, helps form red blood cells and maintain the central nervous system
Vitamin C (ascorbic acid)	An antioxidant that promotes healthy teeth and gums; helps the body absorb iron, maintain healthy tissue, and heal wounds
Vitamin D (the "sunshine" vitamin) Most Vitamin D comes from sunlight	Helps the body absorb calcium for the normal development and maintenance of healthy teeth and bones; helps maintain proper blood levels of calcium and phosphorus
Vitamin E (tocopherol)	An antioxidant that helps the body form red blood cells and use vitamin K
Vitamin K	Without it blood would not stick together (coagulate); some studies suggest that it is important for bone health
Biotin	Essential for the metabolism of proteins and carbohydrates, and in the production of hormones and cholesterol
Niacin (B vitamin)	Helps maintain healthy skin and nerves; also has cholesterol-lowering effects
Folate	Works with vitamin B12 to help form red blood cells; needed for the production of DNA, which con-trols tissue growth and cell function; important during pregnancy to avoid birth defects such as spina bifida
Pantothenic Acid	Essential for the metabolism of food; plays a role in the production of hormones and cholesterol
Riboflavin (vitamin B2)	Works with the other B vitamins; important for body growth and the production of red blood cells
Thiamine (vitamin B1)	Helps the body cells change carbohydrates into energy; essential for heart function and healthy nerve cells

Figure 18. Vitamins perform important functions in the body.

sources of antioxidants, have been found to be healthy (Figure 19). Examples of antioxidants include beta-carotene, lutein, lycopene, selenium, and vitamins A, C, and E. Antioxidant molecules have been shown to counteract oxidative stress in laboratory experiments. However, there is debate as to whether consuming large amounts of antioxidants in supplement form actually benefits health. There is also some concern that consuming antioxidant supplements in excessive doses may be harmful (see discussion on the "Recommended Vitamin Intake").

Phytonutrients

Antioxidants are a type of phytochemical, or **phytonutrients**. Plants must produce these chemicals in order for them to stay healthy. For example, some phytonutrients protect plants from insect attacks, while others protect against radiation from UV rays. Phytonutrients can also provide signif-

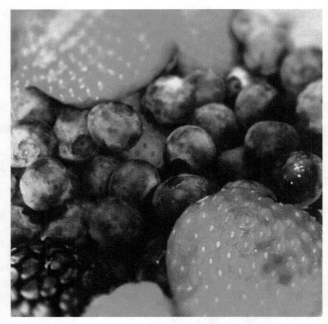

Figure 19. Berries are a common source of antioxidants.

icant benefits for humans who eat plant foods. Phytonutrient-rich foods include colorful fruits and vegetables, legumes, nuts, tea, whole grains and many spices. They affect human health but are not considered nutrients that are essential for life, like carbohydrates, protein, fats, vitamins, and minerals.

Phytonutrients help the body because of their antioxidant and anti-inflammatory properties. They may also enhance immunity and intercellular communication, repair DNA damage from exposure to toxins, detoxify carcinogens, and alter estrogen metabolism. The US Department of Agriculture (USDA) notes that consuming a phytonutrient-rich diet seems to be an "effective strategy" for reducing cancer and heart disease risks.

Many phytonutrients give plants their pigment, so a good way to tell if a fruit or vegetable is rich in phytonutrients can be by its color. Look for deep-hued foods like berries, dark greens, melons, and spices. These foods also are rich in flavor and aroma, which makes them more palatable. But some phytonutrient-rich foods have little color, like onions and garlic, and you don't want to forget these flavor sources. The different types of phytonutrients each do different things and offer different benefits.

Lignans can mimic the effects of estrogen, so lignans are considered phytoestrogens, though they can also affect the body in other ways. Like all phytonutrients, these are found in fruits and vegetables, especially kale, broccoli, flaxseeds, apricots, and strawberries. They are particularly abundant in seeds and whole grains. Lignans are associated with preventing hormone-related cancers because of their estrogen-like activity, and potentially other cancers, such as endometrial and ovarian.

Resveratrol has gotten a good deal of buzz in recent years because large concentrations of it are found in red wine. The best-known source of resveratrol is grapes. You will also find it in peanuts, grape juice, cocoa, blueberries and cranberries. Some studies suggest that resveratrol may help slow cognitive decline and improve insulin sensitivity and glucose tolerance though more research is needed.

Carotenoids are the yellow, orange, and red pigments in plants, such as carrots, yams, sweet potatoes, papaya, watermelon, cantaloupe, mangos, spinach, kale, tomatoes, bell peppers, and oranges. The most common carotenoids are alpha-carotene, beta-carotene, beta-cryptoxanthin, lutein, zeaxanthin and lycopene. Carotenoids contribute to eye health, immune system activity, intercellular communication, and a reduced risk of cancer and cardiovascular disease.

Ellagic acid, also called tannin, is found in raspberries, strawberries, blackberries, cranberries, grapes, pomegranates, and walnuts. The body absorbs this acid rapidly. It can also be produced during the body's process of breaking down larger phytonutrients. Ellagic acid helps in reducing inflammation, reducing blood pressure and arterial plaque, and may have properties that help your body remove carcinogens before they metabolize.

Flavonoids are a very large group of phytonutrients known for its heart benefits, contributions to overall longevity, and reduction of cancer risk. Flavonoids can be found across a large range of foods, such as apples, onions, coffee, grapefruit, tea, berries, chocolate, legumes, red wine, broccoli, cabbage, kale, leeks, tomatoes, ginger, lemons, parsley, carrots and buckwheat.

Recommended Vitamin Intake

When the winter sets in in most of the country, you might find yourself craving some sunshine. After three weeks of straight rain or snow and minimal sun, you might be feeling weak, achy, and a bit gloomy. The weatherman says to start popping vitamin D because the sun will not be out any time soon. Do you run to the drug store, or is there a better way?

Recommended amounts of vitamins vary by person, and the intake amount can be supplemented, but is not considered safe for everyone. Vitamin supplementation should only occur where deficiencies are evident. For example, men over 50 may need a B12 supplement and everyone who lives west of the Cascades in the Pacific Northwest can probably use some additional vitamin D. According to the *2015 Dietary Guidelines for Americans*, individuals should aim to meet their nutrient needs primarily through healthy eating patterns that include nutrient-dense foods. These contain essential vitamins and minerals and also dietary fiber and other naturally occurring substances that may have positive health effects.

It can be pretty difficult to keep track of how much you need of each vitamin. You've seen the list so far, and it's quite substantial. The bottom line is this—eat a large variety of healthy, nutrient-dense foods from all of the five food groups, making sure to get proteins, fruits, vegetables, grains, and dairy. That's it. You will only need to supplement if you have a particular illness or condition (like pregnancy) or have a true vitamin deficiency.

Minerals

Minerals are micronutrients that come from the Earth and can't be made by us. Plants take in minerals from the soil, and we get most of the minerals in our diets from the plants we eat ourselves or from eating the animals that eat them. In some areas, minerals may also be present in the water people drink. Minerals from plant sources can also vary with the mineral content of the local soil.

You need minerals for your body to stay healthy. Your body uses them for many different jobs, including keeping your bones, muscles, heart, and brain working properly, and for producing enzymes and hormones. Most people get the number of minerals they need by eating a wide variety of foods.

There are two kinds of minerals: macrominerals and trace minerals. You need larger amounts of **macrominerals**. They include calcium, phosphorus, magnesium, sodium chloride, and potassium among others. You only need small amounts of **trace minerals** such as iron, copper, iodine, zinc, chromium, and selenium.

Calcium

You have more **calcium** in your body than any other mineral, which is great because it has many important jobs. The body stores more than 99% of its calcium in the bones and teeth to help make and keep them strong. Bone itself undergoes continuous remodeling, with constant resorption and accumulation of calcium into new bone. The calcium not used by the bones is stored throughout the body in blood, muscle, and the fluid between cells. Your body needs calcium to help muscles and blood vessels contract and expand, to secrete hormones and enzymes, and to send messages through the nervous system.

Foods rich in calcium include: dairy products such as milk, cheese, and yogurt; leafy, green vegetables, fish with soft bones that you eat, such as canned sardines and salmon; and calcium-enriched foods such as breakfast cereals, fruit juices, soy and rice drinks, and tofu.

The exact amount of calcium you need depends on your age and other factors. Women need between 1000–1300mg of calcium each day, and men between 1000–1200mg. Growing children and teenagers need more calcium than most adults, but older adults need plenty of calcium to prevent osteoporosis.

The Tolerable Upper Intake Levels (ULs) for calcium established by the Food and Nutrition Board are 2500mg per day for people aged 19–50 and 2000 for those over 50.

Getting too much calcium from foods is rare—excess intakes are more likely to be caused by using calcium supplements. Studies indicate that approximately 5% of women older than 50 years have estimated total calcium intakes (from foods and supplements) that exceed the UL by about 300–365mg.

Sodium Chloride

Sodium occurs naturally in most foods. We often use the words "salt" and "sodium" interchangeably, but they do not mean the same thing. Sodium is a mineral and one of the chemical elements found in salt. Salt (also known by its chemical name, sodium chloride) is a crystal-like compound abundant in nature and used to flavor and preserve food. Many foods, such as milk, beets, shellfish, eggs, and celery naturally contain sodium, as does drinking water, although the amount varies depending on the source.

Sodium is an essential nutrient, and your body needs it in relatively small amounts (provided that substantial sweating does not occur). Sodium supports many bodily functions such as fluid balance, muscle contraction, and nervous system function. As a food ingredient, sodium is used in curing meat, baking, thickening, retaining moisture, enhancing flavor (including the flavor of other ingredients), and as a preservative.

Most of the sodium you consume doesn't actually come from the salt-shaker. It is added to various food products. It flies under the radar with names like monosodium glutamate, sodium nitrite, sodium saccharin, baking soda (sodium bicarbonate), and sodium benzoate. These are all forms of sodium. About 75% of dietary sodium comes from eating packaged and restaurant foods, whereas only a small portion (11%) comes from salt added to food when cooking or eating.

Condiments and seasonings such as Worcestershire sauce, soy sauce, onion salt, garlic salt, and bouillon cubes contain sodium. Processed and cured meats, like bacon, ham, and lunchmeat, tend to be high in sodium. Processed food, like potato chips and crackers, and canned foods like soups and vegetables also contain added sodium. Fast foods generally have high quantities. Even breads, cheese, pasta, and pizza contain added sodium. Check the Nutrition Facts label on foods to learn how much sodium is in a serving (Figure 20)).

Expect health problems to develop in the not-too-distant future if you consistently consume a lot of high-sodium foods. The daily limit for sodium is 2,300mg a day and about 90% of Americans eat too much. Your kidneys control how

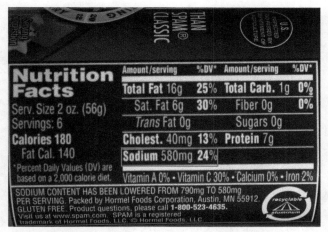

Figure 20. Nutrition Facts labels contain information about dietary content and %Daily Values.

much sodium is in your body. If you have too much and your kidneys can't get rid it, sodium builds up in your blood. This can lead to high blood pressure, which can lead to other health problems.

Potassium

Potassium is a type of electrolyte. It helps your nerves to function, muscles to contract, and your heartbeat to stay regular. It also helps move nutrients into cells and waste products out. A diet rich in potassium helps to offset some of sodium's harmful effects on blood pressure. Most people get all the potassium they need from what they eat and drink.

Foods rich in potassium include:

- Leafy greens, such as spinach and collards

- Fruit from vines, such as grapes and blackberries

- Root vegetables, such as carrots and potatoes

- Citrus fruits, such as oranges and grapefruit

Your kidneys help to keep the right amount of potassium in your body. If you have chronic kidney disease, your kidneys may not remove extra potassium from the blood. Some medicines also can raise your potassium level. If you have one of these issues, you may need a special diet to lower the amount of potassium that you eat.

Iron

Like the other minerals, the body needs **iron** for many functions. For example, iron is part of hemoglobin, a protein that carries oxygen from your lungs throughout your body tis-

sues. It helps your muscles store and use oxygen. Iron is also part of many other proteins and enzymes.

Most of the elemental iron in adults is in hemoglobin. Much of the remaining iron is stored in various forms in the liver, spleen, and bone marrow or is located in muscle tissue. Humans typically lose only small amounts of iron in urine, feces, the gastrointestinal tract, and skin, though loss is greater in menstruating women.

Foods rich in iron include red meat, pork, poultry, seafood, beans, dark green leafy vegetables, dried fruit, iron-fortified cereals, breads, pasta, and peas. Your body absorbs iron best from meat. If you eat a primarily vegetarian diet, you may need to increase your intake of some of these other iron-rich foods. Vitamin C also helps improve the absorption of iron, so eating citrus foods as you eat iron-rich foods can help increase iron levels.

Your body needs the right amount of iron. People in the US usually get adequate amounts of iron from their diets, but infants, young children, teenage girls, pregnant women, and premenopausal women have a higher risk of getting too little. Men need approximately 8mg per day. Women need 18mg per day until around age 50 when their iron needs decrease to 8mg. Pregnant women need more at 27mg per day.

If you have too little iron, you may develop iron deficiency anemia, a common type of anemia. In this condition, the blood doesn't have enough healthy red blood cells. Red blood cells carry oxygen to the body's tissues. Without them, you could find yourself feeling fatigued and short of breath. Causes of low iron levels include blood loss, poor diet, or an inability to absorb enough iron from foods.

Too much iron, however, can damage your body and lead to iron poisoning. This usually occurs from taking too many iron supplements, though some people have an inherited disease called hemochromatosis, which causes too much iron to build up in the body. Sudden intakes of more than 20mg per kg of iron from supplements or medicines can lead to gastric upset, constipation, nausea, abdominal pain, vomiting, and faintness, especially if food not taken with food. In severe cases (e.g., one-time ingestions of 60mg per kg), overdoses of iron can lead to multisystem organ failure, coma, convulsions, and even death. You should see your health care provider for blood screening before taking an iron supplement.

Deficiencies in Vitamins and Minerals

Cases of people having serious shortages in vitamins and minerals aren't as common in the US as they are in countries that lack sufficient access to healthy foods. But the US isn't immune to poverty-linked food concerns. We just don't experience them at the same level. Many of our foods are fortified with nutrients that we need, our school systems work hard to provide children with balanced diets, and our communities frequently strive to help people gain access to food in times of need. However, even those of us who don't struggle to access a healthy diet can sometimes find ourselves coming up short with vitamins and minerals. This happens for a variety of reasons from a poor diet reliant on fast-food drive-thrus, a lack of understanding of what foods are healthy, an illness, poverty, or just inadequate planning.

According to the most recent US Dietary Guidelines, there are 7 important nutrients in food that most Americans aren't getting in sufficient amounts: calcium, potassium, fiber, magnesium, and vitamins A, C, and E. Every vitamin has a purpose in your body. You could begin to feel adverse effects if you consistently don't get enough of a particular vitamin in your diet. Most Americans have access to a variety of foods, so unless you are limiting your diet or have an underlying medical condition, you aren't likely to have a noticeable deficiency.

Certain illnesses, however, could suggest a deficiency. One such illness is anemia. Vitamin deficiency anemia is a lack of healthy red blood cells caused when you have lower than normal amounts of certain vitamins. Vitamins linked to vitamin deficiency anemia include folate, vitamin B-12, and vitamin C. This anemia can occur if you don't eat enough foods rich in these vitamins or if your body has trouble absorbing or processing these vitamins.

Not all anemias are caused by a vitamin deficiency. Other causes include iron deficiency and certain blood diseases (see section on "Iron"). That's why it's important to have your health care provider diagnose and treat your anemia. It can usually be corrected with vitamin supplements and changes to your diet, but it is important to know which deficiency exists.

One of the most common deficiencies is in vitamin D—not many foods have naturally occurring vitamin D. Your body also requires a regular dose of sunlight to get vitamin D generating, which can be a challenge in some areas and at certain times of the year. Vitamin D deficiency impacts your ability to absorb calcium as well, which leads to bone weakness

and diseases or injuries related to bones, such as osteoporosis.

You can fix vitamin and mineral deficiencies primarily with good planning and attention to a healthy diet rich in lean protein, fruits, vegetables, whole grains, and low-fat dairy products, which will be discussed more in this chapter. If you think you may need a supplement for any vitamin or mineral, take a close look at your diet first and the consult your health care practitioner.

Supplements and Safety

Many adults in the US take one or more dietary supplements either every day or occasionally, often without much thought. Supplements are not regulated by the FDA, so what you take over-the-counter may not be effective or may interact with other medications you are taking—and, again, that's if you need it at all.

Today's dietary supplements include vitamins, minerals, herbals and botanicals, amino acids, enzymes, and many other products. They come in traditional tablets, capsules, and powders, as well as in drinks and energy bars. Popular supplements include vitamins D and E; minerals like calcium and iron; herbs such as echinacea and garlic; and specialty products like glucosamine, probiotics, and fish oils (Figure 21).

According to the National Agricultural Library's Food and Nutrition Information Center, you should ask yourself one big question before taking a supplement—Do I really need this? First and foremost, you should try to you're your nutritional needs by eating a variety of foods as outlined in the *2015 Dietary Guidelines for Americans*. Vitamin or mineral supplements are not a replacement for a healthy diet. Remember

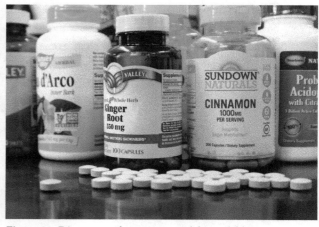

Figure 21. Dietary supplements are widely available.

that in addition to vitamins and minerals, foods also contain hundreds of naturally occurring substances that can help protect your health.

In some cases, vitamin/mineral supplements or fortified foods may be useful for providing nutrients that may otherwise be eaten in less than recommended amounts. If you are already eating the recommended amount of a nutrient, you may not get any further health benefit from taking a supplement. In some cases, supplements and fortified foods may actually cause you to exceed safe levels of intake of nutrients. (Note that fortified foods are those to which one or more essential nutrients have been added to increase their nutritional value.)

The *2015 Dietary Guidelines for Americans* makes these recommendations for certain groups of people:

People over age 50 should consume vitamin B12. This should be in its crystalline form from fortified foods (like some fortified breakfast cereals) or as a supplement. Note that older adults often have a reduced ability to absorb vitamin B12 from foods. However, crystalline vitamin B12, the type of vitamin B12 used in supplements and in fortified foods, is much more easily absorbed.

Women of childbearing age, including adolescents, should eat foods that are a source of iron. The most common source would be from meats, but they could eat iron-rich plant foods (like cooked dry beans or spinach) or iron-fortified foods (like fortified cereals) along with a source of vitamin C.

Women who are pregnant or may become pregnant should consume adequate synthetic folic acid daily. This is possible from fortified foods or supplements in addition to food forms of folate from a varied diet.

Older adults, people with dark skin, and people who get insufficient exposure to sunlight should consume extra vitamin D. This can be gained from from vitamin D-fortified foods and/or supplements.

People who smoke need more vitamin C. This need is due in part to increased oxidative stress. For this reason, it is recommended that these individuals need 35mg more vitamin C per day than people who don't smoke.

The Food and Drug Administration recommends discussing these questions with your health care provider when considering whether you should take a vitamin/mineral supplement:

- Do you eat fewer than 2 meals per day?

- Is your diet restricted? That is, do you not eat meat or dairy products, or eat fewer than five servings of fruits and vegetables per day?

- Do you eat alone most of the time?

- Without wanting to, have you lost or gained more than 10 pounds in the last 6 months?

- Do you take 3 or more prescription or over-the-counter medicines per day?

- Do you have 3 or more alcoholic drinks per day?

If you answer yes to one or more of these questions, it may give you an idea of why you may be deficient. It is also a good idea to speak to your provider to determine what supplements are necessary if you cannot get the vitamin from your diet. The **UL**—the maximum usual daily intake level at which no risk of adverse health effects is expected for most people—is not considered a recommended level of intake. Currently, there is no research demonstrating a benefit for healthy individuals to consume quantities of nutrients above the recommended dietary allowance or adequate intake, except in a few specific cases. In short, you have no real reason to take nutritional supplements unless you have a diagnosed vitamin deficiency and your health care provider recommends them.

Many supplements contain active ingredients that can have strong effects in the body. Always be alert to the possibility of unexpected side effects, especially when taking a new product. Supplements are most likely to cause side effects or harm when people take them instead of prescribed medicines or when people take many supplements in combination. Some supplements can increase the risk of bleeding or, if a person takes them before or after surgery, they can affect the person's response to anesthesia. Dietary supplements can also interact with certain prescription drugs in ways that might cause problems. Here are just a few examples:

- Vitamin K can reduce the ability of the blood thinner Coumadin® to prevent blood from clotting.

- St. John's wort can speed the breakdown of many drugs (including antidepressants and birth control pills) and thereby reduce these drugs' effectiveness.

- Antioxidant supplements, like vitamins C and E, might reduce the effectiveness of some types of cancer chemotherapy.

Keep in mind that some ingredients found in dietary supplements are added to a growing number of foods, including breakfast cereals and beverages. As a result, you may be getting more of these ingredients than you think, and more might not be better. Taking more than you need is always more expensive and can also raise your risk of experiencing side effects. For example, getting too much vitamin A can cause headaches and liver damage, reduce bone strength, and cause birth defects. Excess iron causes nausea and vomiting and may damage the liver and other organs.

Be especially cautious about taking dietary supplements if you are pregnant or nursing. Also, be careful about giving them (beyond a basic multivitamin/mineral product) to a child—your parent was right about having just one. Most dietary supplements have not been fully tested for safety in pregnant women, nursing mothers, or children.

Overdose

In large doses, some vitamins have documented side effects that tend to be more severe. The likelihood of consuming too much of any vitamin from food is remote, but overdose (vitamin poisoning) from vitamin supplementation does occur. At high enough dosages, some vitamins cause side effects such as nausea, diarrhea, and vomiting. You can usually resolve side effects by reducing the dosage. The doses of vitamins differ because individual tolerances can vary widely and appear to be related to age and state of health. The majority of overdoses, though not fatal, happen in children under the age of six.

Water

Nearly every living thing requires **water** to survive. It's impossible to overstate the value of drinking enough water every day for your overall health. Nearly every part of your body contains and relies on water to function, from the transportation of nutrients to the processing of waste, from regulation of body temperature to lubrication of your joints and tissues. Without it, the body simply cannot function effectively. And as an added bonus, plain drinking water has zero calories, so it can also help with managing body weight and reducing caloric intake when substituted for drinks with calories, like regular soda.

Water Storage in the Body

In some organisms, up to 90% of their body weight comes from water. Up to 60% of the adult human body is water. Your brain, heart, lungs, skin, muscles, kidneys, and even bones all contain significant amounts.

Different people have different percentages of their bodies made up of water. Babies have the most, being born at about 78%. By one year of age, that amount drops to about 65%. In adult men, about 60% of their bodies are water. However, fat tissue does not have as much water as lean tissue. In adult women, fat makes up more of the body than men, so they have about 55% of their bodies made of water. Likewise, people who have an excess of body fat will have less water.

It's understandable given the large role of water and its prevalence in the body that you need lots of it for good health. You lose a good portion, close to one liter, each day just from breathing, sweating, and through bowel movements. You lose another 1.5 liters by urinating. You lose even more than these averages if you're physically active.

Men need approximately 3.7 liters (15 cups) of fluid each day, and women 2.7 (11 cups). Some of this water comes from food. However, you should get about 80% of it or more from the liquids you drink. Men should drink 13 cups and women 9 cups each day. You need even more water when you're ill (having vomiting, diarrhea, or running a fever), exercising, or in a hot or humid climate. People with excess body fat have less water in their bodies, as mentioned, and so will need to drink a bit more.

So how do you know if you are getting enough? Many of us experience mild forms of dehydration without even realizing it. Symptoms include but are not limited to: fatigue, headaches, dizziness or lightheadedness, irritability and mood swings, constipation, urinary tract infections, dry skin and chapped lips, and urine that is too yellow in color (it should be light yellow, like lemonade).

Getting Enough Water

Healthy people typically meet their fluid needs by drinking when they are thirsty and drinking with meals. As noted, about 20% of your water intake also comes from foods, with fruits and vegetables serving as better sources of water than grains. Cooked grains, like rice or oats, will have some water injected as part of the cooking process. Fruit, like watermelon, retains plenty of water. Anything you drink contains water as well, though it's good to be mindful of any diuretic side effects of your beverage, which can potentially lead to mild dehydration. Diuretics—like coffee, alcohol, or drinks with added sugar—make you urinate more frequently.

If you think you are not getting enough water, these tips may help:

Carry a water bottle. This is great for easy access when you are at work or running errands.

Keep freezer safe water bottles in the freezer. Take one with you for ice-cold water all day long.

Choose water instead of sugar-sweetened beverages. This can also help with weight management. Substituting water for one 20-ounce sugar sweetened soda will save you about 240 calories.

Choose water when eating out. Generally, you will save money and reduce calories.

Add a wedge of lime or lemon to your water. This can help improve the taste and help you drink more water than you usually do.

Improving Your Nutrition

Assessing your current nutritional habits is a great first step. You may think that you eat fairly healthy but may learn that you aren't eating enough nutrient-dense foods for good health. You may find, as is common for many people, that you take in more food (energy) than you can expend each day. Look at the food diary you've created and consider how much of the Daily Values you are likely taking in and how much energy you're consuming. This can also help you as you plan.

The benefits of healthy nutrition are most apparent in their relationship to body composition (see Chapter 6). Lowering your energy intake (fewer calories) helps create the negative energy balance needed to manage weight and obtain or maintain a healthy proportion of body fat and muscle. Much of this can be done with portion control and the selection of healthy foods, rather than strictly counting calories.

You can improve your nutrition by following some of the recommendations in the first section of this chapter, usually in conjunction with a combination of meal plans and careful assessments of your food's nutrient content. These plans focus on following some basic steps for meeting the established US Dietary Guidelines for nutrition:

Follow a healthy eating pattern across the lifespan. All food and beverage choices matter. Choose a healthy eating pattern at an appropriate calorie level to help achieve and maintain a healthy body weight, support nutrient adequacy, and reduce the risk of chronic disease.

Focus on variety, nutrient density, and amount. To meet nutrient needs within calorie limits, choose a variety of nutrient-dense foods across and within all food groups in recommended amounts.

Limit calories from added sugars and saturated fats and reduce sodium intake. Follow an eating pattern low in added sugars, saturated fats, and sodium. Cut back on foods and beverages higher in these components to amounts that fit within healthy eating patterns.

Shift to healthier food and beverage choices. Choose nutrient-dense foods and beverages across and within all food groups in place of less healthy choices. Consider cultural and personal preferences to make these shifts easier to accomplish and maintain.

Support healthy eating patterns for all. Everyone has a role in helping to create and support healthy eating patterns in multiple settings nationwide, from home to school to work to communities.

Fortunately, several plans are customizable for your individual needs, goals, and preferences. You can approach healthy eating through a structured program, like the ones offered here, or through an approach of your own. This section offers just a few but they should help you on your path toward improving or maintaining nutritional balance in your life.

Setting Goals for Nutrition

You can use the principle of SMART goals for nutrition as well. You may be one of those all or nothing people when it comes to a new meal plan. You may need to ease your way into it, particularly if it is a large change. It's okay to start with small changes. For example, you may have determined that your saturated fat intake far exceeds the recommended amount of 10% per day. Consider some small, achievable changes to begin:

Specific—I want to lower my saturated fat intake

Measurable—From 25% to 20%

Achievable—This is a small step

Relevant—This will reduce my risk of disease

Time-based—I will do this for 2 weeks then make further changes

You might begin by cooking your morning eggs in olive oil instead of butter and using less butter on your vegetables at dinner. You may have more changes needed in your diet and would rather give a structured plan your best effort. That's great too. Don't punish yourself if you have brief lapses. If you have trouble sticking to it, try following it 4 or 5 days a week and giving yourself a bit more flexibility on the other days. Try using some of the tips for converting your favorite meals into healthier versions. Give yourself a pat on the back for good choices and don't throw in the towel if you have a lapse. There are many ways to make gradual but sustainable changes in your nutrition and they don't all have to happen overnight.

Using MyPlate to Plan

USDA's MyPlate is a tool to help you focus on the five food groups that are the building blocks for a healthy diet and help you determine the amounts from different food groups that should be represented in your daily eating plan.

Many individuals remember the Pyramids—the Food Guide Pyramid and MyPyramid—USDA's food guidance symbols before MyPlate, but not many people realize just how long USDA's history of providing science-based dietary guidance to the American public actually is. Starting over a century ago, USDA has empowered Americans to make healthy food choices by providing a number of publications, food guidance symbols, and, more recently, a suite of interactive online tools.

MyPlate (Figure 22) is a visual reminder to find your healthy eating style and build it throughout your lifetime. Everything you eat and drink matters. The right mix can help you be healthier now and in the future.

Eating healthy is a journey shaped by many factors, including our stage of life, situations, preferences, access to food, culture, traditions, and the personal decisions we make

over time. MyPlate offers ideas and tips to help you create a healthier eating style that meets your individual needs and improves your health.

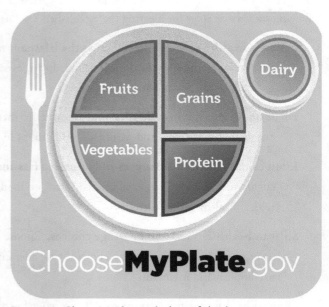

Figure 22. ChooseMyPlate is the latest federal nutrition program.

MyPlate helps you determine the types and portion sizes—based on your age, gender, and level of physical activity—you need for each of the five food groups. These are fruits, vegetables, grains, proteins, and dairy. MyPlate also contains recommendations for oils, but they are not a separate consideration.

Fruits

Any fruit or 100% fruit juice counts as part of the Fruit Group. Fruits may be fresh, canned, frozen, or dried, and may be whole, cut-up, or pureed. In general, 1 cup of fruit or 100% fruit juice, or 0.5 cup of dried fruit can be considered as 1 cup from the Fruit Group. Recommended total daily

Recommended Daily Fruit Amounts		
Women	19–30 years old	2 cups
	31–50 years old	1.5 cups
	51+ years old	1.5 cups
Men	19–30 years old	2 cups
	31–50 years old	2 cups
	51+ years old	2 cups

Figure 23. Recommended fruit amounts per day.

Recommended Daily Vegetable Amounts		
Women	19–30 years old	2.5 cups
	31–50 years old	2.5 cups
	51+ years old	2 cups
Men	19–30 years old	3 cups
	31–50 years old	3 cups
	51+ years old	2.5 cups

Figure 24. Recommended vegetable amounts per day.

amounts and recommended weekly amounts from each vegetable subgroup are shown in the first table (Figure 23).

Vegetables

Any vegetable or 100% vegetable juice counts as a member of the Vegetable Group. Vegetables may be raw or cooked; fresh, frozen, canned, or dried/dehydrated; and may be whole, cut-up, or mashed. Based on their nutrient content, vegetables are organized into five subgroups—dark-green vegetables, starchy vegetables, red and orange vegetables, beans and peas, and other vegetables.

In general, 1 cup of raw or cooked vegetables or vegetable juice, or 2 cups of raw leafy greens can be considered as 1 cup from the Vegetable Group. Recommended total daily amounts and recommended weekly amounts from each vegetable subgroup are shown in these two tables (Figure 24) and (Figure 25).

These amounts are appropriate for individuals who get less than 30 minutes per day of moderate physical activity, beyond normal daily activities. Those who are more physically active may be able to consume more while staying within calorie needs.

Vegetable subgroup recommendations are given as amounts to eat weekly. It is not necessary to eat vegetables from each subgroup daily. However, over a week, try to consume the amounts listed from each subgroup as a way to reach your daily intake recommendation.

Grains

Earlier in this chapter you learned about grains as a form of carbohydrate. Any food made from wheat, rice, oats, cornmeal, barley or another cereal grain is a grain product. Bread, pasta, oatmeal, breakfast cereals, tortillas, and grits are examples of grain products. But there is a difference between whole grains and refined grains.

Recommended Weekly Vegetable Amounts		Dark green vegetables	Red and orange vegetables	Beans and peas	Starchy vegetables	Other vegetables
Women	19–30 years old	1.5 cups	5.5 cups	1.5 cups	5 cups	4 cups
	31–50 years old	1.5 cups	5.5 cups	1.5 cups	5 cups	4 cups
	51+ years old	1.5 cups	4 cups	1 cup	4 cups	3.5 cups
Men	19–30 years old	2 cups	6 cups	2 cups	6 cups	5 cups
	31–50 years old	2 cups	6 cups	2 cups	6 cups	5 cups
	51+ years old	1.5 cups	5.5 cups	1.5 cups	5 cups	4 cups

Figure 25. Recommended vegetable amounts per week.

Recommended Daily Grain Amounts		Daily Recommendation	Daily minimum amount of whole grains
Women	19–30 years old	6 ounce equivalents	3 ounce equivalents
	31–50 years old	6 ounce equivalents	3 ounce equivalents
	51+ years old	5 ounce equivalents	3 ounce equivalents
Men	19–30 years old	8 ounce equivalents	4 ounce equivalents
	31–50 years old	7 ounce equivalents	3.5 ounce equivalents
	51+ years old	6 ounce equivalents	3 ounce equivalents

Figure 26. Recommended grain amounts per day.

Whole grains contain the entire grain kernel — the bran, germ, and endosperm. Examples of whole grains include whole-wheat flour, bulgur (cracked wheat), oatmeal, whole cornmeal, and brown rice. Refined grains have been milled, a process that removes the bran and germ. This is done to give grains a finer texture and improve their shelf life, but it also removes dietary fiber, iron, and many B vitamins. Some examples of refined grain products are white flour, de-germed cornmeal, white bread, and white rice.

Most refined grains are enriched. This means certain B vitamins (thiamin, riboflavin, niacin, folic acid) and iron are added back after processing. Fiber is not added back to enriched grains. Check the ingredient list on refined grain products to make sure that the word "enriched" is included in the grain name. Some food products are made from mixtures of whole grains and refined grains.

Most Americans consume enough grains, but few are whole grains. At least half of all the grains eaten should be whole grains. In general, 1 slice of bread, 1 cup of ready-to-eat cereal, or 0.5 cup of cooked rice, cooked pasta, or cooked cereal can be considered as 1 ounce-equivalent from the Grains Group. Recommended daily amounts are listed in this table (Figure 26).

Proteins

All foods made from meat, poultry, seafood, beans and peas, eggs, processed soy products, nuts, and seeds are considered part of the Protein Foods Group. Beans and peas are also part of the Vegetable Group.

Select a variety of protein foods to improve nutrient intake and health benefits, including at least 8 ounces of cooked seafood per week. The advice to consume seafood does not apply to vegetarians. Vegetarian options in the Protein Foods Group include beans and peas, processed soy products, and nuts and seeds. Meat and poultry choices should be lean or low-fat. Recommended daily amounts are listed in this table (Figure 27).

Most Americans eat enough food from this group, but need to make leaner and more varied selections of these foods. In general, 1 ounce of meat, poultry or fish, 0.25 cup cooked beans, 1 egg, 1 tablespoon of peanut butter, or 0.5 ounce of nuts or seeds can be considered as 1 ounce-equivalent from the Protein Foods Group.

The USDA recommends several strategies for choosing healthy protein sources:

Choose lean or low-fat meat and poultry. If higher fat choices are made, such as regular ground beef (75–80% lean) or chicken with skin, the fat counts against your limit for calories from saturated fats.

Count solid cooking fats as calories. If solid fat is added in cooking, such as frying chicken in shortening or frying eggs in butter or stick margarine, this also counts against your limit for calories from saturated fats.

Choose healthy fish. Select some seafood that is rich in omega-3 fatty acids, such as salmon, trout, sardines, anchovies, herring, Pacific oysters, and Atlantic and Pacific mackerel.

Recommended Daily Protein Amounts		
Women	19–30 years old	5.5 ounce equivalents
	31–50 years old	5 ounce equivalents
	51+ years old	5 ounce equivalents
Men	19–30 years old	6.5 ounce equivalents
	31–50 years old	6 ounce equivalents
	51+ years old	5.5 ounce equivalents

Figure 27. Recommended dairy amounts per day.

Be aware of sodium in processed meats. Processed meats such as ham, sausage, frankfurters, and luncheon or deli meats have added sodium. Check the Nutrition Facts label to help limit sodium intake. Fresh chicken, turkey, and pork that have been enhanced with a salt-containing solution also have added sodium. Check the product label for statements such as "self-basting" or "contains up to __% of __", which mean that a sodium-containing solution has been added to the product.

Choose unsalted nuts and seeds to keep sodium intake low. Many nuts and seeds in stores are salted before packaging, adding unnecessary sodium levels. They taste good without all that salt!

Dairy

All fluid milk products and many foods made from milk are considered part of this food group. Most Dairy Group choices should be fat-free or low-fat. Foods made from milk that retain their calcium content are part of the group. Foods made from milk that have little to no calcium, such as cream cheese, cream, and butter are not. Calcium-fortified soymilk (soy beverage) is also part of the Dairy Group.

In general, 1 cup of milk, yogurt, or soymilk (soy beverage), 1.5 ounces of natural cheese, or 2 ounces of processed cheese can be considered as 1 cup from the Dairy Group. This table lists specific amounts that count as 1 cup in the Dairy Group towards your recommended daily intake (Figure 28).

The USDA recommends several strategies for choosing healthy dairy sources:

Choose fat-free or low-fat milk, yogurt, and cheese. If you choose milk or yogurt that is not fat-free, or cheese that is not low-fat, the fat in the product counts against your limit for calories from saturated fats.

Recommended Daily Dairy Amounts		
Women	19–30 years old	3 cups
	31–50 years old	3 cups
	51+ years old	3 cups
Men	19–30 years old	3 cups
	31–50 years old	3 cups
	51+ years old	3 cups

Figure 28. Recommended dairy amounts per day.

Count added sugars as calories. If sweetened milk products are chosen (flavored milk, yogurt, drinkable yogurt, desserts), the added sugars also count against your limit for calories from added sugar.

Limit lactose in lactose-intolerant individuals. For those who are lactose intolerant, smaller portions (such as 4 fluid ounces of milk) may be well tolerated. Lactose-free and lower-lactose products are available. These include lactose-reduced or lactose-free milk, yogurt, and cheese, and calcium-fortified soymilk (soy beverage). Also, enzyme preparations can be added to milk to lower the lactose content.

Calcium choices for those who do not consume dairy products include:

- Calcium-fortified juices, cereals, breads, rice milk, or almond milk. Calcium-fortified foods and beverages may not provide the other nutrients found in dairy products. Check their labels.

- Canned fish (sardines, salmon with bones) soybeans and other soy products (tofu made with calcium sulfate, soy yogurt, tempeh), some other beans, and some leafy greens (collard and turnip greens, kale, bok choy). The amount of calcium that can be absorbed from these foods varies.

Oils

Oils, though not a food group, provide essential nutrients. Therefore, the USDA includes oils in their food plan. Some commonly eaten oils include canola, corn, cottonseed, olive, safflower, soybean, and sunflower. Some oils are used mainly as flavorings, such as walnut and sesame oil. A number of foods naturally a high oil content, like nuts, olives, some fish, and avocados.

Foods that are mainly oil include mayonnaise, certain salad dressings, and soft (tub or squeeze) margarine with no trans fats. Check the Nutrition Facts label to find margarines with 0 grams of trans fat.

Most oils are high in monounsaturated or polyunsaturated fats, and low in saturated fats. Oils from plant sources (vegetable and nut oils) do not contain any cholesterol. In fact, no plant foods contain cholesterol. A few plant oils, however, including coconut oil, palm oil, and palm kernel oil, contain a lot of saturated fat and for nutritional purposes should be considered to be solid fats. Solid fats are those that are solid at room temperature, like butter and shortening. Many of these are the evil trans fats discussed earlier. Some common fats include butter, milk fat, beef fat (tallow, suet), chicken fat, pork fat (lard), stick margarine, shortening, and partially hydrogenated oil. Recommended daily amounts are listed in this table (Figure 29).

Some Americans consume enough oil in the foods they eat, such as: nuts, fish, cooking oil, and salad dressings. Others could easily consume the recommended allowance by substituting oils for some solid fats they eat.

To use MyPlate and customize your program, simply go to www.choosemyplate.gov and look through the tools, tips, resources, and quizzes available to you. Since record-keeping

Recommended Daily Oils Amounts		
Women	19–30 years old	6 teaspoons
	31–50 years old	5 teaspoons
	51+ years old	5 teaspoons
Men	19–30 years old	7 teaspoons
	31–50 years old	6 teaspoons
	51+ years old	6 easpoons

Figure 29. Recommended oil amounts per day.

is such an important tool for success, you can download and use one of their easy-to-use daily checklists designed to fit a variety of ages and calorie requirements.

Using Nutrition Labels to Plan

Nutrition labels on food provide specific information about serving sizes and daily percentages based on average calorie intakes. With a little practice, these labels can be easy to use. In the sample Nutrition Facts labels in this chapter, we have colored certain sections to help you focus on those areas that will be explained in detail. You will not see these colors on the food labels on products you purchase.

Serving Size

The first place to start when you look at the Nutrition Facts label is the serving size and the number of servings in the package. Serving sizes are standardized to make it easier to compare similar foods using familiar units, such as cups or pieces, followed by the metric amount, e.g., the number of grams.

The size of the serving on the food package influences the number of calories and all the nutrient amounts listed on the top part of the label. Pay attention to the serving size, especially how many servings there are in the food package. Then ask yourself, "How many servings am I consuming?" (e.g., 0.5 serving, 1 serving, or more). In the sample label, one serving of macaroni and cheese equals one cup. If you ate the whole package, you would eat two cups. That doubles the calories and other nutrient numbers, including the %Daily Values as shown in the sample label.

Daily Value

The % Daily Values (%DVs) are based on the Daily Value recommendations for key nutrients but only for a 2,000-cal-

orie daily diet—not 2,500 calories. You may not know how many calories you consume in a day. But you can still use the %DV as a frame of reference whether or not you consume more or less than 2,000 calories (Figure 30).

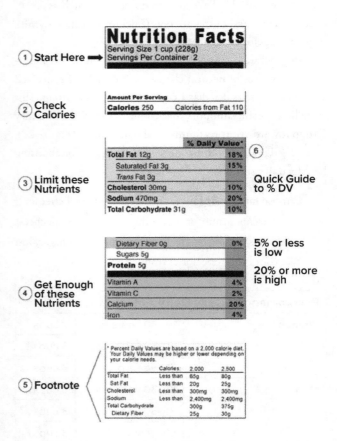

Figure 30. How to read a Nutrition Facts label.

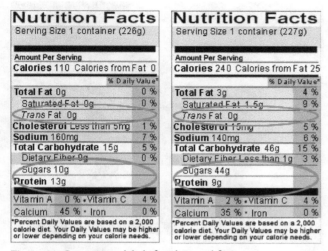

Figure 31. Comparison labels for plain and fruit yogurt.

The %DV helps you determine if a serving of food is high or low in a nutrient. A few nutrients, like trans-fat, do not have a %DV, but trans-fat should be avoided anyway. The %DV also makes it easy for you to make comparisons. You can compare one product or brand to a similar product. Just make sure the serving sizes are similar, especially the weight (e.g. gram, milligram, ounces) of each product. It's easy to see which foods are higher or lower in nutrients because the serving sizes are generally consistent for similar types of foods, except in a few cases like cereals.

Use the %DV and grams per serving to help you quickly distinguish one claim from another, such as "reduced fat" vs. "light" or "nonfat." Just compare the %DVs for Total Fat in each food product to see which one is higher or lower in that nutrient—you don't need to memorize definitions (Figure 31). This works when comparing all nutrient content claims, e.g., less, light, low, free, more, high, etc.

You can use the labels to help you make dietary trade-offs with other foods throughout the day. You don't have to give up a favorite food to eat a healthy diet. When a food you like is high in fat, balance it with foods that are low in fat at other times of the day. Also, pay attention to how much you eat so that the total amount of fat for the day stays below 100% DV.

A %DV is required to be listed if a claim is made for protein, such as "high in protein." Otherwise, unless the food is meant for use by infants and children under 4 years old, none is needed. Current scientific evidence indicates that protein intake is not a public health concern for adults and children over 4 years of age.

No daily reference value has been established for sugars because no recommendations have been made for the total amount to eat in a day. Keep in mind, the sugars listed on the Nutrition Facts label include naturally occurring sugars (like those in fruit and milk) as well as those added to a food or drink. Check the ingredient list for specifics on added sugars.

The Accuracy of Food Labels

Nutrition labels have raised awareness of the energetic value of foods, and represent for many a pivotal guideline to regulate food intake. However, recent data has created doubts on label accuracy. Calories, especially, on food labels can have a wide margin of error, about 20% on either side.

Using Organic Food to Plan

Organic food is produced by methods that comply with the standards of organic farming. Standards vary worldwide, but organic farming in general features practices that strive to cycle resources, promote ecological balance, and conserve biodiversity. Organizations regulating organic products may restrict the use of certain pesticides and fertilizers in farming. In general, organic foods are also usually not processed using irradiation (exposing the food to radiation), industrial solvents, or synthetic food additives.

There is not sufficient evidence to support claims that organic food is safer or healthier than conventionally grown food. While there may be some differences in the nutrient contents of organically- and conventionally-produced food, the variable nature of food production and handling makes it difficult to generalize results. Claims that organic food tastes better are generally not supported by evidence.

However, there is widespread public belief that organic food is safer, more nutritious, and better tasting than conventional food, which has largely contributed to the development of an organic food culture. Consumers purchase organic foods for different reasons, including concerns about the effects of conventional farming practices on the environment, human health, and animal welfare.

In a recent analysis, detectable pesticide residues were found in 7% of organic produce samples and 38% of conventional produce samples. The FDA recommends

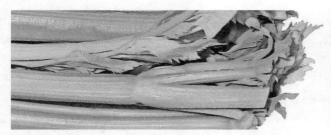

Figure 32. Celery is on the Dirty Dozen list.

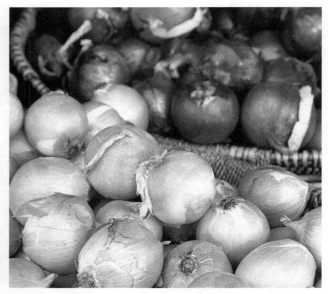

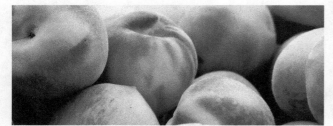

Figure 33. Peaches are on the Dirty Dozen list.

Figure 34. Onions are on the Clean 15 list.

washing produce before consuming, but some produce may retain more chemicals than others. These are respectively called the "Dirty Dozen" and the "Clean 15" and are updated annually.

The fruits and vegetables on **The Dirty Dozen** list, when conventionally grown, tested positive for at least 47 different chemicals, with some testing positive for as many as 67. For produce on the "dirty" list, you could definitely go organic—unless you relish the idea of consuming a chemical cocktail (Figure 32) and (Figure 33). The Dirty Dozen list includes:

- Celery
- Peaches
- Strawberries
- Apples
- Domestic blueberries
- Nectarines
- Sweet bell peppers
- Spinach, kale and collard greens
- Cherries
- Potatoes
- Imported grapes
- Lettuce

All the produce on **The Clean 15** bore little to no traces of pesticides, and are considered safe to consume in non-organic form (Figure 34). This list includes:

- Onions
- Avocados
- Sweet corn
- Pineapples
- Mango
- Sweet peas
- Asparagus
- Kiwi fruit
- Cabbage
- Eggplant
- Cantaloupe
- Watermelon
- Grapefruit
- Sweet potatoes
- Sweet onions

Why are some types of produce more prone to sucking up pesticides than others? Many fruits and vegetables have an outer layer of defense, such as pineapples and corn. Others have no protection between the edible portion and the ground, pesticides, and hands of people picking the produce, such as strawberries.

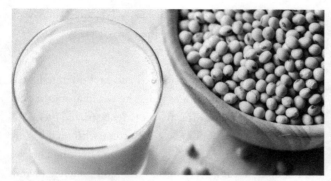

Figure 35. Soy is a good source of protein for meatless diets.

A lot of people choose to eat all organic. However, this can be costly since organic produce tends to be a bit more expensive and can often have a shorter shelf-life. To watch cost, you can focus on eating The Clean 15 from conventional produce and buy organic for The Dirty Dozen. If you want to go organic, try shopping at markets focused on whole foods. These stores often (though not always) offer slightly cheaper prices on organic produce than your local chain.

Meatless and Meat-Restricted Diets

Many diets limit your food intake of certain types of food. Vegetarian diets are probably the most well-known meat-restrictive diet, while also being one of the least understood. Others include vegan, lacto-vegetarian, lacto-ovo vegetarian, flexitarian, and pescatarian. Since a major problem with nutrition in the US is a lack of vegetables in the average diet, reviewing the different types of limited diets (none of which "limit" vegetables) can be a good idea when making your nutrition plan.

It has become very popular to be vegan or vegetarian though many people do not fully understand what this means. Vegetarians avoid the consumption of animals, including seafood and animal flesh. Vegetarians will often still consume dairy products and products that may be made with eggs, such as pasta. There are many variations to this diet. Vegans, for example, will eat absolutely no animal products. They will avoid all meat, dairy, fish, eggs, sometimes even honey, and need to read the label on packaged goods to determine if any animal products are used in the ingredients. Lacto vegetarians will consume dairy, but no meat. Lacto-ovo vegetarians will consume both dairy and eggs. Pescatarians will consume fish. The most recently introduced modification to the vegetarian diet is flexitarian. Many people consider themselves to be primarily vegetarian but choose to consume meat on occasion, making them a bit more flexible. These individuals, in general, avoid meat for health reasons rather than political ones.

Planning is key. Some nutrients should be of particular concern for individuals on these restricted diets because they are mostly found in foods that they do not eat, including Vitamins B-12 and D, Calcium, Iron, and Zinc. A common misperception is that vegetarians lack protein, but as we've learned already, protein is easy to get from plant sources. The FDA offers the following tips for getting enough nutrients and variety on a meat-restricted diet:

Think about protein. Your protein needs can easily be met by eating a variety of plant foods. Sources of protein for vegetarians include beans and peas, seeds (like quinoa), nuts, and soy products (such as tofu, tempeh). Lacto-ovo vegetarians also get protein from eggs and dairy foods.

Bone up on sources of calcium. Some vegetarians consume dairy products, which are excellent sources of calcium (Figure 35) Other sources of calcium for vegetarians include calcium-fortified soymilk (soy beverage), tofu made with calcium sulfate, calcium-fortified breakfast cereals and orange juice, and some dark-green leafy vegetables (collard, turnip, and mustard greens, and bok choy).

Make **simple changes.** Many popular main dishes are or can be vegetarian—such as pasta primavera, pasta with marinara or pesto sauce, veggie pizza, vegetable lasagna, tofu-vegetable stir-fry, and bean burritos.

Enjoy a cookout. For barbecues, try veggie or soy burgers, soy hot dogs, marinated tofu or tempeh, and fruit or veggie kabobs.

Include beans and peas. Because of their high nutrient content, consuming beans and peas is recommended for everyone, vegetarians and non-vegetarians alike.

Try different veggie versions. A variety of vegetarian products look—and may taste—like their non-vegetarian counterparts but are usually lower in saturated fat and contain no cholesterol. For example, try soy-based sausage patties, bean burgers, or falafels (chickpea patties).

Make some small changes at restaurants. Most restaurants can make vegetarian modifications to menu items by substituting meatless sauces or nonmeat items, such as tofu and beans for meat, and adding vegetables or pasta in place of meat. Plan ahead by looking at restaurant menus online when possible.

Nuts make great snacks. Choose unsalted nuts as a snack and use them in salads or main dishes. Add almonds, walnuts, or pecans instead of cheese or meat to a green salad.

Get your vitamin B12. Vitamin B12 is naturally found only in animal products. Vegetarians should choose fortified foods, such as cereals or soy products, or take a vitamin B12 supplement if they do not consume any animal products. Check the Nutrition Facts label for vitamin B12 in fortified products.

It may sound a bit complicated and high-maintenance, and it can be if the person expects the world around them to adapt to their diet. This is true for any restricted diet. The person may end up nibbling iceberg lettuce with no dressing at a restaurant. But it really comes down to making choices and planning ahead. Every person has food preferences and every person should put a little planning into what they eat, regardless of whether or not that includes animal products. Anyone can adapt to a plan and make life easier on themselves and others with a little forethought and personal responsibility for their food. Most people on a restricted diet become very good at this and stay healthy in the process.

Other Dietary Plans

So many diet plans exist today. Grain-free diets in which you eat like your caveman ancestors. Ketogenic diets that focus on increasing fat intake. Diets focused on juicing, bacteria, pre-prepared meals, eating clean, and the list goes on and on. Some make complete sense. Others, as previously discussed, have no supported science behind them. A few have been around for quite some time and are supported by health professionals as providing a balanced, safe approach to a healthy diet.

The DASH Eating Plan

The **DASH** (Dietary Approaches to Stop Hypertension) eating plan is rich in fruits, vegetables, fat-free or low-fat milk and milk products, whole grains, fish, poultry, beans, seeds, and nuts. It also contains less sodium, sugars, fats, and red meats than the typical American diet. This heart-healthy way of eating is also lower in saturated fat, trans fat, and cholesterol and rich in nutrients associated with lowering blood pressure—mainly potassium, magnesium, calcium, protein, and fiber.

The DASH plan does involve monitoring caloric intake, along with sodium and fats. The plan uses the following guideline for calories:

People on DASH are advised to choose and prepare foods with less sodium and salt, and not to bring the saltshaker to the table. It's important to be creative—try herbs, spices, lemon, lime, vinegar, wine, and salt-free seasoning blends—in cooking and at the table. And, because most of the sodium that we eat comes from processed foods, be sure to read food labels to check the amount of sodium in different food products. Aim for foods that contain 5% or less of the Daily Value of sodium. Foods with 20 percent or more are considered high. These include baked goods, certain cereals, soy sauce, and some antacids—many foods have added sodium (see minerals section of this chapter).

The Mediterranean Diet

The Mediterranean Diet contains more fruits and seafood and less dairy than the traditional approach utilized by the FDA. People in Mediterranean countries have eaten this way for many years and have been known to have lower incidence of heart disease and other illnesses, many of which are associated with lower cholesterol levels and more stable blood sugar. The Mediterranean Diet includes

- Eating primarily plant-based foods, such as fruits and vegetables, whole grains, legumes and nuts

- Replacing butter with healthy fats, such as olive oil and canola oil

- Using herbs and spices instead of salt to flavor foods

- Limiting red meat to no more than a few times each month

- Eating fish and poultry at least twice a week
- Drinking red wine in moderation (optional)

There may be health concerns with this eating style for some people, including:

- You may gain weight from eating fats in olive oil and nuts.
- You may have lower levels of iron. If you choose to follow the Mediterranean diet, be sure to eat some foods rich in iron or in vitamin C, which helps your body absorb iron.
- You may have calcium loss from eating fewer dairy products. Ask your health care provider if you should take a calcium supplement.
- Wine is a common part of a Mediterranean eating style but some people should not drink alcohol. Avoid wine if you are prone to alcohol abuse, pregnant, at risk for breast cancer, or have other conditions that alcohol could make worse.

It's Not as Hard as It Seems

College students and busy, working individuals can have crazy schedules that make eating healthy a challenge. Starting a new plan when you already have a full plate can be intimidating. It may be a bit time consuming initially, but even learning to make small, gradual changes can make a world of difference and help you adapt to a new, healthier way of eating.

You may also be concerned about giving up some of your favorite foods. A healthy eating plan that helps you manage your weight includes a variety of foods you may not have considered. If "healthy eating" makes you think about the foods you **can't** have, try refocusing on all the new foods you **can** eat:

Fresh, Frozen, or Canned Fruits. Don't think just apples or bananas. All fresh, frozen, or canned fruits are great choices. Be sure to try some "exotic" fruits, too. How about a mango? Or a juicy pineapple or kiwi fruit! When your favorite fresh fruits aren't in season, try a frozen, canned, or dried variety of a fresh fruit you enjoy. One caution about canned fruits is that they may contain added sugars or syrups. Be sure and choose canned varieties of fruit packed in water or in their own juice.

Fresh, Frozen, or Canned Vegetables. Try something new. You may find that you love grilled vegetables or steamed vegetables with an herb you haven't tried like rosemary. You can sauté vegetables in a non-stick pan with a small amount of cooking spray. Or try frozen or canned vegetables for a quick side dish—just microwave and serve. When trying canned vegetables, look for vegetables without added salt, butter, or cream sauces. Commit to going to the produce department and trying a new vegetable each week.

Calcium-rich foods. You may automatically think of a glass of low-fat or fat-free milk when someone says "eat more dairy products." But what about low-fat and fat-free yogurts without added sugars? These come in a wide variety of flavors and can be a great dessert substitute for those with a sweet tooth.

A new twist on an old favorite. If your favorite recipe calls for frying fish or breaded chicken, try healthier variations using baking or grilling. Maybe even try a recipe that uses dry beans in place of higher-fat meats. Ask around or search the Internet and magazines for recipes with fewer calories—you might be surprised to find you have a new favorite dish!

Cooking

It must apparent to you by now, perhaps painfully so, that you need to eat your vegetables. There are many lonely vegetables longing for homes, often because consumers don't know how to prepare them. For every person who loves kale, there are three others that detest it. The same goes for broccoli, asparagus, squash, and many other foods valued for their nutrition but questioned for their taste. Growing up, it is likely that someone in your home refused to have them on their plate (was it you?). Maybe your parent would make you try it and you would grudgingly swallow a small bite for permission to leave the table. Well, no offense to Mom, but maybe the problem was with the preparation, not the food.

How foods are cooked can have a big impact on their nutrient content and flavor. That's because many vitamins are sensitive to heat and air exposure (vitamin C, the B vitamins, and folate in particular). Loss of nutrients increases as cooking time increases and with higher temperatures (Figure 36).

Cooking methods that minimize the time, temperature, and amount of water needed will help to preserve nutrients. Steaming is a great way to cook vegetables quickly and retain valuable nutrients. Microwave cooking is also good because it uses minimal water, and the cooking time is very short. Stir-frying can quickly cook a variety of vegetables.

It's useful to remember that cooking creates a chemical change in your food, using heat as a catalyst and, in some cases, will alter which nutrients you can more easily digest. In some cases, it makes otherwise inedible foods edible, such as taro, which is full of toxic crystals that need to be broken down before any of the plant can be consumed. Cooking also softens food, making it easier to chew and digest—imagine trying to eat rice without cooking it first!

Here are a few other tricks you can use to preserve nutrients:

- **Leave vegetables in big pieces.** That way, fewer vitamins are destroyed when they are exposed to air.

- **Always cover your pot to hold in steam and heat.** This will also help to reduce cooking time.

- **Use any leftover cooking water.** This is perfect for starting soups and stews, sauces, or vegetable juice drinks.

- **Eat fruits and vegetables raw.** Do this whenever possible in salads and smoothies, or as whole fruits and vegetables.

- **Cook vegetables until crisp.** Don't overcook them.

- **Use as little water as possible when cooking.**

Let's talk a moment more about flavor, since this is often the largest objection. Many vegetables taste better and are better for you when they are steamed. Having said that, if you need to add a touch of olive oil and lemon to your broccoli, sauté your asparagus or kale in a bit of olive oil and garlic, or add pine nuts to your steamed or sautéed spinach, go ahead. Throw some onion into the pot when you cook your green beans—it tastes great and there is no harm done. Even a *tiny* bit of olive oil, butter, salt, and pepper can make a world of difference as long as you aren't loading it with saturated fat (consider the pad of your thumb as a guide on butter).

If you need to store food, you have a lot of options. The best method for storing food while keeping the existing nutrients intact is by freezing. Research suggests there is no significant loss of nutritional value in frozen food, and it can be more convenient and cost effective than fresh if those issues are a factor for you. Canning is another good option, but the process requires cooking the food at a boil for a short time (so it doesn't give you botulism), which can alter the nutritional profile of the food. Older methods of preservation, like fermenting (kimchi, sauerkraut, etc.), drying, curing (usually

Myth	Fact
The only reason to let food sit after it's been microwaved is to make sure you don't burn yourself on food that's too hot.	In fact, letting microwaved food sit for a few minutes ("standing time") helps your food cook more completely by allowing colder areas of food time to absorb heat from hotter areas of food.
Leftovers are safe to eat until they smell bad.	The kinds of bacteria that cause food poisoning do not affect the look, smell, or taste of the food.
Once food has been cooked, all the bacteria have been killed, so I don't need to worry once it's "done".	Actually, the possibility of bacterial growth increases after cooking because the drop in temperature allows bacteria to thrive. Keeping cooked food warmed to the right temperature is critical for food safety.
Marinades are acidic, which kills bacteria-so it's OK to marinate foods on the counter.	Even in the presence of acidic marinade, bacteria can grow very rapidly at room temperatures. To marinate foods safely, it's important to marinate them in the refrigerator.
If I really want my produce to be safe, I should wash fruits and vegetables with soap or detergent before I use them.	In fact, it's best not to use soaps or detergents on produce, since these products can linger on foods and are not safe for consumption. Using clean running water is actually the best way to remove bacteria and wash produce safely.

Figure 36. Common food handling myths and facts.

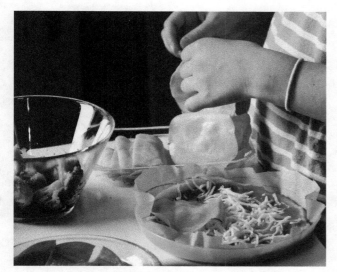

Figure 37. Safe food handling is critical.

meats and cheeses), smoking, storing in oil (like confit or olives), or storing in brine (pickles), have been around longer than recorded history and, like cooking, alter the flavors and nutritional values of your food.

Food Safety

One common challenge for people concerned with their nutrition is food safety, especially since they may be choosing and preparing food in new ways they might be unfamiliar with. This is especially true for people who aren't used to cooking, but want to take advantage of the health benefits of preparing their own food. For years, high schoolers took home economics classes that taught them how to handle, prepare, and store food safely. But many of these programs have disappeared, leaving new generations unprepared in the kitchen. Unless your parents taught you, you may not have learned. You may even be operating under some of the common misconceptions about food safety (Figure 37).

Foodborne illness (sometimes called "foodborne disease," "foodborne infection," or "food poisoning") is a common, costly—yet preventable—public health problem. Each year, 1 in 6 Americans gets sick by consuming contaminated foods or beverages. Many different disease-causing microbes, or pathogens, can contaminate foods, leading to many different foodborne infections. In addition, poisonous chemicals, or other harmful substances can cause foodborne diseases if they are present in food.

The most common food safety concerns can be addressed with common sense healthy food handling, including proper cooking temperature, eliminating cross contamination, and consistent handwashing. Others can be more difficult to avoid because of their connection to food safety issues that occur outside your control.

- Trichinellosis, also called trichinosis, is a disease that people can get by eating raw or undercooked meat from animals infected with the microscopic parasite Trichinella. Most often found in pork though not as commonly as it used to be.

- Botulism is a rare but serious illness caused by a toxin that attacks the body's nerves. You can encounter botulism in improperly canned foods and shellfish. While rare, botulism is potentially lethal and proper food storage and preparation are important factors in its prevention.

- Salmonella, which is bacteria most often found in poultry (including eggs).

These different diseases have many different symptoms, so there is no one "syndrome" that is foodborne illness. However, the microbe or toxin enters the body through the gastrointestinal tract, and often causes the first symptoms there, so nausea, vomiting, abdominal cramps, and diarrhea are common symptoms in many foodborne diseases.

When it comes to many of the vitamin-rich foods—fruits, vegetables, grains, seeds, and beans—there isn't much you have to do to keep yourself safe, though some risks exist. With meats and dairy, however, you do need to pay attention. Food comes from many sources and is handled by many people under many conditions before you bring it to your home, even your produce. Years ago, our livestock for meat in particular were fed and cared for differently. People had to cook pork, for example, thoroughly to avoid trichinosis (in part because we used to let pigs control garbage problems—apparently they'll eat almost anything). Our standards are better now, but food-borne bacteria, like E. coli, salmonella, norovirus, and sometimes even trichinosis are still common. Let the follow guidelines help you avoid most food-borne illness:

- Wash your fruits and vegetables before preparing them.

- Watch for expiration dates, both at the time of purchase and at home.

- Never buy a package of food that has been torn or is leaking.

- Always refrigerate perishable food within 2 hours of purchase, and one hour if it's hot out.

- Cook or freeze meats within 2 days.

- Be sure to wrap meat tightly to avoid leakage and store meat in the refrigerator it has no opportunity to leak on other foods.

- Wash your hands and preparation surfaces before, during, and after cooking.

- Any canned food that is dented, swollen, or has an elevated safety bubble (for jars) should be discarded.

Improper handling of food is the most common reason for foodborne illness, with the major culprit being cross contamination. You can avoid cross contamination easily. First keep your meat and vegetables separated at all times. Do not use the same cutting board for meat preparation as you use for preparing vegetables, and wash your hands after every time you touch meat. If your utensils (like tongs) touch raw meat, make sure you wash them afterwards. As a general rule, wash your hands a lot when preparing food.

The other main contributor to foodborne illnesses is improper cooking temperature. Chicken should be cooked to an internal temperature of 165 degrees Fahrenheit. Beef and pork should reach a minimum internal temperature of 145 degrees. To get the temperature correct, use a meat thermometer. Meat needs to rest for three to five minutes before eating to allow the cooking process to finish.

Food storage can be another major factor contributing to foodborne illnesses. If you are keeping food hot, it needs to hold at or above 145 degrees. If you are keeping it cold, the food needs to be below 45 degrees. Anything in between offers a great environment for bacteria to thrive.

Rapid temperature changes wreak havoc as well. For example, if you stick a pot of hot soup in your fridge with the cover on, you can expect to get sick after eating it the next day. Leave the cover off, so it can cool faster, and give it an occasional stir. That will get the food to a safe temperature faster.

Following these simple guidelines can keep your food safe — make sure you learn them as you learn to prepare your own healthy, delicious meals:

Clean. Wash hands and surfaces often.

Separate. Don't cross-contaminate.

Cook. Cook to the right temperature.

Chill. Refrigerate promptly.

Shopping. Purchase refrigerated or frozen items after selecting your non-perishables. Never choose meat or poultry in packaging that is torn or leaking. Do not buy food past "Sell-By," "Use-By," or other expiration dates.

Storage. Always refrigerate perishable food within 2 hours. Check the temperature of your refrigerator and freezer with an appliance thermometer. Cook or freeze fresh poultry, fish, ground meats, and variety meats within 2 days. To maintain quality when freezing meat and poultry in its original package, wrap the package again with foil or plastic wrap that's recommended for the freezer. Canned foods are safe indefinitely as long as they are not exposed to freezing temperatures, or temperatures above 90 (F).

Preparation. Always wash hands with warm water and soap for 20 seconds before and after handling food. Don't cross-contaminate. Keep raw meat, poultry, fish, and their juices away from other food. After cutting raw meats, wash cutting board, utensils, and countertops with hot, soapy water. Using a solution of 1 tablespoon of unscented, liquid chlorine bleach in 1 gallon of water can sanitize cutting boards, utensils, and countertops. Marinate meat and poultry in a covered dish in the refrigerator.

Thawing. The refrigerator allows slow, safe thawing. Make sure thawing meat and poultry juices do not drip onto other food. For faster thawing, place food in a leak-proof plastic bag. Submerge in cold tap water. Change the water every 30 minutes. Cook immediately after thawing. Cook meat and poultry immediately after microwave thawing.

Cooking. Cook all raw beef, pork, lamb and veal steaks, chops, and roasts to a minimum internal temperature of 145 (F) as measured with a food thermometer before removing meat from the heat source. For safety and quality, allow meat to rest for at least three minutes before carving or consuming.

Serving. Hot food should be held at 140 (F) or warmer. Cold food should be held at 40 (F) or colder. When serving food at a buffet, keep food hot with chafing dishes, slow cookers, and warming trays. Keep food cold by nesting dishes in bowls of ice or use small serving trays and replace them often.

Conclusion

Your next steps should be assessing your food intake based on nutrient content, using the guides available from MyPlate and other sources. Then, you can set SMART goals to achieve healthier nutrition in your life.

Changing your behavior can be difficult no matter what it is. Choosing to eat healthy is a choice, and one that takes much of the same kind of careful planning as a new fitness plan. It doesn't have to happen all at once, though. You might try swapping healthier snacks, eating a healthier breakfast, or planning a meatless dinner once a week. Consider ways you might incorporate more fiber into your diet or make sure that you are getting enough healthy fats and other essential nutrients. Assess your diet every once in a while, to make sure that you are making choices that are meeting your nutrient needs and fueling your body effectively.

Reflection Questions

1. Looking at Figure 1 and Figure 2, how many calories per day are recommended for a person with your height, age, activity level and biological sex?

2. Explain the concepts of energy density and nutrient density, and provide examples of each.

3. What role does each essential nutrients play in the human body?

4. Why are whole grains preferable to refined grains?

5. Describe the impact of the following on overall health and major sources of each: Fiber, added sugar, trans fats, antioxidants

6. What is the difference between saturated and unsaturated fats? What are examples of foods that are high in each type of fat? What type of fat is the most beneficial for health?

7. What is the difference between complete and incomplete protein? What are examples of each?

8. What are health concerns associated with high-protein diets?

9. What are characteristics of people who should consider taking a dietary supplement?

10. Describe how a person can use MyPlate to create a plan for nutrition.

11. Briefly describe habits that can help prevent the spread of foodborne pathogens.

Chapter 8
Stress Management

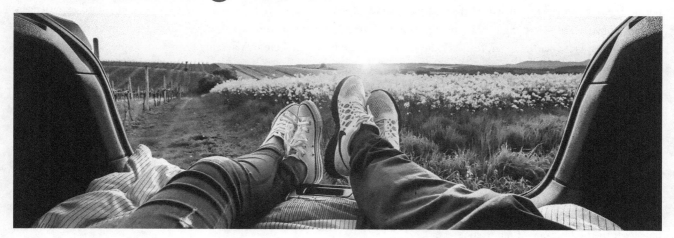

Learning Objectives

1. Explain what stress is and how people can react to it physically, emotionally and behaviorally.

2. What are the different types of stress? How does each type affect health differently?

3. Describe the stress response and how the body changes.

4. Describe techniques for preventing and managing stress.

5. Create a plan for successfully managing the stress in your life.

6. Describe the relationship between stress and illness.

It's your first term in college, and you're realizing that it's not as easy as you thought it would be. You registered for more courses than you could handle, your boss keeps scheduling you to work on days when you're supposed to be in class, your family keeps asking about your grades (You have to keep that scholarship!), and midterm exams are next week. You need to study, but some days it seems like you barely have time to take a shower. And if that's not bad enough— you're broke! Welcome to college, right? You're happy to be here, but can't help but wonder if it's going to be like this all four years.

Everyone feels stress from time to time, and we all react differently to it. But what exactly is stress? How does it affect your health? And what can you do about it? Your brain and body respond to demands in ways that don't always make sense. Any type of demand on you—such as exercise, work, school, major life changes, or traumatic events—can be stressful, sometimes without a logical reason.

It may not seem like it, but some stress can be beneficial by helping people develop the skills they need to cope with and adapt to new and potentially threatening situations. However, the beneficial aspects of stress diminish when the stress is severe enough to overwhelm a person's ability to take care of themselves and their family, or when it begins to impact their health. Healthy ways to cope with stress, combined with getting the right care and support, can put problems in perspective and help stress and its symptoms subside.

One of the most critical elements of healthy emotional wellness is effectively managing your stress before it becomes overwhelming. This chapter begins by defining the different kinds of stress that we experience and some of their common sources. It then describes the ways that stress can affect your health. Finally, this chapter recommends some stress management techniques to help you avoid the potentially dangerous effects of too much stress.

Defining Stress

Have you ever been so nervous that you began to tremble or felt nauseous? Have you gotten so scared that your heart was pounding and you started to sweat? If you have, you've experienced how your body reacts to what your mind experiences. You may have heard of the "fight or flight" reaction to danger, referring to animal's tendency to either fight or run away from danger. When faced with danger, fear, or other trials, your body tries to help by releasing hormones to prepare your body for rapid action like fighting or getting away.

But it doesn't only happen in crisis situations. Stress can be a physical and emotional reaction that people experience as they encounter changes in their life. It's a normal feeling. But long-term, regular stress may put your body in its "fight or flight" state too often. This may contribute to or worsen a range of health problems including digestive disorders, headaches, sleep disorders, asthma, and other physical symptoms, in addition to depression, anxiety, and other mental illnesses.

We all know what it feels like to be stressed. A 2017 American Psychological Association study found most participants reported moderate to high levels of stress—and 44% said their stress levels had increased over the past few years. Concerns about the future of our nation, money, and work are the most commonly reported sources of stress (Figure 1). Fears about job stability were reported by 49% of study participants. Millennials (people born between 1981 and 1996) top the list of individuals with the highest rate of reported stress.

In a study focused on college students who sought counseling on campus, these numbers rose dramatically over a 13-year period, with many students indicating stress and anxiety as a major complaint. The CDC has identified particular stressors college students typically face, including:

- Social and sexual pressures
- The temptation of readily available alcohol, drugs, and unhealthy food
- The challenge of getting enough sleep
- Stress from trying to balance obligations to classes, friends, homework, jobs, athletics, and leadership positions

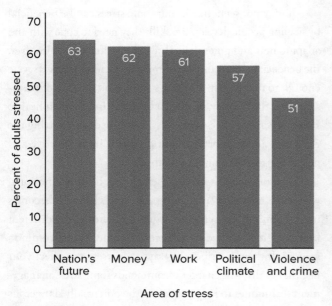

Figure 1. Percentage of adults who experience stress in these areas (Source: APA).

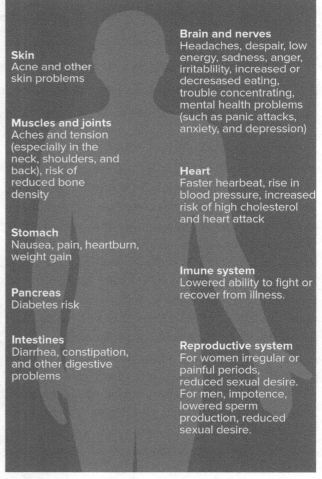

Figure 2. Stress affects many systems in the body.

This list may sound familiar to you. Stress is common and a normal part of life. Some people may cope with stress more effectively or recover from stressful events more quickly than others. Many factors affect the way a person manages their stress. In learning to handle stress, it can be helpful to understand that there are different types of stress—all of which carry physical and mental health risks (Figure 2).

Stressors are those things that cause us to become stressed. A stressor may be a one time or short-term occurrence, or it can keep happening over a long period of time. **Minor acute stressors** are short-lived, like the nerves before a class presentation or the concern that you may run out of gas on the freeway. **Major acute stressors** can be more traumatic, like a traffic accident, an argument with a friend, or experiencing an assault or natural disaster.

Chronic stressors are those that last long-term. This could be the result of routine stress related to the pressures of work, school, family, and other daily responsibilities. Chronic stress could be brought on by a sudden negative life change, such as loss of a job, divorce, or illness. These aren't situations that you can resolve quickly. Often, chronic stress stems from situations that have a high level of demand on you, but over which you have limited ability to make decisions or control the outcome. Some stressors can be both chronic and major acute stressors, such as what soldiers experience during a war.

The body always attempts to maintain a level of **homeostasis**, or balance, within its physiologic systems. As it faces stressors, the body feels threatened and attempts to "right the ship," so to speak, to keep it from tipping or sinking. Stressors can set off a chain reaction of hormone release in the body, primarily hormones that control functions such as heart rate or breathing. The release of these hormones can cause a wide range of physical reactions, including headache, dry mouth, difficulty swallowing, rapid heartbeat, nausea, cold hands, lack of concentration, difficulty sleeping, certain food cravings, and angry outbursts. On top of being behind in school, now you get a headache whenever you think about it! In order to succeed, we have to identify sources of stressors and learn to balance them in our life.

Sources of Stress

Stress can arise from any number of common sources (Figure 3).

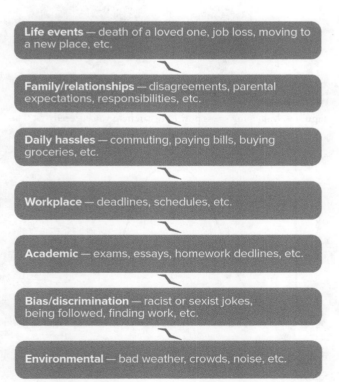

Figure 3. Stress can arise from any number of common sources.

Life events — death of a loved one, job loss, moving to a new place, etc.

Family/relationships — disagreements, parental expectations, responsibilities, etc.

Daily hassles — commuting, paying bills, buying groceries, etc.

Workplace — deadlines, schedules, etc.

Academic — exams, essays, homework dedlines, etc.

Bias/discrimination — racist or sexist jokes, being followed, finding work, etc.

Environmental — bad weather, crowds, noise, etc.

Types of Stress

Your body and mind experience different immediate and long-term affects based on the type of stress. There are six different kinds of stress: eustress, distress, acute stress, episodic acute stress, chronic stress, and traumatic stress.

Eustress is stress that enhances your functions, whether physical or mental, such as through strength training or challenging work. It results from positive, exhilarating, or desired experiences—the type of stress you likely experience with a job promotion, a happy move to a better house, the birth of a child, an inheritance of a large amount of money, or running a marathon.

Eustress is not defined by the cause of the stress, but rather how you perceives that stressor—as a positive challenge instead of a negative threat). This is considered "good stress" or "adaptive stress." Eustress refers to the positive response you have to a stressor, which can depend on whether you feel in control of the change, whether the change is something you want, and convenient location and timing of the stressor. The change may be temporarily stressful because it's new, different, or maybe even unexpected, but you respond to it by being motivated to work through the situation and adapt to its challenges (Figure 4).

Your body doesn't physically differentiate between types of stress and may still release hormones to compensate. For example, if you move into a new apartment, you may be excited about the change, even though you have to pack, unpack, clean, and organize. The stress is there, but it's a positive form. You still have the stressors to push through (the broken plates, the missing shoes, and the box of things you really should have thrown away) but you feel excited and challenged.

Your body and mind need to face challenges, especially ones you can overcome. This gives a sense of meaning and success in your life, improving your overall sense of well-being and your health. Through these situations, you learn how to manage stress in a positive way.

Distress is a negative type of stress. It can be short-term or long-term, and might be something that you struggle to cope with or adapt to. It may even feel overwhelming. Rather than motivating you, it can cause a decrease in your ability to perform.

Any negative stressor can lead to an overall feeling of distress. Just as with eustress, the stressor doesn't define distress. It's defined by the person's reaction to the stressor. Your experiences of eustress or distress depend on your personal expectations for the outcome of the stressor, and the resources you have available to cope with the stress. You experience distress when the resources you would use to handle the stress are exhausted.

In a recent study, over 3% of adults reported experiencing serious psychological distress over a 30-day period. If participants in the study accurately represent the nation as a whole, that's a significant number of people each month that can't handle the level of stress they experience. 3% of adults feel their coping resources are overwhelmed or not readily available. Distress that doesn't get resolved through coping or adaptation may lead to experiences of anxiety or even depression.

Acute Stress

Acute stress is the most common form of stress. We typically associate acute stress with things in our everyday lives such as paying a bill on time, rushing to class, or meeting deadlines. These are the demands and pressures of the recent past and that we anticipate in the near future. Acute stress tends to be short-term stress that resolves without any serious damage to your health. Once you've turned in that essay, paid that bill, or made it to class, the situation is resolved, at least for the moment. When the same things start over again the next day, and the next day, you may begin to experience problems. Acute stress can actually be exciting and thrilling, but too much can make you feel exhausted (Figure 5).

Symptoms of acute stress can include emotional anguish, headaches, back pains and general muscle problems. They may also include irritable bowel syndrome (IBS), dizziness, shortness of breath, chest pains, and heart palpitations. A lot of these symptoms can be triggered by adrenaline, like the rush you get rushing to catch the bus.

Episodic acute stress is when a person experiences acute stress more frequently. People that suffer from this seem to always be in a rush, are overscheduled (even deliberately), or are constantly facing some sort of pressure. They take too much on and tend to not be able to organize themselves or deal with the demands they too often place upon themselves.

Episodic acute stress can affect interpersonal skills. It can make sufferers generally respond in a negative way toward others, causing a deterioration of relationships at home or at work. This type of prolonged overstimulation can lead to persistent tension headaches or migraines, hypertension, and even chest pains. Most of us know at least one person like this. Some of us might even be this person.

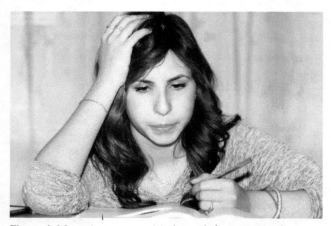

Figure 4. Managing stress positively can help you succeed.

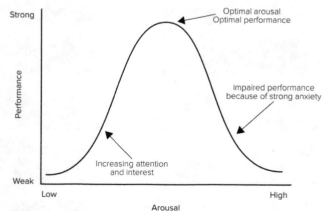

Figure 5. Stress can be good for you when it increases your performance.

Type	Symptoms
Re-living	Experiencing flashbacks, nightmares, and extreme emotional and physical reactions to reminders of the event. Emotional reactions can include feeling guilty, extreme fear of harm, and numbing of emotions. Physical reactions can include uncontrollable shaking, chills or heart palpitations, and tension headaches.
Avoidance	Staying away from activities, places, thoughts, or feelings related to the trauma or feeling detached or estranged from others.
Increased Arousal	Being overly alert or easily startled, difficulty sleeping, irritability or outbursts of anger, and lack of concentration.

Figure 6. Types and symptoms of PTSD.

Chronic Stress

Chronic stress can wear a sufferer down, making them feel "burned-out." It occurs when someone feels that they can't see the end of the demands. Over time, the negative feelings of stress make them feel sad, miserable, and disheartened on a continual basis. Factors like poverty, chronic illness, unhappy relationships, or dissatisfaction with your job can lead to this type of stress.

Individuals experiencing chronic stress may even grow accustomed to feeling badly. They may still notice acute episodes of stress, but they have stopped trying to resolve the source of their chronic stress. They've given up hope and no longer look for answers. Sometimes they form an unhealthy worldview on life, and they feel like they'll never measure up or that the world is only ever cruel and harsh.

This form of stress can be detrimental to your health, particularly when you become acclimated or even comfortable with it. You may not feel any more stressed this month than you did last month because every month is the same. Over time, your body definitely feels the effects of the stress, placing you at greater risk for stroke, heart attack, and depression.

Traumatic Stress

Post-traumatic stress is associated with traumatic events. Traumatic events are marked by a sense of horror or helplessness, or the threat of or actual serious injury or death. Traumatic events affect survivors of trauma, rescue workers, and the friends and relatives of victims or survivors of trauma. Traumatic events may also have an impact on people who witness the event firsthand, or experience the event later in video or a retelling of the event or its impact. These can be traumatic experiences from childhood, war, poverty, major accidents, shootings, violence, sexual assault, or abuse.

A person's response to a traumatic event may vary. Responses include feelings of fear or grief. Physical and behavioral responses include nausea, dizziness, and changes in appetite and sleep patterns. Trauma may also cause a person to withdraw from their daily activities.

Responses to trauma can last for weeks or months before a person starts to feel normal again. Most people feel better within a few months after a traumatic event, but for some, problems last longer or become worse. In some situations, the person may be suffering from **post-traumatic stress disorder** (PTSD).

Post-traumatic stress disorder (PTSD) is an intense physical and emotional response to thoughts about or reminders of the traumatic event that may last for weeks, months, or even years after the event. The symptoms of PTSD fall into three broad types—re-living, avoidance, and increased arousal (Figure 6).

Other symptoms linked with PTSD include panic attacks, depression, suicidal thoughts and feelings, drug abuse, feelings of being estranged and isolated, or not being able to complete daily tasks.

Stress in the US

Since 2007, the American Psychological Association's Stress in America™ survey has examined how stress affects the health and well-being of adults living in the US. In 2017, reported overall stress levels increased slightly, with greater percentages of adults reporting extreme levels of stress than in 2016. Overall, adults report that stress has a negative impact on their mental and physical health, but the number of adults taking action to cope with stress has been on the rise since 2014. 74% of adults feel they have someone they can rely on for emotional support, and nearly 53% exercise or take part in physical activity to cope with stress.

In a recent survey conducted by the American Psychological Association (APA), younger Americans report higher average stress levels on a scale of 1–10 than older individuals. Older adults (age 72 or older) have the lowest stress levels at 3.3, Baby Boomers (age 53-71) are at 3.9, Gen Xers (age 39-52) are at 5.3, and Millennials (18-38) are highest with 5.7. The survey shows that younger groups are more likely to say their stress has increased in the past year, and in fact, the survey revealed Millennials as the only age group with stress levels that increased since 2016. All other groups had reported decreased stress levels.

Higher stress is disproportionately reported by Americans with lower incomes. Survey findings show that Americans whose total reported household income before taxes was less than $50,000 have an average stress level of 5.1, compared to 4.6 for Americans whose households made $50,000 or more. In addition, 25 % of those with a total household income before taxes of less than $50,000 reported they were not doing enough to manage stress compared to 19 % of those above $50,000 (Figure 7).

Race and gender impact stress, as well. Hispanic adults experienced an average stress level of 5.2, and Black adults' overall stress level is at 5.0. This is a significant increase from the 2016 survey, which had Hispanic adults at 5.0 and Black adults at 4.7. White adults showed no increase to their stress level, remaining at 4.7 in both years. Women have reported higher stress levels than men since 2007, and their stress levels increased last year (from 5.0 to 5.1) while men's stress levels went down (from 4.6 to 4.4).

College students and young adults frequently feel high levels of stress during this period of significant transition in life (Figure 8) Roles shift, identities change, and additional stressors make students particularly vulnerable. Students often attend school away from their homes and must meet the expectations that they do well academically while managing a new environment and learning to interact with others on a different level socially, culturally, and intellectually. These stressors continue throughout their time in college as other expectations and pressures arise (Figure 9) Often students work and attend school at the same time, begin long-term relationships, and take on more adult roles requiring maturity. Learning "how to adult"—keeping up with the increased workload, meeting challenges with roommates and romantic partners, and generally being more mature—can be an intensely stressful experience.

However, there is good news. Higher education has been linked to a reduction in psychological distress in both men and women, and these effects persist throughout the aging process, not just immediately after receiving their education. The major mechanism by which higher education plays a role in reducing stress in men is more closely related to labor-market resources (increased chances of getting a well-paying job). This is compared to social resources, the mechanism by which higher education plays a role in reducing stress for women. The process of becoming educated may be stressful, but your body and mind will thank you in the long-term.

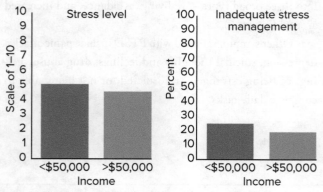

Figure 7. Comparison of reported stress rating and percent of unsuccessful stress management for people with annual incomes below and above $50,000 per year.

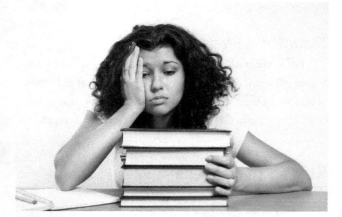

Figure 8. Students frequently report stress from school.

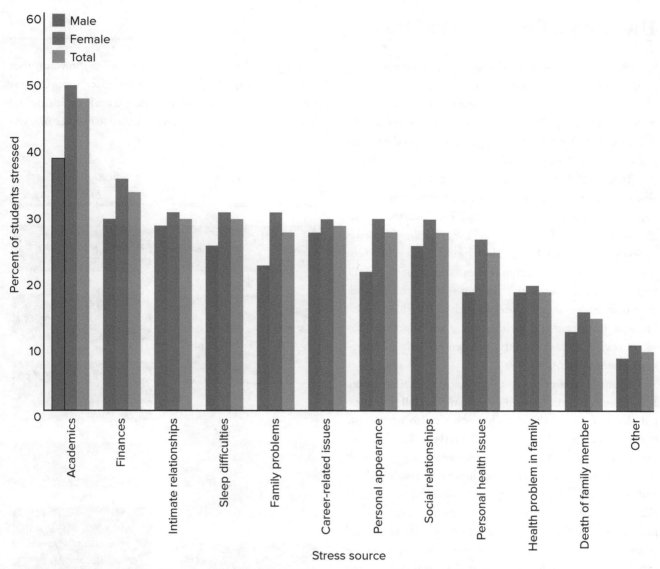

Figure 9. Percentage of male and female students expereiencing the most common sources of stress.

Effects of Stress on the Body and Mind

A stressful situation, regardless of the source, can unleash the flow of stress hormones in an attempt to bring homeostasis to your body, causing your heart to pound, your breathing to quicken, your muscles to tense, and sweat begin to form on your brow. This "**fight-or-flight**" response evolved as a survival mechanism, enabling people and animals to react quickly to life-threatening situations, and either fight off the threat or get to safety. This may be great when you're trying to outrun a bear, but not so great when you're caught in traffic or racing to class, neither of which are life threatening. Sometimes the body can overreact to stressors that require you to neither fight nor flee, depending upon how you see the situation.

Unfortunately, chronic stress can have long-term effects on your physical and psychological health. Over time, this biological battleground, when experienced too often, can take a toll on your body. Chronic stress may contribute to high blood pressure, clogged arteries, and even cause changes in your brain that may contribute to anxiety, depression, and addiction.

The Body's Response to Stress

So, when you feel stress, what happens to make your body do the things it does (Figure 10)? When someone confronts an oncoming form of danger, their eyes and ears send information to the amygdala, an area of the brain that contributes to emotional processing. The amygdala interprets the images and sounds, and if it suspects danger, it sends a distress signal.

Three glands work together to help you cope with a change or a stressful situation. Two are in your brain—the hypothalamus and the pituitary gland. The third, the adrenal glands, are on top of your kidneys. The amygdala first sends a message the hypothalamus. The hypothalamus is like your brain's remote control. It communicates with the rest of the body through the autonomic nervous system. This controls your body's involuntary functions such as breathing, blood pressure, heartbeat, and the dilation or constriction of key blood vessels. It has two parts, the sympathetic and parasympathetic systems.

The hypothalamus sets off a physiological chain reaction. It signals your pituitary gland that it is time to tell your adrenal glands to release the stress hormones called **adrenaline** (epinephrine), **noradrenaline**, and **cortisol**. These chemicals, called catecholamines, pump into your body through the bloodstream, increasing your heart rate and breathing and providing a burst of energy (increase of blood sugar) to take on the problem. Your breathing gets deeper, sending more oxygen to the brain, and heightening your senses and awareness. These chemicals can also control body temperature (which can make you feel hot or cold), keep you from getting hungry, and make you less sensitive to pain. Essentially, your **sympathetic nervous system**, true to its name, "feels sorry for you" and steps in to help.

This reaction can start before you are even fully aware of what's going on. It's instantaneous! You may have heard stories of people completing super-human feats like lifting heavy objects and jumping out of the way of cars without thinking about it because of a rush of adrenaline. That's all thanks to the body's ancient capacity for self-preservation.

Once the danger has passed, the hypothalamus hits the remote control to change the channel again. This time, it activates your **parasympathetic nervous system**, which is like going from heavy metal music videos to public broadcasting of the symphony. This system tells the sympathetic system to calm down, which promotes a "rest and digest" response and calms the body back down.

But what happens when life continues to throw surprises at you? If you have one stressful event after another, your stress response may not be able to stop itself from running overtime, and you may not have a chance to rest, restore, and

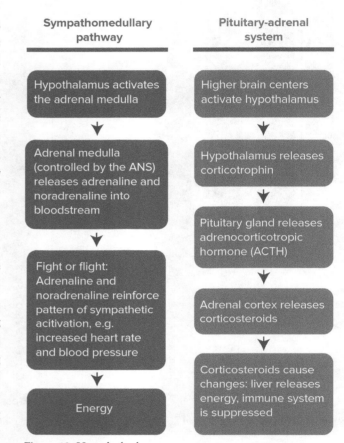

Figure 10. How the body reacts to stress.

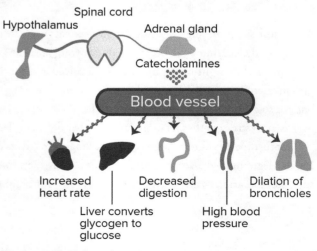

Figure 11. Physiological responses to stress.

recuperate. This can add up. Suddenly, the signs of overload hit you, turning short-term stressors into long-term stress. This means that you may have even more physical signs of stress. Things like a headache, eating too much or not at all, tossing and turning all night, or feeling down and angry all the time, are all signs of long-term stress. These signs will likely start just when you're sure you can't deal with any more.

Long-term stress can affect your health and how you feel about yourself, so it is important to learn to deal with it. No one is completely free of stress. The most important thing to learn about long-term stress is how to spot it. You can do that by paying attention to your body's physiological signals and learning healthy ways to handle them (Figure 11).

The Mind's Response to Stress

Stress has an impact on your emotional state in similar ways to its impact on your physiological responses. Stress, especially when prolonged, can intensify and create strong emotions in people, such as anger and fear. Like all your emotions, there is an appropriate time and place for each, but if it seems like you may be angry all the time, or you feel afraid of things that shouldn't cause fear, take some time to figure out what could be causing these emotional responses.

Anger is a normal emotion for most people, but intense or prolonged anger can jeopardize your employment, relationships, education, freedom, and even your health. This knowledge of anger's effect on health dates back centuries. In Buddhist teachings, anger is considered one of the Three Poisons of the Mind, along with greed and foolishness. Consider what it means to consume poison or for something to be poisonous. It ultimately leads to pain.

Typically, when someone gets angry, they experience responses that are physiological (becoming flushed or having a burst of energy and arousal), cognitive (thoughts occur in response to an event), emotional (feeling afraid, discounted, disrespected, or impatient), and behavioral (sarcasm, swearing, crying, or yelling). You're human, so you probably understand this. You've likely slammed a door or two or mentally stewed over an argument at some point in your life. This is normal. Anger becomes a problem when someone's behavior harms others, which is typically rooted in experiencing anger as a chronic condition. Problem anger may feel like it never goes away and is punctuated by physical violence or a full-on verbal rage. The consequences of long-term anger issues can lead to arrest, injury (to yourself self or others), a negative impact to important relationships, or job loss. Some groups have a higher risk of experiencing problems with anger, including individuals who struggle with substance abuse, traumatic brain injury, PTSD, or personality disorders.

If a person realizes they may have a problem with anger, they should start by taking a moment to think about why,

exactly, they are angry. There are many types of anger (Figure 12). They can ask themselves useful questions like "Have I eaten recently?" or "Is the thing I am angry about my actual issue?" Identifying the problem clearly and reasonably can make an angry person more capable of handling the issue in a healthy way. If the problem is ongoing, it's a good idea to learn more about anger management.

The goal of anger management is to reduce both your emotional feelings and the physiological arousal that anger causes. You can't get rid of or avoid the things or people that enrage you, nor can you change them, but you can learn to control your reactions. Try some of the following tips to help manage periods of anger:

Walk away when you're angry. Count to 10 before you react, then reconsider. If needed, walk even farther, giving yourself time to relax. Exercise can boost endorphins that improve your mood. Chronic anger and stress can be improved with daily exercise, so commit to some form each day.

Anger	Description
Chronic	Prolonged anger, this can impact the immune system and be the cause of other mental disorders.
Passive	Doesn't always come across as anger and can be difficult to identify.
Overwhelmed	Caused by life demands that are too much for an individual to cope with.
Self-inflicted	Directed toward the self and may be caused by feelings of guilt.
Judgmental	Directed toward others and may come with feelings of resentment.
Volatile	Involves sometimes-spontaneous bouts of excessive or violent anger.

Figure 12. Anger is normal but it can be a problem.

Practice relaxation. Breathe deeply. Inhale from the diaphragm (breathing from your chest won't relax you). Really visualize the path of your breath from deep in your core out through your mouth. Slowly repeat a calming word or phrase such as "relax," "you're fine," or "take it easy." Imagine that you're someplace relaxing or more pleasurable to you. Yoga and/or frequent meditation can be a good option to help you relax and remove tension from your body.

Problem-solve realistically. It takes time to solve some problems. Set a plan or approach for how you will solve the problem and how you will face it rather than growing frustrated.

Refocus using logic. Demand logic from yourself. Are you expecting more than is practical from yourself or someone else. Is what you expect reasonable? Practical? Tell yourself "I would like . . . " rather than "I demand . . . " or "I must have . . . " (Figure 13).

Like many horror movie aficionados, you may have learned that there is a certain value in **fear**—we're talking about the sense of power that comes from being able to escape of defeat a monster, the heroic idea of saving yourself and others. In these situations, fear comes with a sense of exhilaration, like being on a rollercoaster. The difference between this type of fear and those that happen in real life is the knowledge that it will end. You know the rollercoaster ride will end with you safely exiting a turnstile. You know the movie ends in 1 hour and 55 minutes, with the heroes (mostly) intact.

In the real world, we have a lot to fear from carcinogens, radiation, new technologies capable of spying on us and dominating the world. Okay, maybe not world domination, but often we fear things we feel unable to control. The sense of worry over one thing or another, whether real or imagined, can extend beyond a particular moment and become overwhelming.

Even when actual danger exists, fear can cloud good judgment. There are hazards to the misperception of risk. The decisions you make when fearful are often over- or under-reactions to the actual risk at hand. Your heightened senses under stress—caused by adrenaline—can make unreal dangers seem real, and real dangers seem insignificant.

Why are so many people afraid so often? We no longer fear death or illness from many diseases like smallpox or measles because of vaccines. In many ways, the world is safer now than it has ever been. Fear is, at its base, a response to risk. In the US, most people have access to food, clean water, and

Tips on Controlling Anger	
Relaxation	Breathe deeply, from your diaphragm. Use imagery. Try non-strenuous, slow exercises.
Cognitive Restructuring	Avoid words like "never" or "always" when talking about yourself or others. Use logic. Translate expectations into desires.
Environmental Change	Give yourself a break. Consider the timing. Avoid what you can.

Figure 13. Ideas for controling anger.

medical care. Those who study risk perception say that our responses to risks aren't simple. They aren't just an internal, rational analysis of the risk, but also intuitive responses that apply our emotions, values, and instincts as we try to determine our level of danger. It helps us understand why our fears often do not match the facts.

The Characteristics of Risk

The risk itself is most often relative the person assessing the situation. What is "risky" to one person may be fun (or not as stressful) to another. Risk perception researchers have determined some consistent characteristics of risk that form the basis of a person's perceptions and their fears.

Trust—The less you trust the people or equipment that is supposed to protect you, the more afraid you will be. This is especially true in situations where your supposed protectors are the same things that are exposing you to risk in the first place. The opposite is true, too: the more you trust, the less you fear.

Dread—Dread is the extreme life-or-death kind of fear, and is relative to the level of risk. This doesn't always have a relationship to reality. There are many things in life that people dread besides actual death. You may dread giving a presentation, leaving your family for long periods, flying, hunting for a new job, attending a funeral, or any number of things about which your mind has determined risk—risk of death, sadness, failure, suffering, and so on.

Control—If you feel you have some control over the level of risk that you will face, it will probably not seem as threatening as if it was determined by someone or something else that you can't control. You may hate riding as a passenger in a car but love to drive—you feel safer when you're in control.

Natural or Man-Made—Risks created by man evoke more fear than natural ones. There is an element of the unknown to something man-made rather than something that has occurred since the beginning of time.

Choice—A risk you choose seems less dangerous than a risk you don't. You may have to give many speeches in class because you chose a Speech and Debate course, but giving a presentation in front of your boss may feel higher risk.

Children—Many creatures have an inherent need to preserve their species and their offspring. People are far less likely to subject their children to risk than themselves.

Uncertainty—There is an old saying that "uncertainty is the mother of fear," or something along those lines. This seems to be true. The greater the uncertainty, the more cautious you are. You feel this way when you don't have all the answers to your questions (What will happen? Will this cause harm?), or the answers are confusing to understand (consider the language of academic journal articles). That feeling of uncertainty contributes to fear.

Novelty—New risks, like artificial intelligence or the Ebola virus, tend to be frightening until you have lived with them for a while and learned enough to put the risks into perspective.

Awareness—The more you are aware of a risk, the more you will likely be concerned about it. When some new unsafe trend gains media exposure, it's more likely to cause concern.

Vulnerability—Any risk seems greater if you think you or someone you care about could be a victim.

Risk-Benefit Trade Off—If you think something risky could also have benefits to you, you're more likely to see the risk as smaller or more worthwhile.

Catastrophic or Chronic—People are more likely to fear a mass attack, plane crash, or natural disaster than something like heart disease. These catastrophic incidents kill many people at once, often in a horrific way. As you've learned in this book, heart disease is the number one killer in the US, but most of us are likely less afraid of it than a large earthquake that could happen any time. This is a good example of the dangers of misperceiving risk. You might stock up on gallons of water and non-perishable food at the grocery store and then visit the drive-thru for a combo meal on the way home.

Phobias

A **phobia** is a strong, irrational fear of something that poses little or no real danger. Many specific phobias exist. Some of us have a fear of heights (acrophobia), enclosed spaces (claustrophobia), spiders (arachnophobia), or even leaving our homes (agoraphobia). If you become anxious and extremely self-conscious in everyday social situations, you could have what is referred to as a **social phobia**. Social phobias affect about 7% of people in the US and 0.5–2.5% of people in the rest of the world. Agoraphobia affects about 1.7% of people, women about twice as often as men. Typical onset of agoraphobia is age 10–17, with rates that get lower as people age. Common phobias involve tunnels, highway driving, water, flying, animals, and blood (Figure 14).

Most commonly, people have specific phobias of spiders, snakes, and heights. Occasionally they are triggered by a

Common Phobias*	Percentage of US Population Affected**
Acrophobia (fear of heights)	7.5%
Arachnophobia (fear of spiders)	3.5%
Aerophobia (fear of flying)	2.6%
Astraphobia (fear of thunder and lightning)	2.1%
Dentophobia (fear of dentists)	2.1%
*Approximately 4–5% of the US population has one or more clinically significant phobias in a given year. **The average age of onset for social phobia is between 15 and 20 years of age, although it can often begin in childhood.	

Figure 14. Phobias are more than just fears. These percentages represent diagnosed phobias in the US.

negative experience with the object or situation. They often begin in childhood but can occur in response to any trigger at any time. Specific phobias affect about 6–8% of people in the Western world and 2–4% of people in Asia, Africa, and Latin America in a given year.

People with phobias most often try to avoid the source of their fear. If they can't, they may experience panic and fear, rapid heartbeat, shortness of breath, trembling, and a strong desire to get away from the thing they're afraid of. Phobias should be treated rather than accepted, as they can lead to additional stress. One common method is exposure therapy, where the person gradually increases their contact with whatever they fear. Say, for example, that you fear snakes. You might begin by reading about snakes and looking at pictures of them, progress to looking at snakes at the zoo for longer and longer periods of time, then touch or handle one in a controlled setting, and so on. Essentially, practice being around them. Medications may not always be useful with phobias or may need to be combined with therapy. It can also be helpful to join a support group for whatever phobia you face.

Is it Fear or Anxiety?

We often conflate the terms "fear" and "anxiety" because the body's response to both of them is similar, if not the same, such as a fast heart rate and shakiness. Fear is a response to risk. **Anxiety,** however, occurs even when the risk is not present. People experiencing anxiety worry about future events. People experiencing fear react to specific, identifiable events. people who are anxious may not even know the source of their anxiety.

It's normal for people to feel anxious in response to stress. Sometimes, however, anxiety becomes a severe, persistent problem that's hard to control and can affect a person's day-to-day life. This is called an **anxiety disorder**. About 12% of people are affected by an anxiety disorder in a given year, and between 5–30% are affected at some point in their life. Anxiety disorders occur about twice as often in females as males, and generally begin before the age of 25. Anxiety disorders cost the US more than $42 billion per year in treatment costs, almost one-third of the country's $148 billion total mental health bill. More than $22 billion of those costs relate to the repeated use of health care services—people with anxiety disorders often seek relief for symptoms that mimic physical illnesses.

Differences in brain chemistry may account for at least part of these differences. The brain system involved in the fight-or-flight response activates more readily in women and stays activated longer than in men, partly as a result of the action of estrogen and progesterone. The neurotransmitter serotonin may also play a role in responsiveness to stress and anxiety. Some evidence suggests that the female brain does not process serotonin as quickly as the male brain. Recent research has found that women are more sensitive to low levels of corticotropin-releasing factor, a hormone that organizes stress responses, making them twice as vulnerable to stress-related disorders.

Diagnosing anxiety disorders can be complicated. With physical illnesses, health care providers can often pinpoint a likely cause. The cause of anxiety disorders is a combination of genetic and environmental factors. Certain factors make a person more at risk for developing a disorder, such as a history of abuse, family history of mental disorders, and poverty. People often have more than one anxiety disorder. They can often occur with other mental disorders, particularly major depressive disorder, personality disorder, and substance use disorder. A co-occurrence with depression is quite common. Nearly half of those diagnosed with depression also have a diagnosis of an anxiety disorder.

There are a number of anxiety disorders, including generalized anxiety disorder, specific phobia, social anxiety disorder, separation anxiety disorder, agoraphobia, and panic disorder. Each disorder differs by the symptoms the person experiences. The most common are specific phobias, which affect nearly 12% of the population, and social anxiety disorders, which affect 10% of the population at some point in their life.

Generalized anxiety disorder (GAD) is characterized by excessive worry about a variety of everyday problems for at least 6 months. For example, people with GAD may excessively worry about and anticipate problems with their finances, health, employment, and relationships. They typically have difficulty calming their concerns, even though they realize that their anxiety is more intense than the situation warrants. Symptoms of GAD vary widely (Figure 15).

Many of us will on rare occasions have what we believe to be a panic attack. We become so overwhelmed with a particular situation that we find ourselves unable to control the sensation of fear or dread, even when our body is telling us we need to calm down. We can usually put our finger on exactly what occurred and why. People with **panic disorder** have recurrent unexpected panic attacks, which include sudden periods of intense fear, even a feeling of impending doom. This may cause the heart to palpitate, pound, or race. They may experience sweating, trembling, shaking, shortness of breath, a sensation of smothering or choking, or other symptoms

Generalized Anxiety Disorder

Restlessness, feeling of being wound up, on edge
Being easily fatiigued
Difficulty concentrating
Irritability
Muscle tension
Difficulty controlling worry
Difficulty sleeping

Figure 15. Some symptoms of generalized anxiety disorder.

Panic Disorder

Sudden, repeated attacks of intense fear
Feeling out of control during attacks
Intense worry about next attack (when and where)
Avoidance of places where past attacks occurred

Figure 16. Some symptoms of panic disorder.

Social Anxiety Disorder

Feeling anxious around people
Difficulty talking with people
Fear of being judged by people
Worrying long before events with other people
Avoiding places where there are people
Difficulty making and keeping friends
Blushing, sweating, trembling around people
Nausea when peope are around

Figure 17. Some symptoms of social anxiety disorder.

(Figure 16). People with panic disorder often cannot say what caused the attack and may not be able to anticipate when the next one will occur.

People with **social anxiety disorder** (sometimes called "social phobia") have a fear of social or performance situations. It isn't unusual for someone to feel a bit awkward or anxious when trying to make a good first impression on someone new. It's also common to dread being in a social environment with someone you don't get along with. A person with a social anxiety disorder, however, actively attempts to avoid social situations out of a genuine fear that people will react negatively to them in some way. Symptoms of social anxiety disorders vary widely (Figure 17)).

For a person with any type of anxiety disorder, the anxiety doesn't go away and can get worse over time. The feelings can interfere with daily activities such as job performance, school, work, and relationships. This makes treatment very important. To be diagnosed, symptoms typically need to be present for at least 6 months, be more severe than would be expected for the situation, and impair the person's regular functioning.

Evaluation of a disorder often begins with a visit to a primary care provider. Some physical health conditions, such as heart disease, an overactive thyroid, or low blood sugar, can imitate or worsen an anxiety disorder. Certain medications can also cause side effects that mimic anxiety disorders. Your health care provider will also look to identify issues with heavy use of caffeine, alcohol, cannabis, or withdrawal from certain drugs. A thorough mental health evaluation is also helpful, because anxiety disorders, as mentioned, often co-exist with other related conditions, such as depression or obsessive-compulsive disorder.

Treatment for Anxiety

Anxiety disorders can generally be treated with psychotherapy, medication, or both. To be effective, **psychotherapy**, or "talk therapy," must be directed at the person's specific anxieties and tailored to their needs. The individual will typically experience some temporary discomfort involved with thinking about confronting feared situations. Therapists will often use other forms of therapy alongside psychotherapy.

Cognitive Behavioral Therapy (CBT) teaches the person different ways of thinking, behaving, and reacting to anxiety-producing and fearful situations. CBT can also help people learn and practice social skills, which is vital for treating social anxiety disorder.

Two specific stand-alone components of CBT used to treat social anxiety disorder are cognitive therapy and exposure therapy. Cognitive therapy focuses on identifying, challenging, and then neutralizing unhelpful thoughts underlying anxiety disorders. Exposure therapy focuses on confronting the fears underlying an anxiety disorder in order to help people engage in activities they have been avoiding. This is used along with relaxation exercises and/or imagery. CBT may be conducted individually or with a group of people who have similar problems. Often, participants receive "homework" to complete between sessions.

Some people with anxiety disorders might benefit from joining a **self-help or support group** and sharing their problems and achievements with others. Internet chat rooms might also be useful, but any advice received over the web should be used with caution. A trusted friend or member of the clergy can also provide support, but they may not necessarily be a sufficient alternative to care from an expert clinician.

Stress management techniques and **meditation** can help people with fears and anxiety disorders calm themselves and may enhance the effects of therapy. You'll learn more about stress management techniques later in this chapter. Since caffeine, certain illicit drugs, and even some over-the-counter cold medications can aggravate the symptoms of anxiety disorders, these should be limited.

For students, test anxiety and nervousness about public speaking is quite common. School can be stressful, particularly when other issues coincide with your studies or when you are struggling with a particular subject. People with learning disabilities or who have had difficulty taking exams in the past can find themselves feeling panicked and paralyzed. Often, this anxiety can be lessened with some preparation, strategy, and stress management techniques. Here are a few tips for overcoming test anxiety (Figure 18).

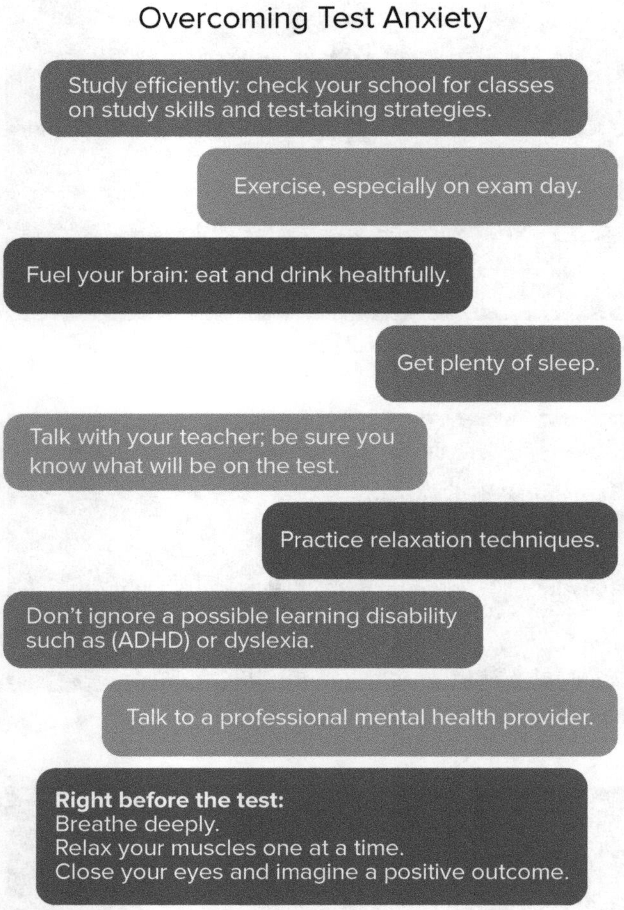

Medications do not cure anxiety disorders, but they may relieve symptoms. They are sometimes used as the initial treatment of an anxiety disorder or only if the person does not respond well enough to a course of psychotherapy. Research shows that patients treated with a combination of psychotherapy and medication often have better outcomes than those treated with only one or the other. The most common classes of medications used to combat anxiety disorders are antidepressants, anti-anxiety drugs, and beta-blockers. Be

Overcoming Test Anxiety

Study efficiently: check your school for classes on study skills and test-taking strategies.

Exercise, especially on exam day.

Fuel your brain: eat and drink healthfully.

Get plenty of sleep.

Talk with your teacher; be sure you know what will be on the test.

Practice relaxation techniques.

Don't ignore a possible learning disability such as (ADHD) or dyslexia.

Talk to a professional mental health provider.

Right before the test:
Breathe deeply.
Relax your muscles one at a time.
Close your eyes and imagine a positive outcome.

Figure 18. Test anxiety can be lessened with these strategies.

aware that some medications work effectively only if taken regularly and that symptoms may recur if the medication is stopped.

Factors that Affect How You Manage Stress

Your best friend has road rage. The littlest "offense" by another driver turns him into a racecar driver. He stays on the offender's bumper until he can pull alongside them, sneer or gesture, and then find a way to box them in so that they can't change lanes. While most people would just assume the person cut them off by accident, he takes personal offense. You've known for years that he just can't stand to not be in control of the situation (and that you should drive whenever you travel together).

You may react one way to a certain stressor, while your friend has a completely different way of handling the same situation. Several factors affect stress for individuals, including their personality type and traits, gender, biological sex,

cognitive patterns, and coping strategies.

According to the American Psychological Association, **personality** refers to individual differences in characteristic patterns of thinking, feeling, and behaving. The study of personality focuses on two broad methods. One is understanding individual differences in particular personality characteristics, such as sociability or irritability. The other is understanding how the various parts of a person come together as a whole.

It is human nature to question aspects of personalities, our own and others. What may seem normal to one person may seem abnormal to another. Character traits, like strength or weakness, shyness or boldness, empathy or apathy, self-confidence or insecurity, and humbleness or narcissism are commonly understood on paper but often relative to the situation and highly variable within a person. What is normal in this situation for this person, and what is pathological? We like to think that we can determine a lot about people based on their "type" of personality.

Personality Types

Over thousands of years, we have developed a variety of categories to help describe personality types ranging from humors (different quantities of four fluids—blood, phlegm, yellow bile, and black bile—determined your personality type up until the nineteenth century) to the Myers-Briggs personality test (which also uses four personality indicators and combinations of those indicators to classify personality). These approaches clearly oversimplify something that can be rather complex. Despite any controversy, classifying stress responses can give people some insight into how they respond to or generate stress. They can use that information to figure out a course of action that will help them deal with stress in a positive way.

In the mid-twentieth century, cardiologists Friedman and Rosenman noticed a particular pattern among their patients. More "intense" people were more likely to have heart disease and high blood pressure. From there, they developed their widely accepted theory of four personality types.

Type A. These are the classic Type A personalities, characterized as driven, highly competitive, self-critical, and deadline focused (always rushing). They may be seen as high achieving but short-tempered and impatient with themselves and sometimes others.

Type B. In theory, Type B individuals are the opposite of Type A. They are more tolerant of others, creative, relaxed, reflective, and have a lower level of stress. They tend to take the "go with the flow" attitude. This could be to the point of a lack of drive and competitiveness, or no sense of urgency to meet deadlines. They can often be seen as more patient and adaptable to what happens around them. They also have a lower incidence of stress and disease.

Type C. The studies and categories have evolved over the years, with additional theorists bringing in additional categories to often include a C and D. Type C individuals have difficulty expressing emotions

and will often suppress them. They tend to avoid conflict and desire social favorability. They often appear pathologically nice, overly compliant, and overly patient, but they may not feel this patience. In fact, they may be angry, but they tend to keep it inside. Type C individuals often suppress their own needs and have difficulty speaking up for themselves. This makes them more prone to stress and stress-related illness, such as depression.

Type D. Individuals with a Type D personality tend to be very negative. They are critical of themselves, tense, and tend to worry a lot. It is frequently referred to as Type Distressed or Type Disease Prone. They tend to be frequently dissatisfied with life, anxious, depressed, and irritable. With this comes a higher risk for stress-related illnesses such as heart disease.

Most people do not fit one particular category, but it's worth noting the characteristics of each type. If you're a clear Type A, you may be on your way to cardiac issues. A Type B may be a bit too unmotivated for some professions and not particularly successful. The gloom and doom personality of Type D and self-effacing nature of Type C present their own complications. Consider the elements of each type that you have in your personality and how it could impact your health. Psychologists look at personality types as a means of determining what characteristics of an individual most likely impact their level of stress.

Personality Traits

Much of your ability to handle and adapt to stress comes down to particular **personality traits**. In particular, they can impact how often you will push your "fight or flight" response to its limits. Some traits can keep you from losing control of your feelings, and building these traits can help you learn to handle stress in a healthy way.

Psychological hardiness is defined as a compilation of attitudes, beliefs, and behavioral tendencies that consist of three components—challenge, control, and commitment. Each boils down to your resilience when faced with difficulty and your ability to cope with stress.

Challenge. Hardy people see problems as challenges and opportunities to overcome an obstacle and succeed. They don't expect life to be easy. They accept change as part of life and are willing to work the problem at hand.

Control. Hardy people do not see themselves as victims of their stressors, nor do they accept them as something that they cannot control. They have an internal locus of control (see Chapter 1) and believe that their actions can improve the situation.

Commitment. Hardy people have a purpose in life. Rather than getting by, they set a course of direction and move forward.

Studies suggest that your level of psychological hardiness is often a predictor of your ability to succeed, adapt, cope, and achieve a mentally healthy well-being. Some of this likely comes from training. It begins in childhood. Children taught to problem-solve as they grow become hardier adults.

However, even if your parents stepped in and managed your issues for you, or played the victim to their stressors themselves, this hardiness can still be learned. For most, it comes down to shifting negative attitudes about yourself. Critical inner voices that are self-defeating or self-destructive can often be part of the problem. When you hear that voice that says, "They aren't treating you fairly," or "Nothing you do works," recognize it as the language of a victim.

It can also help to be honest about the negativity of those around you and how it may influence your thinking. For example, maybe you and your siblings always called your father "Daddy Downer." As far as Daddy Downer is concerned, the world is always horrible, life is out to get him, and he is just keeping his head above water—every day is a race to the grave. Sounds miserable! Did you pick up any of this from your father? You don't need to judge him or change him, but you should try to learn from him, or at least what not to do when it comes to negativity.

Avoid self-soothing behaviors that aren't productive. If you've grown accustomed to making yourself feel better by eating a pan of brownies or drinking excessively, it may be time to find healthier ways that are less about being a victim and more about being in control. Hardiness is about taking responsibility for your life with confidence rather than just letting things happen to you.

Shift-and-persist traits can also be quite valuable when it comes to learning how to manage stress. People with a low socioeconomic status often have more challenges when it comes to access to medical care, safe living environments, and sometimes even having enough healthy food. Studies have shown that people facing such challenges often have a higher risk for disease.

Yet the shift-and-persist trait often thrives in people who face challenges on a daily basis. Children, for example, who grow up in difficult environments often learn to shift (adapt with and to the stress) and persist (hold on to life as something that has meaning), with optimism. They learn to accept that stress and challenges exist and work around them. They stare down adversity and stay focused on positive things in life. This takes them off the road to disease and depression and keeps them on a road that is likely to be healthier.

In fact, your environment and culture can impact the way you view and handle stress. Some cultures promote an independent approach to stress management. Depending on how you were raised or the place you live, you may not feel comfortable asking for help or seeking support. Others may have a large network of individuals, a community of support ready to step in and help them manage. There are pros and cons to both, as we see with the shift-and-persist model and as you will see in a moment.

Gender and Biological Sex

As scientists discover that biological differences between males and females are less distinct than believed, there is, oddly enough, a sex-based component to the "fight or flight" response.

The sympathetic nervous system functions differently in men and women. For men, the fight and flight responses initiate that exact approach. When faced with danger or stress, the hormones circulate and men either stand and fight or seek safety. Women, on the other hand, are more likely to "tend and befriend" (Figure 19) Let's fight that boogey man one more

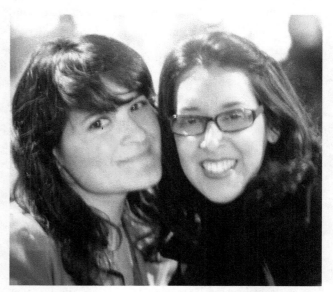

Figure 19. The tend and befriend stress management technique is more common amoung women.

time. He comes up behind your friends, Mary and Jack, with some form of menacing weapon wearing a ridiculously scary mask. Jack prepares to take him on. Mary begins to negotiate. "You don't really need to attack us," she says. "I can help you if you just put the machete down." The stress response specifically builds on attachment care-giving processes in females.

Theories suggest that women release more endorphins during stress that help alleviate pain and make them feel better about social interactions. Women release oxytocin as a stress hormone to combat negative feelings during labor and breastfeeding. There is also a theory that men have an extra gene, called the SRY gene, that increases the amount of norepinephrine released during stress, making the "fight or flight" response stronger than in women. Testosterone and estrogen may play a role as well, with testosterone generating a more intense response.

As you're learned already, that biological sex does make people more or less prone to certain diseases, both mentally and physically. Men are more prone to hypertension, aggressive behavior, and the abuse of drugs. Women tend to have more issues with chronic pain, depression, and anxiety disorders. Much of your risk of disease results from lifestyle choices, but sex hormones likely contributing to some degree. Often, these differences are more prevalent during reproductive years and then diminish after menopause for women.

Environmental issues and socially constructed roles are a significant contributing factor in how your body handles stress and develops health risks associated with stress. Women still take on a greater responsibility for housework caregiving (in addition to jobs outside the home) than their male counterparts. Combine this with full-time work and you can understand how their stress load may be different.

However, while both men and women recognize the impact stress can have on physical health, men appear to be somewhat more reluctant to believe that it's having an impact on their own health. Therefore, men put less emphasis on the need to manage their stress than women do. Men are more likely to see psychologists as unhelpful and are less likely to employ strategies to make lifestyle and behavior changes. Women are more likely than men to say they've tried to reduce stress and implement strategies for behavior change.

Research shows that prolonged periods of stress accompanied by the release of "fight or flight" hormones can decrease proper cell function, contributing to numerous emotional and physical disorders including depression, anxiety, heart attacks, stroke, hypertension, and immune system disturbances that increase susceptibility to infections. It's likely no coincidence that men more often experience these physical illnesses like hypertension, heart disease or attacks, and Type 2 diabetes.

Cognitive Patterns

Many theories attempt to answer why humans react to stress the way they do. Every person is unique in how they respond to a particular stressor, or even whether they view it as a stressor at all. One theory, the **Transactional Model of Stress and Coping**, suggests that individuals, when faced with a stressor, go through a series of steps in an attempt to cope.

First, they conduct a primary appraisal the situation — Is this even significant? Does it impact me? Next, they conduct a secondary appraisal — How can I handle this and reach a favorable outcome? Do I have the resources to cope with this? Last is the specific coping mechanism, which is either problem-based or emotional. In a problem-based approach, the individual senses their ability to cope and handle the situation. In emotion-based coping, the individual may feel as if they don't have the control and may avoid the situation entirely or struggle to deal with it.

The basics of the concept suggest that the stress is between the person and the environment. Stress occurs when a person perceives that the demands exceed their ability to mobilize the resources needed to solve the problem. The essential point is that we all respond differently based on how we measure the stressor and how capable we feel of handling it.

Other theories suggest we take slightly different approaches when we encounter stress. **Attribution Theory** suggests that we naturally try to make sense of the problems around us — it is in our nature to establish a cause and effect relationship, even when one doesn't exist. There are two relevant parts to this theory:

Internal Attribution. We attach the cause of the behavior to some internal characteristic, rather than to outside forces. When we explain the behavior of others we look for internal attributions, such as personality traits. For example, we attribute the behavior of a person to their personality, motives, or beliefs. This could apply to the individual, as well, attributing the problem to his or her own personality.

External Attribution. We attach the cause of behavior to some situation or event outside a person's control rather than to some internal characteristic. When we try to explain our own behavior, we tend to make external attributions, such as situational or environmental features.

For example, say that you took a test and did well on it. With internal attribution, you might be quite proud of yourself and discuss how hard you'd studied and how you earned that "A." If you had done poorly, you would remember how you went out with friends instead of studying and take responsibility for the "D." With external attribution theory, you may blame your success or failures on your instructor, tutor, or textbook. With both forms of attribution, we look for the "Why?" behind the incident, as it is our nature to do.

Understanding theories of how we react to stress can help us cope. They can help us determine what approach we may be taking in our assessment of a stressor and whether or not we are accurate and objective. Sometimes the first step in solving any problem is taking one backward to assess and get perspective.

Coping Strategies

Coping is the process of making a conscious effort to solve personal and interpersonal problems. When it comes to stress, people cope by attempting to solve, minimize, or tolerate the stress they face. To do this, they utilize **coping strategies** (Figure 20). All coping strategies are intended to resolve or reduce the stressor (adaptive) but some can be unhealthy or ineffective (maladaptive). Maladaptive behaviors can hinder or interfere with the individual's ability to adjust to the situation. Often, this occurs in an attempt to reduce anxiety, but the result is not productive.

Say, for example, that you have an argument with a friend. You're really upset and worried that if you attempt to talk to her about it, you may yell or cry. Instead, you avoid her entirely, dodging her phone calls for nearly a month until she gives up. You avoided the anxiety of having an uncomfortable conversation, but you lost a friend in the process.

The term "coping" usually refers to dealing with the stress that comes after being presented with a stressor, but many people also use proactive coping strategies to eliminate or avoid stressors before they occur—strategies that may help you look at a stressor in a different light. How you choose to cope depends upon your personality traits and type, the social context, and the nature of the stressor presented.

According to psychologists, though theories differ on how people cope, there are also some consistencies within these theories related to how we approach the stressor. We

Coping Strategies	Examples of Adaptive Strategies
Self-soothing	Something to touch (stuffed animal, stress ball) Something to hear (music, meditation guides) Something to taste (mints, tea, sour candy) Something to see (snow globe, happy pictures) Something to smell (lotion, candles, perfume)
Distraction	Taking your mind off of the problem with activities such as puzzles, books, artwork, crafts, knitting, crocheting, sewing, Sudoku, music, or movies
Opposite action	Doing something opposite of your impulse that is consistent with a more positive emotion
Affirmations and inspiration	Looking at motivational statements, drawing motivational images, or watching or reading something funny
Emotional awareness	Identifying and expressing your feelings with a list or chart of emotions, journal writing, drawing, or art
Mindfulness	Using tools for centering and grounding yourself in the present moment, such as meditation, relaxation recordings, yoga, breathing exercises, or grounding objects (like a rock or paperweight)
Crisis plan	Developing a contact list of supports and resources for when coping skills aren't enough, including family, friends, therapist, hotline, crisis team/ER, 911

Figure 20. Common coping strategies.

tend to approach them in three distinct ways—through how we appraise the problem, how we problem-solve, and how we use our emotions as we strategize.

Appraisal-focused strategies attempt to change the way you look at the stressor and approach it differently, sometimes questioning your goals and values. **Problem-focused strategies** strive to deal with the cause of the stressor, work through the problem, and in doing so remove the source of the stress or learn skills to manage it. **Emotion-focused strategies** focus on the emotions you are having due to the stressor and attempt to modify them. This could be by releasing the emotions, distracting themselves, or actively trying to manage their mental state. Let's look at some specific emotion-focused strategies.

Be positive. Think of every situation in life as a learning experience and be positive regardless of what happens. For example, if you failed to perform well in an exam, don't be intimidated by it when you face it again. Rather, be positive and find better ways to prepare for it. The next time around, you will do better. Negative emotions will only prevent you from dealing with situations effectively.

Don't let stressful events get the better of you. This is easier said than done, but once you realize that you're dealing with a stressful situation, quickly find a remedy. If you have to deal with several stressful situations at the same time, just step back for a minute, take deep breaths, and motivate yourself to deal with one issue at a time. Take control of the situation and you've already solved half the problem.

Communicate with others. Bottling up your emotions will only increase stress levels and could lead to a big outburst. Always maintain good communication channels with the people around you. Talk or confide in someone about your stressful situation and discuss ways in which you can handle it. This will give you the comfort and strength needed to deal with difficult situations.

Be accepting. Accept the fact that no one is perfect. Mistakes will always be made and it is impossible to control everything. Once you are accepting of yourself and others around you, you'll find that a lot of self-made stress is relieved.

Acknowledge mistakes. Mistakes are simply the steping stones to a better future. Don't get disappointed with yourself or put yourself down when you make mistakes. Rather, learn from your mistakes so that your future decision making will be better.

Acknowledge success. Success can also be a huge stressor since it sets up expectations to keep performing at exceptional levels to maintain that success. Learn from your success and build on your competence to avoid unwanted pressures.

Be disciplined. Follow a good discipline in whatever you do. When you are consistent in your efforts you will be able to handle any situation with confidence.

A typical person may engage in a mixture of these strategies when attempting to cope with a stressor. Their skill at this can change over time as they become more accustomed to actively learning to cope, or as they perceive a strategy as effective or ineffective.

Adaptive vs. Maladaptive Strategies

Sometimes it seems like you just can't get ahead. Some days, it feels like if one more thing happens, you're going to "lose it." How you manage stress may have something to do with this. **Adaptive** or positive coping strategies reduce stress and help the person learn from the situation. Seeking support from a friend, taking care of your health, meditating, getting enough sleep, and maintaining a sense of humor are all examples of adaptive coping strategies. Sometimes coping strategies can be proactive. The person anticipates a particular situation to be stressful and determines ahead of time how they will cope with it. Adaptive coping strategies include:

Support—Talk to a friend, counselor, or family member for advice or assistance. Talk to someone who can do something concrete.

Accept—Accept that it has happened and that you must adapt and/or address it. Take responsibility for the problem if you are in control of it.

Reinterpret positively—Decide what you can learn from it. See it as an opportunity for growth.

Restraint—Give yourself time to think about it rather than making a hasty decision, possibly making the stressor worse.

Plan—Develop a plan to cope with either the stress or the stressor.

Suppress—Suppress any competing activities. Give yourself breathing room to concentrate on the situation.

Maladaptive or negative coping strategies might work to make you feel better, but the result is dysfunctional and non-productive. They may offer a quick fix that either enables you to disassociate the source of stress from the symptoms or create another source of stress. Either way, you don't learn to cope with the stress productively. The relief is short lived. This often occurs when you ignore or avoid a certain stressor, or use alcohol, drugs, or some other mechanism in an attempt to forget about it. Maladaptive coping strategies to avoid include:

Don't avoid—Escaping or avoiding the problem by turning to other activities to take your mind off of it.

Don't disengage—Giving up trying to cope.

Don't seek just emotional support—Looking for sympathy rather than assistance.

Don't vent—Focusing on letting the emotions out and venting but not on adapting or resolving once the emotions are out.

Don't deny—Refusing to believe that it is happening.

Don't use alcohol or drugs—Using substances to forget the situation or make yourself feel better.

The first list above focuses on skills that actively manage stress, the source of the stress, or both. The second list probably sounds familiar, though. How many times have you vented to a friend, felt better, and then ignored the problem at hand? This may be fine if the source of the stress was someone who cut you off in traffic. But what if it's something larger? What if you lose your job? Going out with friends for a few drinks and complaining about your boss may make you feel better in the moment, but once that's done, you still need an adaptive strategy that will be more productive. Otherwise, the problem remains unresolved, which can often lead to greater stress.

High Stress Is a Health Risk

Stress, and long-term or chronic stress in particular, can negatively affect several dimensions of wellness. Your body adapts to changes in state, including those changes caused by stress. **Chronic stress** is stress that lasts for a longer period of time. You may have chronic stress if you have money problems, an unhappy marriage, or trouble at work. Any type of stress that goes on for weeks or months is chronic stress. If you don't find ways to manage stress, it may lead to health problems. Many signs of too much stress can point to a need to improve stress management. A few to look out for are:

- **Skin**—Your skin is breaking out in acne. Stress hormones cause acne to appear.

- **Hair**—Your hair is shedding. It is common to have hair that falls out or that is thinning all over during periods of stress.

- **Weakness**—Your blood sugar feels low. High stress levels can affect your levels, making you feel weak and shaky.

- **Aches**—You feel achy and sore. This is especially true when you internalize all of your stress. This can also lead to headaches.

- **Fainting**—You've experienced a fainting spell. When your blood pressure drops, it can make you feel woozy during times of stress.

Physiological Reactions

The fight or flight hormones released during stress make your brain more alert, cause your muscles to tense, and increase your pulse. These reactions are good in the short term because they can help you handle the situation causing stress. Your body does this to protect itself.

Chronic stress causes your body to stay alert, even if no immediate danger exists. Over time, this puts you at risk for health problems, including high blood pressure, heart disease, diabetes, obesity, depression or anxiety, skin problems such as

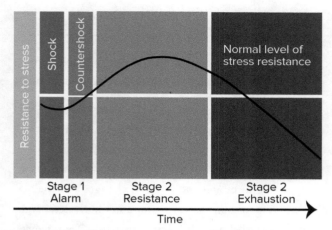

Figure 21. Seyle's path through the stages of stress.

acne or eczema, or menstrual problems. If you already have a health condition, chronic stress can make it worse.

General Adaptation Syndrome (GAS) theorizes that during the fight or flight response, the body enters 3 different stages—alarm, resistance, and exhaustion (Figure 21). The initial stage is **alarm**—the body responds first by setting off that wonderful chain reaction of hormones, preparing you to react. The second stage is **resistance**. Your hormone levels are still high and your body still in a ready state, but you are no longer alarmed (at least not at the same level). At this point, is ready to fight or flee (resist the stress). What you aren't able to do is take on an additional stressor very easily. The third stage is **exhaustion**. Once the body has remained in this ready state for a time, it begins to fatigue and become apathetic to the stress. This is the state that can lead to illness. Your body isn't meant to stay in this heightened state and other bodily systems begin to weaken, such as your immune system.

Allostatic load refers to the overload the body experiences when it reaches this state of exhaustion. **Allostasis** refers to the body's attempt to create a new and poorer form of homeostasis. Homeostasis occurs when the body is comfortable with its environment—everything is as it should be. If you spend too much time under stress, the body reaches a new normal, allostasis, in an attempt to adapt in the aftermath of

a response to stress.

Short-term, sporadic stress can have an impact on health as well. Have you ever gotten sick to your stomach before a test or speech, or taken a sudden fall and found yourself dizzy even though you didn't hit your head? The body can overreact at times, or just over-work in an attempt to help out. Imagine what it does during major acute stress, like an earthquake or a large argument with a friend.

Stress can start to interfere with your ability to live a normal, productive life. Over time, this can become dangerous. Studies suggest that sudden emotional stresses, particularly anger, can trigger heart attacks, arrhythmias and even sudden death. This happens primarily in people who already have heart disease, but often people don't know they have a problem until acute stress causes a heart attack or other serious medical issues. The longer the stress lasts, the harder it is on your mind and body. Fatigue and irritability are just the tip of the iceberg.

Some emotional effects are less serious, like fatigue or irritability. Others can be much more serious and even dangerous. Contact your health care provider if you experience any of these symptoms:

- Stress that is overwhelming or affecting your health
- New or unusual symptoms
- Feelings of panic, such as dizziness, rapid breathing, or a racing heartbeat
- You're unable to work or function at home or at your job
- Fears that you cannot control
- Memories of a traumatic event

Your provider may refer you to a mental health care provider. You can talk to this professional about your feelings, what seems to make your stress better or worse, and why you think you are having this problem. Call a suicide hotline immediately if you are having thoughts of suicide.

Depression

Sadness is a normal human emotion, but these feelings usually pass with a little time. People often use the term "depression" as a catch-all word for feeling sad, but the two aren't the same. **Depression**—also called "clinical depression" or a "depressive disorder"—is a mood disorder that causes distressing symptoms that affect how you feel, think, and handle daily activities, such as sleeping, eating, or working (Figure 22). Depressed people are often sad, but you can be sad without being depressed. To be diagnosed with depression, symptoms must be present most of the day, nearly every day for at least two weeks. Over 5% of Americans 12 years and older report being depressed. That number climbs to almost 10% of adults aged 40–59.

Some symptoms of depression include persistent sad, anxious, or "empty" mood; feelings of hopelessness or pessimism, guilt, worthlessness, or helplessness; loss of interest or pleasure in hobbies or activities; decreased energy, fatigue, or being "slowed down;" difficulty concentrating, remembering, or making decisions; difficulty sleeping, early-morning awakening, or oversleeping; appetite and/or weight changes; thoughts of death or suicide or suicide attempts; restlessness or irritability; and aches or pains, headaches, cramps, or digestive problems without a clear physical cause or that do not ease even with treatment.

Depression can be a serious medical illness and is an important public health issue. It can cause suffering not only for depressed individuals but their families and the communities in which they live. The economic burden of depression, including workplace costs, direct health care costs, and indirect costs to families is estimated to be over $200 billion annually.

The two most common forms of depression are major depression and persistent depressive disorder. These two forms of depression have different patterns of depressive symptoms:

Major depression—having symptoms of depression most of the day, nearly every day for at least 2 weeks that interfere with your ability to work, sleep, study, eat, and enjoy life. An episode can occur only once in a person's lifetime, but more often, a person has several episodes.

Persistent depressive disorder (dysthymia)—having symptoms of depression that last for at least 2 years. A person diagnosed with this form of depression may have episodes of major depression along with periods of less severe symptoms.

Other forms of depression are slightly different in their patterns or symptoms, or they may develop under unique circumstances:

Perinatal or Postpartum Depression is much more serious than the "baby blues" that many women experience after giving birth, which is known to accompany the hormonal and physical changes and the new responsibility of caring for a newborn that can be overwhelming. I?An estimated 10–15% of women experience postpartum depression after giving birth. Some women begin to see these mood changes during pregnancy, long before the birth of the child.

Bipolar disorder is different from depression. The reason it is included in this list is because someone with bipolar disorder experiences episodes of extreme low moods (depression). But a person with bipolar disorder also experiences extreme high moods (called "mania").

Seasonal Affective Disorder (SAD) is a type of depression that comes and goes with the seasons, typically starting in the late fall and early winter and going away during the spring and summer.

Psychotic Depression occurs when a person has severe depression plus some form of psychosis, such as delusions or hallucinations.

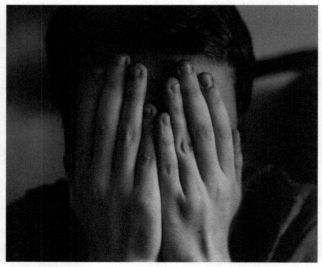

Figure 22. Depression is a serioius condition.

Depression affects different people in different ways. Women have depression more often than men, possibly due to biological, lifecycle, and hormonal factors. Women with depression typically have symptoms of sadness, worthlessness, and guilt. Men with depression more often exhibit symptoms of tiredness, irritability, and sometimes anger. They may lose interest in work or activities they once enjoyed, have sleep problems, and behave recklessly, including misusing drugs or alcohol. Many men do not recognize their depression and fail to seek help.

Older adults with depression may have less obvious symptoms, or they may be less likely to admit to feelings of sadness or grief. They more often have medical conditions, such as heart disease, which may cause or contribute to depression. Younger children with depression may pretend to be sick, refuse to go to school, cling to a parent, or worry that a parent may die. Older children and teens with depression may get into trouble at school, sulk, and be irritable. Teens with depression may have symptoms of other disorders, such as anxiety, eating disorders, or substance abuse.

Depression Treatment

The first step in getting the right treatment should be a visit to a health care provider or mental health professional, such as a psychiatrist or psychologist. Your health care provider can do an exam, interview, and lab tests to rule out other health conditions that may have the same symptoms as depression. Once diagnosed, depression can be treated with medications, psychotherapy, or a combination of the two. If these treatments do not reduce symptoms, brain stimulation therapy may be another treatment option to explore.

Medication called antidepressants can work well to treat depression, many of which are designed to alter the levels of neurotransmitters (signaling chemicals) in the brain — essentially, they try to put your brain in a happier state. They can take 2–4 weeks to work and can have side effects (drowsiness, nausea, insomnia), but many side effects may lessen over time.

Psychotherapy helps by teaching you new ways of thinking and behaving, and changing habits that may be contributing to depression. Therapy can help you understand and work through difficult relationships or situations that may be causing your depression or making it worse.

Brain Stimulation Therapies (such as Electroconvulsive Therapy) are sometimes used when medications and therapy prove unsuccessful on their own. Brain stimulation therapies involve activating or inhibiting the brain directly with electricity. These types of therapies are less frequently used than medication and psychotherapies, but they hold promise for treating certain mental disorders that do not respond to other treatments.

In addition, people experiencing depression can add **self-help techniques**. These are often learned through research, support groups, or medical guidance. Approaches like improving diet, getting exercise, and making sure to seek out positive social interactions can help you help yourself. Talking to people in your close social group, like friends and family, is a good idea and can help alleviate some of the burden of depression. In fact, being alone too much can have severe negative effects. If self-help is your preferred technique, here are some suggestions for success:

Stick to your treatment plan. Don't skip psychotherapy sessions or appointments. Even if you're feeling well, don't skip your medications. If you stop, depression symptoms may come back, and you could also experience withdrawal-like symptoms. Recognize that it will take time to feel better.

Pay attention to warning signs. Work with your health care provider or therapist to learn what might trigger your depression symptoms. Make a plan so that you know what to do if your symptoms get worse. Contact your health care provider or therapist if you notice any changes in symptoms or how you feel. Ask relatives or friends to help watch for warning signs.

Avoid alcohol and recreational drugs. It may seem like alcohol or drugs lessen depression symptoms, but in the long run they generally worsen symptoms and make depression harder to treat. Talk with your health care provider or therapist if you need help with alcohol or substance use.

Simplify your life. Cut back on obligations when possible and set reasonable goals for yourself. Give yourself permission to do less when you feel down.

Don't become isolated. Try to participate in social activities and get together with family or friends regularly. Support groups for people with depression can help you connect to others facing similar challenges and share experiences.

Structure your time. Plan your day with a list of daily tasks, use sticky notes as reminders, or use a planner to stay organized.

Don't make important decisions when you're down. Avoid decision-making when you're feeling depressed, since you may not be thinking clearly.

Be active and exercise. This releases mood-enhancing endorphins, boosts energy, and helps prevent other illnesses that can exacerbate depression

Reach out to family and friends. Rely on your support group, especially in times of crisis, to help you weather rough spells.

Get treatment at the earliest sign of a problem. Avoid worsening depressive episodes by seeking help before issues get out of control. Self-help should never be seen as exclusive to your treatment plan.

Consider getting long-term maintenance treatment. Think of maintenance treatment as filling a gap in your self-help, should one occur. This can help prevent a relapse of symptoms you thought were improved.

In addition to seeking help or treatment, try to do things that you used to enjoy. Remember to go easy on yourself, give yourself some time to see improvements. The resources at the end of this chapter offer more information on how to get help with depression.

Major depression is one of the most common mental disorders in the US. According to the World Health Organization, major depression also carries the heaviest burden of disability among mental and behavioral disorders. Specifically, major depression in the US accounts for 3.7% of all disability-adjusted life years and 8.3% of all years lived with disability.

Special Concern: Self-Injury and Suicide

Depression and forms of mental illness can sometimes feel overwhelming. Many people living with depression struggle with thoughts of suicide. The risk factors for suicidal behavior are complex. People of all genders, ages, and ethnicities can be at risk. Each suicide takes a substantial toll on individuals, families, and communities far beyond what the victim could anticipate. In the past, suicide was addressed by providing mental health services to people who were already experiencing or showing signs of suicidal thoughts or behav-

ior. But we now understand that we have to address many problems before they get too far and increase access to as many resources as possible to avoid tragedies. As with many other illnesses and diseases that have the potential to end badly, suicide is preventable.

Most suicidal individuals give **warning signs** or signals of their intentions. The best way to prevent suicide is to recognize these warning signs and know how to respond if you spot them. In addition to the signs and symptoms for depression, major warning signs for suicide include:

- Talking about killing or harming oneself

- Talking or writing a lot about death or dying

- Increasing substance use

- Big changes in eating or sleeping patterns

- Seeking out things that could be used in a suicide attempt, such as weapons and drugs

- Loss of interest in day-to-day activities

- Neglecting his or her appearance and hygiene

- Decreased energy, fatigue, or being "slowed down"

- Thoughts of death or suicide or suicide attempts

A subtler, but equally dangerous, warning sign of suicide is hopelessness. Studies have found that hopelessness is a strong predictor of suicide. People who feel hopeless may talk about "unbearable" feelings, predict a bleak future, and state that they have nothing to look forward to. These signals are even more dangerous if the person has a mood disorder, such as depression or bipolar disorder, suffers from alcohol dependence, has previously attempted suicide, or has a family history of suicide.

If you believe that a friend or family member may be suicidal, you can play a preventative role by pointing out the alternatives, showing that you care, and getting a health care provider or psychologist involved. If the threat may be imminent, do not hesitate to call 911. If the threat is not imminent, let the person express their feelings. Be cautious of using judgmental language and encourage them to seek professional help. Check on them, or send someone else to check on them, if you question the severity of the situation. Most communities have psychiatric staff available in emergencies to assess questionable situations and your local police can provide you with that information. Above all, do not ignore their behavior.

The resources at the end of this chapter offer more information and assistance.

Special Concern: Violence

Violence and abuse can take many forms—physical, emotional, verbal, and sexual. It can happen to anyone by anyone and can be a significant form of stress. One of the most common types of violence is **intimate partner violence** (IPV). In fact, one in every four women and one in every nine men are victims of either sexual violence, physical abuse, and/or stalking by an intimate partner. The term "intimate partner violence" describes physical, sexual, or psychological harm by a current or former partner or spouse. This type of violence can occur among heterosexual or same-sex couples and does not require sexual intimacy.

Persons with certain risk factors are more likely to become perpetrators or victims of intimate partner violence. Those risk factors contribute to IPV but might not be direct causes. Not everyone who is identified as "at risk" becomes involved in violence. Some risk factors for IPV victimization and perpetration are the same, while others are associated with one another. For example, childhood physical or sexual victimization is a risk factor for future IPV perpetration and victimization. A combination of individual, relational, community, and societal factors contribute to the risk of becoming an IPV perpetrator or victim. Stress can increase the risk and side effects of violence.

Being abusive is not a clear-cut issue of problems with anger management. Abuse is about power. Understanding the multilevel intersecting factors below that contribute to abuse can help you identify various opportunities for prevention. People experiencing these risk factors are statistically more likely to be the perpetrators of abuse. This is known as the cycle of abuse (Figure 23). It's not a guarantee of that behavior, but just as other health risks disproportionately affect people (disparities), so does abuse.

The factors that put someone at higher risk can be related specifically to the individual, their relationship with the victim or abuser, and even the community in which they live. Increased risk, to a certain extent, can be affected by:

History—Past experiences with child abuse, domestic abuse, or other forms of physical or emotional aggression, whether as a victim or perpetrator, which can affect how someone defines, tolerates, or responds to violence

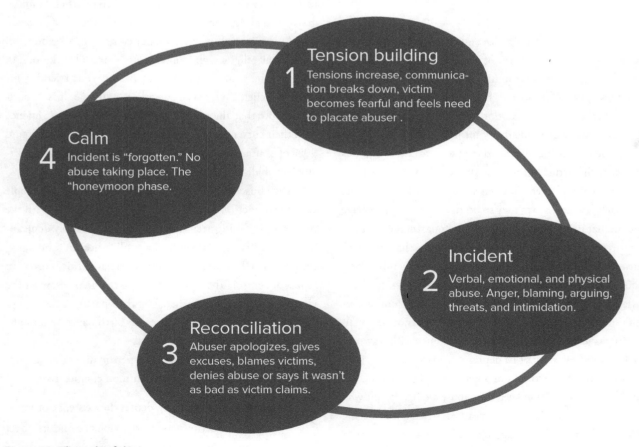

Figure 23. The cycle of abuse.

Personality Traits—Low self-esteem, emotional dependence or insecurity, depression, anger and hostility, controlling, jealousy, possessiveness, anti-social behavior or isolation, borderline personality disorder, and being of young age

Lifestyle—Heavy drug or alcohol abuse and elevated stress

Socioeconomic Status and Environment—Lower levels of income and education, poverty, or living in an area with low social capital (i.e. overcrowding, a lack of resources or support, a community tolerance toward aggression or unwillingness to intervene)

Ideologies—A strict belief in gender roles, such as that a man should work and make decisions, and a woman should tend to children and cook, indicating a culture of dominance or power imbalance

Relationships—Marital conflict, increased stress related to finances, power imbalances, unhealthy family dynamics, divorce or separation, or other forms of instability

It's important to recognize signs of abuse in victims. People experiencing any form of abuse often don't realize it themselves or may attempt to hide it from friends out of fear for their safety or fear of judgment. Abuse takes on many forms, whether physical, emotional, or psychological. Warning signs of abuse can take many forms.

People who are being abused may seem afraid or anxious to please their partner, go along with everything their partner says and does, and even check in with them often to report where they are and what they're doing. They might receive frequent, harassing phone calls from their partner; talk about their partner's temper, jealousy, or possessiveness; have frequent injuries, with the excuse of "accidents;" frequently miss work, school, or social occasions, without explanation; dress in clothing designed to hide bruises or scars (e.g. wearing long sleeves in the summer or sunglasses indoors); show major personality changes (e.g. an outgoing person becomes withdrawn or have lower self-esteem); or be depressed, anxious, or suicidal.

Isolation of the victim from others is a very common tactic of an abuser who wishes to keep their abuse hidden. People who are being isolated by their abuser may be restricted from seeing family and friends, rarely go out in public without their partner, or have limited access to money, credit cards, or transportation.

The impact of violence on an individual's health can be severe. In addition to the immediate injuries from an assault, the person may suffer from chronic pain, gastrointestinal disorders, psychosomatic symptoms, and eating problems, often from the stress of a difficult situation. Although psychological abuse is often considered less severe than physical violence, all forms of intimate partner violence can have devastating physical and emotional health effects. Domestic violence, for example, is associated with mental health problems such as anxiety, post-traumatic stress disorder, and depression. Women who are abused suffer an increased risk of unplanned or early pregnancies and sexually transmitted diseases, including HIV/AIDS. As trauma victims, they are also at an increased risk of substance abuse.

Pregnant women are particularly vulnerable to attacks, and thus may more often experience medical difficulties in their pregnancies. Recent research has called for increased study of pregnancy-associated deaths. Women who are abused are more likely to have a history of sexually transmitted disease infections, vaginal and cervical infections, kidney infections and bleeding during pregnancy, all of which are risk factors for pregnant women. Abused women are more likely to delay prenatal care and are less likely to receive antenatal care. In fact, partner abuse may be a larger risk than other common gestational health concerns, such as hypertension and diabetes.

Anyone can abuse others. They come from all groups, all cultures, all religions, all economic levels, and all backgrounds. They can be your neighbor, your pastor, your friend, your child's teacher, a relative, a coworker—anyone. It is important to note that the majority of abusers only show violence with their current or past intimate partners. One study found 90% of abusers do not have criminal records and are generally law-abiding outside the home.

The abuse can often fly under the radar of the people around the victim. Often, it becomes a mind game, with the perpetrator making accusations of flirting, possibly demeaning or humiliating the victim in public, or even sabotaging the person's efforts at home, work, or school. This is often an aspect of control. They may control all the finances, what the victim wears, force sex or disregard their partner's unwillingness to have it, sabotage or disregard birth control methods, and so on, in an effort to dominate.

There is no typical, detectable personality of an abuser. However, they do often display common characteristics:

Denial—An abuser often denies the existence or minimizes the seriousness of the violence and its effect on the victim and other family members.

Objectification—An abuser objectifies the victim and often sees them as their property or sexual objects.

Low Self-Esteem—An abuser has low self-esteem and feels powerless and ineffective in the world. He or she may appear successful, but internally, they feel inadequate.

Blaming—An abuser externalizes the causes of their behavior. They blame their violence on circumstances such as stress, their partner's behavior, a "bad day," or on alcohol, drugs, or other factors.

Masking—An abuser may be pleasant and charming between periods of violence and is often seen as a "nice person" to others outside the relationship.

Support and Prevention of Violence

One of the things you can do if you suspect someone you know is a victim of abuse is to maintain contact with that person. Abusers often try separating their victims from friends and family, making them feel like they have no support network. Make sure you are supportive—it won't help to try and make someone feel guilty or bad if they don't leave the relationship. Many factors can make a victim return to an abuser multiple times. Abusers often tell victims that if they attempt to leave the relationship they will be killed, making any attempt to leave a potential for increased violence. The important thing is that you remain available for your friend or family member. However, if you know someone may be in immediate physical danger, call 911.

You can take steps to help. Each of us has the power to reach out to someone we love and tell them that abuse is not their fault. Love shouldn't hurt, and safety is possible. Check the resources at the end of this chapter for more advice and assistance.

Benefits of Stress Management

The risks of not managing stress should be apparent by now, but what about the benefits? Research suggests that individuals who learn to manage stress do much more than just avoid disease, particularly in comparison to people who haven't learned to manage it. Exercise, healthy eating, relaxation, and positive thinking all help to improve your overall wellness, but stress management has its own set of physical and psychological benefits (Figure 24):

Physical Benefits	Psychological Benefits
Lower blood pressure	Improved self esteem
Reduced risk of heart attack and stroke	Reduced anxiety levels
Reduced osteoporosis risk	Reduced risk of depression
Lower risk for certain cancers	Less reliance on alcohol
Better immune system	Improved coping skills
Fewer colds and flu	Reduced anger levels
Lower risk of type 2 diabetes	Improved relationships
Reduced risk of intestinal problems	Greater optimism
Higher energy levels	Greater efficiency at work
Improved sleep pattern	Improved concentration and memory
Improved cholesterol profile	Increased feeling of control
Reduced back pain	Improved decision making
Reduced muscle tension	Reduction in mood swings

Figure 24. Managing stress has many benefits.

Improving How You Manage Stress

With each form of wellness, we've asked you to assess where you are and determine where you need to go, setting goals and creating a plan. Many aspects of your health, like weight, blood pressure, percent body fat, and even flexibility, are objective and concrete—easy to assess and measure. Stress can be somewhat abstract because it's subjective, based on your perceptions and emotions. Your health care provider might consider stress as a likely cause of a concrete, tangible problem, but only you can really define your stress (and sometimes it's difficult even for you). The improvement section of this chapter will focus primarily on assessment along with strategies and tools to help you manage various aspects of stress.

Perceived Stress Scale

A good plan for managing stress begins with assessing your stress level and anticipated stressors in your life. A variety of tools can help you assess you level of stress, many of which are best used with the aid of an expert. One commonly used way to assess stress is with the **Perceived Stress Scale (PSS)**. You've learned in this chapter that stress and your ability to cope with it is relative more to your perception of the stressor than the stressor itself. Understanding how you perceive stress can help you determine your risk for negative, health-related impacts and take appropriate strategies to manage it (Figure 25).

You can find a sample PSS questionnaire on pages 216-217. The questions in the scale ask about your feelings and thoughts during the last month). For each question, you will estimate how many times you thought of felt a certain way, whether never, very often, or somewhere in between. Some of the questions seem similar, but there are differences between them. Be sure to answer each question. Don't worry about how many times you've answered a particular way—it's best to answer fairly quickly and avoid the urge to count or adjust your answers before you're done.

Your perception of what is happening in your life is most important. Consider the idea that two individuals could have the exact same events and experiences in their lives for the past month. Depending on their perception, their total score on the PSS could put one of those individuals in the low stress category and put the second person in the high stress category.

Keep a Daily Stress Log

Another way to determine your typical stressors is by keeping a log of your daily stress for a week or two. For example, for each time during the day that you felt stressed in any way, make an entry on a log or in a journal. Include the time and place it began (and how long it lasted), what triggered the stress, how you felt, your level of tension (measured on a scale of 1–4, from slight to intense), and how you responded or coped (Figure 26). This can help you determine the

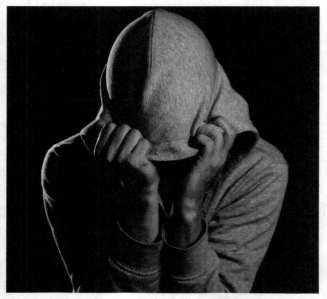

Figure 25. Managing stress can eleminate overwhelming moments.

Time and Duration	Place	Source of Stress or Trigger	How I Felt	Tension Level 1–4*	How I Coped or Responded to the Situation
8:00–8:30 a.m.	Car on the way to school	Traffic	Anxious; I was very late and worried I'd miss my test; my heart was pounding	3	I blew my horn a lot at people, swore at them. I didn't really calm down until 5 minutes into the test even though I made it on time.

Figure 26. A daily stress log helps identify stressors.

types of situations that cause the most stress, whether your response is proportionate to the stressor, and if you could have handled it differently.

There are many techniques to effectively manage your stress and limit its negative effects, from preventative measures to reduce stress before it occurs to active stress management techniques that are useful during and after stress experiences.

Setting Goals for Managing Stress

Because stress can be less tangible than, for example, poor flexibility, it can be a bit more challenging to measure, monitor, and improve. But once you've determined how you perceive stress, the types of stressors you typically face, and how you normally respond to them, you can begin to see how to plan ways of improving your stress.

Like any form of wellness, you cannot expect to change drastically overnight. You can, however, plan to improve in certain areas and practice many of the techniques and tools you will learn about over the next few pages of this chapter. The areas you choose will be based upon your current ways of managing stress and the stressors you typically face. Consider this scenario, for example. You kept a daily log for a bit and determined that you often feel stressed from trying to keep up with assignments for your classes. It's now clear to you that you need to manage your time better. One problem is that you often stay up late watching TV, trying to decompress, but end up oversleeping and starting the day behind.

You may find that after 2 weeks, you are more caught up on your work but still a bit behind. There may be many things contributing to your problem with time management, such as procrastination or agreeing to do things for others that you don't have time to do. You may need to set a few SMART goals for this concern. In fact, you may need to set several small goals for different stressors to help you change the patterns and approaches that impact your level of stress.

Specific—I want to manage my time better
Measurable—By keeping a consistent sleeping pattern
Achievable—This Is a small goal
Relevant—This will improve my grades and reduce stress
Time-based—For 2 weeks, and then I will reassess

The tools and techniques that follow in this chapter will help you find ways to manage your stress by being proactive, taking care of your mind and body, and using efficient coping strategies. Consider these as you plan ways to improve how you manage stress in your life.

Time Management

First, let's look at some effective tools to manage one common form of stress before it happens—a busy schedule. There never seem to be enough hours in the day to get everything done. Between work, school, chores, errands, and family commitments, you could fill 24 hours with tasks.

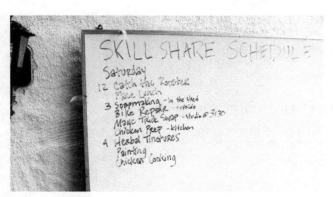

Figure 27. Manage your time to avoid stressful situations.

Time management becomes increasingly important when your workload is heavy. It enables you to arrange your schedule for many of the things you want and need to do and to decide which things are urgent and which can wait. Learning how to manage your time, activities, and commitments can be hard. But doing so can make your life easier, less stressful, and more meaningful (Figure 27). There are three parts to time management—prioritize tasks and activities, control procrastination, and manage commitments.

Prioritize Tasks

You're sitting at the kitchen table staring at the screen of your laptop. You know this paper won't write itself, but you become distracted by the large pile of laundry sitting in the basket a few feet away. You tell yourself you'll be able to concentrate better if the clothes get folded, so you tackle those. You head

Perceived Stress Scale

The Perceived Stress Scale (PSS) is a classic stress assessment instrument. The tool, originally developed in 1983, remains a popular choice for helping us understand how different situations affect our feelings and perceived stress. The questions in this scale ask about your feelings and thoughts during the last month. In each case, indicate how often you felt or thought a certain way. Although some of the questions are similar, there are differences between them. You should treat each one as a separate question. The best approach is to answer each question quickly. Don't try to count up the number of times you felt a certain way. Instead, choose what you think is a fair and reasonable estimate.

For each question, choose from the following choices:					
0 – never	1 – almost never	2 – sometimes	3 – fairly often	4 – very often	
1. In the last month, how often have you been upset because of something that happened unexpectedly?					
2. In the last month, how often have you felt that you were unable to control the important things in your life?					
3. In the last month, how often have you felt nervous and stressed?					
4. In the last month, how often have you felt confident about your ability to handle your personal problems?					
5. In the last month, how often have you felt that things were going your way?					
6. In the last month, how often have you found that you could not cope with all the things that you had to do?					
7. In the last month, how often have you been able to control irritations in your life?					
8. In the last month, how often have you felt that you were on top of things?					
9. In the last month, how often have you been angered because of things that happened that were outside of your control?					
10. In the last month, how often have you felt difficulties were piling up so high that you could not overcome them?					

Determining Your PSS Score

You can determine your PSS score by following these directions:

First, reverse your scores for questions 4, 5, 7, and 8. On these 4 questions, change the scores like this:

$$0 = 4, 1 = 3, 2 = 2, 3 = 1, 4 = 0.$$

Now add up your scores for each item to get a total. My total score is _____.
Individual scores on the PSS can range from 0 to 40 with higher scores indicating higher perceived stress:

- Scores ranging from 0–13 are considered low stress.
- Scores ranging from 14–26 are considered moderate stress.
- Scores ranging from 27–40 are considered high perceived stress.

The PSS is important because your perception of what is happening in your life is most important. Two individuals could have the exact same events and experiences in their lives for the past month. Depending on their perception, their total score could put one of those individuals in the low stress category and put the second person in the high stress category.

Disclaimer: The scores on the following self–assessment do not reflect any particular diagnosis or course of treatment. They are meant as a tool to help assess your level of stress. If you have any further concerns about your current well being, you may contact EAP and talk confidentially to one of our specialists.

	Urgent	Non-Urgent
Important	Quadrant 1: Examples: Things due today or tomorrow, dealing with emergencies or crises	Quadrant 2: Examples: Long-term projects, planning ahead, studying in advance, getting started early
Non-Important	Quadrant 3: Examples: Interruptions, distractions, fun events that come up, social invitations	Quadrant 4: Examples: Time wasters, busy work, procrastination activities, aimless internet browsing

Figure 28. Covey's task prioritizer sorts the tasks in your life into prioritized quadrants.

back toward the table but notice that there are several dishes in the sink, so you tackle those. Finally, you sit back down to get to work, but you end up spending 30 minutes on social media and watching online videos of cats. The paper is due tomorrow.

People often become overwhelmed because they have too many tasks and no plan for how to approach them. One common tactic in this situation is to complete things that are less urgent because they are less difficult and end up pushing later tasks into a stressful situation. If this happens to you, start by making a list of all your tasks and activities for the day or week. Then, rate these tasks by how important or urgent they are.

One method for doing this is offered by Steven Covey in his book *The 7 Habits of Highly Effective People*. Covey's method focuses on breaking tasks into categories based on importance and urgency (Figure 28). Consider the importance, urgency, and "due date".Quadrant 1 should be your highest priority, followed by quadrant 2. These get first priority because of their importance. Quadrants 3 and 4 are typically the tasks that draw your time away from more meaningful tasks. Some of them may be quite fun and can offer a nice break, but you don't want to spend too much time in those quadrants until the first two quadrants have been cleared. You may have some tasks from quadrants 3 and 4 in your schedule with the majority being from quadrants 1 and 2.

ABC Analysis

A technique that has been used in business management for a long time is the categorization of large data into groups. These groups are often marked A, B, and C—hence the

name. Items to be done are ranked by priority "A" status items would be of most importance, followed by "B" and "C" in descending importance (Figure 29). To further refine the prioritization, some individuals choose to then force-rank all "B" items as either "A" or "C". ABC analysis can incorporate more than three groups.

Control Procrastination

Somewhere in this world is someone who never procrastinates on their tasks. We've never met them. Most of us struggle with procrastination to some degree. When it adds stress to our lives, it becomes a problem—procrastination becomes yet another stressor we have to handle. Fortunately, there are some ways to do that. The Academic Success Center at Oregon State University offers the following tips:

Make a plan. Set goals and make use of a weekly schedule and a to-do list. These can keep you organized and help you stay committed to completing your tasks.

Find motivation. Think of one or two good reasons for getting tasks done early and write those reasons down. You may often allow yourself to procrastinate by thinking "I can do this later." When that thought comes up, make sure you have an answer for why it's important to complete the task now.

Make it easier on yourself. Schedule a date and time for starting your task, be specific about what you will accomplish, and find a location that is conducive to accomplishing your task.

"A" Status—"Must Do"	High priority, very important, critical items, with close deadlines or high level of importance to them
"B" Status—"Should Do"	Medium priority, quite important over time, not as critical as "A" items, but still important to spend time doing
"C" Status—"Nice to Do"	Low priority at this time, low consequences if left undone at this moment

Figure 29. ABC analysis helps you prioritize items on your to-do list.

Identify your procrastination tendencies and your excuses. If you know that cleaning is a technique you use to procrastinate from homework, plan ahead for this. Set aside time for each task, pay attention when you get distracted, and redirect yourself to the reasons you want to complete the task now.

Learn to say "no" when distractions arise. There will always be things that threaten to interrupt your productivity. Saying "no" to interruptions or distractions can keep you on track as you complete your task.

Be patient. Procrastination is something you work to overcome over time by developing better habits. There will be areas of your life and times during the term when it will be harder to overcome this challenge. Recognize when you are making positive choices and reward your successes.

Manage Commitments

Your Type A friend thinks that the only way things get done is if he does them himself. This can actually be a form of narcissism. Really, some people can do things better than you can—if you can let them. And sometimes they *should* do them. Can your 5-year-old do his own laundry? Probably not. Can he put his dirty clothes in the hamper and pick up his own toys? Absolutely!

Sometimes you also need to be honest with yourself about which of your commitments fall into the "important" or "must do" categories. Was it really important for you to become the secretary of your sorority during your busiest term? Did you need to go shopping with a friend the day before your essay was due just because she broke up with her boyfriend (again)? You should be supportive, but could you have invited her to study with you instead? It's great, and even relaxing, to be a good friend and a good member of your community. But sometimes you need to learn to say no to more commitments, especially if saying yes means taking on more than you can handle.

Cognitive Strategies

Most of us occasionally say defeatist phrases to ourselves that, rather than offering a solution, make us feel worse or even encourage us to give up on a resolution.

"I can't do it."

"It will never work."

"I'm lousy at this."

You may not realize how significantly your language to yourself can impact your emotions and behaviors, and ultimately your level of stress. You can, however, change the way you talk to yourself utilizing **cognitive strategies** to help you manage stress.

Therapists teach cognitive strategies to their clients to encourage them to shift negative self-talk to language that is positive, more likely to reduce stress, and that will enable individuals to better manage their lives. They do this through a process of recognition, restructuring, and refocusing.

Step One: Recognize Negative Thoughts

Start by recognizing the negativity you encourage in yourself by recognizing some common forms of **negative thinking**. These include filtering, personalizing, catastrophizing, and polarizing.

Filtering occurs when you highlight all the negative parts of a situation and filter out all of the positive ones. For example, you got stuck in heavy traffic on your way home from work. You took a detour on some side streets to avoid it, stopped at a great market you'd never been to, and managed to pick up something unique for dinner. You were only 15 minutes later getting home than you had planned, but that night at dinner while everyone is happy with the food, you focus only on being late and getting stuck in traffic.

Personalizing is when you automatically blame yourself when something bad happens. For example, a friend you haven't seen in a while comes into town and doesn't call you. You assume it's because he doesn't like you and doesn't want to see you.

Catastrophizing happens when you automatically anticipate the worst. For example, if you got a "C" on an exam the first week of the term and just know that the class will be too difficult for you and you will fail.

Polarizing things as either black or white, good or bad, right or wrong can also be negative. If you aren't perfect, you're a failure. If you aren't smart, you're dumb. If he doesn't call today, he must not be interested in you. Polarizing leaves no option for gray areas.

Step Two: Restructure Your Thoughts

When you hear the negative self-talk, rephrase it to reflect positive thinking. Here are some common examples of negative self-talk, with their positive thinking alternatives ((Figure 30).

Step Three: Refocusing on the Present

It's easy to feel overwhelmed from getting bogged down with too many things at once. Your future responsibilities can creep into your present worries. Take time to set priorities and determine what needs to be done now, handled today or this week (see section on "Time Management). Focus on the moment. Competitive athletes often have periods of "mental blocks." Gymnasts, for example, who have performed the same skill many times will suddenly start freezing up. They mount the bars or the beam and when they try to begin a skill, they stop, over and over again. Sports psychologists have them break each move into steps and talk their way through each skill. This keeps them focused on what they are supposed to be doing at that moment, not on the dismount that is six skills in the future. Long-term goals are fine, but you cannot complete them if you ignore the little steps in life along the way.

We've talked a lot about setting SMART goals. This applies to nearly everything in life. Are you being realistic about what you can accomplish? Are you breaking goals into short-term and long-term? For example, it's great to have a goal to be a columnist for the *New York Times* and win a Pulitzer Prize for journalism. First you need to write a great article for your school newspaper, pass your journalism class, take several more, do

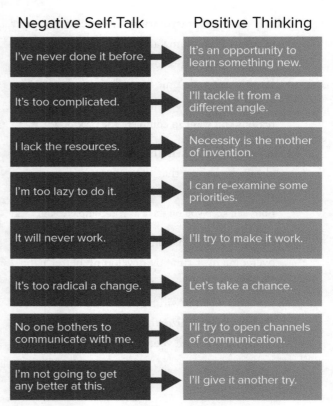

Negative Self-Talk	Positive Thinking
I've never done it before.	It's an opportunity to learn something new.
It's too complicated.	I'll tackle it from a different angle.
I lack the resources.	Necessity is the mother of invention.
I'm too lazy to do it.	I can re-examine some priorities.
It will never work.	I'll try to make it work.
It's too radical a change.	Let's take a chance.
No one bothers to communicate with me.	I'll try to open channels of communication.
I'm not going to get any better at this.	I'll give it another try.

Figure 30. Use positive self-talk to encourage positive stress management.

well, get a degree and a job at a local paper, and so on. Very few people win a Pulitzer Prize. You might, but it isn't a particularly realistic thing to focus on and shouldn't be a source of pressure. Lofty goals like this may give you the tendency to see small setbacks as goal-threatening rather than opportunities to learn.

ABCDE Model for Effective Thought Remodeling

The **ABCDE model** (Figure 31) provides a way for people to examine their internal processes by learning to break down events into clear steps. The idea is to take the mystery out of the situation. You are responsible for the images and thoughts in your mind and the emotions they generate. You can work yourself into a frenzy over a situation, giving yourself a stomachache. Or, you can attach new meanings and interpretations that help you deal with something positively. This gives you power over your emotions. You can do this with five steps, ABCDE.

For practice, think about a recent event that resulted in a strong emotional reaction. This should be an event where you would wish you had responded differently. Consider each of the five steps of the ABCDE model and write down your own experience each step of the way.

"A"—Adversity or Activating Event

Consider the event that triggered the emotional response in you, whatever happened right before you began feeling an emotion such as anxiety, sadness, or anger. When you become more mindfully aware of events that typically trigger strong emotional responses, you can learn to watch out for these events in the future and be better prepared to deal with them more effectively.

Example: A friend asks you if he can borrow your car again.

"B"—Beliefs

People often try to establish meaning for why something occurs. For the moment, avoid labeling your beliefs as "right" or "wrong" and simply recognize them. Some beliefs are irrational and create maladaptive emotional responses and generate problems. A belief is generally "irrational" when it lacks clear evidence, is overgeneralized, or is otherwise based on faulty reasoning.

Example: "He just hangs out with me to use my car."

"C"—Consequences

Consequences are more than just the outcome of the event. They can take behavioral and emotional forms. Sometimes you observe them externally, such as noticing that another person is angry with you or ignoring you. Other times, consequences are internal, such as experiencing anxiety or sadness.

Example: Regret, disappointment, and withdrawal from the friend. Refusal to hang out with the friend that borrows your car.

"D"—Disputing

This step involves actively disputing harmful belief systems through mindfully examining, questioning, and challenging them. First, locate the harmful beliefs in your stream of consciousness in such a way that you can examine them carefully. Then prepare to enter the "disputation phase" by asking yourself the following six questions:

- Does this belief fit with reality?
- Does this belief support the achievement of reasonable/constructive interests and goals?
- Does this belief help foster positive/healthy relationships?
- Does this belief make you feel better or worse?
- Does this belief seem reasonable and logical given the context in which it occurred?
- Is this belief generally detrimental or generally helpful?

These questions can help you separate realistic from dysfunctional thinking. Through mindfully examining your beliefs in this way, you are also increasing your own self-awareness and insight into the ways that you tend to think and behave.

Example:

- No, there are plenty of times when we've hung out and he hasn't asked to use my car.
- No, this belief actually defeats my interest in overcoming the anxiety related to his requests.
- No, my emotional reaction only served to harm the friendship.
- No, the belief that he's using me makes me feel weak and gullible.
- No, my friend really does need a car at times and can't afford one, and it really doesn't matter if he borrows mine.
- In this case, it's generally detrimental. It only costs time and emotional energy, with no beneficial return.

"E"—Effects

Notice the effects that result from actively examining and disputing faulty thinking. Once you become realistically aware of your emotionally charged beliefs about a situation, you can begin to adjust your line of thinking based upon more rational and reasonable beliefs.

Example: I know he's been down on his luck, and by using my car he may be able to improve his situation.

Keep in mind that the ABCDE model will not set aside normal, healthy emotions, such as appropriate loss, regret, realistic fears, or frustration. Not all emotions need to be changed. If your friend never calls you except when he wants the car, does not thank you, does not pitch in for gas, and does not respect your vehicle, your response might be rational, and it may teach you to set healthy boundaries. Quite often, emotions prove incredibly valuable and useful tools that, providing you with important information about the situation. Other times, when emotional responses are causing unnecessary suffering or are based in faulty thinking, mindfully applying the ABCDE model can shed light on a situation where you feel struck.

Figure 31. The ABCDE model.

Problem Solving Skills

You can't solve a problem successfully until you understand it. If you're so overwhelmed with a particular problem that you choose to just ignore it or worry over it rather than try to fix it, try taking time to analyze the problem. Write down a brief description of the problem you want to solve. Then ask yourself these questions:

- What is happening?

- Where and when is it happening?

- Is it happening around certain people or in specific situations?

- How do I feel about it?

Be specific and focus on issues rather than on whose fault it is. Now consider its severity and how much time you need to solve it realistically:

- Is the problem really that big? Would others think so?

- Will this matter in two years?

- Would solving it improve my life?

- Do I have control over any aspect of the situation?

You can't change everything. Focus on issues you can realistically change and that will improve your level of stress. Pick your battles.

Think about solutions, of all the ways you might solve your problem. Now isn't the time to judge whether one solution is better than another. Recall past problems that were similar that you were able to solve. Could a similar solution work for this problem, too? Don't be afraid to ask others for advice, particularly those that may be knowledgeable in the area.

If you're still having trouble, maybe your problem is too complicated. Break the problem down into smaller parts you can more easily handle. Then, brainstorm some ideas for taking on each part. Which has the most potential? Ask yourself:

- Do I realistically think it will solve the problem?

- How will using this solution make me feel in the end?

- What are the possible positive and negative consequences of this path?

Take another couple of minutes to think through your decision. Ask yourself:

- Do I have the resources and the drive to carry out this plan? Can I complete it?

- Will it create any new problems?

- What might go wrong? Can I adjust the plan to prepare for it?

A good long-term solution may temporarily create new problems. That doesn't mean you should give up the plan, just that you need to be ready to make adjustments or even switch to a plan B.

Healthy Relationships and Social Support

Hugs, kisses, and caring, supportive conversations are key ingredients of close relationships. Scientists have found that your links to others can have powerful effects on your health. Social connections—whether with romantic partners, family, friends, neighbors, or others—can influence your biology and well-being.

Wide-ranging research suggests that strong social ties can be linked to a longer life. In contrast, loneliness and social isolation may also be linked to poorer health, depression, and increased risk of early death. Studies have found that having a variety of social relationships may help reduce stress and heart-related risks. Such connections might improve your ability to fight off germs or give you a more positive outlook on life. Physical contact—from hand-holding to sex—can trigger the release of hormones and brain chemicals that not only make you feel great and reduce stress but also have other biological benefits.

Any behavior that is positive and promotes deepening trust and closeness between people is considered a **pro-social** maintenance behavior. The more pro-social behaviors evident in a relationship, the more likely for strong bonds to be formed, and the relationship to prosper and continue. Positivity, openness, task sharing, supportiveness, humor, and working together are all examples of pro-social behavior. Here are some ways to nurture your friendships:

Be kind. This most-basic behavior, emphasized during childhood, remains the core of successful, adult relationships. Think of friendship as an emotional bank account. Every act of kindness and every expression of gratitude are deposits into this account, while criticism and negativity draw down the account.

Listen. Ask what's going on in your friends' lives. Let the other person know you are paying close attention through eye contact, body language and occasional brief comments such as, "That sounds fun." When friends share details of hard times or difficult experiences, be empathetic, but don't give advice unless your friends ask for it.

Be open. Build intimacy with your friends by opening up about yourself. Being willing to disclose personal experiences and concerns shows that your friend holds a special place in your life and deepens your connection.

Show that you can be trusted. Being responsible, reliable and dependable is key to forming strong friendships. Keep your engagements and arrive on time. Follow through on commitments you've made to your friends. When your friends share confidential information, keep it private.

Make yourself available. Building a close friendship takes time — together. Make an effort to see new friends regularly, and to check in with them in between meet-ups. You may feel awkward the first few times you talk on the phone or get together, but this feeling is likely to pass as you get more comfortable with each other.

Manage your nerves with mindfulness. You may find yourself imagining the worst of social situations and feel tempted to stay home. Use mindfulness exercises to reshape your thinking (focus on the present and identify your feelings). Each time you imagine the worst, pay attention to how often the situations you're afraid of actually take place. You may notice that the scenarios you fear usually don't happen.

Keep some perspective. When difficult situations do happen, remind yourself that your feelings will pass, and you can handle them until they do.

Relax. Yoga and other mind-body relaxation practices also may reduce anxiety and help you face situations that make you feel nervous.

Sometimes, social bonds feel more like restrictions. People can get into patterns of disrespectfulness, impatience, intolerance, being judgmental and using language and behavior toward each other that adds to stress. Improve the positive aspects of your relationships starting with how you behave within your social networks, whether it is to treat those around you more respectfully or react to the anti-social behavior of others in a productive way. We've all heard the golden rule — treat others the way you want to be treated. There are many healthy ways to do this and, hopefully, reap the benefits of pro-social behavior in return. If your relationships don't build you up, it may be time to end them.

Surround yourself with supportive, positive people who respect you and your goals whenever possible. Supportive people make you feel good about yourself because they sincerely care about your well-being. They are also understanding of your experiences.

It's a good idea, for example, to make friends with people who are in college with you, because they can understand your time allowances and the goal you are working toward. You can find new friends in your classrooms and by doing things like joining clubs. Shared hobbies can be a great way enhance your social circles, and people who share your interests are likelier to be as excited and supportive of your successes as you are.

Spiritual Wellness

Spirituality means more than a belief in a god. There are many different religions and belief systems that invest in the idea of a higher power. This higher power can mean many different things to different people. But, many of the habits of spiritual people can be good for our health.

Meditation and prayer often take on similar forms — they involve internal reflection and release. For people who pray, it is often because they've taken the opportunity to be thankful, look for support or strength, consider the world and people around them, and release their problems to a higher power. In other words, they de-stress! You do not have to believe in a higher power to embrace your spiritual side. Taking time to meditate, reflect, and release negative energy out into the universe can be a positive, relaxing experience.

For many people, part of spirituality is a larger consideration for the environment and the community. Taking time to volunteer at a homeless shelter, planting trees, or simply helping out your neighbor can make you feel good about your purpose in life. That's a large part of what it means to be spiritual—identifying a sense of purpose.

Embrace your spiritual side in whatever form that takes. You'll enjoy a more relaxed, grateful, and reflective attitude on the people and world around you. Emphasizing the role of spiritual wellness in your life can help improve your self-esteem, give meaning to the activities you choose, and help you foster positive relationships.

Helping the Mind by Helping the Body

Setting goals, as described in every chapter in this book, can be used to also help manage stress. The school term has just begun and the pace is already picking up. It's your last few classes before transferring to a four-year university and you want that transcript to be pristine. The nursing program only takes students with a 4.0 and you have Biology this term. Your tendency might be to forget everything else in your life but that biology class. However, let's look at some active techniques that can be used to manage stress while it is happening. Here are some tips for good self-care:

Avoid drugs and alcohol. They may seem to be a temporary fix to feel better, but in the long run drugs and alcohol can create more problems and add to your stress—instead of taking it away.

Find support. Seek help from a partner, family member, friend, counselor, health care provider, or clergyperson. Having someone with a sympathetic, listening ear and sharing about your problems and stress really can lighten the burden.

Connect socially. After a stressful event, it is easy isolate yourself. Make sure that you are spending time with loved ones. Consider planning fun activities with your partner, children, or friends.

Take care of yourself. Eat a healthy, well-balanced diet. Exercise regularly. Get plenty of sleep. Give yourself a break if you feel stressed out—for example, treat yourself to a therapeutic massage. Maintain a normal routine.

Stay active. You can take your mind off your problems with activities like helping a neighbor, volunteering in the community, and taking the dog on a long walk. These can be positive ways to cope with stressful feelings.

Physical Activity

This text has devoted many pages to the merits of physical exercise, from contributing to a healthy body composition to avoiding disease. But it is also vital for your mental health and can reduce stress. Studies suggest that it is very effective at reducing fatigue, improving alertness and concentration, improving sleep, elevating and stabilizing mood, enhancing self-esteem, and enhancing overall cognitive function (Figure 32).

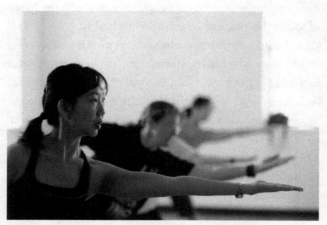

Figure 32. Meditation amd yoga are just two techniques to improve stress management.

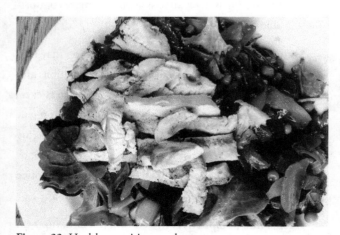

Figure 33. Healthy nutrition can boost your energy.

You've learned a lot about the body's reaction to stress. Exercise and other physical activities produce endorphins — chemicals in the brain that act as natural painkillers — which in turn can reduce stress. It also gives you energy. You often feel a sense of fatigue when stressed, and that burst of energy may be just what you need to rally your internal resources. Finally, let's not forget that illness is a stressor, maybe one of the largest ones. When you stay healthy and keep your heart pumping efficiently, you reduce your risk of chronic illnesses that can lead to chronic stress.

Nutrition

It may sound strange, but the foods you eat can impact your stress level (Figure 33). No, not just the three energy drinks you consumed that now have you anxious and jittery. The bag of potato chips that you hurriedly chased down with the sugary soda for lunch the last few days on your lunch break are impacting your stress as well. Worry and overwork can lead to unhealthy lifestyle habits, which causes more stress, leading to a very harmful cycle. When you are facing a very tight deadline at work or school, you might make poor choices about what to eat, relying on sugar and caffeine to get you through the day.

Unfortunately, these food choices can create more stress in the long run, as well as other problems. Here is a list of common bad habits people sometimes indulge in when overwhelmed and worried:

Drinking too much caffeine. You may find yourself drinking several cups of coffee, soda, or energy drinks.

Eating unhealthy foods. Increased levels of cortisol make people tend to crave foods high in fat, sugar, and salt. This combined with a busy schedule often leads to foods with poor nutritional value.

Skipping meals. When you are juggling a dozen things at once, eating a healthy meal often drops down in priorities. You might find yourself skipping breakfast because you're running late or not eating lunch because there's just too much on your to-do list. Sometimes, we get so busy we simply forget to eat.

Mindless snacking. Stress also makes us prone to emotional eating, where we eat despite not being hungry but eat because it feels comforting.

Forgetting water. It's easy to forget to drink your water. A good portion of Americans drink no water, and get water only from soda or coffee.

Fast food. So many drive-thrus, so little time. It's easier to just drive through a fast food place or go to a restaurant than to go home and cook something. Unfortunately, this gets expensive and is often unhealthy.

Crash diets. Stress often leads to weight gain, which can lead to people to look for a quick fix in their busy schedule. Some people intentionally eat less food than they need or try dangerous fad diets in order to lose the excess weight. Diets that aren't balanced with fruits and vegetables, protein, and healthy carbohydrates can often be bad for your health in the long run, even if they look attractive short term.

Eating nutrient-rich food and a balanced diet and making sure you stay hydrated, are two simple practices that can keep your stress levels healthy and manageable. The bottom line, as you learned in Chapter 7, is that healthy food has a positive impact on our health, can help our self-esteem, and can prevent the stress of increased body fat and illness.

Sleeping Habits

People often don't treat the need for sleep with respect. You love when you get enough but often see it as something you can catch up on later when stress subsides. Sleep is a necessary human function that allows the brain to recharge and the body to rest. Your body needs sleep to repair muscle and consolidate memory. Sleep is so crucial that even slight sleep deprivation or poor sleep can affect memory, judgment, and mood.

In addition to feeling fatigued and sluggish, chronic sleep deprivation can contribute to health problems, from obesity and high blood pressure to safety risks while driving. Research suggests that most Americans would be happier, healthier, and safer if they were to sleep an extra 60 to 90 minutes per night. Here are a few tips for improving your sleep habits:

Keep a consistent sleep schedule. Get up at the same time every day, even on weekends or during vacations.

Set a bedtime. Try picking a time that is early enough for you to get at least 7 hours of sleep.

Establish a routine. Make sure to include something to help you relax, like a warm bath.

Use your bed only for sleep and sex. Don't use electronics or watch TV in bed.

Make your bedroom quiet and relaxing. Keep the room at a comfortable, cool temperature, and decorate with comforting items.

Reduce screen time. Turn off electronic devices at least 30 minutes before bedtime.

Don't eat a large meal before bedtime. If you are hungry at night, eat a light, healthy snack.

Exercise. Regular exercise and a healthy diet improve your sleep quality.

Lower your caffeine intake later in the day. Avoid consuming caffeine in the late afternoon or evening.

Reduce your fluid intake before bedtime. Lower the chances of waking up to urinate by slowing your fluid intake before bed. That means not drinking alcohol before bedtime, too.

As you can see, most of your healthy sleep routines overlap with other stress-reducing practices. What you gain from healthy sleep patterns are lowered stress levels, improved immune system health, improved cardiac health, and higher cognitive function.

People's sleep needs vary by age and amongst individuals. Sleep is considered to be adequate when you have no daytime sleepiness or dysfunction. You know you are getting enough sleep when you are able to wake up on your own and feel rested, usually at least 6–7 hours.

Relaxation

How many times have you heard someone say "just relax"? If it was only that simple. The good news is that relaxation can actually be learned and practiced. Relaxation techniques include a number of practices, such as progressive relaxation, guided imagery, meditation, biofeedback, self-hypnosis, and deep breathing exercises. They may be varied but tend to have a common goal—to produce the body's natural relaxation response, characterized by slower breathing, lower blood pressure, and a feeling of increased well-being. Meditation and practices that include meditation with movement, such as yoga and tai chi, can also promote relaxation.

Breathing Exercises

Deep breathing exercises are usually done by breathing deeply through the nose (filling the lungs) and slowly exhaling through the mouth. Physically, it should feel like you are filling up with air, starting from the belly and moving up above the heart. You can count to help stay focused on breathing. Imagine that your inhalation fills you with energy and positive thoughts, while exhalation lets out stress and negative thoughts. To practice deep breathing, you can try diaphragmatic breathing (Figure 34). The technique is pretty simple:

- Lie on your back on a flat surface or in bed, with your knees bent and your head supported. You can use a pillow under your knees to support your legs. Place one hand on your upper chest and the other just below your

rib cage. This will allow you to feel your diaphragm move as you breathe.

- Breathe in slowly through your nose so that your stomach moves out against your hand. The hand on your chest should remain as still as possible.

- Tighten your stomach muscles, letting them fall inward

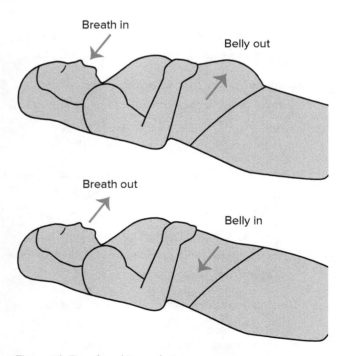

Figure 34. Deep breathing technique.

as you exhale through pursed lips. The hand on your upper chest must remain as still as possible.

- When you first learn the diaphragmatic breathing technique, it may be easier for you to follow the instructions lying down. As you gain more practice, you can try the diaphragmatic breathing technique in a seated position.

You can do this breathing exercise while sitting in a chair:

- Sit comfortably, with your knees bent and your shoulders, head, and neck relaxed.

- Breathe in slowly through your nose so that your stomach moves out against your hand. The hand on your chest should remain as still as possible.

- Place one hand on your upper chest and the other just below your rib cage. This will allow you to feel your diaphragm move as you breathe.

- Tighten your stomach muscles, letting them fall inward as you exhale through pursed lips. The hand on your upper chest must remain as still as possible.

Note: You may notice an increased effort will be needed to use the diaphragm correctly. At first, you'll probably get tired while doing this exercise. But keep at it, because with continued practice, diaphragmatic breathing will become easy and automatic.

At first, practice this exercise 5 to 10 minutes, 3 or 4 times per day. Gradually increase the amount of time you spend doing this exercise, and perhaps even increase the effort of the exercise by placing a book on your abdomen.

Progressive Muscle Relaxation

Progressive muscle relaxation (PMR) is a recognized technique for the reduction of stress and anxiety. Muscle tension accompanies anxiety—you can reduce anxiety by learning how to release the tension in your muscles.

Try reclining in a dark room and following a simple progression through your muscles. Start by tensing and relaxing the muscles in your toes and progressively working your way up to your neck and head. You can also start with your head and neck and work down to your toes. Tense your muscles for at least 5 seconds, and then relax them for 30 seconds, and repeat. Here are three more specific progressive muscle relaxation techniques:

Autogenic relaxation. Autogenic means something that comes from within you. In this relaxation technique, you use both visual imagery and body awareness to reduce stress. You repeat words or suggestions in your mind that may help you relax and reduce muscle tension. For example, you may imagine a peaceful setting and then focus on controlled, relaxing breathing, slowing your heart rate, or feeling different physical sensations, such as relaxing each arm or leg one by one.

Progressive muscle relaxation. In this relaxation technique, you focus on slowly tensing and then relaxing each muscle group. This can help you focus on the difference between muscle tension and relaxation. You can become more aware of physical sensations. In one method of progressive muscle relaxation, you start by tensing and relaxing the muscles in your toes and progressively working your way up to your neck and head. You can also start with your head and neck and work down to your toes. Tense your muscles for about five seconds and then relax for 30 seconds, and repeat.

Visualization. In this relaxation technique, you may form mental images to take a visual journey to a peaceful, calming place or situation. To relax using visualization, try to incorporate as many senses as you can, including smell, sight, sound and touch. If you imagine relaxing at the ocean, for instance, think about the smell of salt water, the sound of crashing waves and the warmth of the sun on your body. You may want to close your eyes, sit in a quiet spot, loosen any tight clothing, and concentrate on your breathing. Aim to focus on the present and think positive thoughts.

Meditation

Meditation is a mind and body practice that has a long history of use for increasing calmness and physical relaxation, improving psychological balance, coping with illness, and enhancing overall health and well-being. Mind and body practices focus on the interactions among the brain, mind, body, and behavior. There are many types of meditation, but most have these elements in common:

- A quiet location with as few distractions as possible

- A specific, comfortable posture (sitting, lying down, walking, or in other positions)

- A focus of attention (a specially chosen word or set of words, an object, or the sensations of the breath)

- An open attitude (letting distractions come and go naturally without judging them).

Many studies have investigated meditation for different conditions, and there's evidence that it may reduce blood pressure as well as symptoms of irritable bowel syndrome and flare-ups in people who have had ulcerative colitis. It may ease symptoms of anxiety and depression, and may help people with insomnia.

In modern guided meditation, or mindfulness, you might be instructed to sit comfortably in a chair with your eyes "softly focused" on nothing in particular. Then you would be instructed to take several deep breaths—in through the nose and out through the mouth. After a few breaths, you close your eyes and begin to breath normally, focusing on the sensations in your body. If you start to get distracted by stressful thoughts, you could focus on your breathing, counting them in tens, with the odd number on the inhale and the even number on the exhale. After about 10 minutes, open your eyes and recognize the feeling of relaxation you have before stretching and carrying on with your day.

This process can be as short as just a few minutes. If you feel you need to "ground" yourself and relax, a brief meditation exercise can provide a short break from a chaotic time.

Other Relaxation Techniques

Other techniques include journaling, creativity, music, practicing gratitude, massage, humor, and other outlets. If you experience depression, for example, keeping a daily log of good experiences or moments of pleasure and happiness can be a useful tool that provides evidence to your depressed mind that you experience good things. Learning to paint, craft, or play music can provide you with relaxing activities that also give you a sense of self-satisfaction.

Important Resources for Depression, Anxiety, Violence and Suicide Prevention

This chapter has focused a great deal on many of the issues in life that can lead to stress, the side effects of stress, and how you can improve your stress levels. Often times people need help to do this or face a situation that is out of their control, even dangerous. It's important to understand that no one is alone. There are individuals, instructors, and agencies available to help.

Resources for Anxiety and Depression

Most college campuses have counseling offices that can be a good first step. These departments often have access to local resources, mental health professionals, and a wealth of information ranging from self-help to structured programs. Campus resources most often come at no additional charge to the student.

In addition to campus resources, psychiatric help is often available from local resources in your area:

- The Substance Abuse and Mental Health Services Administration (SAMHSA) can help you locate local professionals in your area: 1-877-SAMHSA7 (1-877-726-4727)

- The National Alliance on Mental Illness (NAMI) also has a help line that can connect you with local branches: 1-800-950-NAMI (6264).

- The Anxiety and Depression Association of America (ADAA) offers web resources for people suffering from these conditions and their supporters at: adaa.org

Resources for Domestic Violence

- The National Domestic Abuse Hotline: 1-800-799-7233
- TTY: 1-800-787-3224

Resources for Suicide Prevention

If you're thinking about suicide, are worried about a friend or loved one, or would like emotional support, the National Suicide Prevention Lifeline is available at all times across the US. You can contact:

- 1-800-273-TALK (8255), or go to www.suicidepreventionlifeline.org where you can also chat live

- En español: 1-888-628-9454

- TTY: 1-800-799-4TTY (4889)

The following websites can also offer advice or assistance:
- Centers for Disease Control and Prevention: www.cdc.gov/violenceprevention

- CDC Facebook Page on Violence Prevention: facebook.com/vetoviolence

- National Institute for Mental Health: nimh.nih.gov

- Substance Abuse and Mental Health Services Administration: samhsa.gov

- Suicide Prevention Resource Center: www.sprc.org

- Preventing Suicide: A Global Imperative: www.who.int/mental_health/suicide-prevention/world_%report_2014/en/

Resources for Sexual Assault, Dating Violence, Domestic Violence, Harassment or Discrimination Stalking

Students with these concerns can information and resources at the following links:

- The National Domestic Violence Hotline: http://www.thehotline.org/resources/

- The National Coalition Against Domestic Violence: https://ncadv.org/resources

- The Family and Youth Services Bureau: https://www.acf.hhs.gov/fysb/resource/help-fv

Conclusion

Your next steps should be to assess your stress levels and anticipated stressors, make a plan for how you will avoid experiencing stress using preventative management techniques, and manage the unavoidable stress in your life with active stress management tools.

This chapter covered the basics of stress and how it is processed by the body and brain. You learned about the different kinds of stress and its sources, as well as how widespread stress is among adults in the US. You also saw several techniques for identifying and managing the stress in your life and were provided with a list of resources for addressing situations where you may feel out of control. You're not alone, and help is available, no matter the seriousness or cause of the situation.

Reflection Questions

1. What is the difference between eustress and distress? How does each affect the body differently?

2. In what ways can mental or cognitive factors affect an individual's perception of stress?

3. What impact can gender dynamics have on the stress response?

4. Identify and describe three possible consequences of excessive stress on wellness.

5. When do you think anger in an appropriate emotion? When can it become a problem?

6. What is the cycle of abuse? What are the key elements of each point?

7. Describe a positive coping habits that might improve your wellness.

8. What role does physical wellness play in managing stress?

Chapter 9
Chronic Disease

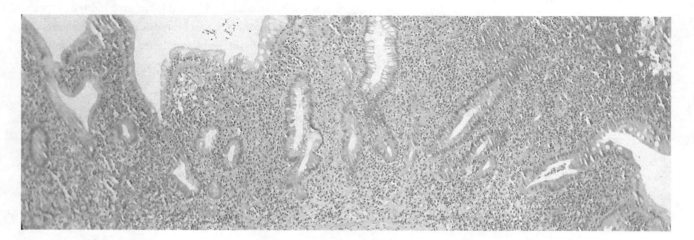

Learning Objectives

1. Discuss the major forms of cardiovascular disease and how they develop.

2. Explain what cancer is and how it develops.

3. Describe the controllable and uncontrollable risk factors associated with cardiovascular disease, cancer and diabetes.

4. Identify the steps you can take to reduce your personal risk of developing cardiovascular disease, cancer and diabetes.

Eight of the top ten causes of death for Americans are chronic diseases. A chronic disease is any disease that lasts longer than 3 months. If you consider how miserable you feel with a simple cold that lasts a few weeks, imagine living with an illness on a daily basis for several years, even decades. The potential restrictions to your daily activities could easily impact the overall quality of your life. Some chronic diseases can't be prevented with vaccines or cured by medication, nor do they just disappear over time. They often develop slowly and take time to reverse, if they can be reversed at all. These conditions affect millions of Americans each year (Figure 1).

These were the top 10 causes of death in the US in 2016:

- Heart disease: 633,842

- Cancer: 595,930

- Chronic lower respiratory diseases: 155,041

- Accidents (unintentional injuries): 146,571

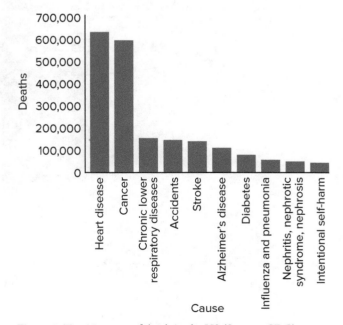

Figure 1. Top 10 causes of death in the US (Source: CDC).

- Stroke (cerebrovascular diseases): 140,323

- Alzheimer's disease: 110,561

- Diabetes: 79,535

- Influenza and pneumonia: 57,062

- Nephritis, nephrotic syndrome, nephrosis: 49,959

- Intentional self-harm (suicide): 44,193

It's more common for older adults to contract these diseases, but the risk has been rising among younger people as unhealthy behaviors become the norm, especially with regard to nutrition and fitness. Your body can become susceptible to disease for many reasons, and yes, some of those are out of your control. Many chronic diseases, however, can be prevented or better managed with improved nutrition and fitness habits, and common-sense lifestyle choices.

In earlier chapters, we talked about Chuck in his recliner, who starts a fitness program and improves his lifestyle before any chronic diseases can take hold. But his story could have gone very differently. It's not hard to imagine what would happen to Chuck if he never decided to start his jogging routine. As you'll see in this chapter, his risk for heart disease, certain cancers, and diabetes increases due to his continued poor nutrition, lack of physical activity, and unhealthy body composition.

This chapter begins by explaining several types of cardiovascular disease, cancer, and diabetes, the top three leading causes of death in the US. The chapter then shifts its focus to behaviors that can help you prevent these diseases in your life, starting by assessing your risks for chronic diseases and then recommending behaviors to lower those risks.

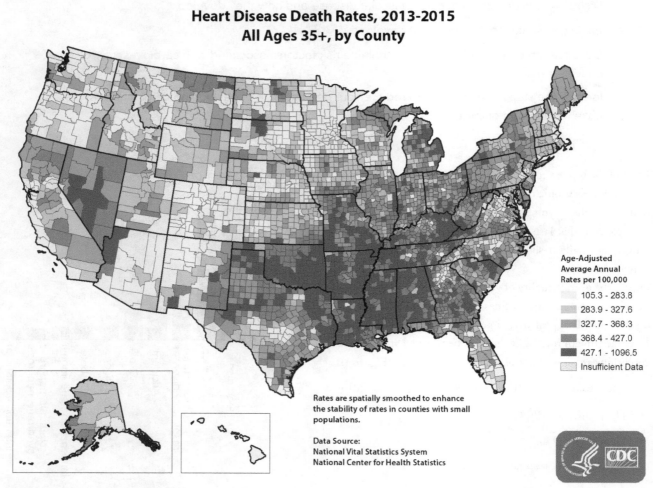

Heart Disease Death Rates, 2013-2015
All Ages 35+, by County

Age-Adjusted
Average Annual
Rates per 100,000

- 105.3 - 283.8
- 283.9 - 327.6
- 327.7 - 368.3
- 368.4 - 427.0
- 427.1 - 1096.5
- Insufficient Data

Rates are spatially smoothed to enhance the stability of rates in counties with small populations.

Data Source:
National Vital Statistics System
National Center for Health Statistics

Figure 2. Heart disease map of the US.

Cardiovascular Diseases

Cardiovascular diseases involve narrowed or blocked blood vessels, dysfunctional heart muscles and valves, or irregular heart rhythm. Heart disease is the number one cause of death in the US, causing nearly 24% of all deaths nationwide. In fact, about 80 million Americans suffer from some form of it, and more than 600,000 of those people die each year. Scary, right? The disease does not discriminate—it attacks men and women equally, claiming credit for one in four deaths for both sexes. Approximately half of all victims had no knowledge they were ill before their death (Figure 2).

The mortality rates are scary enough, but heart disease has also become quite costly to treat. Annually, about one in every six US health care dollars is spent on cardiovascular disease.

Types of Cardiovascular Disease

The heart is a complex organ that plays a large role in many functions of the body. This small yet mighty warrior has a complicated anatomy when you consider the number of other systems in the body it can affect and the sheer magnitude of what can happen when it doesn't work properly (Figure 3). Understanding the risks and symptoms of various cardiovascular diseases is important for living your longest, fullest life possible.

Coronary artery disease (CAD) is the most common type of heart disease and claims 370,000 victims each year in the US. It is the single leading cause of death in the nation.

CAD develops in two major ways—atherosclerosis and arteriosclerosis—both of which inhibit blood flow in the arteries.

Atherosclerosis occurs when plaque (a hardened byproduct of cholesterol, fat, calcium, and other substances) accumulates in the walls of the arteries that feed blood to the heart and other parts of the body (Figure 4). The plaque partially blocks the artery's flow, creating a narrower passage for the blood to navigate. When the heart cannot get enough blood, the person may experience chest pain (see "angina pectoris"), the most common symptom of CAD (Figure 5). Unfortunately, a heart attack is the first symptom of CAD for some people. This is an obvious risk, since a first heart attack can still result in death.

Atherosclerosis is a form of arteriosclerosis. **Arteriosclerosis** occurs when the artery walls thicken, stiffen or harden. We commonly refer to this as "hardening of the arteries." It can happen through fatty buildup, calcification of the artery walls, or thickening of the muscular wall of the arteries from long-term high blood pressure (this is one muscle area you

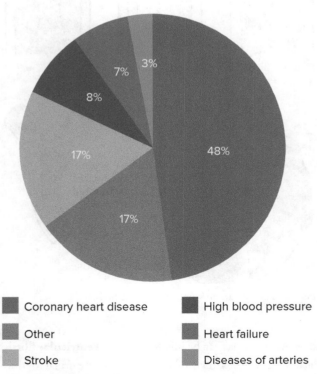

Coronary heart disease

Other

Stroke

High blood pressure

Heart failure

Diseases of arteries

Figure 3. Comparing all types of heart disease.

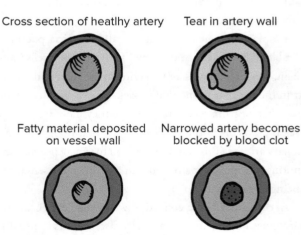

Cross section of heatlhy artery

Tear in artery wall

Fatty material deposited on vessel wall

Narrowed artery becomes blocked by blood clot

Figure 4. Development of atherosclerosis.

Normal artery

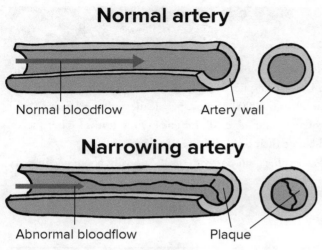

Normal bloodflow   Artery wall

Narrowing artery

Abnormal bloodflow   Plaque

Figure 5. Plaque buildup on the sidewall of an artery.

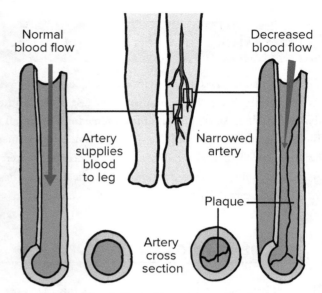

Figure 6. Blood flow is blocked in an atherosclerotic artery.

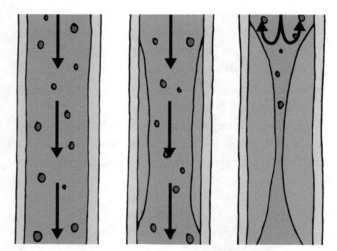

Figure 7. Blood clots cause serious problems.

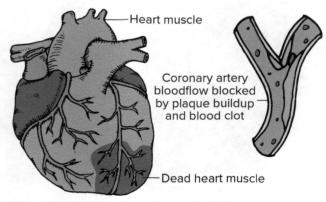

Figure 8. Blood can no longer flow to the body.

don't want to increase). This can also be quite common among older adults since arteries, which are normally flexible, begin to stiffen with age. High cholesterol levels in the blood, a lack of exercise, and smoking can accelerate the hardening process.

Atherosclerosis and arteriosclerosis impact your body differently depending on which arteries experience the most narrowing or hardening. If your coronary artery narrows, you might experience the symptoms of CAD already mentioned. If the peripheral artery narrows, you'll likely experience **peripheral artery disease** (PAD), which impacts blood flow to your legs, arms, head, and stomach. The legs are most commonly affected in people with PAD (Figure 6). People with PAD often experience pain, cramping, or tiredness in these extremities.

Restrictions in the cerebral artery impact blood flow to the brain. This can result in blood clots, known as **aneurysms**, forming in the narrowed passages (Figure 7). If one ruptures or cuts off the flow entirely, it can cause a stroke. The restriction of the blood flow alone, even without a clot, can cause headaches, blurred vision, facial pain, and dementia (particularly in older adults).

People experience a condition called **angina pectoris** when blood flow to the heart is low. This could be a sensation of pain, pressure, fullness, or squeezing in the chest or discomfort in the neck, arm, shoulders, back, or jaw. Women often have different pains than men because they more frequently develop problems in the smaller arteries that branch off the coronary arteries. This could cause them to experience nausea, vomiting, sharp chest pain, abdominal pain, and a sensation of being out of breath.

Arrhythmia is the condition when the heart beats in an irregular manner, beats unusually fast, or beats unusually slow. Arrhythmias can be life threatening. **Ventricular fibrillation** is a type of arrhythmia that causes an abnormal rhythm

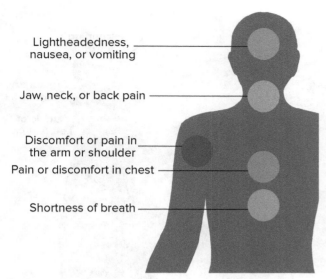

Lightheadedness, nausea, or vomiting

Jaw, neck, or back pain

Discomfort or pain in the arm or shoulder

Pain or discomfort in chest

Shortness of breath

Figure 9. Warning signs of heart attack.

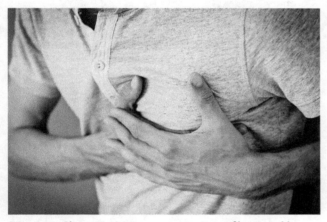

Figure 10. Chest pain is a common symptom of heart problems.

that must be corrected by electric shock (defibrillator) or the person will die. Other types of arrhythmias may not be quite as serious but can lead to other issues, such as **atrial fibrillation**. This arrhythmia can cause a rapid, irregular beat in the upper chambers of the heart. This can lead to the formation of clots, increasing the risk of stroke or heart attack (Figure 8).

That's a lot of ways the heart can experience damage. Someone in the US has a **heart attack** (myocardial infarction) every 43 seconds. That's nearly 735,000 heart attacks each year. A heart attack occurs when a portion of the heart does not get enough blood. The longer the person stays in this state, the more damage it will cause to the heart itself, forming other potentially fatal problems. It's good to be aware of the warning signs of a heart attack, and seek immediate medical assistance if you suspect someone (including yourself) may be having one (Figure 9).This would not be a situation to schedule an appointment with a health care provider or attempt to

drive yourself or someone else to the emergency room as this can be life threatening and time is critical (Figure 10). If you survive the heart attack, your life will most certainly change significantly. At minimum, you will have to undergo a change in lifestyle, such as diet, exercise, and stress management. For some individuals, it could mean medications to prevent blood clots and frequent laboratory tests, lengthy hospitalization, and even risky surgery to prevent problems from worsening.

Heart attacks aren't the only danger of heart disease. The heart can also undergo a deterioration in which it essentially fails to thrive. This is known as **heart failure**. Heart failure sounds as though the heart has stopped beating, but what it means is that the heart is no longer pumping enough blood to support the other organs in your body. The heart's complexity means any one of its many parts might cause failure to another part of the body (Figure 11). Sometimes failure affects only the right side of the heart, responsible for pumping blood to the lungs. A person may experience shortness of breath (particularly when lying flat), fatigue, and a cough that is worse when lying down. In most cases, it affects both sides of the heart. Sufferers will experience shortness of breath and swelling of their ankles, legs, feet, liver, and abdomen, as well as pain in their neck area.

Heart failure primarily occurs as the result of diseases that damage the heart such as CAD, but can also be caused by hypertension and diabetes. Heart failure can develop suddenly or over time. Approximately 5.7 million adults in the US have heart failure, and of these, about half will die within 5 years of being diagnosed. Identifying your personal symptoms for any heart diseases should not replace diagnosis by a health care professional. There are lots of different tests for heart problems that can be performed to check your heart health, including:

Electrocardiogram (**ECG** or **EKG**)—Electrodes are placed on the skin to detect and record the heart's electrical signals. The test can show problems with heart rate or rhythm and detect underlying damage to the heart.

Exercise Stress Test—An electrocardiogram that is performed while the person is exercising on a treadmill or stationary bike. The test monitors the response to exercise and detects problems with the cardiovascular system during physical effort.

Coronary Angiography—A catheter is threaded through the artery, typically in the leg, and dye is injected into the arteries of the heart; special X-rays are then used to identify blockages. A similar procedure can be done to visualize the brain's blood vessels.

Blood Tests—In addition to checking cholesterol and glucose levels, blood samples can be analyzed for enzymes and proteins in the blood that indicate heart muscle damage.

Chest X-ray—Ionizing radiation creates pictures of the heart, lungs, and blood vessels that can be used to determine the size and shape of the heart as well as to detect fluid buildup or damage.

Echocardiogram—A small device called a transducer transmits ultrasound waves into the chest, which are converted into computerized images of the heart. The test can show the heart's size, structure, and motion, as well as blood volume, speed. and direction of blood flow.

Nuclear Scan, Positron Emission Tomographic (PET) Scan—In both tests, small amounts of radioactive tracer materials are injected into the bloodstream. Special imaging equipment monitors blood flow to the heart, as well as the heart's efficiency in pumping blood, and checks for heart muscle damage.

Computed Tomography (CT) Scan—A special X-ray machine takes cross-sectional images that are used to create three-dimensional models of organs. Scans can be used to detect problems in the blood vessels in both the heart and the brain.

Magnetic Resonance Imaging (MRI)—A special scanner uses radio waves, magnets, and a computer to create images of organs and tissues. MRIs can evaluate the condition of the heart and blood vessels and detect the presence and size of aneurysms and malformed blood vessels that are potential causes of hemorrhagic stroke.

Electroencephalogram (EEG)—Electrodes are placed on the scalp, and the electrical activity of the brain is monitored for any indication of problems.

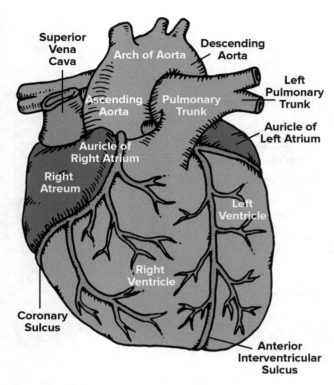

Figure 11. The complex anatomy of the heart.

Congenital Heart Conditions

Many other heart diseases can occur though not all of them are within your control. Some are congenital, meaning they are present at birth. Others can occur as a result of other illnesses.

Cardiomyopathy can be inherited or acquired as the result of another disease or drug. With cardiomyopathy, the heart becomes enlarged, rigid, or thick. In some cases, the tissue is replaced with scar tissue. Cardiomyopathy can be caused by alcohol abuse. As the disease progresses, the heart becomes less effective at pumping blood, leading to heart failure, arrhythmias, or heart valve problems.

Heart valve problems exist when one or more of the valves in your heart (tricuspid, mitral, pulmonary, or aortic) do not function properly. Each valve has a flap that opens and closes as the heart beats, responsible for distributing blood through the heart's chambers and through the body. A faulty or damaged valve may not open fully or may let blood back into the chamber (regurgitation) when it is supposed to be pumping through. This causes the heart to work harder.

Heart valve problems can be congenital, caused by aging, or result from damage from an infection. Many people live with valve problems a long time without noticing them, though others will have noticeable difficulties and will need to have the valve replaced. Valve issues can lead to other heart diseases, like heart failure or stroke.

Some **heart murmurs** are actually an issue with a heart valve (sometimes congenital). A murmur is an abnormal sound, like a "whoosh" noise, between heartbeats. They can occur when the blood flows more rapidly through the heart than normal. A person with a heart murmur may experience shortness of breath, blue coloration to the skin, a chronic cough, dizziness, or fainting. Many heart murmurs cause no trouble to the person. Some can occur during childhood or pregnancy and then resolve. Treatment, if necessary at all, depends on the cause of the murmur.

Varicose veins offer yet another indication that blood is not moving properly through the body. These bluish, spider web-like veins are visible through the skin. They typically occur in the legs. When the valves in your veins become weakened or damaged, blood can begin to pool in the area, causing veins to swell. Some will swell just a little and be simply appear strange. Others will swell to the point of pain, bulging, clotting, or ulceration on the skin. Painful veins may need to be surgically removed.

Varicose veins can be quite common and are usually harmless, occurring often during pregnancy, in people who stand for long periods of time, after trauma to the leg, or when there is a prolonged lack of movement. Being overweight or obese increases your risk for varicose veins. Heredity can sometimes play a role in whether or not you develop varicose veins

Stroke

Stroke, or cerebrovascular accident (CVA), is the fifth leading cause of death in the US and affects 795,000 people each year. Strokes lead to a significant source of disability for many Americans.

There are two different types of strokes, ischemic stroke and hemorrhagic stroke. An **ischemic stroke** can happen when the blood flow to the brain becomes blocked. Sometimes this blockage is just temporary, resulting in a transient ischemic attack (TIA). These are often called "mini-strokes," but the term "warning stroke" might be better. People who suffer from a TIA have a high risk for a more severe blockage in the future. A **hemorrhagic stroke** occurs when a blood vessel in the brain leaks or ruptures causing leaked blood to exert pressure on brain cells, damaging them (Figure 12).

Your brain needs oxygen in order to do its job controlling your movements, emotions, memories, language, and nearly everything you do. Your blood carries oxygen to your brain. When it can't, the cells in that part of your brain begin to die or become permanently damaged, resulting in long-term disability and, potentially, death. The nature of the disability depends on the part of the brain that is affected and what part of the body it controls. Some stroke victims experience problems with speech or swallowing, a loss of control on one side of the body, or difficulty managing their emotions. They may experience problems with sudden and uncontrollable crying, laughing, or swearing—these emotional outbursts may not align with how they actually feel.

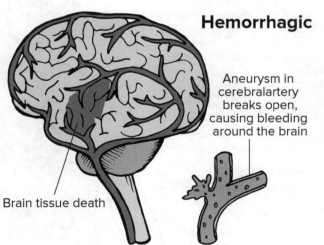

Hemorrhagic

Aneurysm in cerebralartery breaks open, causing bleeding around the brain

Brain tissue death

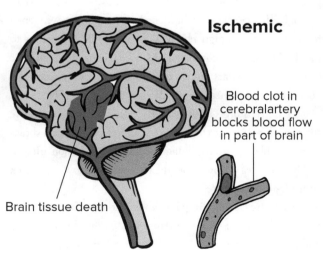

Ischemic

Blood clot in cerebralartery blocks blood flow in part of brain

Brain tissue death

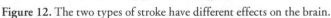

Figure 12. The two types of stroke have different effects on the brain.

Strokes are one of the possible effects of heart diseases like CAD and atrial fibrillation (arrhythmia). Essentially, any disease that can lead to an interruption in the normal flow of blood to the brain—whether through arterial plaque, leakage, or clotting—can lead to a stroke.

According to the National Institute of Neurological Disorders and Stroke (NINDS), some of the most common signs and symptoms of a stroke are:

- Sudden numbness in the face, arms, or legs

- Sudden confusion, and sudden difficulty speaking or understanding others

- Sudden difficulty seeing in one or both of your eyes

- Sudden difficulty with balance, walking, or coordination

- Sudden extreme headache with no apparent cause

As with a heart attack, every minute is critical. If you or someone you know seems to be having a stroke, call 911. Use the FAST test to quickly determine if a person has possibly suffered a stroke (Figure 13).

Stroke Treatment

Generally, three treatment stages for stroke are recommended by the NINDS: prevention, therapy immediately after the stroke, and post-stroke rehabilitation. Therapies to prevent a

F	Face: Ask the person to smile. Does on side of the face droop?
A	Arms: Ask the person to raise both arms. Does one arm drift downward?
S	Speech: Ask the person to repeat a simple phrase. Is their speech slurred or strange?
T	Time: If you see any of these signs, call 911 immediately.

Figure 13. Use the FAST test to quickly identify possible signs of stroke.

first or recurrent stroke are based on treating an individual's underlying risk factors for stroke, such as hypertension, atrial fibrillation, and diabetes. Acute stroke therapies try to stop a stroke while it is happening by quickly dissolving the blood clot causing an ischemic stroke or by stopping the bleeding of a hemorrhagic stroke. Post-stroke rehabilitation (physical, occupational, and speech therapy) helps individuals overcome disabilities that result from stroke damage. Medication or drug therapy is the most common treatment for antithrombotics and thrombolytics, which are intended to keep clots from forming and causing another stroke.

Strokes often recur. About 25% of people who recover from their first stroke will have another within 5 years, so proper post-stroke treatment is important to reduce the risk of reoccurrence.

High and Low Blood Pressure

Hypertension, otherwise known as sustained high blood pressure, is a form of cardiovascular disease in which the pressure of the blood in your body's vessels is higher than normal. This can lead to hardened arteries and a weakened heart. Over time, high blood pressure can be dangerous to the body, causing complications like aneurysms, chronic kidney disease, heart attack, cognitive changes, eye damage, heart failure, peripheral artery disease, and stroke (Figure 14).

Hypertension is known as "the silent killer." One in five sufferers don't realize they have it. Often hypertension shows no noticeable symptoms, though occasionally a person affected will have nausea or vomiting. The only way to know is to check your blood pressure regularly.

This disease even impacts young adults. The results of studies vary, but anywhere from 4–11% of adults in their mid-to-late twenties and early thirties have high blood pressure.

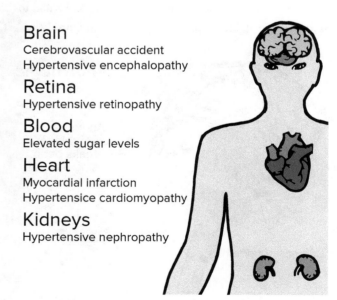

Brain
Cerebrovascular accident
Hypertensive encephalopathy

Retina
Hypertensive retinopathy

Blood
Elevated sugar levels

Heart
Myocardial infarction
Hypertensice cardiomyopathy

Kidneys
Hypertensive nephropathy

Figure 14. High blood pressure impacts several areas of the body.

Part of this may be because health care providers now document an "elevated" or "pre-hypertension stage" that wasn't previously recognized. Research has shown that blood pressures even in this stage can begin to impact the heart's function.

Hypertension has two types, primary and secondary. People with **primary hypertension** have no known cause for the disease. It can occur gradually over several years. **Secondary hypertension** stems from some other underlying condition, like a congenital defect in your blood vessels, kidney or thyroid problems, atherosclerosis, or medications that can cause increased pressure. Alcohol and drug abuse can also cause hypertension because they can damage the heart. Secondary hypertension can increase in seriousness suddenly and dramatically. Anything that causes blockage in your arteries can increase your risk of developing hypertension.

Hypertension is determined by measuring the pressure in your blood. During a blood pressure test, a cloth is wrapped around your upper arm, strapping it in tight. Air is pumped into the cloth until your arm feels uncomfortably snug. The pump and cloth are called a **sphygmomanometer**, but it feels

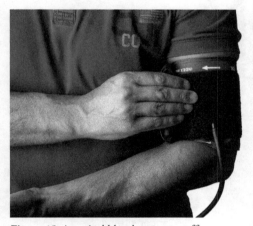

Figure 15. A typical blood pressure cuff.

BLOOD PRESSURE CATEGORY	SYSTOLIC mm Hg (upper number)		DIASTOLIC mm Hg (lower number)
NORMAL	LESS THAN 120	and	LESS THAN 80
ELEVATED	120 – 129	and	LESS THAN 80
HIGH BLOOD PRESSURE (HYPERTENSION) STAGE 1	130 – 139	or	80 – 89
HIGH BLOOD PRESSURE (HYPERTENSION) STAGE 2	140 OR HIGHER	or	90 OR HIGHER
HYPERTENSIVE CRISIS (consult your doctor immediately)	HIGHER THAN 180	and/or	HIGHER THAN 120

Figure 16. Blood pressure ranges based on systolic and diastolic pressure.

a little like a friendly boa constrictor (Figure 15). The resulting numbers on the test might be something like 110 over 70 (110/70), which tells you everything is great. But great for what? Those numbers sound more like a speeding ticket than something related to your health. These numbers are the systolic and diastolic readings.

The **systolic** reading is the first or top number of the reading, and indicates how much pressure your blood is exerting against the walls of your arteries when your heart beats. Systole occurs when your ventricles contract and push blood out of the heart. The **diastolic** reading is the second or bottom number of the reading and indicates how much pressure your blood is exerting against the walls of your arteries when your heart is resting (between beats). Diastole occurs when the ventricles relax, allowing blood to be pumped in.

So what is a healthy blood pressure? You've heard that high blood pressure is bad, but what is considered high? You were right, 110/70 is good—healthy numbers for adults of any age are a systolic reading below 120 and diastolic reading below 80. It's normal for blood pressures to change when you sleep, wake up, or are excited or nervous. It's also normal for your blood pressure to increase during activity. However, once the activity stops, your blood pressure should return to your normal baseline range. Hypertension has varying degrees, ranging from "elevated" (which indicate hypertension could become a problem) to a hypertensive crisis requiring emergency medical care (Figure 16).

Blood pressure starts out low in infants and gradually rises as children grow into adults. A baby with a reading of 80/45 would be normal, but this would be cause for alarm in an adult. It's possible to have low blood pressure. **Hypotension** means a systolic reading below 90 and a diastolic below 60. This can occur during pregnancy, after a prolonged period of bed rest, from blood loss following trauma, or as the result of a severe infection or allergic reaction. It could also be the cause of something more chronic, such as a heart problem. Health care providers typically become concerned about chronic hypotension when it coincides with other symptoms such as nausea, dizziness, fatigue, clammy skin, and blurred vision.

Cancers

Unfortunately for most of us, cancer is not an unfamiliar word. You might have been forced to talk about cancer more times than you would like. Maybe you've walked or run in support of cures, donated money to research, given up a potentially hazardous food because of its association with the disease or, even worse, known someone who has fought cancer. **Cancer** is the term used for a number of diseases in which abnormal cells divide uncontrollably and invade other parts of the body through the blood and lymph systems. This may be caused by a DNA change in the cells, or some kind of damage to them. Hundreds of different types of known cancers exist, and they can occur in many parts of the body (Figure 17).

It may seem like hardly a day goes by where you don't hear something about cancer. This isn't surprising, since cancer is the number two cause of death in the US, responsible for nearly 23% of deaths nationwide. The Agency for Health care Research and Quality estimates that the direct medical costs (total of all health care costs) for cancer in the US in 2014 were $87.8 billion.

How Cancer Develops

Your body is made up of cells. Your first cells began dividing when you were conceived. Those cell divided and divided into more and more cells. Certain cells join together to form parts of the body, like a toe or eye. They have a set of instructions in their DNA telling them exactly which other cells to match up with to create the perfect union. They know when to stop dividing and when to die. Some are meant to replicate as others die (such as skin cells) and others aren't (such as if you lose a toe).

When their DNA is affected, cells become abnormal and no longer understand their instructions. They can either divide and replicate too much within their area, or they can spread to other parts of the body where they don't belong. Your immune system can handle a few abnormal cells, but if they grow too rapidly, they begin to form lumps or growths called tumors.

Benign tumors don't spread and usually don't pose a problem unless they get too large and interfere with comfort

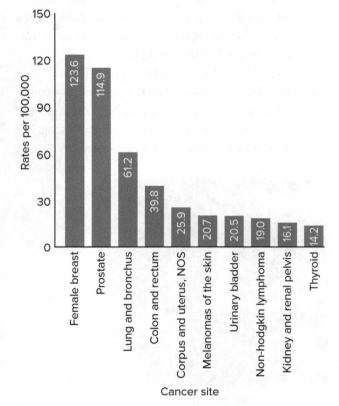

Figure 17. Top 10 US cancer sites in the body.

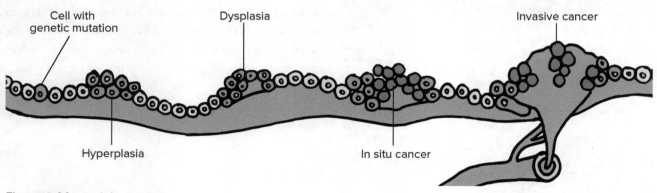

Figure 18. Metastasis in progress.

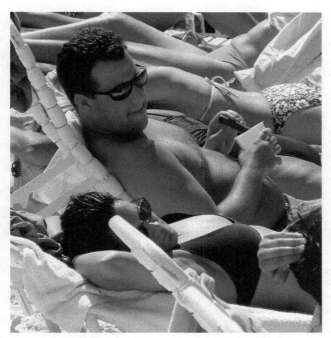

Figure 19. Excessive sun exposure can cause skin cancer.

tobacco, poor nutrition (or the consumption of a carcinogenic food), and a lack of physical activity all relate to lifestyle carcinogens. Other carcinogens are the result of exposure to things like pollution, ultra-violet rays (skin cancer), workplace hazards (such as asbestos or coal dust), or radiation, just to name a few (Figure 19).

Types of Cancer

Cancer comes in many forms based on how and where they develop in the body, and each type has a different effect on the body.

Carcinoma—This type develops in epithelial tissues, linings—such as the skin. Any part of your body with this type of tissue can be affected, such as the colon, breast, lung, or prostate. You have many parts of the body lined with epithelial cells.

Sarcoma—This type forms in bones and in soft and connective tissues like blood vessels, muscles, tendons, and ligaments.

Lymphoma—This type affects the lymph system, more specifically lymphocytes—your white blood cells, part of the immune system responsible for fighting disease.

Myeloma—This type impacts another type of immune cell, your plasma cells. The abnormal cells form tumors in bones any place in the body.

Leukemia—This type originates in the blood-forming tissues of your bone marrow, causing abnormal blood cells (white or red) to develop. They accumulate in the blood and marrow, leaving little room for normal cells. The body has trouble getting enough oxygen to its cells, controlling bleeding, and fighting infection.

or another part of the body. These tumors are non-cancerous. They are like the neutered house cat that eats too much. He stays home, binge-eating treats and getting chubby, but he doesn't bother anyone but his owner. These tumors can, however, become malignant over time in some cases.

Malignant tumors are invasive and considered cancerous. They spread to other parts of the body (**metastasize**), destroy the surrounding tissue, and cause more tumors to grow (Figure 18). They are like the un-neutered tomcat that runs free in the neighborhood, tearing up kids' toys and making "friends" with other cats. Before you know it, the neighborhood is filled with stray kittens looking for food and homes.

Sometimes cancers begin after exposure to an environmental factor known as a **carcinogen**, a substance capable of causing abnormal cell division. You come into contact with many carcinogens voluntarily through your lifestyle, with or without your knowledge. For example, smoking or chewing

Cancer Detection and Diagnosis

Detecting cancer isn't always simple. The symptoms of cancer vary greatly depending on the type and location of the disease. Symptoms for breast cancer, for example, would include swelling of any part of the breast, dimpling, changes

in shape, discharge, pain, or finding a lump in your breast. Symptoms of colon cancer might include changes in bowel movements (such as diarrhea), blood in the stool, or abdominal pain. The symptoms, to a large extent, are specific to the location of the disease. Look for signs from the "CAUTION" test and see a health care professional if you experience any of these possible warning signs of cancer (Figure 20).

But for many cancers, symptoms don't present right away, if they do at all. Symptoms could be similar to the symptoms of common and less serious illnesses. Someone with colon cancer, for example, could easily assume they have the flu or irritable bowel syndrome. For that reason, it's important to have an annual physical, complete any tests recommended by your health care provider, and notify them if your symptoms don't improve.

Just as there are multiple cancers and multiple symptoms, there are many ways of detecting and diagnosing the disease, including biopsy, imaging procedures, and lab tests. Your health care provider will most often begin with laboratory tests, such as blood and urine samples, to determine the count of your white and red blood cells. This tells them if your body is attempting to fight something off, and is a good place to start looking for clues.

They may also look for **tumor markers**, usually particular proteins (or an increase in them) or patterns of genes, which might indicate that cancer could be developing within your body. These serve as red flags to show a need for further testing. Imaging tests are also quite common. X-rays, ultrasounds, mammograms, and MRIs, among other types of procedures, help health care providers see inside your body to determine if a tumor or other issue is present and how large or advanced the abnormal cells have become. They commonly complete biopsies of abnormalities. Surgeons take a small sample of the abnormal growth from the patient and test it to determine if it is benign or malignant, the type of cancer, and to plan the best treatment.

Change in bowel or bladder habits

A sore that does not heal

Unusual bleeding or discharge

Thickening or lump in breast or elsewhere

Indigestion or difficulty in swallowing

Obvious change in wart or mole

Nagging cough or hoarseness

Figure 20. Use the CAUTION test to identify possible warning signs of cancer.

Early Screening

Last year your Aunt Phyllis was diagnosed with breast cancer. She underwent a few rounds of chemotherapy and a month of radiation. Her hair fell out, and she spent several months not feeling so great, but everyone kept saying "Thank goodness they caught it in time!" The thing is, you visited her after her third chemotherapy treatment, and it didn't seem like there was anything good about it. She looked like she was in a lot of pain, like the treatment was making things worse. Yet by the time it was all over, you had spent many hours in the oncology center with her. You were able to realize what it all meant. You saw many people in different stages of the disease. It's true, Aunt Phyllis really was fortunate—she survived in part because a routine mammogram found the tumor during early screening rather than after it had advanced.

With so many different forms of cancer, it's no surprise

Type of Screening	Gender	Age	Frequency
Mammogram	Female	40–44	Optional annual screenings
		45–54	Annually
		55 and up	Every 2 years
Colonoscopy for colon cancer	Male & Female	50 and up	Every 10 years
Stool sample for colon cancer	Male & Female	50 and up	1–3 years depending on type
Pap smear for cervical cancer	Female	21–65	Every 3 years or co-tested with HPV every 5 years for age 30–65
HPV test for cervical cancer	Female	30–65	Every 5 years
Chest CT scan for lung cancer	Either if smoking	55–74	Annually
Rectal exam & PSA for prostate cancer	Men	40 and up	Depending on risk factors

Figure 21. Cancer screening tests should be performed by your health care provider according to several risk factors.

that we screen differently depending on the type and the person's risk factors. The tests you need often depend on your age, gender, family history, and any illnesses or other risk factors you may have. It also depends on the form of cancer health care provider is looking for. It could be done with lab work, imaging, or something a bit more invasive like a colonoscopy. The chart of cancer screening tests can give you a basic guide of the types of screenings and how often they are recommended for different people (Figure 21).

Not all tests have set guidelines for completion. Imaging procedures pose their own risk of excessive radiation exposure, even though the radiation is often low-dose. Other invasive procedures pose risks, too. Someone in good health with no family history may choose to screen less often to avoid unnecessary risk. A person who is physically compromised or experiencing other illnesses may not be a good candidate for these types of screenings. Often, blood work or stool samples will be done initially before more aggressive screening measures.

For some cancers, self-exams may detect problems. Women, for example, should do monthly self-exams on their breasts. If done routinely, she can become very aware of what her breast area is like when normal and can easily notice if something abnormal begins to form. Self-exams can also be a proactive approach for skin cancer. Checking your body for moles of an irregular shape or color, or moles that change shape can help you address an issue while it is still in the early stages of developing into something potentially dangerous.

It helps to begin by determining your risk. You should try to learn your family history of cancer, understand your personal risks related to your health and lifestyle, and ask your health care provider about which screenings you should routinely perform, whether medically and through self-exam.

Staging

Cancer is partially identified by its stage. Stage refers to the extent of the cancer, such as the size of the tumor and if it has spread (metastasized). This can help your health care provider plan the best treatment for you. A cancer is always referred to by the stage it was given at diagnosis, even if it gets worse or spreads. New information about how a cancer has changed over time gets added on to the original stage. So, the stage doesn't change, even though the cancer might.

Health care providers utilize many staging systems. Some may be used for multiple types of cancer. Others are specific to a particular type. Most staging systems include information about, where the tumor is located in the body, the cell type (such as, adenocarcinoma or squamous cell carcinoma), the size of the tumor, whether the cancer has spread to nearby lymph nodes, whether the cancer has spread to a different part of the body, and the appearance of the cancer cells in comparison to healthy cells (tumor grade).

Cancer Treatment

Research and treatment for cancer have come a long way over the years, giving many people a greater chance of surviving cancer. The best treatment plan will depend on the type and stage of the cancer. Some people with cancer will have only one treatment, but most people have a combination of treatments, such as surgery to remove a part of the body or the cancer, along with chemotherapy, radiation therapy, or both. Others might also have immunotherapy, targeted therapy, or hormone therapy.

Chemotherapy is a form of intense drug treatment using drugs designed to stop the growth of cancer cells, either by killing the cells or by stopping them from dividing. Chemotherapy may be given by mouth, injection, infusion, or directly on the skin, depending on the type and stage of the cancer being treated. It may be given alone or with other treatments, such as surgery or radiation therapy. Some patients may receive

chemotherapy for several weeks or months, while others may try various forms of chemo over a period of years. Cancer is by no means easy to cure, and many cells resist treatment.

The side effects of chemotherapy can also become burdensome, particularly for patients already in a weakened state. These drugs don't kill just cancer cells. They don't differentiate between a rapidly growing cancer cell and a rapidly growing healthy one. Many of your cells are meant to die and regenerate often, such as those in your mouth, hair, intestines, finger nails and so on, and these healthy cells also grow rapidly. As a result, patients often experience hair loss, nausea, mouth sores, and fingernail or tooth loss in addition to a great deal of fatigue when undergoing treatment.

Radiation therapy is like a high-powered X-ray, but without the pictures. Radiologists use radiation in lower doses to look for broken bones and dental cavities. But radiation cancer treatment requires the use of high-energy radiation from X-rays, gamma rays, neutrons, protons, and other sources to kill cancer cells and shrink tumors. Radiation may come from a machine outside the body (external-beam radiation therapy), or it may come from radioactive material placed in the body near cancer cells (internal radiation therapy or brachytherapy). Systemic radiation therapy uses a radioactive substance that travels in the blood to tissues throughout the body.

The cancer cells die slowly and continue dying for a while after treatment is finished. Patients often need several doses given close together. For example, a patient may have to receive radiation 5 days per week for a month or more. As with chemotherapy, there can be side effects as the healthy cells nearby the cancerous ones also become damaged. Fatigue, swelling, skin damage, and hair loss are just a few, though it does vary depending on the location of the cancer.

Immunotherapy is a type of biological therapy that uses substances to stimulate or suppress the immune system to help the body fight cancer, infection, and other diseases. Some types of immunotherapy only target certain cells within the immune system, while others affect the immune system in a general way.

Targeted therapy uses drugs or other substances to identify and attack specific types of cancer cells with less harm to normal cells. Some targeted therapies block the action of certain enzymes, proteins, or other molecules involved in the growth and spread of cancer cells. Other types of targeted therapies help the immune system kill cancer cells or deliver toxic substances directly to cancer cells. Targeted therapies may have fewer side effects than other types of cancer treatment.

Hormone therapy adds, blocks, or removes hormones. In cancer treatment, it is used to slow or stop the growth of certain cancers (such as prostate and breast cancer) if hormones are a contributing factor. Synthetic hormones or other drugs may be given to block the body's natural hormones. Surgery may be needed to remove the gland that makes a certain hormone.

The effectiveness of these treatments varies with how early the cancer is detected, the overall health of the patient, and the type and aggressiveness of the cancer cells.

Diabetes

Diabetes has also become a familiar term to us over the past several years. Diabetes causes 3% of all deaths in the US, ranking at number 7 on the top causes of death. Its prevalence is also expensive to the nation. The American Diabetes Association reports that annual costs for diabetes treatment in the US totals over $176 billion.

To produce energy, nearly all of the food you consume breaks down into glucose in your body. Insulin, a hormone secreted by the pancreas, aids this glucose in getting into your cells. In some people the pancreas does not make insulin at all or not enough to deal with the glucose, leaving too much of it in the blood. Diabetes develops when a person's glucose level in their blood is too high and their body cannot make enough insulin to balance it out.

There are four different types of diabetes:

Pre-Diabetes—The blood sugar level is too high but not high enough to be considered diabetes. A person with prediabetes can have many of the same complications as diabetes and is at risk for diabetes if nothing within their body changes to lower the blood sugar.

Type 1—The body does not produce insulin. The immune system attacks and destroys the cells in the pancreas that make it. It is usually diagnosed in children and young adults, although it can appear at any age. People with Type 1 diabetes need to take insulin every day to stay alive.

Type 2—The body does not produce insulin well. A person can develop Type 2 diabetes at any age, even during childhood. However, this type of diabetes occurs most often in middle-aged and older people.

Gestational—The body experiences a temporary problem producing enough insulin while pregnant. This usually goes away after birth.

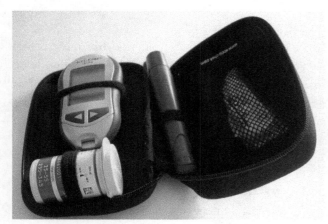

Figure 22. A typical blood insulin testing kit.

Diabetes can take a large toll of the body. This abundance of sugar can cause serious damage to your eyes, kidneys, nerves, and heart. The impact to the nerves and to the circulatory system can make a person prone to skin sores that can be difficult to heal and may even lead to amputation of a limb. As if this wasn't enough, the risk of stroke also increases for a person with diabetes.

Managing Type 2 diabetes

Healthy eating, physical activity, and insulin injections are the basic therapies used to manage diabetes. The amount of insulin taken must be balanced with food intake and daily activities. Blood glucose levels must be closely monitored through frequent blood glucose testing (Figure 22).

Many people with Type 2 diabetes can manage their blood sugar through diet and exercise, and by maintaining a healthy body composition, sometimes eliminating the need for insulin. Others require oral medication, insulin, or both to control their blood glucose levels.

Healthy eating with diabetes means following a meal plan that will help you manage your blood glucose, blood pressure, and cholesterol. This means planning carbohydrate intake. Choose fruits, vegetables, beans, whole grains, chicken or turkey without the skin, fish, lean meats, and nonfat or low-fat milk and cheese. Drink water instead of sugar-sweetened beverages (some people even have difficulty tolerating artificial sweeteners). Choose foods that are lower in calories, saturated fat, trans-fat, sugar, and salt. Your health care provider or a dietician will typically give you a food plan that will help you balance the 5 food groups in a way that helps control blood sugar levels.

Regular physical activity, as mentioned throughout this text, is important in managing your body's systems and keeping your body composition healthy. Work up to the recommended 150 minutes of moderate or 75 minutes of vigorous-intensity exercise each week.

The risk of acquiring other chronic diseases can be quite high if you have diabetes. You can manage your diabetes, reduce these risks, and live a long and healthy life by taking care of yourself each day.

Reducing Your Risk for Chronic Diseases

Assessing your risk for chronic diseases is a matter of comparing your current state to the recommendations for preventing these diseases. If any of your assessments show a need for improvement in a specific area, the other chapters in this book can help you create a targeted plan for improvement to that aspect of your wellness.

Many diseases, as you've learned, have factors that may be beyond your control. But it's important to understand both what puts you at risk and what you have the ability to manage. Your risk for disease can be assessed by determining whether certain risk factors apply in your life. You can potentially lower some of the risk by making healthy decisions in the controllable risk factors following.

Assessing Risks for Heart Disease

You've learned that heart disease has become a wide-spread problem. So many of the choices you make can impact other aspects of health and particularly the health of your heart. Chapter 3 discusses how the heart works in detail—remember this is your engine, responsible for keeping you running smoothly and efficiently. You don't have any control over your heredity, age, biological sex, and ethnicity, all of which can play a role in your risks for heart disease.

Heredity—Certain risks can be inherited genetic traits and make you predisposed to certain diseases, such as high blood pressure and cardiomyopathy. Hypertrophic cardiomyopathy, a condition in which the heart muscle is thickened, is thought to be the most common inherited or genetic heart disease. Several genetic disorders are associated with increased risk of premature heart attacks. A relatively common disorder is familial hypercholesterolemia, which causes high levels of "bad" cholesterol beginning at birth. About one out of 500 people in the US inherit this condition (Figure 23).

Age—As you get older, your risk for atherosclerosis (hardening of the arteries) increases. Genetic or lifestyle factors cause plaque to build up in your arteries over time. By the time you're middle-aged or older, enough plaque may have built up to begin causing signs or symptoms. In men, the risk increases after age 45. In women, the risk increases after age 55.

Biological Sex—The varying levels of risk between male and female adults are due to differences in their reproductive qualities and different types of hormones. Heart disease is the number one killer for both sexes, but women have one risk factor that men don't—menopause. It is theorized that estrogen helps support heart health. As it declines, a woman's risk of heart disease can increase.

Ethnicity—Even when studies adjust for socioeconomic class, some ethnicities still have higher risks. Almost half of all African Americans have cardiovascular disease, compared to one-third of whites. Hispanics and Latinos, though they have a higher risk for other diseases than whites, are 25% less likely to die of heart disease (though this could be due to under-reporting of the illness). Asian immigrants tend to have lower rates of heart disease, but their children raised in the US experience many of the same issues as whites, suggesting that environmental issues play a larger role.

Controllable Risks

Other behaviors that impact your risk, like tobacco use, physical activity, cholesterol levels, blood pressure, body composition, and others, can be changed. Consider what risks you can manage and which choices you make that might be putting you at higher risk for heart disease.

Tobacco Use—The chemicals in tobacco cause buildup in the body's arteries, giving the blood a smaller passageway. It limits the flow of blood through the arteries forcing the heart to work harder, putting a strain on it and the rest of the body. If the buildup becomes

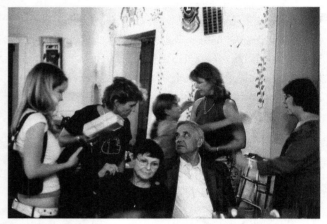

Figure 23. Family medical histry is a good predictor of some chronic diseases.

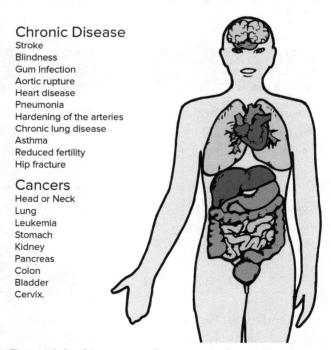

Chronic Disease
Stroke
Blindness
Gum Infection
Aortic rupture
Heart disease
Pneumonia
Hardening of the arteries
Chronic lung disease
Asthma
Reduced fertility
Hip fracture

Cancers
Head or Neck
Lung
Leukemia
Stomach
Kidney
Pancreas
Colon
Bladder
Cervix.

Figure 24. Smoking can contribute to many chronic diseases.

too great, the artery can become totally blocked and the risk of heart attack increases significantly. Smoking speeds up the accumulation of plaque from high cholesterol and robs your body of good cholesterol, putting you at even greater risk of forming dangerous blockages and clots. The nicotine in tobacco products also increases your heart rate and blood pressure. Even occasional smoking and second- hand smoke increases your risk (Figure 24). More information about quitting smoking and its benefits can be found in Chapter 11.

Lack of Physical Activity — As covered in previous chapters, many of the positive aspects of your health can be lost through lack of usage. Muscles atrophy, tendons and ligaments become inflexible, you lose agility and mobility when weight is gained, and your heart does not receive the aerobic benefits it needs to stay healthy (Figure 25). Have you ever parked your car for a month or so without starting it? If you have, you likely found that you had a dead battery. The heart functions in a similar way. It may not die as quickly, but it does experience the side effects of a sedentary lifestyle. Blood needs to pump in your body in the same way that a car's engine needs to rev. Physical activity improves circulation, improves cholesterol, improves the elasticity of arteries, helps control high blood pressure, diabetes, and body weight. It helps you avoid so many of the risk factors that contribute to heart disease, such as overweight or obesity, high cholesterol, and hypertension, and keeps your engine running.

High Cholesterol — Cholesterol levels are primarily impacted by two factors — diet and physical activity. Most often when we discuss cholesterol, we focus on the structures in the body that carry cholesterol — lipoproteins. The body contains different types of lipoproteins. The ones you hear about most often are the **low-density lipoproteins** (LDL) and **high-density lipoproteins** (HDL). Health care providers consider LDL as the "bad" cholesterol or "less desirable cholesterol" because cholesterol carried by LDL's do not move freely through the arteries and can lead to plaque buildup that results in heart disease and stroke. HDL, in contrast, absorbs cholesterol and helps it travel to the liver where it can be processed. Physical activity, of course, plays a significant role. Research shows that exercise lowers LDL numbers and raises HDL. The American Heart Association advocates for a healthy diet low in saturated fats, free of trans fat (a chemical form of fat engineered to lengthen food shelf life and shorten yours), and high in fruits, vegetables, lean protein, fiber, whole grains, oats, and nuts (Figure 26).

High Blood Pressure — Sustained high blood pressure (hypertension) has higher risks for certain individuals, such women over 45, blacks, and people with a family history of hypertension. Your systolic (top number) should be below 120 and your diastolic (bottom number) below 80. Adults should have their blood pressure checked every two years if they have healthy blood pressure, and more frequently if their blood pressure is high. Diet, physical activity, tobacco

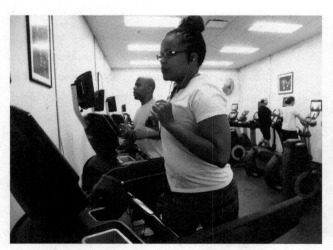

Figure 25. Regular physical activity can help prevent disease.

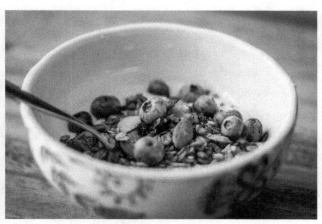

Figure 26. Healthy food choices improve the body's function.

use, and stress can all play a negative role on blood pressure levels (Figure 27).

Overweight/Obesity—A person with a Body Mass Index (BMI) between 25–29 is considered overweight, and obese if above 30. Many of the factors that cause someone to be overweight or obese are the same factors that contribute to heart disease. Inactivity, a high fat diet (and high cholesterol levels), and visceral fat (abdominal fat) all contribute to stress on the heart and arteries. Visceral fat and poor cholesterol levels go hand-in-hand as a troubling tag-team to clog arteries and damage vital organs. Women tend to store fat on their hips and thighs, while men tend to store belly fat. Belly fat, which can be an indicator of visceral fat, is a greater risk. A healthy body composition remains your first line of defense.

Diabetes—The longer a person suffers from diabetes, the larger the impact to their heart. High levels of blood sugar can damage your blood vessels and the nerves that work with your heart, leading to atherosclerosis and other forms of heart disease. People with diabetes are also more likely to have issues with high cholesterol and high blood pressure. In fact, heart disease is the most common cause of death for people with diabetes.

Psychological and Social Factors—These can also impact heart health in their connection to stress, personality type, chronic hostility and anger, suppressing psychological distress, depression and anxiety, social isolation, low socioeconomic status, and alcohol use (Figure 28). The common thread among most of these is stress. People who have difficulty managing anger, anxiety, depression, etc., experience fight or flight hormones for an extended period of time can damage their body. They often tend to have less concern for their health and lower motivation to manage it effectively. Some may even drink more alcohol than recommended, which causes a temporary increase in heart rate. People with lower socioeconomic status tend to have more stress and, therefore, need to pay closer attention to how they manage it.

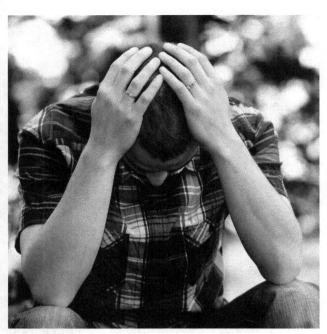

Figure 27. High blood pressure can stem from stress.

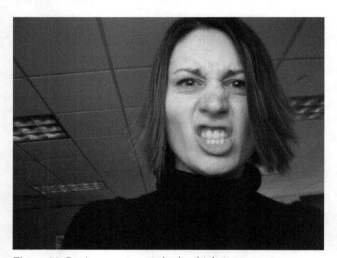

Figure 28. Persistent anger can lead to high stress.

Metabolic Syndrome—This is a term the medical field uses for a group of risk factors or traits that contribute to heart disease and other health problems. These include many of the issues already discussed, such as obesity, high cholesterol and triglycerides, high blood pressure, and high blood sugar. When these are in check, your body is more likely to function as it should and your risk of heart disease is lower.

Sleep apnea—Untreated sleep apnea can increase your risk for high blood pressure, heart attack, or stroke. This is a common disorder in which you have one or more pauses in breathing or shallow breaths while you sleep.

Alcohol Use—Heavy drinking can damage the heart muscle and worsen other CHD risk factors. Men should have no more than 2 drinks containing alcohol a day. Women should have no more than one drink containing alcohol a day. More information on alcohol consumption can be found in Chapter 11.

Assessing Risks for Cancer

While it's true that some cancers have no single cause that health care providers can pinpoint, we do know a lot about what can contribute to your risk of cancer. Many of these risks can be managed, but some of them can't. You don't have any control over your heredity, age, biological sex, and ethnicity, all of which can play a role in your risks for cancer.

Heredity—There are certain inherited genetic mutations that result in an increase in some cancers, called Hereditary Cancer Syndrome (Figure 29). Scientists don't yet have a perfect understanding of how cancer and genetics relate, but your family history of cancer plays an important role in determining which kinds of cancer screenings you should get.

Age—Natural aging is a significant risk factor in most cancers in general, but especially in certain types of cancer such as breast, colon, and prostate cancer. Half of all cancer diagnoses occur in people with an average age over 66. However, cancer can happen at any age.

Biological Sex—Hormones can also contribute to cancer growth, particularly in women. Menopausal women who undergo hormone replacement therapy for estrogen are at a higher risk for developing breast cancer. Cancer mortality rates, however, tend to be higher among men than women. Some forms may strike a particular sex more often than another (Figure 30).

Ethnicity—African American women have a higher incidence of aggressive breast cancers than other ethnicities, and African American men have a higher rate of prostate cancer. Native Americans and Alaskan Natives have higher rates of kidney cancer. Asians and Pacific Islanders show a higher risk of liver cancer. Hispanic and African American women also see greater risk of cervical cancers. It's uncertain why some ethnicities are more prone to certain forms of cancer aside from socioeconomic factors.

Figure 29. Heredity plays a role in your risk for chronic disease.

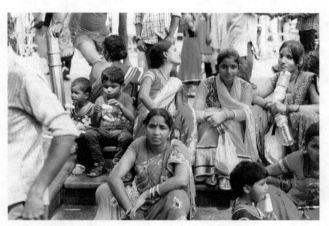

Estimated Cancer Deaths in the US in 2016

	Males 314,290	Females 281,400	
Lung & bronchus	27%	26%	Lung & bronchus
Prostate	8%	14%	Breast
Colon & rectum	8%	8%	Colon & rectum
Pancreas	7%	7%	Pancreas
Liver & intrahepatic bile duct	6%	5%	Ovary
Leukemia	4%	4%	Uterine corpus
Esophagus	4%	4%	Leukemia
Urinary bladder	4%	3%	Liver & intrahepatic bile duct
Non-Hodgkin lymphoma	4%	3%	Non-Hodgkin lymphoma
Brain & other nervous system	3%	2%	Brain & other nervous system
All other sites	24%	24%	All other sites

Figure 30. Estimated US cancer deaths by gender.

Controllable Risks

Now for the good news. You can reduce your risk of cancer by using many of the same strategies used to prevent other chronic illnesses. If you manage your body composition, get plenty of exercise, avoid harmful substances, and eat a healthy diet, you're well on your way (Figure 31). But these aren't the only things that can help you avoid higher risks for cancer.

Alcohol Use—More than 2 drinks of alcohol per day can increase your risk for cancers of the mouth, throat, esophagus, larynx, liver, and breast. It does this in a few different ways. One is that the body converts alcohol into a chemical called acetaldehyde, which damages DNA and hinders the body's cells from repairing the damage. Alcohol also impairs the body's ability to break down and absorb a variety of nutrients that may be associated with cancer risk, including vitamin A, nutrients in the vitamin B complex (such as folate), vitamin C, vitamin D, vitamin E, and carotenoids. In addition, it increases the risk of breast cancer by increasing blood levels of estrogen. For more information on alcohol use and abuse, see Chapter 11.

Infections—Approximately 16% of new cancer cases can be connected to infectious disease. Certain infectious agents such as viruses, bacteria, and parasites can cause chronic inflammation, which may increase your risk of cancer. Some viruses can disrupt signaling that normally keeps cell growth and proliferation in check. Also, some infections weaken the immune system, making the body less able to fight off other cancer-causing infections. And some viruses, bacteria, and parasites also cause chronic inflammation, which may lead to cancer. You can lower your risk of infection from some infectious agents by getting vaccinated, not having unprotected sex, and not sharing hypodermic needles. For more information on infectious diseases, see Chapter 10.

Radiation—Radiation from certain sources, like radon, X-rays, and gamma rays increase your risk of cancer by damaging DNA structure. The affected cells become abnormal and can become cancerous at a higher rate. Sunlight, sunlamps, and tanning booths give off ultraviolet (UV) radiation and should be avoided without protection. UV radiation damages skin cell's DNA, which may lead to skin cancer. For more information on radiation, see Chapter 12.

Stress—There is little evidence that stress directly causes cancer. Long-term stress does weaken your immune system. Those great yet pesky fight or flight hormones we keep mentioning disrupt your immune system, which is why you often get a cold when stressed or suffering from sleep deprivation. This puts your body at risk for viruses and bacteria, some of which may be dangerous, as mentioned earlier.

Stress can also impact your decision-making in the other risk factors above, leading to cancer indirectly. Stressed individuals often focus on immediate issues and tend to put off healthy lifestyle changes in lieu of solving other concerns. This can become a difficult cycle since people manage stress better when healthy and, certainly, a disease like cancer could add even more stress. For more information on stress management, see Chapter 8.

Chemicals and Toxic Environments—Exposure to chemicals in your environment can cause cancer, as well (environmental carcinogens). The highest risks are associated with radon radiation in basements, cigarette smoking, and pollution. The National Toxicology Project publishes a list of known human carcinogens every few years. For more information on environmental health, see Chapter 12.

Assessing Risks for Diabetes

Earlier in this chapter, you learned that Type 1 diabetes can only be managed, not prevented. Other types of diabetes can be prevented. Your 50-year-old neighbor, James, was overweight and inactive. He's been quite the junk-food junky for years. You remember when you were a kid, James used to have you mow his lawn for $10 every weekend. James would then give you the money to walk down to the convenience store and pick up a case of soda for him. He'd always give you enough to get yourself a candy bar, too. You didn't mind—every kid likes to make a buck. Until the job went away. James suddenly started mowing his own lawn! And the trips to the corner? Gone! Turns out his health care provider diagnosed him with Type 2 diabetes. James learned to manage his diabetes through nutrition and physical activity. James found out that he could manage his risk (and still get you to help him pull weeds for some extra money).

Changes like the ones James made are possible, but not every risk factor is under your control. You don't have any control over your heredity, age, biological sex, and ethnicity, all of which can play a role in your risks for diabetes.

Heredity—Diabetes can run in families due to genetic factors. Type 1 diabetes can be inherited, caused by an autoimmune disorder, or the result of environmental factors. A predisposition to Type 2 diabetes can also be inherited.

Age—Adults 45 and older are more likely to develop Type 2 diabetes. Research suggests that insulin resistance is more common due to muscle loss. As you age, fat can build in your muscles and liver, contributing to this resistance.

Biological sex—Men are at a greater risk for developing Type 2 diabetes due to a higher incidence of visceral fat than women.

Ethnicity—American Indians and Alaskan Natives are at a higher risk at 15.9%, followed by blacks, Hispanics, Asian Americans, and whites.

Certain Health Conditions—Other health conditions, such as history of gestational diabetes or having given birth to a baby over nine pounds, polycystic ovary syndrome (PCOS), and acanthosis nigricans—dark, thick, and velvety skin around your neck or armpits, can increase risk.

Controllable Risks

The usual suspects are in place here with risks for diabetes, too. As you might expect by now, your general health is impacted by the same set of factors, and diabetes risk is no different.

Overweight and obesity—A BMI over 25 increases your risk for diabetes.

Low HDL Cholesterol—HDL cholesterol is the "good" kind, so low levels of HDL or high levels of triglycerides can increase risks.

High Blood Pressure—High blood pressure is most often a result of lifestyle choices and can be lowered with improved nutrition and physical activity.

Physical Inactivity—Over and over, we have recommended fitness training to increase your physical activity, and lowering your risk for diabetes is yet another reason to strive for healthy physical fitness.

History of Heart Disease or Stroke—Most heart diseases and stroke risk are preventable, so making healthier decisions overall can help you avoid multiple chronic diseases.

Depression—Clinical depression may not be preventable, but it can be managed. See Chapter 8 for more information.

Online Resources for Lowering Risks

American Heart Association—Healthyforgood.heart.org
Centers for Disease Control—CDC.gov/cholesterol
The Franklin Institute—FI.edu/heart-engine-of-life

National Stroke Association—Stroke.org
American Diabetes Association—Diabetes.org

Conclusion

Your next steps should be to use the recommendations for each risk area to assess your own risk of developing a chronic disease. Using that information, you can create a plan for improving your wellness to lower those risks and live a healthier, longer life.

This chapter has looked closely at some of the life-threatening diseases that can be caused by poor health and fitness. We covered the causes, symptoms, and some treatments for disease, but most importantly, we explored several ways you can act now to avoid these diseases altogether. We all want to live longer, fuller lives, and understanding the consequences of unhealthy decisions can provide some of the motivation that may be lacking for you to make a change. Consider implementing lifestyle strategies that can reduce your risk for chronic disease, including habits in your diet, physical activity, stress, substance use, or other areas that may need attention.

Reflection Questions

1. What are the different types of cardiovascular disease? What are characteristics of each?

2. How does cancer develop? Describe the process of cancer development, tumor development and metastasis.

3. Identify a type of cancer that concerns you. How is this type of cancer screened?

4. Briefly describe the scope of diabetes in the US, as a public health problem.

5. What should a person with diabetes to do stay healthy?

6. Consider your own personal risk for cardiovascular disease, cancer or diabetes. What uncontrollable risks do you have? What controllable risks do you have? How concerned are you about your personal risk for this type of disease?

7. What can you do to reduce your risk for chronic disease?

Chapter 10
Infectious Disease

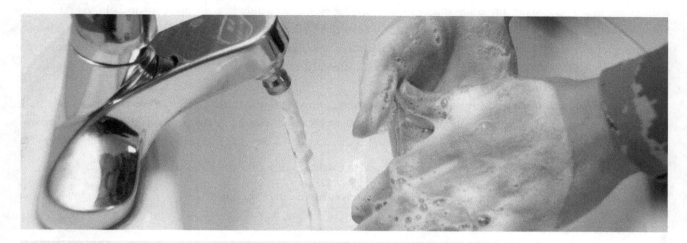

Learning Objectives

1. Describe types of pathogens and how each affects the body.

2. Describe the chain of infection.

3. Discuss the major sexually transmitted infections and identify their transmission, symptoms and treatment.

4. Describe how sexually transmitted infectious affect overall wellness.

5. Identify strategies for preventing STIs.

You and your friend stop for smoothies after an early-morning workout. You get some form of fruity concoction and she goes with a kale-filled, green, chunky mixture that looks like it came from a swamp. She's always trying to persuade you to join in her love of kale and makes yet another attempt. "Just taste it. It won't hurt you. It's good for you!" Little does she know that it's not your aversion to the leafy super-food that's causing you to hesitate—it's the residue on her straw! She thinks she's offering you healthy food, but you see it as a microscopic threat. All you can think about are the millions of bacteria that could be crawling around on that tiny piece of plastic. And so, you politely decline her offer.

Your friend and her straw may have been germ-free, but you have every right to be cautious. Infections are nothing to sneeze at. An **infection** is a disorder caused by the invasion of a disease-causing agent into your body. Dangers from infection surround you all the time, but most infectious diseases can be prevented with healthy strategies including engaging in good hygiene, protecting yourself against pathogens, and practicing safer sexual activity.

This chapter introduces the basics of infection and infectious diseases and how most of them can be prevented. It then turns to the dangers of sexually transmitted infections (STIs) and the importance of practicing safer sexual activity.

Defining Infectious Disease

No one goes through life without "catching a bug," not even your friend who drinks kale smoothies (though to be fair, she really is giving it a good shot). Infectious diseases accounted for over $120 billion in economic costs in 2014. As infectious diseases spread and new forms of them arise—and they do—the US feels the burden physically and financially. Consider the common flu. In a typical year, 5–20% of the US population contracts influenza (flu). Tens of thousands are hospitalized, and thousands die from flu-related illness. This costs an estimated $10.4 billion in direct medical expenses and an additional $16.3 billion in lost earnings annually.

Infectious diseases are caused by microorganisms. Microorganisms are tiny living things found everywhere—in air, soil, and water. You can get infected by touching, eating, drinking or breathing something that contains these germs. Microorganisms can also spread through animal and insect bites, kissing, and sexual contact. The main kinds of microorganisms are:

Bacteria—one-celled germs that multiply quickly and may release chemicals which can make you sick

Viruses—capsules that contain genetic material and use your own cells to multiply

Fungi—primitive plants, like mushrooms or mildew

Protozoa—one-celled animals that use other living things for food and a place to live

Helminths—intestinal worms transmitted through soil

These are all forms of **pathogens.** A pathogen is the first link in the chain of disease. Anything that causes disease is considered a pathogen. It's important to remember that not all microorganisms are pathogens. Some bacteria, affectionately referred to as "good" bacteria, keep your body functioning properly. Some bacteria that live in your digestive tract, for example, aid in the digestion of food and help your body process the things you eat. The microbes we focus on in this chapter are the pathogens—the ones you don't want in your body.

Pathogens

We normally think of pathogens in hostile terms—as invaders that attack our bodies. But a pathogen or a parasite, like any other organism, is simply trying to live and procreate. Living at the expense of a host organism (that's us) is a very attractive strategy, and it's possible that every living organism on Earth is subject to some type of infection or parasitism. Your body makes a great living space for a pathogen. It's a nutrient-rich, warm, and moist environment that remains at a uniform temperature and constantly renews itself. It's not surprising that many microorganisms have evolved the ability to survive and reproduce inside us.

Bacteria

Bacteria are living things that have only one cell. Under a microscope, they look like balls, rods, or spirals. They are so small that a line of 1,000 could fit across the width of a pencil eraser. Most bacteria won't hurt you—fewer than 1% of the different types make people sick. Many are helpful. Some bacteria help to digest food, destroy disease-causing cells, and give the body needed vitamins. In fact, bacteria are used in making healthy foods like yogurt and cheese. But infectious bacteria can make you ill. They reproduce quickly in your body, and many give off chemicals called toxins or enzymes, which can damage tissue and give your immune system real problems.

Some bacteria that cause disease can only replicate inside the cells of the human body. These are called **obligate pathogens.** Others replicate in an environmental space such as water or soil and only cause disease if they happen to encounter a susceptible host. These are called **facultative pathogens**. Many bacteria are normally benign but have a latent ability to cause disease in someone with a compromised immune system. These are called **opportunistic pathogens**.

Some bacterial pathogens can be fussy in their choice of host and will only infect a single species or a group of related species, whereas others prove less picky about where they live. We call them generalists. *Shigella flexneri*, a bacterium that causes epidemic dysentery (bloody diarrhea) in areas of the world lacking a clean water supply, will only infect humans and other primates. On the other hand, the closely related bacterium *Salmonella enterica*, a common cause of food poisoning in humans, can also infect many other vertebrates including chickens and turtles. A champion generalist is the opportunistic pathogen *Pseudomonas aeruginosa*, which is capable of causing disease in plants as well as animals. Other well-known bacteria that can harm us are Lyme disease, pneumonia, tuberculosis, E. coli, listeria, meningitis, gonorrhea, chlamydia, and syphilis.

For bacterial infections, a health care provider will prescribe medications including antibiotics. Bacteria are very adaptable, and the widespread overuse of antibiotics since their discovery has cause many types of bacteria to become resistant to antibiotics.

Viruses

Viruses are very tiny microorganisms that contain just one or two molecules of RNA (ribonucleic acid) and DNA inside of a protein coating. Viruses cause some of the most familiar infectious diseases such as the common cold, flu, and warts. They also cause more severe illnesses such as HIV/AIDS, smallpox, influenza, mononucleosis, measles, mumps, rabies, polio, hepatitis, and Ebola. Each virus is different, and can cause different symptoms to appear, even if they seem similar at first like the cold and flu viruses (Figure 1).

You probably associate a virus with the runny nose and cough you get with the flu or the chicken pox. But what's actually happening in your body when you have a virus? Viruses invade living, normal cells and use those cells to multiply themselves and reproduce. This can kill, damage, or change the invaded cells, making you sick. Different viruses attack specific cells in your body such as your liver cells, cells in your lungs, or blood cells. When a virus enters your system, you may not always get sick from it. Your immune system may be able to fight it off.

For most viral infections, treatments can only help with symptoms while you wait for your immune system to fight

Symptom	Cold	Flu
Fever	Rare	High (100–102°F), can last 3–4 days
Headache	Rare	Intense
General aches, pains	Slight	Usual, often severe
Fatigue, weakness	Mild	Intense, can last up to 2–3 weeks
Extreme exhaustion	Never	Usual, starts early
Stuffy nose	Common	Sometimes
Sneezing	Usual	Sometimes
Sore throat	Common	Common
Cough	Mild to moderate	Common, can become severe
Complications	Sinus, congestion or earache	Bronchitis, Pneumonia. You may need to go to a hospital
Prevention	Regular hand washing and avoid ill people	Flu vaccine once per year, regular hand washing, avoid ill people, antiviral drugs oseltamivir (Tamiflu) and zanamivir (Relenza)
Treatment	Over the counter products ease symptoms	Over the counter products to ease symptoms, prescription treatments Oseltamivir (Tamiflu) or Zanamivir (Relenza) within 24–48 hours after symptoms start, Peramivir (Rapivab) for some cases taken by IV

Figure 1. Comparing cold and flu symptoms.

off the virus. Antibiotics do not work for viral infections, though vaccines can help prevent you from getting many viral diseases, such as measles.

Fungus

If you have ever had athlete's foot or a yeast infection, you've had an infection from a **fungus or fungi**. A fungus is a primitive organism that can be single- or multi-celled, such as mushrooms, mold, and mildew. Fungi live in air, in soil, on plants, and in water. Some live in the human body, on the skin, on and inside animals, and on many indoor surfaces. Common fungal infections are thrush, athlete's foot, meningitis, ringworm, and yeast infections.

Some fungi reproduce through tiny spores in the air. You can inhale the spores, or they can land on your skin. As a result, fungal infections often start in the lungs or on the skin. Fungi are everywhere. Approximately 1.5 million different species of fungi exist on Earth, but only about 300 of those are known to make people sick.

Anyone can get a fungal infection, even healthy people. You come in contact with fungal spores every day, usually without getting sick. However, for people with weak immune systems, these fungi are more likely to cause an infection.

Protozoa

Protozoa are microscopic, one-celled organisms that can be free-living or parasitic in nature. They have the ability to multiply in humans, which contributes to their survival and enables serious infections to develop from just a single organism. Transmission of protozoa occurs through the protozoa's environment. That means that protozoa that live in a human's intestine gets transmitted to another human through a fecal-oral route. Protozoa ends up in human waste, and is transferred, for example, through contaminated food or water or person-to-person contact. Protozoa that live in the blood or tissue of humans are transmitted to other humans by an arthropod vector such as the bite of a mosquito or sand fly.

Examples of protozoa include malaria, trichomoniasis (trich), toxoplasmosis, and naegleriasis. Some parasitic infections are rare, but deadly, like naegleriasis (brain-eating amoeba). This is contracted through warm, freshwater ponds or rivers and poorly chlorinated pools or hot tubs. Others, like toxoplasmosis, are much more common and are contracted through poorly prepared foods and contact with cat feces.

Toxoplasmosis is considered to be a leading cause of death attributed to foodborne illness in the US. More than 30 million men, women, and children in the US carry the toxoplasma parasite, but very few have symptoms because the immune system usually keeps the parasite from causing illness. However, women infected with toxoplasma during pregnancy and anyone with a compromised immune system can experience severe consequences from it. This is why you may have heard that pregnant women should not change a cat's litter box.

Helminths

Helminths are among the larger parasites. The word "helminth" comes from the Greek word for "worm." If this parasite—or its eggs—enters your body, it makes a home in your intestinal tract, lungs, liver, skin, or brain, where it lives off your body's nutrients. These free-loading helminths include tapeworms and roundworms.

Soil-transmitted helminths (STH) refer to the intestinal worms—such as whipworms, Ascaris, or hookworms—infecting humans through contaminated soil. This occurs mainly in areas with warm and moist climates where sanitation and hygiene are poor, including in temperate zones during warmer months. These STH's are considered Neglected Tropical Diseases (NTD) because they inflict tremendous disability and suffering yet can be controlled or eliminated.

Soil-transmitted helminths live in the intestine and their eggs transmit through the feces of infected persons. If an infected person defecates outside (near bushes, in a garden, or field) or if the feces of an infected person is used as fertilizer, the eggs deposit on the soil. Ascaris and hookworm eggs become infective as they mature in soil. People become infected with Ascaris and whipworm when eggs are ingested. This can happen by putting contaminated hands in the mouth or by consuming vegetables and fruits that have not been carefully cooked, washed, or peeled. Most hookworm eggs do not infect humans, but their mature worms do. The eggs hatch in soil, releasing larvae (immature worms) that mature into a form that can penetrate the skin of humans. People acquire hookworm infections primarily by walking barefoot on contaminated soil. One kind of hookworm, *Anclostoma duodenale*, can also be transmitted through the ingestion of its larvae.

People with light soil-transmitted helminth infections usually have no symptoms. Heavy infections can cause a range of health problems, including abdominal pain, diarrhea, blood and protein loss, rectal prolapse, and problems with physical and cognitive growth. These infections are treatable with medications prescribed by a health care provider.

Infection vs. Infectious Disease

There's a difference between infection and disease. Infection is like having an unwanted guest in your house. The uninvited pathogen doesn't just visit, they move right into their new home in your body and begin to set up for a long stay, producing many new friends. In response, your immune system gets busy. Your body calls in the police, a force of white blood cells, antibodies, and other mechanisms that try to kick out the offending squatters. Most of the time, the police succeed quickly, and the infection is over before you were even aware of it.

Disease occurs when the cells in your body are damaged—as a result of the infection—and signs and symptoms of an illness appear. Your unwelcome house guest hosts a large, messy party and trashes your house. The police are still on it, and they bust up the party and rid your body of whatever is causing the infection over time. For instance, in fighting off the common cold, your body might react with fever, coughing, and sneezing. But the party still left some damage, and it takes more time and energy to repair and clean up. Not every infection will lead to disease, but some do.

Chain of Infection

Each infection goes through a series of steps that progress in seriousness (Figure 2). The traditional model of infection, called the epidemiologic triad, says that infections result when the infectious microbe (pathogen) leaves its reservoir or host (human body, soil, air, or water) through a portal of exit (mouth or intestines) and is conveyed by some mode of transmission (the droplets on your friend's smoothie straw). It enters a new host through an appropriate portal of entry (your mouth, for example) to infect a susceptible host (you).

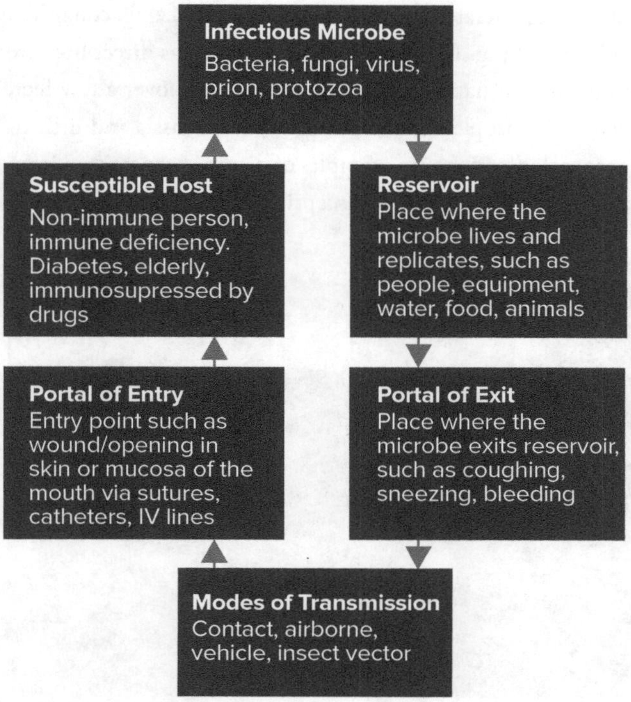

This sequence is sometimes called the **chain of infection**. Each of the links must be present in the right order for an infection to develop.

Understanding how infectious diseases spread will help you protect yourself from contracting and spreading these illnesses to others. If you know how the chain works and where each connection is made, you can take action break the chain.

Reservoir

The **reservoir** of an infectious agent is the habitat in which the agent normally lives, grows, and multiplies. Reservoirs include humans, animals, and the environment. The reservoir may or may not be the source from which an agent is transferred to a host. For example, the reservoir of *Clostridium botulinum* is soil, but the source of most botulism infections is improperly canned food containing *C. botulinum* spores.

Many common infectious diseases have **human reservoirs**. Diseases transmitted from person to person without intermediaries include sexually transmitted diseases, measles, mumps, streptococcal infection, and many respiratory pathogens. This is not always a bad thing. Because humans were the only reservoir for the smallpox virus, for example, naturally occurring smallpox was eradicated after the last human case was identified and isolated.

Human reservoirs may or may not show the effects of illness. A **carrier** is a person who has the pathogen and the capability to transmit it to others. There are a few different types. **Asymptomatic carriers** seem healthy—they never

Infectious Microbe
Bacteria, fungi, virus, prion, protozoa

Susceptible Host
Non-immune person, immune deficiency. Diabetes, elderly, immunosupressed by drugs

Reservoir
Place where the microbe lives and replicates, such as people, equipment, water, food, animals

Portal of Entry
Entry point such as wound/opening in skin or mucosa of the mouth via sutures, catheters, IV lines

Portal of Exit
Place where the microbe exits reservoir, such as coughing, sneezing, bleeding

Modes of Transmission
Contact, airborne, vehicle, insect vector

Figure 2. The chain of infection.

experience symptoms despite being infected. **Incubatory carriers** can transmit the agent during the incubation period before clinical illness begins. **Convalescent carriers** are those who have recovered from their illness but remain capable of transmitting microbes to others. **Chronic carriers** continue to harbor a pathogen for months or even years after their initial infection.

One notorious carrier was Mary Mallon, or Typhoid Mary, an asymptomatic chronic carrier of *Salmonella Typhi* (the causative agent of typhoid fever). While working as a cook in New York and New Jersey in the early 1900s, she unintentionally infected dozens of people. Authorities eventually isolated her in a hospital on an island in the East River where she died 23 years later. It sounds odd now that a person would be isolated in such a way. However, Mary, not understanding the chain of infection, continued to work as a cook (infecting more people) even after being instructed to find a new profession. This led authorities to step in and permanently remove her from the chain.

Carriers commonly transmit disease because they do not realize they are infected, and consequently take no special precautions to prevent transmission. **Symptomatic** carriers know of their illness and may be less likely to transmit infection because they're too sick to be out and about, they take precautions to reduce transmission, or they receive treatment that limits their disease.

Humans can also acquire diseases that have **animal reservoirs**. Many of these diseases transmit from animal to animal, with humans as incidental hosts. The term "zoonosis" refers to an infectious disease transmissible under natural conditions from vertebrate animals to humans. Long recognized zoonotic diseases include brucellosis (cows and pigs), anthrax (sheep), plague (rodents), trichinellosis/trichinosis (swine), tularemia (rabbits), and rabies (bats, raccoons, dogs, and other mammals). Recent examples of zoonosis in North America include West Nile encephalitis (birds), and monkeypox (prairie dogs). Many newly recognized infectious diseases in humans, including HIV/AIDS, Ebola infection, and SARS, are thought to have emerged from animal hosts, although those hosts have not yet been identified.

Plants, soil, and water can also be reservoirs (**environmental reservoirs**) for some infectious agents. Many fungal agents, such as those that cause histoplasmosis, live and multiply in the soil (from bird and bat droppings). Outbreaks of Legionnaire's disease often can be traced back to reservoirs that are the water supplies in cooling towers and evaporative condensers.

Portal of Exit

The **portal of exit** is the path by which a pathogen leaves its host or reservoir, which usually corresponds to the site where the pathogen is found. For example, the portal of exit for influenza and tuberculosis is the respiratory tract. For cholera, the portal of exit is feces, for scabies it's skin lesions, and for conjunctivitis (pink eye) it's the infected eye. Some blood borne agents can exit their host by crossing the placenta from mother to fetus (rubella, syphilis, toxoplasmosis), while others exit through cuts or needles in the skin (hepatitis B) or are exit through the bite of arthropods like mosquitos (malaria).

An infectious agent may be transmitted from its natural reservoir to a susceptible host in different ways, both direct and indirect.

Modes of Direct Transmission

In direct transmission, an infectious agent transfers from a reservoir to a susceptible host by direct contact or droplet spread. **Direct contact** occurs through skin-to-skin contact, kissing, and sexual intercourse (Figure 3). Direct contact also refers to contact with soil or vegetation harboring infectious organisms. Infectious mononucleosis ("mono" or "kissing disease") and gonorrhea, for example, spread from person to person by direct contact. Hookworm spreads by direct contact with contaminated soil.

Droplet spread refers to liquid spray with relatively large, short-range, aerated droplets produced by sneezing, coughing, or even talking. Droplet spread is classified as direct because transmission happens through direct spray over a few feet, before the droplets fall to the ground. Pertussis and meningococcal infections are examples of diseases transmitted from an infectious person to a susceptible host by droplet spread.

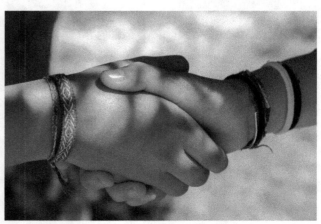

Figure 3. Handshakes are one mode of direct transmission.

Modes of Indirect Transmission

Indirect transmission refers to the transfer of an infectious agent from a reservoir to a host by suspended air particles, inanimate objects (vehicles), or animate intermediaries (vectors).

Airborne transmission occurs when dust or droplet nuclei (tiny, dried residue of droplets suspended in air) carry infectious agents. Airborne dust includes material that has settled on surfaces and gets re-circulated by air currents, as well as infectious particles blown from the soil by the wind. In contrast to droplets that fall to the ground within a few feet, droplet nuclei can stay suspended in the air for a long time and be blown over great distances (Figure 4). Measles, for example, has occurred in children who came into a health care provider's office after a child with measles had left because the measles virus was still suspended in the air.

Vehicles that may indirectly transmit an infectious agent include food, water, biological products (blood), and fomites (inanimate objects such as handkerchiefs, bedding, or surgical scalpels). A vehicle may passively carry a pathogen, as food or water may carry the hepatitis A virus. The vehicle may also provide an environment in which the agent grows, multiplies, or produces toxin, as improperly canned foods provide an environment that supports production of botulinum toxin by *Clostridium botulinum*.

Vectors, such as mosquitoes, fleas, and ticks, may carry an infectious agent through purely mechanical means or may support growth or changes in the agent. Examples of mechanical transmission are flies carrying Shigella (which leads to a stomach infection) on their appendages, mosquitoes carrying Malaria and Zika, ticks carrying Lyme disease, and fleas carrying *Yersinia pestis* (the agent of plague) in their gut.

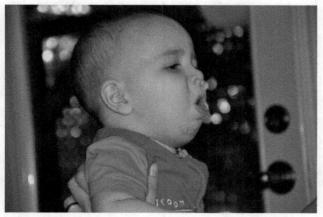

Figure 4. Airborne infectious agents are transmitted indirectly.

Portal of Entry

The **portal of entry** refers to how a pathogen enters its susceptible host. The portal of entry must provide access to tissues in which the pathogen can multiply or a toxin can act. Often, infectious agents use the same portal to enter a new host that they used to exit the source host. For example, the flu virus exits the respiratory tract of the source host and enters the respiratory tract of the new host. But some pathogens that cause gastroenteritis follow a so-called "fecal-oral" route because they exit the source host in feces, travel on inadequately washed hands to a vehicle such as food, water, or utensil, and enter a new host through the mouth. Other portals of entry include the skin (hookworm), mucous membranes (syphilis), and blood (hepatitis B, HIV).

Host

The final link in the chain of infection is a susceptible **host**. In human infectious diseases, we're talking about people. In humans, these factors include:

- **Genetic makeup**—An individual's genetic makeup may either increase or decrease their susceptibility to infection. For example, people with the sickle cell trait seem to be at least partially protected from a particular type of malaria.

- **Specific immunity**—Some individuals may have protective antibodies that shield against a specific agent. Such antibodies develop in response to a previous infection, vaccines, or toxoids (toxins that have been deactivated but retains their capacity to stimulate production of toxin antibodies). These antibodies may be acquired by transfer from mother to fetus or from being injected with antitoxin.

- **Nonspecific factors**—Some factors that defend against infection include the skin, mucous membranes, gastric acidity, cilia in the respiratory tract, the cough reflex, and the immune system.

Infection of the host begins when an organism successfully enters the body, grows, and multiplies. This is referred to as **colonization**. A colony of infection can either stay located at the port of entry, or it may migrate and spread its infection to other parts of the body, causing systemic infection in different organs. Some pathogens grow within your cells while others grow freely in bodily fluids.

Types of Infection

Most of the time you come into contact with a pathogen, you don't become ill. Your immune system works and fights the germ. Disease only arises if your protective immune mechanisms aren't up to the task and the organism inflicts damage on you, its host. Not all infectious agents cause disease in all hosts, either because of the host or the nature of the pathogen. For example, less than 5% of individuals infected with polio develop the disease. On the other hand, some infectious agents can be highly virulent. The pathogens causing mad cow disease and Creutzfeldt-Jakob disease invariably kill all the animals and people that it infects.

Different pathogens react differently to their new environment, even if some have similarities. We categorize infections by how quickly they settle in, how they treat their new home, and how long they stick around.

Acute

An **acute infection** has a rapid onset and relatively brief period of symptoms, often resolving within days, though it could be six months depending on the pathogen and your general health. Bouts of the flu, sinus infections, and even Ebola are good examples of acute infection. The disease itself could be sudden, severe, and fairly miserable—even fatal in some people—but you won't live with it long-term.

Often an acute infection may cause little or no clinical symptoms, called an **inapparent** infection. The poliovirus that affected so many people years ago is a good example. Over 90% of people infected had no symptoms. During an inapparent infection, the pathogens reproduce enough in the host to call on your antibodies, but not enough to cause disease. This might sound like good news, but inapparent infections can be problematic because the disease can spread easily this way. During the polio epidemic in the US, the quarantine of paralyzed patients did not stop the spread of the disease because most of the infected individuals had no symptoms and continued with their lives, unknowingly spreading the disease to others.

Acute infections begin with an **incubation** period. This is the time it takes for the person to become ill after the initial infection. Sometimes the incubation is short like influenza, which incubates in just a few days, while other infections like HIV (a chronic infection) can incubate for several years. In some cases, a person can be contagious during the incubation period, while in others the person can't transmit the infection to others until symptoms begin. The amount of time a person remains contagious depends on the infection and the person.

Sometimes a **prodrome**—an early sign or symptom—can indicate the onset of a disease before specific symptoms develop. These can be specific to a particular disease, such as the tingling that occurs just before getting a cold sore. Or they can be more general like the feeling you get when it seems like you are "fighting a bug," just before getting the full set of cold symptoms.

Acute viral infections often lead to epidemics of disease involving millions of individuals each year, such as influenza and measles. When a vaccine for the virus doesn't exist or is unavailable, these infections can be difficult to control. Between the incubation period and the time a person feels symptoms, they've already spread it to someone else. This can be an even larger problem in crowded areas, like college campuses and health care facilities.

After the symptoms begin to fade, your body enters a stage of **convalescence**, where you start regaining energy. Acute symptoms subside slowly during this time as your immune system wins the battle against the disease. This takes a variable amount of time depending on the infection severity and the overall health of the individual. Yet with some infections, a person could be a convalescent carrier, spreading the disease despite their own improvement.

Acute infections need treatment, but as we've seen, it can be hard to know when they are serious. Look at this set of symptoms and treatment suggestions for common infectious diseases that are all acute infections (Figure 5).

Chronic Infection

In contrast to acute infections, a **chronic infection** lasts for long periods, and can occur when the immune system does not clear the primary infection. Varicella-zoster virus (chicken pox), measles virus, hepatitis, and HIV-1 are all examples of chronic infections. Acute infections can become chronic in people whose immune systems are unable to fight off the pathogen.

Infections can go through periods where the virus lays dormant (or latent) then returns under the right circumstances, like the virus that causes chicken pox. Shingles is a great example of a **latent infection**. People often get chicken pox when they are young. It can resurface later in life in the form of shingles, a painful, blistery rash. The reason why people

Illness (Pathogen)	Symptoms	Home Treatment	When to Seek Medical Care
Common cold (Over 200 different viruses)	Runny nose, nasal congestion, mild cough, sore throat, low-grade fever, sneezing	Usually resolves on its own; fluid, rest, and over-the-counter medications to treat symptoms; avoid alcohol and tobacco	Worsening symptoms after third day, difficulty breathing, stiff neck
Influenza (Influenza A or B virus)	Sudden-onset fever, extreme fatigue, headache, body aches, cough	Usually resolves on its own; same home treatment as for colds; prescription anti-virals available	Difficulty breathing, severe head-ache or stiff neck, confusion, fever lasting more than 3 days; new, localized pain in ear, chest, sinuses; people at high risk for complications should contact a health care provider if they develop flu symptoms
Bronchitis (different viruses or bacteria)	Cough that may start out dry and later produce mucus; sore throat, fever	Usually resolves on its own; same home treatment as colds	Shortness of breath, high fever, shaking chills (signs of pneumonia); wheezing and cough that last more than 2 weeks; people at high risk for complications should check with a health care provider
Mononucleosis (Epstein-Barr virus)	High fever, swollen glands, severe sore throat, fatigue; nausea, vomiting, and loss of appetite can occur	Usually resolves on its own; rest, fluids; avoid contact sports until symptoms resolve due to risk of spleen rupture	Fever lasting more than 3 days; symptoms lasting longer than 7-10 days; severe abdominal pain (possibly indicating ruptured spleen)

Figure 5. Common illnesses and their symptoms and treatments.

with herpes don't have sores on their mouths all their life is because the herpes virus that causes cold sores (HSV-1) goes repeatedly dormant over time. A latent infection can be difficult to treat with drugs and other therapies.

Many sexually transmitted diseases go through periods of latency, where individuals have no symptoms and the infection lays dormant in their bodies. This is likely the biggest reason that STIs are a hidden epidemic. People can spread the disease if the dormant infection reactivates before symptoms appear.

People with chronic infections are considered carriers. They serve as reservoirs of the infection and will likely always carry it around. In populations with a high population of carriers, the disease is said to be **endemic**, such as HIV is in certain parts of Africa.

The Immune System

Your **immune system** is a complex network of cells, tissues, and organs that work together to defend against germs. It helps your body to recognize these invaders. Its job is to keep them out, or if it can't, to find and destroy them. An example of this principle can be found in **immune-compromised** people, including those with genetic immune disorders, immune-debilitating infections like HIV, and even pregnant women, who are susceptible to a range of microbes that typically don't cause infection.

The immune system can distinguish between normal healthy cells and unhealthy cells by recognizing a variety of "danger" cues called **danger-associated molecular patterns** (DAMP's). Cells may be unhealthy because of infection or because of cellular damage caused by non-infectious agents like sunburn or cancer. Infectious microbes, such as viruses and bacteria, release another set of signals recognized by the immune system called **pathogen-associated molecular patterns** (PAMP's).

Your immune system first recognizes these signal, then responds to address the problem. Problems arise, like infection, if an immune response can't be activated when needed. Different problems, such as allergic reactions or autoimmune disease, can occur if the immune system responds without a real threat or doesn't turn off when danger passes.

All immune cells come from precursors in the bone marrow and develop into mature cells in different parts of the body. Your skin, for example, is usually the first line of defense against germs. Skin cells produce and secrete important antimicrobial proteins, and immune cells can be found in specific layers of the skin. Your bloodstream also serves as another important helper. Immune cells constantly circulate throughout the bloodstream, patrolling for problems.

Mucosal tissue also pitches in to help defend the body against infection. Mucosal surfaces are prime entry points for pathogens, and specialized immune hubs are strategically located in mucosal tissues like the respiratory tract and gut. For instance, Peyer's patches, similar to lymph nodes, live in the small intestine and monitor the presence of intestinal bacteria, working to prevent the growth of anything pathogens.

The Lymphatic System

Perhaps the biggest player in this defensive strategy is the **lymphatic system**. The lymphatic system is a network of vessels and tissues composed of lymph, an extracellular fluid, and lymphoid organs, such as lymph nodes. The lymphatic system serves as a conduit for travel and communication between tissues and the bloodstream. Immune cells travel through the lymphatic system and converge in lymph nodes found throughout the body.

Lymph nodes provide a communication hub where immune cells sample information brought in from the body. For instance, if adaptive immune cells in the lymph node recognize pieces of a microbe brought in from a distant area,

they will activate and replicate themselves. These adaptive immune cells then leave the lymph node to circulate and address the pathogen. When you're sick, a health care provider might check for swollen lymph nodes, which can indicate an active immune response to some threat.

The lymph system gets help from other organs, including the thymus and spleen. Your thymus is in your chest behind your breastbone. T lymphocytes grow and multiply in the thymus. Your spleen is located behind your stomach. It helps the lymphatic system by processing information from the bloodstream. Specific areas of the spleen enrich immune cells, and when they recognize a blood borne pathogen, they will activate and respond accordingly.

The real workers of your immune system are the **white blood cells.** These cells constantly patrol the body, looking for invaders in your bloodstream. They stay on the lookout for **antigens**, proteins found on the surface of invading substances (pathogens). Each antigen is unique to its pathogen. There's a different antigen for every cold that you've ever had.

When an antigen enters your body, your immune system produces **antibodies** to fight against it. And it's quite an impressive fight. Lymphocytes (a type of white blood cell) recognize the antigen as being uninvited and produce a gang of antibodies specific to destroying that antigen. Then they attack the antigen. White blood cells can also produce chemicals called **antitoxins**, which destroy the toxins (poisons) some bacteria produce when they have invaded the body (Figure 6)

Once a person has had a disease, they don't normally catch it again because the body produces **memory cells** specific to that antigen. The memory cells can very quickly recognize the microbe that caused the disease and rapidly make the correct antibody if the infection is detected again.

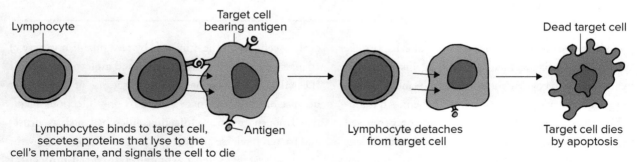

Figure 6. How white blood cells attack viruses.

Preventing Infections

Some part of the world experiences one or more form of infectious outbreak almost every year. From super-strength flu strains to Ebola virus, it can be a bit frightening to think of your body as vulnerable to some new and scary bug. But there are ways to limit your risk and minimize your exposure. Good hygiene, safer sexual health, and routine vaccination are keys to preventing many infections. It takes a lot of individual and group effort to effectively prevent and control infections.

Public Health

Disease knows no borders. It might seem like the Ebola outbreaks we read about are far away, but in today's interconnected world, a disease threat anywhere in the world can become a health threat in the US. We know that disease exploits even the smallest gap that will let it spread and grow. With the ease and speed of global travel, along with rapidly expanding commerce and trade, the need to shut down the exploitable gaps available to infectious disease in the US is more important than ever before.

The Centers for Disease Control monitors not only what happens here in the US but also what happens abroad. The most effective way to protect US citizens (the CDCs job) from known and unknown health threats is to stop those events that occur overseas before they can spread here. To do this, the CDC operates in the more than 60 countries, working with ministries and departments of health and other partners on the front lines where outbreaks occur. They work with an array of partners, including the World Health Organization (WHO) and its 194 member-nations. The WHO directs and coordinates global health strategies, tactics, and priorities. The global activities of these agencies have largely protected the US from major health threats such as Ebola, Zika, and pandemic influenza. This has only been possible by helping other countries build their capacity to prevent, detect, and respond to their own health threats. This work protects the US because it strengthens countries' ability to respond to disease threats as close to their source as possible.

Protecting Yourself: Vaccines

Even the US has challenges when it comes to controlling the spread of infection. Much of this control comes through education. Knowledge of common infection control practices and vaccinations are the primary ways that citizens can help keep themselves healthy.

For a few weeks after birth, babies have some protection from germs that cause diseases. This protection passes to them from their mother through the placenta before birth, and through antibodies in breastmilk. After a short period, this natural protection goes away. After this brief period, infants can be protected by vaccines.

Vaccines help protect against many diseases that used to be much more common, including tetanus, diphtheria, mumps, measles, pertussis (whooping cough), meningitis, and polio. Many of these infections can cause serious or life-threatening illnesses and can lead to life-long health problems. Because of widespread vaccination, many diseases that once threatened thousands of lives are now extremely rare.

Vaccines are our most effective and cost-saving tools for disease prevention. For each group of children in the US who receive the recommended 13 vaccines, approximately 42,000 lives are saved, 20 million cases of disease are prevented, $13.6 billion in direct costs are saved, and $68.9 billion in direct plus indirect (societal) costs are saved.

How Vaccines Work

The primary method of controlling viral disease is by vaccination, which is used to prevent outbreaks by building immunity to a virus. Vaccines are prepared with live viruses, killed viruses, or molecular subunits of the virus. This essentially creates a memory cell that makes attacking any future infection easier for your body.

Vaccines (immunizations) essentially boost your immune system and prevent serious, life-threatening diseases. They "teach" your body how to defend itself when germs, such as viruses or bacteria, invade it. They do this by exposing you to a very small, very safe amount of a virus or bacteria that has been weakened or killed. Your immune system then learns to recognize and attack the infection if you are exposed to it later in life. As a result, you will not become ill, or you may have a milder infection. This is a natural way to deal with infectious diseases.

Vaccines can be also used to treat an active viral infection. By giving the vaccine, immunity is boosted without adding more disease-causing virus. Another way of treating viral infections is the use of the antiviral drugs. These drugs have a limited success of curing viral disease, but can be used to control and reduce symptoms for a wide variety of viral diseases.

Four types of vaccines are currently available:

- **Live virus vaccines** use the weakened (attenuated) form of the virus. The measles, mumps, and rubella (MMR) vaccine and the varicella (chickenpox) vaccine are examples.

- **Killed (inactivated) vaccines** are made from a protein or other small pieces taken from a virus or bacteria. The flu vaccine is an example.

- **Toxoid vaccines** contain a toxin or chemical made by the bacteria or virus. They make you immune to the harmful effects of the infection, instead of to the infection itself. The diphtheria and tetanus vaccines are examples.

- **Biosynthetic vaccines** contain manmade substances very similar to pieces of the virus or bacteria. The Hib (*Haemophilus influenzae* type B) conjugate vaccine is an example.

Staying Up-to-Date on Vaccinations

The protection from some vaccines can wear off or the viruses or bacteria that the vaccines protect against can change so that your resistance is not as strong. As you get older, you may also be at risk for vaccine-preventable diseases due to your age, job, hobbies, travel, or health conditions.

The CDC recommends some ongoing vaccination for adults in addition to several other vaccines that infants and children all need. All adults should get the influenza vaccine every year to protect against seasonal flu, the Tetanus-Diphtheria (Td) vaccine every 10 years to protect against tetanus,

and the Tdap vaccine once instead of the Td vaccine to protect against tetanus and diphtheria plus pertussis (whooping cough) and during each pregnancy for women.

Other vaccines you need as an adult are determined by factors such as age, lifestyle, job, health condition, and the vaccines you have had in the past. Vaccines you need may include those that protect against shingles, human papillomavirus (which can cause certain cancers), pneumococcal disease, meningococcal disease, hepatitis A and B, chickenpox (varicella), measles, mumps, and rubella.

Special Concern: Vaccine Safety

Some people worry that vaccines may be harmful, especially for children. They may ask their health care provider to wait, or even choose not to have them vaccinated. Overwhelming scientific consensus has shown that vaccines are safe. US organizations including the American Academy of Pediatrics, the CDC, and the National Institutes of Health and Medicine, just to name a few, all conclude that vaccines are not dangerous.

Even if vaccines were dangerous, their benefits to society far outweigh any potential risks. The choice not to vaccinate out of fear can lead to dangerous consequences, like the resurgence of diseases that have long been eradicated. This has already occurred on a small scale in multiple recent outbreaks of mostly eradicated diseases like measles.

It's hard to blame a parent who feels concern for the safety of their child. That's normal, and we shouldn't downplay their concern. We believe that education is key to understanding complex health issues, which is why we cover how vaccines work in this book. It's true: vaccines such as the measles, mumps, rubella, chickenpox, and nasal spray flu vaccines contain live, weakened viruses. But unless a person's immune system is weakened, it is unlikely that a vaccine will give the person the infection. Pregnant women and people with weakened immune systems should not receive these live vaccines. Your health care provider can tell you the right time to get these vaccines.

Some parents also show concern for additives in vaccines. Thimerosal is a preservative that was found in most vaccines in the past, one that people feared could cause brain problems, including autism. Today, only one third of flu shots still have thimerosal, no other vaccines commonly used for children or adults contain thimerosal, research done over many years has not shown any link between thimerosal and autism or other medical problems, and allergic reactions are rare and are usually to some other component of the vaccine.

Much of the concern between vaccines and autism arose largely in response to a discredited 1997 study of the measles-mumps-rubella (MMR) vaccine, which started an anti-vaccine movement in the US and other parts of the world. These myths about vaccines continue to exist despite a lack of scientific evidence to support them.

Protecting Yourself: Good Self Care

Many additional strategies can help you avoid infection. Most seem like common sense, but people often only pay attention to them when the person next to them on the bus starts coughing. Be consistent at all times with these basic infection control procedures. You may find that you escape the next round of flu.

> **Wash your hands frequently.** Use soap and water that is as hot as you can stand. Thoroughly lather all surfaces of your hands and make sure to wash under your fingernails (Figure 7).
>
> **Stay home if you are sick.** It's easier said than done, sometimes, but going out and contacting other people when you're can spread disease. In some instances, you may be legally required to stay home. In many states, someone working with food is required to stay home if they have diarrhea, for example.

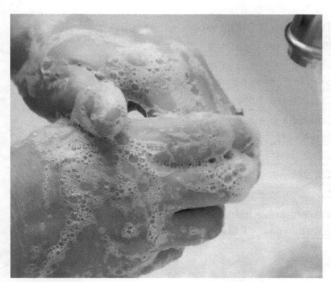

Figure 7. Washing hands helps prevent infection.

> **Use single-use tissues and dispose of them immediately after use.** Once you have used a tissue, it becomes a vehicle for spreading disease. Also, it's gross to leave used tissues lying around.
>
> **Wash your hands after coughing, sneezing, or using a tissue.** If you cough or sneeze into your hands, they become coated in infectious materials, and anything you touch becomes a vehicle for spreading disease.
>
> **Don't touch your eyes, nose, or mouth.** It's pretty tough to avoid touching door handles, chairs, or handrails in public places, so you should assume you're contacting contagions. Touching these surfaces after you would be just like shaking hands with the people who touched it before you. Your eyes, nose, and mouth all have mucous membranes, which are thin enough to make it easy for pathogens to pass into your system, so don't ever touch these areas of your body without washing your hands first.
>
> **Don't share cups, glasses, dishes, or cutlery.** Your kale smoothie-sharing friend may be offended, but people can be contagious before and after being visibly sick, making their cups and cutlery vehicles for infection.
>
> **Be careful how you cover your sneeze or cough.** We are taught to cover our mouth when we cough and sneeze, which is a good thing—it keeps pathogens from spreading through the air in droplets. However, doing it in your hands is a bad idea, since it makes your hand a vehicle for any pathogens in your system. A better practice is to sneeze or cough into your shoulder or elbow, which comes into contact with fewer surfaces than your hands.

Sexually Transmitted Infections (STIs)

Sexually transmitted infections (STIs) are among the most common infections in the US, with over 20 million new cases each year. Half of these new cases are among 15–24-year-olds. STIs can be dangerous when left untreated. In most cases, they can be prevented by practicing "safer" sex. The "safest" sex practice is not having sex with other people (abstinence). But other methods offer ways to have **safer sex**, such as only having sex within a mutually monogamous relationship and using barriers, like condoms, the correct way, consistently with each new sex act.

STIs are more common than most people think (Figure 8). For example, human papillomavirus (HPV) is so common that nearly all sexually active men and women contract the virus at some point in their lives. The CDC estimates that the annual costs of treatment for STIs is over $16 billion.

Sexually transmitted infections are diseases passed from person to person via sexual contact. With most STIs, this occurs by fluid exchanges during oral, anal, and vaginal sex, but some diseases can be transmitted via non-genital skin-to-skin contact. Many STIs don't exhibit external symptoms, so people may spread them unknowingly to their partners. Others exhibit noticeable symptoms like open sores or breaks in the skin. These transmit infection particularly without proper protection.

Some STIs can be treated if detected early, while others can be chronic, incurable, and even life-threatening (e.g. HIV and herpes). The problem is that people with STIs are frequently too embarrassed to talk to a health care provider because STIs carry an unfortunate social stigma. STIs can also lead to depression that may keep a victim from seeking treatment. Despite the stigma, it's important to regularly test for infection if you are sexually active (even if married) and seek treatment as soon as an infection is discovered.

In 2014, people between age 15–24 accounted for the highest rates of chlamydia and gonorrhea, almost two thirds of all reported cases (Figure 9). This is despite them being a relatively small portion of the sexually active population. Additionally, previous estimates suggest that young people in this age group acquire half of the estimated 20 million new STIs diagnosed each year (Figure 10).

STI	Estimated Annual Incidence	Estimated Prevalence*	Treatment if Diagnosed
Trichomoniasis	1.1 million	n/a	Curable with antibiotics
HPV infection	14 million	20 million	Vaccine-preventable; incurable but often resolves on its own; can cause cancer
Chlamydia	2.8 million	1.9 million	Curable with antibiotics
Genital herpes	750,000	45 million	Chronic and incurable; treatments can reduce symptoms and outbreaks
Gonorrhea	820,000	n/a	Curable with antibiotics
Syphilis	55,000	n/a	Curable with antibiotics
HIV infection	41,000	1.2 million	Chronic and potentially fatal; treatable but incurable
Hepatitis B	19,000	1.25 million	Vaccine-preventable; incurable but often resolves on its own; can cause fatal liver disease

Figure 8. Common STI incidence in the US.

There are several reasons for this. Young people often underestimate their risk. There's truth to the stereotype that young people feel that they are invincible. As a result, they're more likely to participate in risky sexual behavior. They're also statistically more likely to have their sexual activity affected by alcohol or substance abuse, leading to unsafe sexual behaviors like "forgetting" to use protection. Finally, younger people simply have more sex, so their potential for exposure to STIs is subsequently higher.

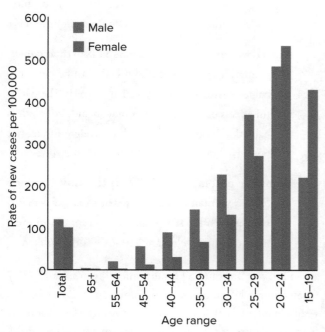

Figure 9. Chlamydia and gonorrhea cases in the US (Source: CDC).

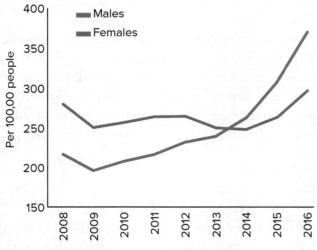

Figure 10. Healthy People 2020 goals for STI incidence.

Gender and STIs

Some people have a greater risk than others for acquiring an STI. People limited to "abstinence only" education have a higher infection rate than people who have had a more comprehensive education. The old saying holds true—knowledge is power, or in this case, protection. Studies suggest that women who only learn abstinence and promise to wait for sex until marriage, and women who haven't made the same pledge, both become sexually active at the same rate. But the women who haven't been properly educated on safer sex practices, contract STIs at a higher rate than their peers and are more likely to become pregnant earlier.

It is easier for men to transmit STIs to women than the other way around, too. The structural differences in the reproductive system creates more chances for women to retain pathogens in their reproductive areas than men (Figure 11) Women experience a different type of risk than men when it comes to STIs. Their bodies do not show the same signs and symptoms and the impact can be more severe. According to the CDC:

A woman's anatomy can place her at a unique risk for STI. The lining of the vagina is thinner and more delicate than the skin on a penis, so it's easier for bacteria and viruses to penetrate. The vagina is a good environment (moist) for bacteria to grow.

Women are less likely to have symptoms of common STIs—such as chlamydia and gonorrhea. If symptoms do occur, they can go away even though the infection may remain.

Female Reproductive Anatomy

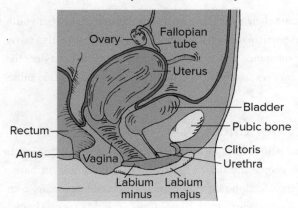

Male Reproductive Anatomy

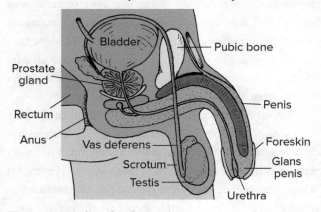

Figure 11. Female and male sexual anatomy.

Women are more likely to confuse symptoms of an STI for something else. Women often have discharge even when healthy or think that burning/itching may be related to a yeast infection. Men usually notice symptoms like discharge because it's unusual.

Women may not see symptoms as easily as men. Genital ulcers (like from herpes or syphilis) can occur in the vagina and may not be easily visible, while men may be more likely to notice sores on their penis.

STIs can lead to serious health complications and affect a woman's future reproductive plans. Untreated STIs can lead to pelvic inflammatory disease, which can result in infertility and ectopic pregnancy. Chlamydia (one of the most common STIs) results in relatively few complications in men.

Women who are pregnant can pass STIs to their babies. Genital herpes, syphilis and HIV can be passed to babies during pregnancy and at delivery. The harmful effects of STIs in babies may include stillbirth (a baby that is born dead), low birth weight (under five pounds), brain damage, blindness, and deafness.

Human papillomavirus (HPV) is the most common STI in women and is the main cause of cervical cancer. While HPV is also very common in men, most do not develop any serious health problems.

Each year untreated STIs cause infertility in at least 24,000 women in the US, and untreated syphilis in pregnant women results in infant death in up to 40% of cases. The fact that many women go untreated, unknowingly, presents an increased risk of transmission for both genders. The good news is that regular pap screenings can catch many infections before they progress. Also, HPV now has a vaccine for both men and women to reduce the risk of contracting related cancers.

This section provides information on the 7 most common STIs in the US, including a description of what their symptoms are, how they are diagnosed, and how they are treated. Some of these sections are more complex than others, just as some STIs are more complex than others. They are listed below in descending order of total new infections each year.

Human Papillomavirus (HPV)

Human papillomavirus (HPV), commonly known as genital or anal warts, is the most common STI in the US (Figure 12). There are approximately 20 million current cases of HPV and 6 million new cases each year. It transmits easily via vaginal, oral, or anal intercourse, but can also be transmitted skin-to-skin, which reduces the effectiveness of condoms somewhat (still—mostly protected is always better than unprotected!). HPV can be passed even when an infected person has no signs or symptoms.

HPV often goes away on its own and does not cause any health problems. In other cases, the individual develops warts or even cancer, not necessarily in that order. The strains of HPV

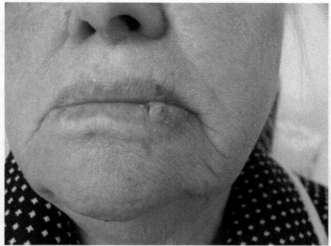
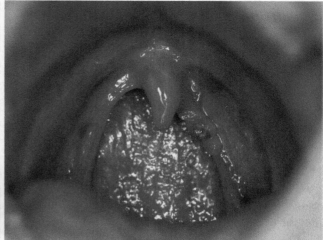

Figure 12. HPV symptoms on the face and throat.

connected to cancer are different than the strains that cause warts. HPV could lead to cancer without first producing warts as a symptom. These cancers include cervical, vulva, penis, anus, and even cancer in the back of the throat or base of the tongue and tonsils (propharyngeal cancer). Cancer often takes years or even decades to develop after a person first gets HPV.

When genital warts occur, they may appear as a small bump or group of bumps in the genital area. They can be small or large, raised or flat, or shaped like a cauliflower and can appear anywhere in or around the genitals. Most people with HPV do not know they're infected and never develop symptoms or health problems from it. Unless warts develop, a person may only find out once they've developed more serious problems.

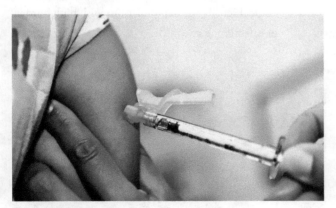

Figure 13. HPV vaccine being administered.

Diagnosis and Treatment

A health care provider can usually diagnose warts by looking at the genital area. Women often learn of HPV through an abnormal Pap test result (during cervical cancer screening). Women should get their first Pap test within three years of becoming sexually active DNA tests conducted on cells from your cervix can recognize the DNA of the high-risk varieties of HPV that have been linked to genital cancers. There is no other test that detects someone's "HPV status."

The virus itself has no treatment. However, the health problems resulting from HPV can be treated. Fortunately, we have recently developed a vaccine for the HPV virus, which is the most effective preventative measure available. This vaccine protects against the types of HPV that cause about 70% of cervical cancers and 90% of genital warts cases.

The HPV vaccine is safe and effective when given in the recommended age groups. The CDC recommends that all boys and girls age 11–12 get two doses of HPV vaccine. Males can receive the vaccine through age 21 and females through age 26, if they did not get vaccinated when they were younger. Everyone within the age group should be vaccinated, regardless of gender or sexual orientation. It is even recommended for men and women with compromised immune systems (including those living with HIV/AIDS) up to age 26 (Figure 13).

Chlamydia

Chlamydia (caused by the bacteria *Chlamydia trachomatis*) is a common STI that can infect both men and women. The US has more than 1.5 million reported cases of chlamydia. It transmits through vaginal, anal, or oral sex. Women can contract it in the cervix, rectum, or throat, men in the urethra (inside the penis), rectum, or throat. Women can potentially experience long-term effects from the infection, including pelvic inflammatory disease and permanent damage to a woman's reproductive system, making it difficult or impossible for her to get pregnant later on.

Chlamydia can also pose many problems during pregnancy. You can pass the infection to your baby during delivery, leading to pneumonia, lung infections, and eye infections that can cause blindness in newborns. Chlamydia can also cause a potentially fatal ectopic pregnancy (pregnancy that occurs outside the womb) or make it more likely to deliver your baby too early. Health care providers often screen for chlamydia during pregnancy check-ups.

Men do not experience long-term effects as often as women, but if their infection goes untreated, they can sustain scarring of the urethra and infection in the epididymis (the tube that carries sperm). This can lead to pain, fever, and in rare cases, infertility.

Most people who have chlamydia have no symptoms, but it can still damage their reproductive system. If symptoms occur, they may not appear until several weeks after you have sex with an infected partner. Symptoms in women include abnormal vaginal discharge; a burning sensation while urinating; pain during intercourse; and in advanced cases, lower abdominal pain, nausea and fever. Symptoms in men include discharge from the penis, difficulty or burning pain while urinating, redness or swelling at the opening of the urethra, itching at the urethra, and pain or swelling in one or both testicles.

Men and women can also get infected with chlamydia in their rectum. This happens either by having receptive anal sex, or by spread from another infected site (such as the vagina). Symptoms, if present, include rectal pain, discharge, and bleeding. Since chlamydia can be transmitted through oral, anal, or vaginal sex, correctly using barriers like condoms is the only way for sexually active people to reduce risk of infection.

Diagnosis and Treatment

If you experience symptoms, you should visit your health care provider right away (Figure 14). Your health care provider will perform a urine and/or swab test (Pap test for women). Chlamydia is treated with antibiotics. Repeat infection with chlamydia, or a gonorrhea infection occurring at the same time, can be common. You should be tested again about three months after you're treated, even if your sex partner was also treated.

Individuals with higher risk factors should be regularly tested for chlamydia. Use the following list to identify your risk factors and the recommend frequency of testing for chlamydia:

Women— Screen all sexually active women under 25 years of age and sexually active women over 25 years of age if they have increased risk for other factors. Retest approximately 3 months after previous treatment.

Pregnant Women— Screen all pregnant women under 25 years of age and pregnant women aged 25 and older if they have increased risk for other factors. Retest during the 3rd trimester for women under 25 years of age or at risk. Pregnant women with chlamydia infection should have a test-of-cure 3-4 weeks after treatment and be retested within 3 months.

Men— Consider screening young men in high prevalence clinical settings or in populations with high burden of infection (e.g. MSM).

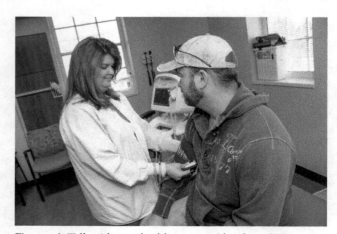

Figure 14. Talk with your health care provider about STIs.

Men Who Have Sex with Men (MSM) — Screen at least annually for sexually active MSM at sites of contact (urethra, rectum) regardless of condom use. Retest every 3–6 months if they have increased risk for other factors

Persons with HIV — For sexually active individuals, screen at first HIV evaluation, and at least annually thereafter. More frequent screening for might be appropriate depending on individual risk behaviors and the local epidemiology.

Gonorrhea

Nearly 400,000 cases of **gonorrhea** are reported in the US every year. The most common of newly infected population is young adults age 15–24. Like many other STIs, it is transmitted through vaginal, oral, or anal sex, leading to infections in the genital tract, mouth, or anus.

Gonorrhea does not always cause symptoms. In men, gonorrhea can cause pain when urinating and discharge from the penis. If untreated, it can cause swelling of the testicles and problems with the prostate. In women, the early symptoms of gonorrhea (if present at all) are often mild. Later, it can cause bleeding between periods, pain when urinating (often mistaken for a bladder infection), and increased discharge from the vagina. If untreated, it can lead to pelvic inflammatory disease, which can cause problems with pregnancy and infertility. As with many STIs, gonorrhea can be passed to a child from an infected mother during birth and can cause infections in the eyes, blood, and joints of newborns. This is a rare but serious risk.

Rectal infections in both men and women can also go unnoticed. When present, symptoms include anal itching, soreness, bleeding, or discharge and pain during bowel movements.

Untreated gonorrhea can cause serious and permanent health problems in both women and men. Rarely, untreated gonorrhea can spread to your blood or joints, which can be life threatening. In women, untreated gonorrhea can cause pelvic inflammatory disease, scar tissue blocking the fallopian tubes, ectopic pregnancy, infertility, and long-term pelvic or abdominal pain. In men, gonorrhea can cause a painful condition in the tubes attached to their testicles. In rare cases, this may cause infertility.

Diagnosis and Treatment

Your health care provider will diagnose gonorrhea with lab tests and treat it with antibiotics. However, treating gonorrhea has become more difficult because drug-resistant strains are increasing. Correct use of condoms greatly reduces, but does not eliminate, the risk of catching or spreading gonorrhea.

Your health care provider will prescribe antibiotics to treat a gonorrhea infection. As with many commonly occurring bacteria, it's becoming harder to treat some gonorrhea, as drug-resistant strains are increasing. If your symptoms continue for more than a few days after receiving treatment, you should return to a health care provider to be checked.

Syphilis

In 2015, the US had 23,872 reported cases of primary and secondary syphilis, with men representing the vast majority of cases at 21,547. **Syphilis** is caused by the bacteria *Treponema* pallidum, and is transmitted by direct contact with a syphilis sore during vaginal, anal, or oral sex. You can find sores on or around the penis, vagina, or anus, or in the rectum, on the lips, or in the mouth. Syphilis has multiple stages — primary, secondary, latent, and tertiary. These stages can be overlapping and have different signs and symptoms associated with each stage.

During the **primary stage** of syphilis, you may notice a single sore or multiple sores. The sore is the location where syphilis entered your body. Sores are usually (but not always) firm, round, and painless. The lack of pain causes it to easily go unnoticed. The sore usually lasts 3–6 weeks and heals regardless of whether or not you receive treatment. Even after the sore goes away, you must still receive treatment. This will stop your infection from moving to the secondary stage.

During the **secondary stage**, 2–10 weeks after infection, you may have skin rashes and/or mucous membrane lesions. Mucous membrane lesions are sores in your mouth, vagina, or anus. This stage usually starts with a rash on one or more areas of your body. The rash can show up when your primary sore is healing or several weeks after the sore has healed. It can look like rough, red, or reddish-brown spots on the palms of your hands and/or the bottoms of your feet. The rash usually won't itch and is sometimes so faint that you won't notice it.

Other symptoms can include fever, swollen lymph glands, sore throat, patchy hair loss, headaches, weight loss, muscle aches, and fatigue. The symptoms from this stage will go away whether or not you receive treatment. Without the right treatment, your infection will move to the latent and possibly tertiary stages of syphilis.

The **latent stage** of syphilis is a period of time when there are no visible signs or symptoms of syphilis. If you do not receive treatment, you can continue to have syphilis in your body for years without any signs or symptoms, making the risk of transmission greater.

Most people with untreated syphilis don't enter its **tertiary stage**. However, when it does happen it can affect many different organ systems. These include the heart and blood vessels, and the brain and nervous system. Tertiary syphilis is very serious and occurs 10–30 years after your infection began. In tertiary syphilis, the disease damages your internal organs and can result in death.

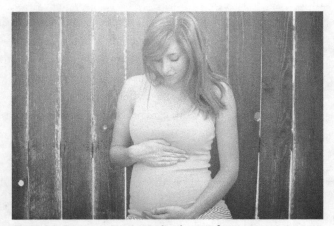

Figure 15. Pregnant women and unborn infants can experience severe complications from untreated STIs.

Like most STIs, if you are pregnant and have syphilis, you can give the infection to your unborn baby (Figure 15). This can lead to low birth weight or make it more likely you will miscarry, deliver your baby too early, or deliver a stillborn baby. Health care providers typically screen for syphilis during the first trimester of pregnancy because the impact to the child can be severe and potentially fatal, and because it can be treated in time if found early. An infected baby may be born without signs or symptoms of disease. However, if not treated immediately, the baby may develop serious problems within a few weeks. Untreated babies can have health problems and birth defects or developmental delays such as cataracts, deafness, or seizures.

Diagnosis and Treatment

Most of the time, a blood test is used to screen for syphilis. Some health care providers will diagnose syphilis by testing fluid from a syphilis sore. Syphilis can be cured with the right antibiotics from your health care provider. However, treatment might not undo any damage that the infection has already done, which is why it's important to get tested if you think you may have been exposed.

Individuals with higher risk factors should be regularly tested for syphilis:

Pregnant Women—Screen all pregnant women at the first prenatal visit. Retest early in the third trimester and at delivery if at high risk.

Men Who Have Sex with Men (MSM)—Screen at least annually for sexually active MSM at sites of contact (urethra, rectum, pharynx) regardless of condom use. Retest every 3–6 months if at increased risk.

Persons with HIV—For sexually active individuals, screen at first HIV evaluation, and at least annually thereafter.

More frequent screening for might be appropriate depending on individual risk behaviors and the local epidemiology.

Herpes

Herpes simplex virus (HSV) is transmitted through skin-to-skin contact. There are varying forms of the herpes virus, including herpes simplex virus type 1 (HSV 1) and herpes simplex virus type 2 (HSV 2), each with various effects. These viruses form either oral or genital herpes.

Oral herpes (such as cold sores or fever blisters on or

around the mouth) is usually caused by HSV-1 (Figure 16). Most people are infected with HSV-1 during childhood from non-sexual contact. For example, people can get infected from a kiss from a relative or friend with oral herpes. More than

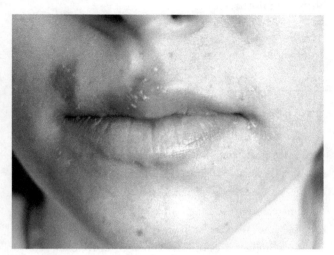

Figure 16. An oral herpes outbreak.

	Prevalence (%)
Total	**16.2%**
Age Group (Years)	
14–19	1.4%
20–29	10.5%
30–39	19.6%
40–49	26.1%
Reported Number of Lifetime Sexual Partners	
1 partner	3.9%
2–4 partners	14.0%
5–9 partners	16.3%
10+ partners	26.7%

Figure 17. Herpes risks rise with age and number of partners.

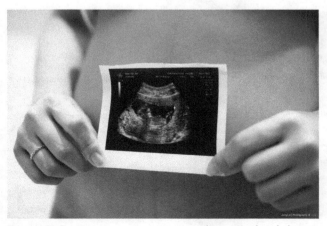

Figure 18. Pregnant women can transmit herpes to their babies.

half of the population in the US has HSV-1, even if they don't show any signs or symptoms. HSV-1 can also be spread from mouth to genitals through oral sex. This is why some cases of genital herpes are caused by HSV-1.

Genital herpes (such as sores appearing as one or more blisters on or around the genitals, rectum, or mouth) is usually caused by HSV-2. It may start with a tingling feeling, then red bumps, and then blisters or red sores. The blisters break and leave painful sores that may take weeks to heal. People often refer to these symptoms as "having an outbreak." The first time someone has an outbreak they may also have flu-like symptoms such as fever, body aches, or swollen glands.

Repeat outbreaks of genital herpes can happen often, especially during the first year after infection, though they are usually shorter and less severe than the first outbreak. Although the infection can stay in the body for the rest of your life, the frequency of outbreaks tends to decrease over the years.

You should be examined by a health care provider if you or your sexual partner notice symptoms, such as an unusual sore, a smelly discharge, burning when urinating, or, for women specifically, bleeding between periods. Most people who have herpes have no or very mild symptoms. Even without signs of the disease, it can still be spread to sexual partners.

Your health care provider can often diagnose genital herpes by simply looking at your symptoms, or they can take a sample from a sore and test it for herpes.

Living with Herpes

Herpes can't be cured—it's a chronic infection. Both topical and oral medications are available that can shorten outbreaks and reduce the chance that you will pass the infection on to a sexual partner. Your likelihood of contracting herpes increases with the number of sexual partners you have (Figure 17).

Some people who get genital herpes have concerns about how it will impact their overall health, sex life, and relationships. Talk to a health care provider about those concerns, but it's important to recognize that while herpes is not curable, it can be managed. Since a genital herpes diagnosis may affect how you will feel about current or future sexual relationships, it's important to understand how to talk to sexual partners about STIs.

Herpes sores can be quite painful and can be severe in people with suppressed immune systems. If you touch your sores or the fluids from the sores, you may transfer herpes to another part of your body, such as your eyes, so immediate and thorough hand-washing is imperative to prevent the spread of infection. Herpes symptoms may also be present in areas that can't be protected by a condom, which makes the risk of transmission greater. Remember, herpes spreads from skin-to-skin contact!

HSV can be transmitted during delivery, so pregnant women are usually monitored towards the end of pregnancy, and a C-section may be performed. Research suggests that women who contract herpes during the latter part of pregnancy have a higher risk of transmitting it to their baby (Figure 18). It can also be transmitted in utero and can cause premature birth and miscarriage.

HIV and AIDS

HIV stands for **human immunodeficiency virus**. This virus can lead to **acquired immunodeficiency syndrome**, or **AIDS**. Unlike some other viruses, the human body can't get rid of HIV completely, even with treatment.

We first began hearing about **HIV** and **AIDS** as a nation back in the 1980s. We knew little about how the disease transmitted and viewed the disease as a death sentence. Today, we have learned about the disease so that we can prevent its spread and offer treatments to those affected. Yet it still remains a significant threat in certain populations. Gay and bisexual men, for example, have the highest rates of infection. They accounted for 70% of all new HIV infections. There were over 6,000 deaths in 2015 attributed directly to HIV. It was the ninth leading cause of death for those aged 25–34 and ninth for those aged 35–44.

An estimated 1.1 million people in the US were living with HIV at the end of 2015, the most recent year for which this data is available (Figure 19). Of those people, about 15%, or 1 in 7, did not know they were infected. There are a disproportionate number of people affected who are African American (44%), sex workers, or living in prison. People aged 20–29 also have higher rates of infection—in 2016, over 14,000 (over 35%) of new cases came from this age group. Worldwide, there were about 2.1 million new cases of HIV in 2015. About 36.7 million people are living with HIV around the world, and as of June 2016, 17 million people living with HIV were receiving ART.

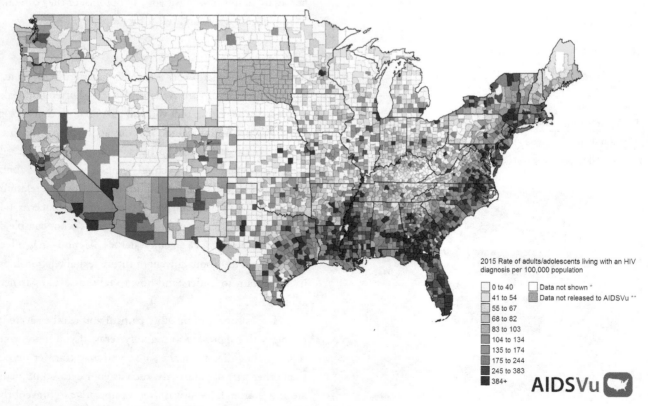

2015 Rate of adults/adolescents living with an HIV diagnosis per 100,000 population

- 0 to 40
- 41 to 54
- 55 to 67
- 68 to 82
- 83 to 103
- 104 to 134
- 135 to 174
- 175 to 244
- 245 to 383
- 384+
- Data not shown *
- Data not released to AIDSVu **

AIDSVu

Figure 19. AIDS affects parts of the US differently.

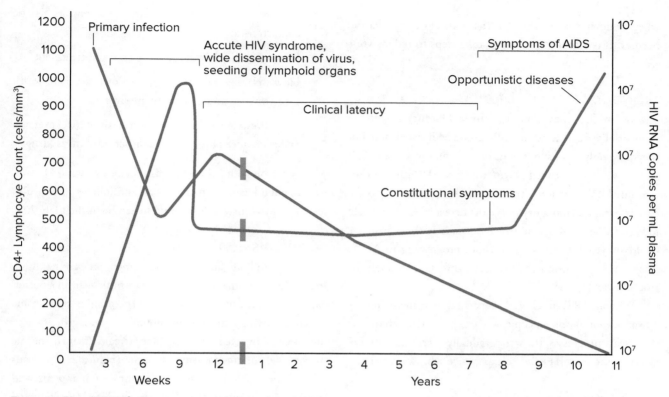

Figure 20. How HIV infection progresses over time.

No effective cure currently exists, but with proper medical care, HIV can be controlled. The medicine used to treat HIV is called antiretroviral therapy (ART). If taken correctly every day, this medicine can dramatically prolong the lives of many people infected with HIV. The medicine keeps them healthy, slows or prevents the advancement of the disease to AIDS, and greatly lowers their chance of infecting others. Before the introduction of ART in the mid-1990s, people with HIV could progress to AIDS in just a few years. Today, someone diagnosed with HIV and treated before the disease is far advanced can live nearly as long as someone who does not have HIV.

Though we know more about the illness, and have methods of treatment, HIV can still be intimidating. HIV attacks the body's immune system, specifically the CD4 cells (T cells). These cells help the immune system fight off infections. Remember those white blood cells we talked about earlier that fight off invaders? HIV reduces the number of these cells in the body, making the person at greater risk for other infections or infection-related cancers. This can get worse over time, making any infection, even normally non-threatening ones, harder to fight. Opportunistic infections or cancers take advantage of the person's weakened immune system and

settle in, signaling that the person has AIDS, the last stage of HIV infection.

There are three stages of HIV infection: acute HIV infection, clinical latency, and AIDS (Figure 20).

Stage 1: Acute HIV Infection

The first sign of infection usually occurs within two to four weeks after infection in the form of what seems like a severe flu for most people. Symptoms can include fever, swollen glands, sore throat, rash, muscle and joint aches and pains, and headache. This is called "acute retroviral syndrome" (ARS) or "primary HIV infection," the body's first attempt to fight the infection. People who suspect they may have come into contact with HIV should seek medical care right away.

Your body uses your cells against you during this early stage, hijacking your CD4 cells to replicate and destroying them in the process. This can happen rapidly. Your immune system will eventually bring the level of virus in your body down to what's called a "viral set point." This is a relatively stable level of virus in your body. Your CD4 cell count will begin to increase, but may not return to normal levels. ART may be particularly beneficial to your health during this stage.

You have a high risk of transmitting HIV at this stage,

whether during sex or through the sharing of hypodermic needles. It is essential for you to take steps to reduce your risk of transmission.

Stage 2: Clinical Latency

The disease then moves into the **clinical latency stage**. The virus still lives and continues to reproduce in the person, but they have only mild symptoms, or no symptoms at all. This stage is sometimes called "asymptomatic HIV infection" or "chronic HIV infection." The virus continues to grow slowly, even if standard laboratory tests can't detect it. ART can help to keep the virus under control and may help the person live for many years in this stage without progressing to AIDS. They can still transmit the disease at this stage, though the risk is lower.

Without ART, the clinical latency stage last approximately 10 years, though some people may progress more rapidly. As the disease progresses, the virus gradually overtakes the CD4 cells and the person begins to experience symptoms again.

Stage 3: AIDS

Stage 3 of HIV infection occurs when the immune system has taken too much of a beating and opportunistic infections easily and rapidly invade the body. People with AIDS commonly experience chills, fever, sweats, swollen lymph glands, weakness, and weight loss. The viral load is high, and the person can be very infectious.

Normal ranges of CD4 cells are between 500 and 1600 cell per cubic millimeter. A person is considered to have AIDS when the number of CD4 cells fall below 200 cells per cubic millimeter of blood (200 cells per cubic millimeter). Opportunistic illnesses also suggest a progression to AIDS. These include certain forms of pneumonia, toxoplasmosis, and Kaposi's sarcoma—regardless of your CD4 count.

Without treatment, people with AIDS typically survive for about 3 years. A serious opportunistic illness can bring that number down to 1 year. This is why ART is so important for people with AIDS. It can improve their symptoms and prolong life at any stage, but the earlier, the better. Most people receiving ART from the early stages of the disease live nearly as long as someone without HIV thanks to the therapy stopping the disease progression.

Many factors can affect how quickly people progress through the stages. These include:

- Genetic makeup
- Their health before they were infected

- How much virus they were exposed to and its genetic characteristics
- How early they began receiving care and treatment
- How well they take their medications, see their health care provider, and care for themselves
- Their lifestyle choices, such as a healthy diet, exercise, and avoidance of tobacco and other substances (drugs).

A person with HIV who was previously in good health, makes good health-related choices, and follows their health care providers instructions could live to be in their late 70's.

Transmission

Only certain body fluids—blood, semen, pre-seminal fluid, rectal fluids, vaginal fluids, and breast milk—from a person who has HIV can transmit HIV. These fluids must come in contact with a mucous membrane or damaged tissue or be directly injected into the bloodstream (from a needle or syringe) for transmission to occur (Figure 21). Mucous membranes are found inside the rectum, vagina, penis, and mouth. According to the CDC, in the US, HIV is spread mainly by:

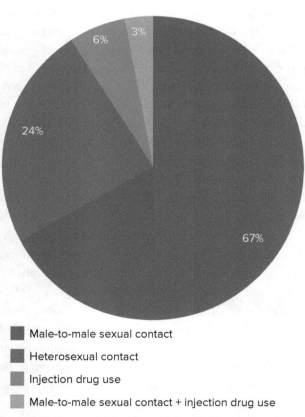

- Male-to-male sexual contact
- Heterosexual contact
- Injection drug use
- Male-to-male sexual contact + injection drug use

Figure 21. Some activities have a higher likelihood of causing HIV transmission.

Sharing needles—Sharing syringes, rinse water, or other equipment (works) used to prepare drugs for injection with someone who has HIV is extremely likely to transmit the disease. HIV can live in a used needle for up to 42 days depending on temperature and other factors.

Sex—Having anal or vaginal sex with someone who has HIV without using a condom or taking medicines to prevent or treat HIV is a very high risk for transmission. For the HIV-negative partner, receptive anal sex is the highest-risk sexual behavior, but you can also get HIV from insertive anal sex. Either partner can get HIV through vaginal sex, though it's less risky than receptive anal sex.

Less commonly, HIV may be spread by:

New mothers with HIV—HIV can be transmitted from mother to child during pregnancy, birth, or breastfeeding. The risk can be higher if a mother is living with HIV and not taking medicine.

Contaminated objects—A risk mostly for health care workers, being stuck with an HIV-contaminated needle or other sharp object can transmit the disease.

In extremely rare cases, HIV has been transmitted by:

Oral sex—Putting the mouth on the penis, vagina, or anus of an infected person. In general, there's little to no risk of getting HIV from oral sex. But transmission of HIV, though extremely rare, is theoretically possible if an HIV-positive man ejaculates in his partner's mouth during oral sex.

Blood transfer—Receiving blood transfusions, blood products, or organ/tissue transplants contaminated with HIV, is a risk. However, the risk is extremely small because of rigorous testing of the US blood supply and donated organs and tissues.

Open wounds—Contact between broken skin, wounds, or mucous membranes and HIV-infected blood or blood-contaminated body fluids may cause transmission.

Because of certain myths and stigma surrounding AIDS since the 1980s, there is a lot of fear regarding how safe it is to be around someone with HIV or AIDS. HIV is *not* transmitted by hugging, shaking hands, sharing toilets, sharing dishes, or closed-mouth kissing with someone who is HIV-positive. It can't be transmitted by saliva, tears, or sweat that is not mixed with the blood of an HIV-positive person. And mosquitoes, ticks, or other blood-sucking insects can't carry HIV, nor can it be transmitted through the air.

HIV Diagnosis and Treatment

The only way to positively diagnose HIV is through testing. The CDC recommends that everyone between ages 13–64 get tested for HIV at least once as part of routine health care. Knowledge is power with HIV just as it is with other STIs.

Three types of tests are available: antibody tests, combination or fourth-generation tests, and nucleic acid tests (NAT). HIV tests may be performed on blood, oral fluid, or urine (Figure 22). Most HIV tests, including most rapid tests and home tests, are antibody tests. Antibodies are produced by your immune system when you're exposed to viruses like HIV or bacteria. HIV antibody tests look for these antibodies to HIV in your blood or oral fluid. In general, antibody tests that use blood can detect HIV slightly sooner after infection than tests done with oral fluid.

Many home tests are available and can offer quick results, such as the **rapid antibody screening test**, the OraQuick HIV

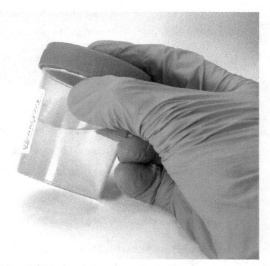

Figure 22. Most STI tests are done by urinalysis.

test, and the Home Access HIV-1 Test System (Figure 23). A person can get their results as quickly as 20 minutes for oral fluid tests, or a few days for blood.

There is a window period of 21–84 days during which an infected person's body makes enough antibodies for an antibody test to detect HIV. Nearly all HIV-positive people will develop enough antibodies during the ARS period to detect the infection. Individuals who suspect they were exposed to HIV but receive a negative result during this window should re-test after 3 months.

Someone with a positive result will need to take a follow-up test. Their best choice is to do this through their health care provider. Most labs will retest samples for accuracy. Health care providers routinely utilize two tests. A combination, or fourth-generation, test looks for both HIV antibodies and antigens. **Combination screening tests** are now recommended for testing done in labs and are becoming more common in the US. A **nucleic acid test** (NAT) looks for HIV in the blood. It looks for the virus and not the antibodies to the virus. The test can give either a positive/negative result or an actual amount of virus present in the blood (known as a viral load test). This test is very expensive and not routinely used for screening individuals unless they recently had a high-risk exposure or a possible exposure with early symptoms of HIV infection.

It's important to follow the routine screening guidelines as a matter of habit when it comes to HIV and other STIs. Prompt identification and treatment makes all the difference in both prevention and proper treatment. Individuals who know themselves to be at higher risk should talk to their health care provider about how often they should be screened:

> **Women**—Screen all women aged 13-64 years (opt-out), and all women who seek evaluation and treatment for STIs

> **Pregnant Women**—Screen all pregnant women should be screened at first prenatal visit (opt-out). Retest in the third trimester if at high risk.

> **Men**—Screen all men aged 13-64 (opt-out), and all men who seek evaluation and treatment for STIs.

> **Men Who Have Sex with Men (MSM)**—Screen at least annually for sexually active MSM if HIV status is unknown or negative and the patient himself or his sex partner(s) have had more than one sex partner since most recent HIV test.

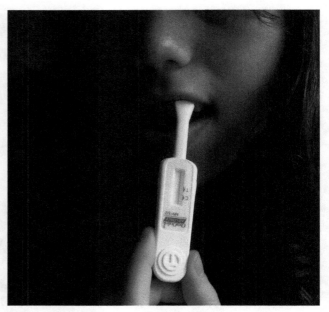

Figure 23. Oral tests are available for HIV.

We talked briefly about ARTs and their importance, but let's look a bit more closely at how they work. HIV is a type of virus called a retrovirus, and the drugs used to treat it are called antiretrovirals (ARV). These drugs are always given in combination with other types ARV's. This combination therapy is referred to as antiretroviral therapy (ART). ART prevents the virus from multiplying, reducing the amount of HIV in the body. This gives the immune system a chance to recover and fight off other infections and certain HIV-related cancers. This also reduces the risk of HIV transmission.

HIV and Pregnancy

Perinatal HIV transmission, also known as mother-to-child transmission, can happen at any time during pregnancy, labor, delivery, and breastfeeding. Approximately 8,500 women living with HIV give birth annually. The CDC recommends that all women who are pregnant or planning to get pregnant take an HIV test as early as possible before and during every pregnancy. This is because the earlier HIV is diagnosed and treated, the more effective HIV medicines will be at preventing transmission and improving the health outcomes of both mother and child.

Because of the advances in health care, many women with HIV deliver without transmitting the disease to the child. Rates of mother-to-child transmission have declined by more than 90% since the early 1990s. With proper medication during pregnancy, and for the baby for its first 4–6 weeks of life, the risk of transmitting HIV can be 1% or less.

The risk of transmission can also be lessened by having a

C-section delivery (in some cases), not breastfeeding, and not pre-chewing the baby's food. Babies born with HIV should start treatment early because the disease can progress more rapidly in children than adults.

It is important that all women who are pregnant or trying to get pregnant encourage their partners to also get tested for HIV. The CDC suggests that women who are HIV-negative but have an HIV-positive partner talk to their health care provider about taking HIV medicines daily, called pre-exposure prophylaxis (PrEP), to protect themselves while trying to get pregnant, and to protect themselves and their baby during pregnancy and while breastfeeding.

Looking Toward a Solution

No current vaccine is able to prevent HIV infection or treat those who have it, though scientists are working to develop one. They are building on a study from 2016 that found some potential for a vaccine to be effective with HIV. The National Institute of Health (NIH) supported a clinical trial to test a modified HIV vaccine. This current vaccine trial, called HVTN 702, is testing whether an experimental vaccine regimen safely prevents HIV infection among South African adults. The goal with this study is to develop a safe and effective vaccine that can be used worldwide to reduce the risk of infection, lower rates of transmission, and help control the pandemic, especially in high-risk populations.

Viral Hepatitis

Hepatitis A, hepatitis B, and hepatitis C are diseases of the liver caused by three different viruses. Each can cause similar symptoms, but they have different modes of transmission and can affect the liver differently. Hepatitis A appears only as an acute or newly occurring infection and does not become chronic. People with hepatitis A usually

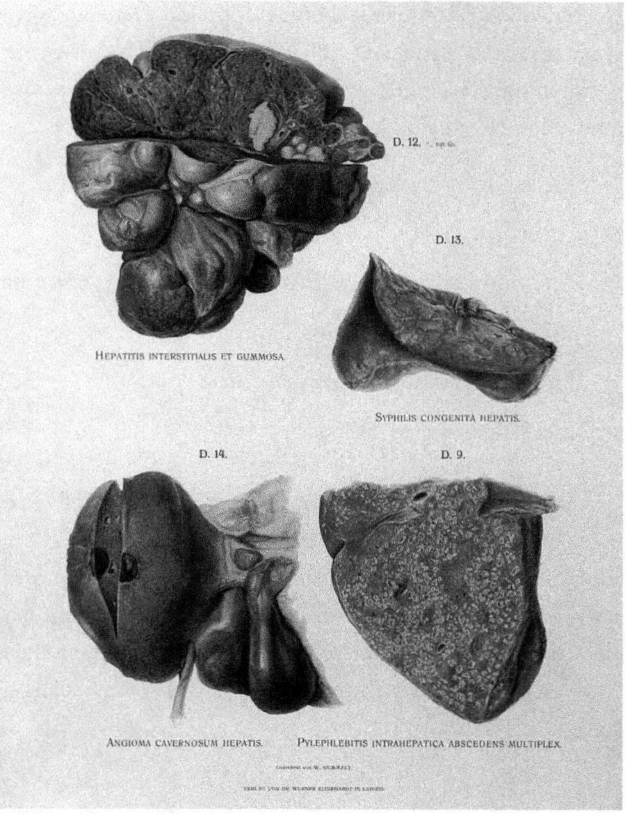

Figure 24. Many STIs affect the shape and function of the liver.

improve without treatment. Hepatitis B and hepatitis C can also begin as acute infections, but in some people, the virus remains in the body, resulting in chronic disease and long-term liver problems. Vaccines can prevent hepatitis A and B. However, there is not a vaccine for hepatitis C. If a person has had one type of viral hepatitis in the past, it's still possible to get the other types.

In 2015, 48 states in the US submitted reports of acute hepatitis B virus (HBV) infection, 40 submitted reports of acute hepatitis C virus (HCV) infection, 40 submitted reports of chronic HBV infection, and 40 submitted reports of chronic HCV infection.

Hepatitis A is caused by the hepatitis A virus (HAV) and is highly contagious. It usually transmits by the fecal-oral route, either through person-to-person contact or consumption of contaminated food or water. HAV does not result in chronic infection. More than 80% of adults with hepatitis A have symptoms, though the majority of children do not show symptoms or have an unrecognized infection. Antibodies produced in response to HAV last for life and protect against reinfection.

Hepatitis B is a liver infection caused by the hepatitis B virus (HBV). It transmits when blood, semen, vaginal fluid, or another body fluid from an infected person enters the body of someone who is not infected. This can happen through sharing needles, syringes, or other drug-injection equipment; through sexual contact; or from mother to baby at birth. This virus transmits even more easily than HIV, so even sharing razors or toothbrushes with someone infected can be risky.

For some people, HBV is an acute illness, but for others, it can become a long-term, chronic infection. Risk for chronic infection relates to the person's age at infection—approximately 90% of infected infants become chronically infected, compared with 2–6% of adults. Chronic HBV can lead to serious health issues, like cirrhosis or liver cancer (Figure 24).

Hepatitis C is a blood-borne infection caused by the hepatitis C virus (HCV). Most people become infected with HCV by sharing needles or other equipment to inject drugs. It can be a short-term illness for some but for 70–85% of people who become infected, it becomes a long-term, chronic, potentially fatal infection. No vaccine protects against hepatitis C. The best way to prevent it is by avoiding behaviors that can spread the disease, especially injecting drugs.

Many people with hepatitis don't have symptoms and don't know they have the infection. If symptoms occur with an acute infection, they can appear anytime from 2 weeks to 6 months after exposure. Symptoms of chronic viral hepatitis can take decades to develop. Acute symptoms of hepatitis that show up after 1–6 months can include: fever, fatigue, loss of appetite, nausea, vomiting, abdominal pain, dark urine, grey-colored stools, joint pain, and jaundice.

Diagnosis, Treatment, and Prevention

Health care providers diagnose hepatitis with a blood test. No medication can treat acute hepatitis. Individuals must manage their symptoms, much like tending to the flu. Diet, exercise, and the avoidance of substances can also help, particularly when sleep patterns are disrupted. In chronic cases of hepatitis, regular monitoring for signs of liver disease progression is required. Some patients may be treated with antiviral drugs.

The best way to prevent hepatitis A and B is by getting vaccinated. Because of how easily hepatitis B transmits, vaccination against HBV is routinely given to infants as a preventative measure.

Pelvic Inflammatory Disease

Pelvic inflammatory disease is an infection of a woman's reproductive organs primarily caused by untreated chlamydia and gonorrhea. This can occur when bacteria from the vagina or cervix travel to your womb, fallopian tubes, or ovaries. Bacteria can enter your body during a medical procedure such as: childbirth, endometrial biopsy (removing a small piece of your womb lining to test for cancer), insertion of an intrauterine device (IUD), miscarriage, or abortion. Untreated PID can cause scar tissue blocking the fallopian tubes, ectopic pregnancy, infertility, and long-term pelvic or abdominal pain.

In the US, nearly 1 million women have PID each year. About 1 in 8 sexually active girls will have PID before age 20. You are more likely to get PID if you have an STI and don't get treated, have more than one sex partner, have a sex partner who has sex partners other than you, have had PID before, douche regularly, or use an intrauterine device (IUD) for birth control. However, the small increased risk is mostly limited to the first three weeks after the IUD is placed inside the uterus by a health care provider.

Diagnosis and Treatment

There are no tests for PID. A diagnosis is usually based on a combination of your medical history, physical exam, and other test results. You may not realize you have PID because your symptoms may be mild, or you may not experience any symptoms. However, if you do have symptoms, you may notice:

- Pain in your lower abdomen
- Fever
- An unusual discharge with a bad odor from your vagina
- Pain or bleeding when you have sex
- Burning sensation when you urinate
- Bleeding between periods

Screening for chlamydia and gonorrhea, and getting treatment for these infections if present, can help prevent PID in addition to safer sex practices. PID can be treated if diagnosed early. However, treatment won't undo any damage that has already happened to your reproductive system. The longer you wait to get treated, the more likely it is that you will have complications from PID.

Safer Sex

The transmission of STIs can be prevented by practicing safer sexual activity. "Safer" sex means exactly that: you are less likely to receive or transmit an STI if you educate yourself on your and your partners' risk factors, communicate with partners, and get tested regularly when you are sexually active.

The Only "Safe" Sex

Abstinence is the safest way to avoid STIs. If you aren't having sex with other people, then you aren't at risk for STIs. That makes sense, right? Abstinence is the idea that you wait to have any kind of sex with another person until you are in a committed, monogamous relationship. Once you are in a mutually monogamous relationship, where both partners remain dedicated to monogamy, your risk levels are much lower. This is especially true if neither partner has been very active sexually prior to this relationship.

Formal abstinence education is often misleading, and studies have found that people who haven't learned about risks will sometimes narrowly define "sex" as "vaginal intercourse" in order to preserve "virginity." This approach causes young people who become sexually active to engage in high-risk sex activities, like unprotected anal intercourse, which is a direct cause for the high rate of infection in places where abstinence-only sex education is taught. This is in addition to the higher prevalence of unsafe sex among young people who have only learned abstinence-only sex education.

Condoms and Barriers

Condoms have been around for a very long time. They are basically a sealed sheath that covers the penis and were originally used to prevent pregnancy, though now we use them to control the spread of infection. Although the materials used to make condoms have been pretty creative over the years, modern condoms are primarily made from latex, polyurethane, polyisoprene, nitrile, or gut (like sausage casings). The latter variety only protects against pregnancy and are not safe for use against STIs.

Correctly using male condoms and other barriers like female condoms and dental dams, during every sex act, can reduce (though not eliminate) the risk of STIs, including HIV

and viral hepatitis. They can also provide protection against other diseases that may be transmitted through sex like Zika and Ebola. Using male and female condoms correctly, every time, can also help prevent pregnancy. However, male and female condoms should not be used at the same time as they could cause breakage to each other.

Male condoms fit over the penis and usually have a reservoir at the tip to catch ejaculate. Female condoms look like a tube with an opening at one end and are inserted into the vagina. Dental dams are latex sheets that are placed over women's genitals for safer oral sex.

Correctly Using Male Condoms

Male condoms are the most readily available barrier method and one of the easiest to use. Correct use is key. Condom failure is almost always due to user error.

First make sure you haven't been carrying around a condom in your wallet for months. Heat, wear and tear, and age are all factors that can cause condom failure—condoms have expiration dates! Always use a fresh condom with each new sex act (even if no ejaculation occurred).

When opening the condom, do not use anything sharp, including your teeth. Most condom packages are easy to open. After opening it, look to see which way it's going to roll ((Figure 25). Pinch the tip of the condom and place it at the tip of the

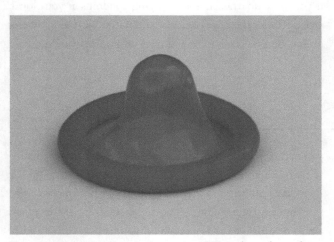

Figure 25. A common protection against STIs is the male condom.

penis. Once it's placed, roll the condom all the way down to the base of the penis. You are receiving no protection from the condom if you don't roll the condom all the way down to the base.

When finished with the condom, remove the it by pulling from the tip and either tie a knot in it (like a balloon) or wrap it in some tissue and throw it away. Never attempt to reuse a condom.

You may have to use lubricant with condoms, because friction has a "drying" effect. If so, use water or silicone-based lubricants. Petroleum or oil-based lubricants break down the latex and increase likelihood of breakage. If a condom ever breaks, stop sexual activity immediately and put on a new condom.

The FC2 "Female" (frequently referred to as "internal") condom offers many advantages for people who want to ensure protection from pregnancy or sexually transmitted infection (Figure 26). The internal condom is a strong, thin, and flexible nitrile sheath inserted into the vagina (up to 4 hours) prior to sex. It has a flexible inner ring for easy insertion and is absolutely latex-free. It is pre-lubricated with a slick silicone-based lubricant, but additional lubricant can be used as well.

Latex condoms can be easy to acquire at grocery and drug stores. Although rare, latex allergies may make regular condoms unusable. There are also "traditional" style condoms designed to fit over a penis that are made from polyurethane, polyisoprene, and synthetic resins. These are latex-free and some people like them for the relative thinness of the material along with the higher level of heat transfer, which combine to create a more "natural" feeling. These materials are less flexible than latex, so correct sizing is important.

Used correctly with every new sex act, condoms have a success rate close to 100% for protecting against infection and avoiding pregnancy. For preventing pregnancy, they have the additional benefit over hormonal birth control of providing protection against STIs.

Condoms have some other benefits as well. They come

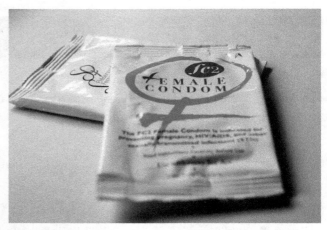

Figure 26. Another protection against STIs is the female condom.

in a wide variety of shapes, textures, thicknesses, and styles, making them something that can "spice things up" a little. Men who want to last longer can experiment with different condom thicknesses until they find something that gives them the effect they want.

Some people complain that they don't like the feeling of wearing a condom, or that putting one on kills the mood. Both of these are easy problems to fix. A drop or two of lubricant in the tip of the condom before putting it on makes it feel almost like there is no condom. The "mood killer" probably has more to do with where the condom is located, than the act of putting it on. Put the condom in an easily accessible location to reduce how much time it takes to get the condom and put it on.

Most resistance to condom use is purely psychological—if you feel like they are a hassle, or that condoms aren't sexy, that's exactly what they will be. If you think condoms are sexy and easy-to-use (while they protect you from infection), you will have no problem using condoms correctly and effectively. Also, if you are embarrassed about buying condoms at your local grocery store, there are plenty of alternative ways to get them online. Some sites even offer advice on finding the right fit.

Staying Safe

Limiting your risk of contracting or transmitting STIs includes limiting your number of sexual partners, communicating about your health, and practicing safer sexual activities. It's a simple statistical likelihood that your chance of contracting an STI increases as your number of partners increases. If you are sexually active with multiple

partners, it's important to communicate and protect yourself (and them).

Communication means talking about health concerns, sharing information, and setting boundaries. It's important to be upfront and honest about your sexual activity with your partner(s), so everyone can make informed decisions.

For example, if one person isn't being monogamous, and they are sexually active with someone who thinks the relationship *is* monogamous, that's unethical. One person in the equation isn't able to make informed decisions about his or her sexual health.

If you already have, or end up contracting an STI, it's your ethical (and in some states, legal) obligation to inform partner(s) so that they can quickly seek treatment and decide whether they are comfortable with the risk of contracting an STI. For example, herpes (HSV-2) is transmittable during a flare up, but otherwise isn't a problem. It's even less of a problem when a person with HSV-2 is using treatments that control outbreaks. Therefore, someone who is aware that it's a relatively low risk to date someone with herpes might choose to do so. But it should be their decision.

Communicating safe sex boundaries is important as well. If you tell a man that you require he wear a condom during sex, and he balks, makes excuses, or refuses, then you know that he isn't a safe sexual partner. Or you may discover that you have different safer sex expectations. He may prefer condoms for any kind of genital contact and require oral barriers in addition to condoms for vaginal or anal sex. Figuring out where your boundaries are beforehand is an important first step to having a useful conversation about safer sex.

No Age Limit on Safer Sex

Even though most new STIs are in younger people, older adults can be just as susceptible to infections. Safer sex has no age limit. In a recent survey of single people over 45, only one in five reported using condoms every time—32% of women and 12% of men. While STIs are by far most common among those under 30, those in their 50s are still at risk. Syphilis, for example, is the most prevalent STI in people over 45, though the percentages are low.

Older singles also neglect condoms because they're less likely to have sex involving the main route of STI transmission—vaginal intercourse. Interest in sex often fades with age. Erectile medications are not as effective as we see on television, and menopausal changes can take the fun out of intercourse as it becomes uncomfortable or impossible. As a result, older couples adapt to sex without intercourse—hand massage, oral sex, and sex toys. As we've learned, however, many STIs can infect the mouth and throat.

Public-health authorities insist that older adults need to continue condom use. As people continue to live longer and more actively, older adults' STI rates have risen. Since 2005, their risk of syphilis has jumped 67% and chlamydia 40%.

Likewise, someone's youth does not make them less likely to become infected or infect others. Young people have such a high rate of STIs for a variety of reasons. You may think that a partner's sexual inexperience makes them safe. But as we've learned here, there are many ways to acquire and transmit infections that can have a serious impact on your health. No wonder health experts recommend consistent condom use for *anyone* who has sex, at least until they are in a monogamous relationship and have been tested for STIs.

These actions increase your risk of contracting an STI:

Having unprotected sex. This includes vaginal or anal penetration by an infected partner who isn't wearing a latex condom, improper or inconsistent use of condoms, and oral sex without a latex condom or dental dam.

Having sexual contact with multiple partners. The more people you have sexual contact with, the greater your risk. This is true for concurrent partners as well as monogamous consecutive relationships.

Having a history of STIs. Having one STI makes it much easier for another STI to take hold.

Being forced to have sexual intercourse or sexual activity. Dealing with rape or assault can be difficult, but it's important to be seen as soon as possible. Screening, treatment, and emotional support can be offered.

Abusing alcohol or using recreational drugs. Substance abuse can inhibit your judgment, making you more willing to participate in risky behaviors.

Injecting drugs. Needle sharing spreads many serious infections, including HIV, hepatitis B and hepatitis C.

Being young. Half of STIs occur in people between age 15–24.

Men who request prescriptions for drugs to treat erectile dysfunction have higher rates of STIs. Be sure you are up to date on safe sex practices if you ask your health care provider for one of these medications.

Are There Any Sexual Activities to Avoid?

The short answer is no. Different sexual activities have different levels of risk, and this question can only really be answered by consenting partners who have taken the time to educate themselves and determine their boundaries. If the activity is too far outside your comfort zone in terms of risk, it's something you can choose to avoid. As noted above, unprotected anal sex presents the highest level of risk for transmitting STIs, whereas activities like kissing or mutual masturbation present the least amount of risk.

The discovery of treatment-resistant gonorrhea elevates the risk of unprotected penile oral sex, which was previously considered moderate- to low-risk activity. Some S&M practices that include the possibility of blood are extremely high-risk and require the same precautions one would expect in a medical setting.

Screening

Getting regularly tested and screened for STIs is a major part of preventing the spread of infection. It's a good practice to get tested after each new partner and people in monogamous relationships should consider being tested at least once a year.

STI screening requires blood and urine samples, or Pap tests, and results come back within a couple of days. Some tests, like herpes, may require special request as HSV-2 screenings aren't necessarily a part of the regular screening process (Figure 27).

Early diagnosis is vital for avoiding the more serious complications of sexually transmitted infections. Not only are most infections preventable via safer sex practices, many are relatively harmless when detected quickly. It's kind of a no-brainer when we put it that way.

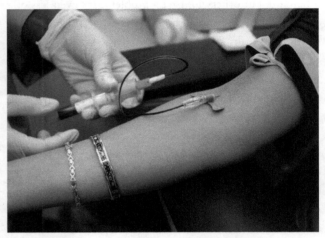

Figure 27. Many STIs can be detected through blood tests.

Resources for Diagnosis and Treatment of STIs

Most medical insurance covers STI screening. You can also utilize one of the following agencies to gain more information or find local agencies that can help:

- The US Department of Health and Human Services—HIV.gov: www.hiv.gov/hiv-basics

- The Centers for Disease Control: www.cdc.gov/std/

- Planned Parenthood: www.plannedparenthood.org/

Planned Parenthood is an excellent resource for comprehensive sexual health services for women and men. They offer a sliding scale for testing services and low-cost or free STI prevention measures, like condoms.

Conclusion

Your next steps should be to become more aware of risk factors for infection in your life. If you find that your risks in certain areas are high, practice more caution and take action to combat the spread of infectious diseases in that area. Your chances of contracting and transmitting an STI depend on your individual decisions about safe sex. If you are sexually active, make sure you communicate with each of your partners about your concerns. Protect yourself and your partner from potential infection by practicing safe sex.

Reflection Questions

1. What are the different types of pathogens? Briefly describe each.

2. Identify the components of the chain of infection.

3. Identify an infectious disease that concerns you, and describe this pathogen based on the chain of infection.

4. How does the lymphatic system work to prevent infectious disease?

5. What are three things you could do to reduce the spread of infectious disease?

6. What are three serious consequences associated with sexually transmitted infectious?

7. In what ways might an STI diagnosis impact the different dimensions of wellness, other than physical?

8. What is meant by the phrase "safer sex"?

Chapter 11
Substances

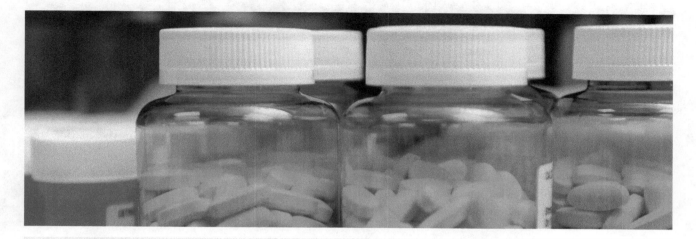

Learning Objectives

1. Define and discuss the concepts of addictive behavior.

2. Describe the major categories of psychoactive drugs.

3. Discuss the short and long-term effects different substances can have on health, including alcohol, tobacco, marijuana, opioids, and caffeine.

4. Describe strategies for drinking alcohol responsibly and in moderation.

5. Discuss how drug abuse can be prevented and treated.

Last night you came home late to find your roommate passed out on the floor with his foot resting in the remnants of what looks to have been a pepperoni pizza. He'd been out with friends and had clearly drank more than he should have. In fact, he reeked of alcohol, had a half-eaten slice of pizza in his hand, and when you tried to wake him he mumbled something about calling his ex-girlfriend (never a good idea). You decided to let him sleep it off right where he was. Fearing he would die the cliché rock-star death and choke on his own vomit, you roll him over on his side and put pillows behind his back. It might be your first term in college, but this isn't your first rodeo. Along with adjusting to classes, homework, and independent life, you've also learned the realities of substance use.

Any substance (other than food) that causes a physiological or chemical change in the body when ingested is considered a drug. Some drugs are used medicinally, but some are used recreationally. You probably use the antihistamine in your bathroom medicinally, while the alcohol your roommate consumed was most definitely recreational. We use the term "substance" collectively in this chapter to refer to alcohol, tobacco, and any drugs that are used in a non-therapeutic manner.

Substance misuse and abuse can have a negative impact on wellness, particularly when the use of these substances results in addiction or dependence. Substance abuse and addictions, including problems with prescription drugs, cost Americans more than $700 billion a year in increased health care costs, crime, and lost productivity. Alcohol, illicit drugs, and prescription drugs contribute to 90,000 deaths every year in the US. An additional 480,000 deaths in the US can be linked to tobacco each year.

This chapter defines what substances are and how they can impact your health. It then introduces the concepts of substance abuse and addiction, focusing on the inherent dangers of substance use that lead to addiction. Then, this chapter examines several different drugs that have addictive properties, addressing the prevalence of addiction and abuse, the short- and long-term effects of each drug, and recovery and treatment options for addiction.

Defining Substances

The terminology seems straight forward, but people often have their own idea of what constitutes a "drug." The FDA defines a **drug** as a "substance intended for use in the diagnosis, cure, mitigation, treatment, or prevention of disease," or a "substance (other than food) intended to affect the structure or any function of the body." By this definition, over-the-counter medicine, prescription medications, and illicit drugs would all qualify. These drugs can be consumed, inhaled, injected, or ingested. Note the word "substance" in the description of a drug. **Substance** is a broader term to encompass anything that impacts your physiology. This includes both legal and illegal drugs, but also things like alcohol, nicotine, and caffeine.

When we hear the words "drug" or "substance," the word "abuse" often follows, or maybe another word with a negative connotation. The association has become common because the misuse and abuse of drugs has become common, but this connotation is due, at least in part, to our loose definitions of what a drug or substance is and what constitutes misuse and abuse.

What Is Misuse?

Not all drug use is harmful. Prescription and over-the-counter medications have a medicinal purpose. If used according to their directions, these drugs can help with any number of psychological and physiological ailments. All substances have the potential to be misused or abused. Think about the cup of coffee you probably consumed with breakfast. It may have helped you wake up a bit, but too much coffee can have negative effects, too.

The line between misuse and abuse can be a bit thin at times, but they are not the same. Many of us have misused a substance at one time or another, probably unintentionally. Not all of us have crossed the line from misuse to abuse.

Your cousin, Dave, recently had his wisdom teeth removed. The oral surgeon gave him a prescription for Oxycodone "just in case" the pain could not be resolved with the extra-strength ibuprofen he also prescribed. The procedure had gone well, and Dave took the ibuprofen for a few days with only a little discomfort. He didn't need the Oxycodone this time, so he decided to save it, "just in case." After all, it's not easy to get pain killers this strong, and he'd heard that people would lie, cheat, and steal to get their hands on it. A few weeks later, Dave had a rotten headache that he couldn't shake, and he reached for the bottle of Oxycodone. This is not the intended use of the prescription drug, and constitutes misuse.

Drug misuse is a broad term. It often involves prescription drugs being used in ways other than they were intended, such as taking a drug for non-medical reasons, taking a drug that was not prescribed for you, or taking a drug at a higher dose than recommended. Examples of drug misuse include taking Vicodin for a headache or Xanax for nausea. This kind of misuse can be a result of people self-diagnosing a problem, or discovering that a prescription drug has side effects that help with something other than its purpose. This is dangerous.

Misuse can happen with any drugs, even those purchased over-the-counter. If you use cold medicine like a sleeping pill, take four acetaminophen at a time instead of two because "you're tall," or chase a few ibuprofen with a beer in anticipation of the headache you plan to have — none of these examples sound like the instructions on the drug's packaging. Drugs come with warnings for a reason — mixing drugs or using them for some other purpose than intended can have dire consequences. The most commonly misused drugs are prescription drugs like opioids (painkillers), depressants (sleeping pills, anti-anxiety medications), and stimulants (ADD medications). These can be misused for many reasons, particularly among teens (Figure 1).

Prescription drug misuse has become a large public health problem. It can lead to addiction and even death from overdose. Being aware of the active ingredients and possible drug interactions is vital to making sure the drugs are safe and effective.

What Is Substance Abuse?

People use many substances for medical and practical reasons. It becomes **substance abuse** when they use substances that are illegal or use legal substances inappropriately. For example, when a person takes drugs for the express purpose of producing pleasure, alleviating stress, and altering or avoiding reality, it's considered abuse. The drug may be used to experience euphoria, relaxation, or otherwise "getting high."

Drugs and other substances capable of such mood-altering feats impact wellness because they often substitute a synthetic, temporary solution for the long-term, natural effects of other wellness-increasing activities. This is why many people will continue to use the substance, regaining the high or low that they desire.

Substance abuse is a harmful pattern of use that persists, continually or intermittently, despite negative consequences. Those negative consequences can include both the harmful effects experienced by the user and those that impact others and their safety. Issues such as drugged or drunk driving, violence, stress, child abuse, homelessness, crime, harm to unborn babies, and job loss are just a few of the ways substance abuse can impact you and those around you.

For example, in many states, marijuana is now legal, but it's still a very commonly abused drug. Your friend praises this plant like it's an organic super-food, a cure for any ailment. But unfortunately, he spent more time "healing" himself than studying last term and failed his math class for the second time. Many drugs are legal, even medicinal, but when one shifts your priorities away from a productive, healthy life, you've entered the realm of abuse. Some other commonly abused drugs include methamphetamine, anabolic steroids, cocaine, heroin, inhalants, opioids (like Oxycodone), and club drugs (like ecstasy).

Substance abuse is a serious public health problem that affects almost every community and family in some way. Each year it causes millions of serious illnesses or injuries among Americans. According to the Drug Abuse Warning Network, 5.1 million people visited the emergency room for drug-related issues in 2011. Nearly half of these visits (49%) occurred because of drug misuse or abuse, with 1.2 million visits due to illicit drugs (Figure 2).

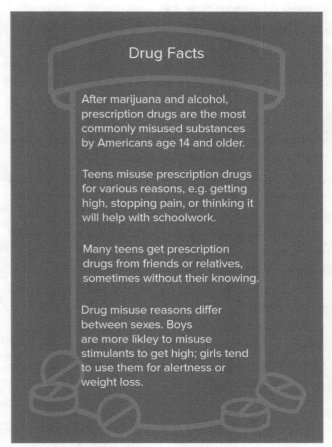

Drug Facts

After marijuana and alcohol, prescription drugs are the most commonly misused substances by Americans age 14 and older.

Teens misuse prescription drugs for various reasons, e.g. getting high, stopping pain, or thinking it will help with schoolwork.

Many teens get prescription drugs from friends or relatives, sometimes without their knowing.

Drug misuse reasons differ between sexes. Boys are more likley to misuse stimulants to get high; girls tend to use them for alertness or weight loss.

Figure 1. Drug misuse is common among teens.

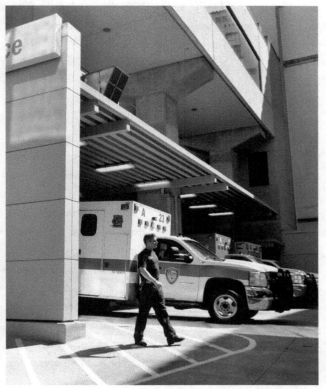

Figure 2. Half of drug-related emergencies are causeed by misuse.

Psychoactive Drugs

Psychoactive drugs are the substances we typically think of when we talk about drugs. **Psychoactive** substances alter the user's mental processes, affecting things like cognition, mood, awareness, and behavior. They act on the central nervous system, modifying the brain's normal, everyday activity and disrupting the communication between neurons (brain cells). Abusing them can have serious short- and long-term effects on the brain.

Psychoactive drugs are classified into four groups: hallucinogens, stimulants, opioids, and depressants. We'll discuss some of these at greater length later in this chapter, but for now, let's look at the basics.

Hallucinogens

The term psychoactive drug might immediately make you think of **hallucinogens**, like LSD and psilocybin mushrooms. Hallucinogens change your brain and behavior in extreme ways. These "psychedelic" drugs (like you might envision from the 1960s), significantly alter the user's perception of reality, including their awareness of surrounding objects and conditions, their thoughts, and their feelings. These cause hallucinations that can be visual, auditory, or even emotional. Hallucinogens are illegal drugs. Some examples include DMT, LSD (D-lysergic acid diethylamide), peyote (mescaline), ayahuasca, and psilocybin (4-phosphoryloxy-N, N-dimethyltryptamine).

Stimulants

Not all psychoactive drugs are illegal, which is one reason we often have difficulty defining "drugs." Stimulants are a good example. A **stimulant** is a substance that increases the physiological and nervous activity of the body. Stimulants can affect alertness, attention, and energy, as well as elevate blood pressure, heart rate, and respiration. Historically, stimulants have been used to treat asthma and other respiratory problems, obesity, neurological disorders, and a variety of other ailments (such as Attention Deficit Disorder). Stimulants increase wakefulness, motivation, and aspects of cognition, learning, and memory. Some can even trigger dopamine releases that give the user a heightened sense of happiness or well-being. Not so bad, right?

Yes and no. Ritalin and Adderall, for example, are stimulants used by prescription for Attention Deficit Disorder. They are also some of the most commonly abused drugs. They can be a great help for someone with a medical need who takes them according to directions, but some people take these drugs to enhance mental performance without the advice of a health care provider. Caffeine and nicotine are other examples of legal stimulants that are commonly abused.

Examples of illegal stimulants include cocaine, amphetamines, and methamphetamines. These probably sound more like "drugs" to you. They can be a much more dangerous substance than your cup of coffee, but all stimulants have the potential to do damage if abused.

Opioids

Opioids are chemicals in the body that help relieve pain by attaching to nerve cells called opioid receptors—they're painkillers. Your body produces some opioids naturally. They act on many places in the brain and nervous system, including the **limbic system**, which controls emotions. Here they can create feelings of pleasure, relaxation, and contentment. Opioids also affect the **brainstem**, which controls things your body does automatically, like breathing. Here they can slow breathing, stop coughing, and reduce feelings of pain. Opioids affect the **spinal cord**, too, which receives sensations from the body before sending them to the brain. Here also they can decrease feelings of pain, even after serious injuries.

The body often does not produce enough to manage serious pain, so pharmaceutical companies manufacture opioids like Vicodin, Oxycodone, or morphine, which health care providers often prescribe to manage pain. These medications act on opioid receptors in both the spinal cord and brain to reduce the intensity of pain-signal perception. They also affect brain areas that control emotion, which can further diminish the effects of painful stimulation. You may have heard these referred to as **narcotics**. Ironically enough, the word "narcotic" comes from the Greek word for "stupor," which should give you a rather large hint about how important it is to follow your health care provider's instructions for these medications. These opioids are a legal form of narcotic, though they are still commonly misused and abused. Examples of illegal opioids include heroin and opium.

Depressants

Central nervous system (CNS) depressants, better known simply as **depressants**, are substances that can slow brain activity. This property makes them useful for treating anxiety, seizures, and sleep disorders. It also makes them commonly misused or abused by individuals looking to relax.

This class of drug includes tranquilizers, sedatives, and hypnotics. Some, like alcohol, sleeping pills (Ambien, Lunesta), Xanax, and Valium are legal when used responsibly. Illegal forms include Rohypnol and GHB, though many other synthetic depressants circulate through illegal channels. Examples include street drugs like barbs, benzos, downers, Liquid X, phennies, or roofies.

Abuse of Psychoactive Substances

Many psychoactive substances have legal uses, but abusing them *is* illegal. That's why the pharmacist asks you for your identification when picking up a prescription for many drugs—using them without medical reason and prescription is against federal and state laws. Abuse of psychoactive drugs is widespread in the US, and rates for some drugs are on the rise (Figure 3).

Abusing prescription drugs is as dangerous as abusing cocaine or heroin. That is one reason why many come with warning labels telling people not to drive or operate heavy machinery. Your brain may not think or respond rationally when under the influence of these substances. Using too much, even of a good thing, can have serious effects on your brain.

Many people like the feeling brought on by even a temporary alteration in the brain—what we call **intoxication**. This is really a type of poisoning, though most individuals seek it for the high or low feeling they experience as a result. It causes a marked reduction in your physical and mental capacities that people often find enjoyable. If you consider other uses for the word "intoxicating," you'll find that we often attach the term to enjoyable things we like to be overwhelmed by, like a comforting aroma or pleasant setting. However, any intoxication we receive from drugs is short-lived and generally followed by unpleasant side effects.

Even legal substances that don't require a prescription have the potential to harm. An excess of caffeine and nicotine, for example, can have significant mood-altering effects. Think about the headache you get when you don't have that daily dose of caffeine or consider the times that you know you've had way too much. You probably didn't feel too great and the people around you probably weren't having much fun either.

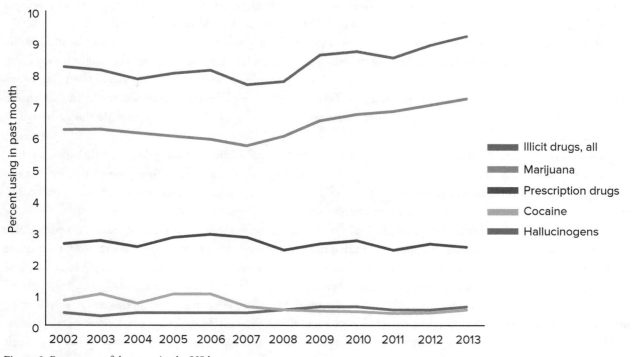

Figure 3. Percentage of drug use in the US by type.

Drug Use Impacts Public Health

The use of substances and illegal drugs has grown into a common problem (Figure 4). Our nation pays a high price in dollars and lives for these misused and abused substances. Abuse of tobacco, alcohol, and illicit drugs exacts more than $740 billion annually in costs related to crime, lost work productivity, and health care. In illness and injury alone, smoking costs approximately $168 billion, alcohol costs $27 billion, illicit drugs cost $11 billion, and prescription opioids cost $26 billion.

Many people die each year from overdose and other injuries sustained due to substance usage. Opioid-related deaths in the US have quadrupled since 1999. Approximately 64,000 people die every year from drug overdose, including 33,000 from opioid overdose, 18,000 of which were from prescription opioids. That could be because as many as 1 in 4 people who receive long-term prescription opioids for non-cancer pain struggle with addiction. There has been a growing trend of "pill mills" and "doctor shopping" to feed this addiction. In the US, non-medical use of these drugs has risen to 12 million people, making them the second most common form of illicit drug use after cannabis in 2010. New data has shown this to be an upward trend, though firm numbers are not yet available.

Type	Health Care	Overall	Year Estimate Based On
Tobacco	$168 Billion	$300 Billion	2010
Alcohol	$27 Billion	$249 Billion	2010
Illicit Drugs	$11 Billion	$193 Billion	2007
Prescription Opioids	$26 Billion	$78.5 Billion	2013

Figure 4. Treatment for drug use and abuse costs billions each year.

Dependence and Addiction

Misuse and abuse can lead to dependence or addiction. **Drug dependence** develops when the neurons in your brain adapt to the repeated drug exposure and can only function normally in the presence of the drug. Your body can develop a **tolerance** for the drug, needing more and more of it to obtain the same effect. This often leads to overdose as users have to take more and more to get high, finally reaching their body's upper threshold. This can occur by accident or by inevitability.

When the drug is withdrawn from their system, users experience a physiological reaction. These can be mild or life threatening depending on the drug and the level of dependency. If you miss that cup of coffee, you might have a lousy headache. But miss a few days of drinking alcohol when your body is dependent, and you may experience vomiting, sweating, agitation, shaking, hallucinations, and even seizures. This is known as **withdrawal syndrome**. In the case of heroin, for example, withdrawal can be very serious, and many users will return to using the drug just to avoid the severe symptoms of withdrawal.

Dependence is a physical condition. Addiction is a disease. The National Institute of Drug Abuse (NIDA) defines drug **addiction** as a chronic, relapsing brain disease that is characterized by compulsive drug seeking and use, despite harmful consequences. Addiction is characterized by an inability to stop using a drug; failure to meet work, social, or family obligations; and, depending on the drug, tolerance to its effects and withdrawal syndrome when it's removed.

Drugs change the structure and function of the brain, which is why we consider addiction a disease. This compulsive behavior can be much like other compulsive disorders in that the addict may be willing to do anything to fulfill their desire for it, even when they're aware that it's detrimental to them or others. The changes in their brain can last a long time and are often why you see and hear about harmful or unusual behaviors in people who abuse drugs.

Physical dependence can happen with the chronic use of many drugs—including many prescription drugs, even if taken as instructed. It doesn't necessarily mean the person will become addicted. Physical dependence does, however, often accompany addiction because the compulsion generally leads to heavier and heavier use of the drug. This distinction can be difficult to understand. People taking prescription painkillers correctly, for example, often need to increase their dosage due to their increased tolerance or underlying medical issues. It does not mean they abuse the drug or will necessarily become addicted.

Understanding Addiction

According to the NIDA, your brain is wired to repeat life-sustaining activities by associating those activities with pleasure or reward. Whenever this reward circuit is activated, the brain notes that something important is happening that needs to be remembered and teaches you to do it again and again without thinking about it. Because abusing drugs stimulates the same circuit, you learn to abuse drugs in the same way.

The NIDA explains that for the brain, the difference between normal rewards and drug rewards can be described as the difference between someone whispering into your ear and someone shouting into a microphone. You turn down the volume on a radio that is too loud. Your brain reacts in a similar manner when it adjusts to the overwhelming surges in dopamine (and other neurotransmitters) caused by drugs. It produces less dopamine or reduces the number of receptors that can receive signals. As a result, dopamine's impact on the reward circuit of the brain of someone who abuses drugs can become abnormally low, and that person's ability to experience *any* pleasure is reduced.

A person who abuses drugs eventually feels flat, lifeless, and depressed, and they may even become unable to enjoy the things they used to. They need to keep taking drugs just to try and bring their dopamine levels back up to normal, which only makes the problem worse. Also, the person will often need to take larger amounts of the drug to produce the familiar dopamine high because their brain has built up a tolerance to the lower amounts.

In general, people initially take drugs voluntarily, but with continued use, a person can have serious difficulty controlling their impulses. This struggle with self-control is a tell-tale sign of addiction. Brain imaging studies of people with addiction show physical changes in areas of the brain that are critical to judgment, decision making, learning, memory, and behavior control.

Many people don't understand why or how other people become addicted to drugs. They may mistakenly think that people who use drugs lack moral principles or willpower and that they could stop their drug use simply by choosing to. In reality, drug addiction is a complex disease, and quitting takes more than good intentions or a strong will. Drugs change the brain in ways that make quitting hard, even for those who want to.

Risk Factors for Addiction

As with any other disease, vulnerability to addiction differs from person to person, and no single factor determines whether a person will become addicted to drugs. In general, the more risk factors a person has, the greater the chance that taking drugs will lead to abuse and addiction. Protective factors, on the other hand, reduce a person's risk of developing addiction. Risk and protective factors may be influenced by:

Biology— Genes account for about half of a person's risk for addiction. Gender, ethnicity, and the presence of other mental disorders may also influence risk for drug use and addiction.

Environment—A person's environment includes many different influences, from family and friends to economic status, and general quality of life. Factors such as peer pressure, physical and sexual abuse, early exposure to drugs, stress, and poor parental guidance can greatly affect a person's likelihood of drug use and addiction.

Development— The earlier that drug use begins, the more likely it will progress to addiction. This is particularly problematic for teens. Because areas in their brains that control decision-making, judgment, and self-control are still developing, teens may be especially prone to risky behaviors, including trying drugs.

Method of Administration— Smoking a drug or injecting it into a vein increases its addictive potential. Both smoked and injected drugs enter the brain within seconds, producing a powerful rush of pleasure. However, this intense "high" can fade within a few minutes, taking the abuser down to lower, more normal levels, leading to more repeated use.

Long-Term Effects on the Brain

The NIDA suggests that the same sort of mechanisms involved in the development of tolerance can eventually lead to profound changes in neurons and brain circuits, with the potential to severely compromise the long-term health of the

The Limbic System

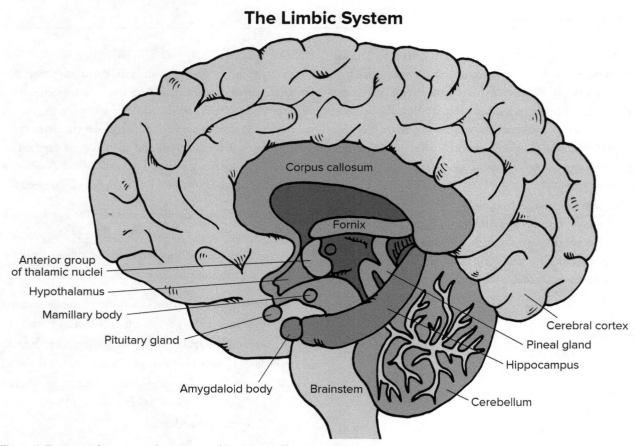

Figure 5. Drugs can have many short-term and long-term affects on the complex anatomy of the brain.

brain (Figure 5). For example, glutamate is a neurotransmitter that influences the reward circuit and the ability to learn. When the optimal concentration of glutamate is altered by drug abuse, the brain attempts to compensate for this change, which can cause impairment in cognitive function.

Long-term drug abuse can also create a type of "muscle memory" or unconscious habit. Constant use can condition the body and brain to expect the behavior and trigger uncontrollable cravings when the person experiences changes in their daily routine. This learned "reflex" is difficult to break and can affect a person who used drugs even after many years of abstinence. Long-term cigarette smokers, for example, often crave not only the nicotine, but also the feel of the cigarette in their fingers and mouth — they will often use pencils or other similar objects to keep their hands busy and mimic the behavior even after the nicotine cravings have passed.

Though this chapter is about substance abuse primarily, it is important to note that you can become addicted to many things, such as gambling, Internet usage, work, exercise, sex, and so on. These are called **process addictions**, or behavioral addictions. Anything capable of stimulating your brain can be addictive. Whenever a habit becomes an obligation — the

person must complete it fulfill a need — it becomes an addiction. How many times have you watched a friend stay up all night playing videogames with an excuse that their online community "needed them?" How many times have you become anxious because you didn't have your phone? These seem minor initially, but over time they can become significant.

Addiction is a lot like other diseases, such as heart disease. Both disrupt the normal, healthy functioning of the underlying organ, have serious harmful consequences, and are preventable and treatable. But, if left untreated, they addiction and the consequences can last a lifetime.

Drug Addiction Impacts Mental Health

Chronic use of some drugs can lead to both short- and long-term changes in the brain, which can lead to mental health issues including paranoia, depression, anxiety, aggression, hallucinations, and the impairment of cognitive function. People with substance addictions often have a diagnosis of mental illness as well. Compared with the general population, people addicted to drugs are roughly twice as likely to suffer from mood and anxiety disorders, with the reverse also true.

In 2015, an estimated 43.4 million (17.9%) adults age

18 and older experienced some form of mental illness (other than a developmental disorder). Of these, 8.1 million had both a substance use disorder and another mental illness. Although substance use disorders commonly occur with other mental illnesses, it's often unclear whether one helped cause the other or if common underlying risk factors contribute to both disorders.

Signs of Drug Dependency or Addiction

Drug dependency and addiction have some common symptoms. You may notice increased drug-seeking behaviors or irritability, anxiety, depression, and restlessness, particularly when the drug is not available. Other symptoms or behaviors include:

- Feeling that you have to use the drug regularly — whether daily or several times throughout the day

- Having intense urges for the drug

- Needing more and more of the drug to get the same effect

- Making sure that you maintain a supply of the drug

- Spending money on the drug, even when you can't afford it

- Not meeting obligations and work responsibilities, or cutting back on social or recreational activities because of drug use

- Doing things to get the drug that you normally wouldn't do, such as stealing or prostitution

- Driving or doing other risky activities when you're under the influence of the drug

- Focusing more and more time and energy on getting and using the drug

- Trying to quit and failing

- Experiencing withdrawal symptoms when you attempt to stop taking the drug

Drug Addiction Treatment

As with most other chronic diseases, such as diabetes, asthma, or heart disease, treatment for drug addiction generally isn't a cure. However, addiction can be treated and successfully managed. People recovering from an addiction will be at risk for relapse for years and possibly for their whole lives. Research shows that combining addiction treatment medicines with behavioral therapy ensures the best chance of success for most patients. Treatment approaches tailored to each patient's drug use patterns and any co-occurring medical, mental, and social problems can lead to continued recovery.

Treatment involves many steps, depending upon the nature of the drug and the level of addiction. This could include detoxification (ridding the body of the drug), behavioral therapy and counseling, assessment of any co-existing mental illness, and long-term monitoring. With severe dependence, some drugs have potentially lethal withdrawal symptoms that require a person trying to break their dependence to seek medical intervention. Sometimes drugs need to be used as well to help ease withdrawal symptoms. Methadone, for example, is often used to treat heroin addiction because it provides a similar effect on the body as the opiate (though legal) and allows treatment centers to wean the person off the illicit drug.

Results from NIDA-funded research have shown that prevention programs involving families, schools, communities, and the media prove effective at preventing or reducing drug use and addiction. Although personal events and cultural factors affect drug use trends, when young people view drug use as harmful, they tend to decrease their drug use rates. Therefore, education and outreach from teachers, parents, health care providers, and cultural influencers are key in helping people understand the possible risks of drug use.

Addiction and Dependence Stigma

Like many mental health issues, addiction can be hard for people who don't experience it to understand. They want the person to "choose" to quit or "suck it up," not realizing that it's just not that simple. They can also grow frustrated or hurt. A person with addiction is hard to predict, will do and say hurtful things, and be compelled by their addiction to make decisions that harm themselves and others. Treatment is labor-intensive and can take a long time, which can be frustrating for the close friends or family of someone with addiction. It can take a depth of patience to help an addict that many people just don't have.

People often worry over whether addiction is a disease or a result of choices. Addiction often occurs amidst a perfect storm of genetic predisposition (disease) and environmental factors. The compulsive behavior of a person with addiction tells us that they have limited control of their actions and their choices are more in line with the kind of choices a person with bipolar disorder or acute social anxiety might make. To make different choices, a person suffering from bipolar disorder needs lifelong treatment and can expect to suffer episodes despite treatment, which appears similar to what we see among people suffering from addiction.

Alcohol

People most often think of "hard" illegal drugs like crystal meth and heroin when they think of substance abuse. As we've covered so far there are a wide variety of substances, many of which are legal for over-the-counter medical and recreational use. Alcohol is one of the most common addictive substances.

You probably understand why people drink—it's usually to socialize, celebrate, or relax. Some people drink to the point of sedation in a futile attempt to manage a seemingly unmanageable problem. Alcohol often has a strong effect on people—and throughout history, we've struggled to understand and manage alcohol's power. Why does alcohol cause us to act and feel differently? How much is too much? Considering how common drinking alcohol is, why do some people become addicted while others do not (Figure 6)?

Here's what we know. Alcohol's effects vary from person to person, depending on a variety of factors, such as how much and how often you drink, your age, your biological gender, your health, and your family history. While drinking alcohol is not necessarily a problem for everyone—drinking too much can cause a range of consequences and increase your risk for a variety of problems.

Age	Lifetime Abstainer	Former Regular	Current Regular
16–44	22.3%	3.3%	56.6%
45–64	16.7%	7.6%	51.8%
65–74	21.8%	10.4%	41.6%
75+	30.9%	12.3%	29.6%

Figure 6. Alcohol use is common throughout life.

Alcohol Content

First, let's take a look at what's actually in alcoholic drinks. **Ethyl alcohol** (ethanol) is the alcohol such as beer or wine. It's made from the fermentation or chemical breakdown of sugars by yeasts, using plants and grains such as corn, wheat, and barley, or grapes (for wine). Ethanol can be produced by milling the grains and then fermenting them with yeast (wine is similar but requires the grapes to be stored under the right conditions). During the fermentation process, the starches of the grains (or the sugar in the grapes) are turned into alcohol.

Alcoholic drinks come in two types—fermented and distilled. Examples of fermented drinks include beer, malt liquor, wine, cider, mead, etc. Beer and cider have a lower alcohol content by volume (usually below 10%) than wine and mead (which can get up to 20% in the case of fortified wines and some meads) (Figure 7). Distilled alcohols basically take fermented alcohol and refine it by a process called distillation, which uses heat to remove water from the original source to create a drink with higher alcohol percentage (usually 40% or more). This percentage is taken when the alcohol is at 60 degrees Fahrenheit and multiplied by two—this is the alcohol's "proof." Examples of distilled alcohol are vodka, whiskey, tequila, and rum.

Regular Beer (5% alc/vol)	Malt Liquor (7% alc/vol)	Table Wine (12% alc/vol)	80-proof Distilled Spirits (40% alc/vol)
12 fl oz = 1 16 fl oz = 1 ⅓ 22 fl oz = 2 40 fl oz = 3 ⅓	12 fl oz = 1.5 16 fl oz = 2 22 fl oz = 2.5 40 fl oz = 4.5	750 ml (a regular wine bottle) = 5	a shot (1.5-oz glass/50-ml bottle=1) a mixed drink or cocktail = 1 or more 200 ml (a "half pint") = 4.5 375 ml (a "pint" or "half bottle") = 8.5 750 ml (a "fifth") = 17

Figure 7. Common alcohol containers and how many equivalent "drinks" they each contain.

The Effects of Alcohol on the Body

As soon as you take a drink, the alcohol enters your stomach and small intestine. Small blood vessels carry it from these organs into the bloodstream. Approximately 20% of alcohol is absorbed through the stomach, and most of the remaining 80% is absorbed through the small intestine. Enzymes in the liver then break down the alcohol.

Understanding the rate of metabolism is critical to understanding the effects of alcohol. For the average person, the liver processes one standard drink in one hour. Consume any more than this, and your system becomes saturated. The additional alcohol will accumulate in the blood and body tissues until it can be metabolized. This is why drinking large amounts quickly (like taking shots and playing drinking games) can result in high **blood alcohol concentrations** (BAC) that last for several hours, causing drunkenness and potentially risky behavior. BAC is the amount of alcohol in your blood by volume. Driving with a blood alcohol concentration of .08% or more, for example, is considered dangerous and illegal (Figure 8).

The effects of alcohol can be felt as quickly as 5–10 minutes after you begin drinking. Your mood and thought processes become altered, your kidneys have to work overtime, and with a high enough BAC your breathing can slow, you can lose consciousness, or even die (Figure 9).

Not everyone metabolizes alcohol the same. There are different factors that affect the way your body processes alcohol that have a direct impact on our BAC, such as:

Age—The amount of water in your body goes down with age, which affects your body's metabolism process. You also have lower muscle mass with age, and muscle absorbs alcohol.

Biological sex—Women have higher BAC's after consuming the same amount of alcohol as men. This has been attributed to women's smaller amount of body water, lower muscle mass, and lower activity of alcohol-metabolizing enzymes in the stomach, causing a larger proportion of the ingested alcohol to reach the blood.

Weight—In general, people who weigh less have less water in their bodies and are able to drink less.

Physical fitness level—The health of your liver, your hydration level, and the amount of fat in your body affect alcohol metabolism. If you're in better physical health, your body metabolizes it more efficiently.

Number of Drinks		Body Weight in Pounds								Driving Condition
		100	120	140	160	180	200	220	240	
0	Male	.00	.00	.00	.00	.00	.00	.00	.00	Only Safe Driving Limit
	Female	.00	.00	.00	.00	.00	.00	.00	.00	
1	Male	.06	.05	.04	.04	.03	.03	.03	.02	Driving Skills Impaired
	Female	.07	.06	.05	.04	.04	.03	.03	.03	
2	Male	.12	.10	.09	.07	.07	.06	.05	.05	
	Female	.13	.11	.09	.08	.07	.07	.06	.06	
3	Male	.18	.15	.13	.11	.10	.09	.08	.07	
	Female	.20	.17	.14	.12	.11	.10	.09	.08	Legally Intoxicated
4	Male	.24	.20	.17	.15	.13	.12	.11	.10	
	Female	.26	.22	.19	.17	.15	.13	.12	.11	
5	Male	.30	.25	.21	.19	.17	.15	.14	.12	
	Female	.33	.28	.24	.21	.18	.17	.15	.14	

Subtract .01% for each 40 minutes of drinking.
1 drink = 1.5 oz. 80 proof liquor, 12 oz. 5% beer, or 5 oz. 12% wine.
Fewer than 5 persons out of 100 will exceed these values.

Figure 8. Blood alcohol concentrations by number of drinks, weight, and gender.

BAC Level	Effects
0.02	Light to moderate drinkers begin to feel relaxed.
0.04	Most drinkers begin to feel relaxed.
0.06	Judgment is impaired. Legally drunk in some states.
0.08	Judgment is further impaired. More likely to do things that you would not do when sober. Legally drunk in all states.
0.10	Reaction time and muscle control are impaired. A person drinking at this level is 10x more likely to cause a fatal car crash. Normal social drinkers rarely reach this level.
0.12	Vomiting for most people.
0.15	Balance and movement are substantially impaired. Difficulty walking or talking. Heavy drinkers with substantial tolerance may learn to look sober at this level. One half-pint of whiskey is circulating in the blood stream. 25x more likely to cause a fatal car crash.
0.20	Blackout and memory loss. A person driving at this level is 100x more likely to cause a fatal car crash.
0.30	Loss of consciousness and passing out. Being able to remain conscious at this level indicates a tolerance that is a serious risk factor for health problems.
0.40–0.60	FATAL: Causes paralysis to brain area that controls breathing and heart rate. This can happen when someone drinks a lot, passes out and the alcohol in the stomach continues to be absorbed into the blood stream. Drinking contests are frequent cause of lethal overdose.

Figure 9. Blood alcohol concentrations and their effects.

Eating before drinking—Drinking alcohol after a meal that includes fat, protein, and carbohydrates allows the body to absorb the alcohol about 3 times more slowly than when alcohol is consumed on an empty stomach.

Drinking quickly—The faster you drink, the higher your BAC.

Using drugs or prescription medicines—Certain medications can speed up the feeling of intoxication or can have dangerous affects when mixed with alcohol.

Knowing how much alcohol constitutes a "standard" drink can help you determine how much you are drinking and understand the associated risks. One standard drink contains about 0.6 fluid ounces or 14 grams of pure alcohol, but drinks come in different sizes and their relative content is not always easy to identify without help (Figure 10).

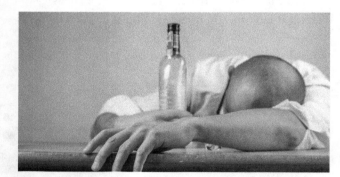

Figure 10. Binge drinking often results in "passing out."

Consequences of Drinking Too Much

The higher your BAC, the more impaired you become by alcohol's effects. These effects can be short-term, including reduced inhibitions, slurred speech, confusion, motor impairment, blacking out, and risky or violent behaviors. It can lead you to overeat (get the munchies), get into arguments, drunk-dial former love interests, and say things you don't mean and do things you wouldn't normally do.

One of the first consequences that comes to mind about the effects of alcohol is the notorious hangover! A hangover is largely the result of dehydration. Alcohol consumption leads to increased urination, which leads to less water in the body. This makes your mouth dry and your head ache (Figure 11). Alcohol also causes your blood sugar to fall, which can result in that weak, tired, and shaky feeling. Some alcohols also contain other chemicals that can lead to headaches and irritate your stomach lining. Some champagnes, for example, have arsenic to make them bubble. Even some of the chemicals that naturally form during the fermentation process can contribute to that miserable feeling of having socks on your teeth and a pounding in your brain. This is typically resolved within a day with water intake, sleep, and over-the-counter headache medicine.

But there are other consequences that can be quite serious and can occur from even one night of heavy drinking. These can be the direct physical result of a high BAC or the indirect result of a decreased mental capacity. These include alcohol poisoning, coma, unintended pregnancy, sexual abuse, breathing problems, and death, including suicide and homicide. Car crashes and other accidents, often fatal, are quite common. Alcohol-related crashes alone account for over 10,000 deaths per year.

People who drink too much over a long period of time may experience long-term effects that can significantly impact their health, such as:

Alcohol use disorder (**AUD**)—This is a chronic relapsing brain disease characterized by compulsive alcohol use, loss of control over alcohol intake, and a negative emotional state when not using. AUD may result in Wernicke-Korsakoff syndrome, a brain disorder due to thiamine (vitamin B1) deficiency. Lack of vitamin B1 is common in people with alcohol use disorder.

Heart disease—Drinking a high amount over a long time or too much on a single occasion can damage the heart, causing problems including cardiomyopathy, arrhythmias, stroke, and high blood pressure.

Liver damage—Heavy drinking takes a toll on the liver and can lead to liver inflammations, including steatosis (fatty liver), alcoholic hepatitis, fibrosis (thickening or scarring), and cirrhosis (Figure 12).

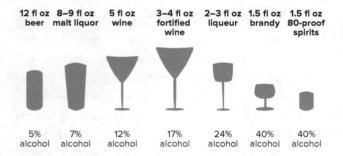

12 fl oz beer	8–9 fl oz malt liquor	5 fl oz wine	3–4 fl oz fortified wine	2–3 fl oz liqueur	1.5 fl oz brandy	1.5 fl oz 80-proof spirits
5% alcohol	7% alcohol	12% alcohol	17% alcohol	24% alcohol	40% alcohol	40% alcohol

Figure 11. Common serving sizes of different types of alcohol.

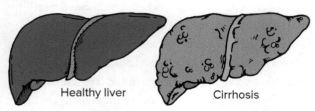

Figure 12. A liver affected by cirrhosis can't function properly.

Pancreas damage—Alcohol causes the pancreas to produce toxic substances that can eventually lead to pancreatitis, a dangerous inflammation and swelling of the blood vessels in the pancreas that prevents proper digestion.

Cancer—Drinking too much alcohol can increase your risk of developing certain cancers, including cancers of the mouth, esophagus, throat, liver, and breast.

Compromised immune system—Excessive alcohol use can weaken your immune system. Chronic drinkers are more likely to contract diseases like pneumonia and tuberculosis than people who do not drink too much. Drinking a lot on a single occasion slows your body's ability to ward off infections—even up to 24 hours after getting drunk.

Excessive Drinking and Public Health

Excessive alcohol use leads to approximately 88,000 deaths and 2.5 million years of potential life lost each year in the US from 2006–2010, shortening the lives of those who died by an average of 30 years. Further, excessive drinking was responsible for 1 in 10 deaths among working-age adults aged 20–64 years. The economic costs of excessive alcohol consumption in 2010 were estimated at $249 billion.

But when does drinking become excessive? When do we cross the line from fun, responsible drinking toward something dangerous and unhealthy? For women, **low-risk drinking** is defined as no more than 3 drinks on any single day and no more than 7 drinks per week. For men, it is defined as no more than 4 drinks on any single day and no more than 14 drinks per week (Figure 13). Research shows that only about 2 in 100 people who drink within these limits have AUD.

On the other hand, binge drinking is the most common, costly, and deadly pattern of excessive alcohol use in the US. Three-quarters of the total cost of alcohol misuse is related to

	Safe limit on any **single day**	Safe limit in any **single week**
Women	3 🍸🍸🍸	7 🍸🍸🍸🍸🍸🍸🍸
Men	4 🍸🍸🍸🍸	14 🍸🍸🍸🍸🍸🍸🍸 🍸🍸🍸🍸🍸🍸🍸

Figure 13. Low-risk drinking has strict limits.

binge drinking. The National Institute on Alcohol Abuse and Alcoholism defines **binge drinking** as a pattern of drinking that brings a person's blood alcohol concentration (BAC) to 0.08% or above. This typically happens when men consume 5 or more drinks or women consume 4 or more drinks in about two hours. However, most people who binge drink are not alcohol dependent. When done on a regular basis, long-term effects can set in, even for younger individuals like college students (Figure 14).

Binge drinking is a major public health problem. 1 in 6 US adults binge drink about four times a month, consuming about 8 drinks per binge. Binge drinking is most common among younger adults aged 18–34 years, but is reported into higher age groups. It's twice as prevalent among men than women. Binge drinking is more common among people with household incomes of $75,000 or more than among people with lower incomes. People with lower incomes binge drink in lower numbers, but those that do binge more often and consume more drinks. Over 90% of US adults who drink excessively report binge drinking in the past 30 days. Most people younger than age 21 who drink report binge drinking, usually on multiple occasions.

Heavy drinking is defined as consuming 8 or more drinks per week for women and 15 or more for men. In short, the more drinks on any day and the more heavy-drinking days over time, the greater the risk—not only for an alcohol use disorder, but also for other health and personal problems. About 1 in 4 people who exceed these limits already have an alcohol use disorder, and the rest are at greater risk for developing these and the other problems in this chapter.

Alcohol Poisoning

Some people getting a kick out of watching people get drunk. Some think it's even funnier when a person passes out from drinking. But there is nothing funny about that person then vomiting while unconscious and suffocating on their own vomit. Neither is the poisoning of the respiratory center in the brain very funny. Both of which can result in death.

Everyone should know about the dangers of an alcohol overdose—also referred to as **alcohol poisoning**. Sadly enough, too many college students say they wish they had sought medical treatment for someone they thought was just drunk. Many end up feeling responsible for alcohol-related tragedies that could have easily been prevented.

Common myths about sobering up include drinking black coffee, taking a cold bath or shower, sleeping it off, or walking it

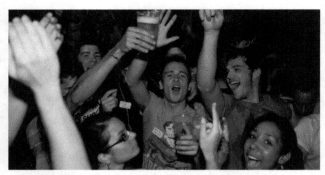

Figure 14. College campuses are known for binge-drinking.

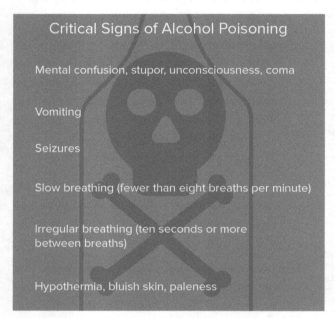

Critical Signs of Alcohol Poisoning

Mental confusion, stupor, unconsciousness, coma

Vomiting

Seizures

Slow breathing (fewer than eight breaths per minute)

Irregular breathing (ten seconds or more between breaths)

Hypothermia, bluish skin, paleness

Figure 15. Be aware of these signs that indicate someone may have alcohol poisoning.

off. These are just myths, and they don't work. The only thing that reverses the effects of alcohol is time—something you may not have if you are suffering from an alcohol overdose. And many different factors affect the level of intoxication of an individual, so it's difficult to gauge exactly how much is too much.

Alcohol depresses nerves that control involuntary actions, such as breathing and the gag reflex (which prevents choking). A fatal dose of alcohol will eventually stop these functions. It is common for someone who drank excessive alcohol to vomit since alcohol is an irritant to the stomach. There is then the danger of choking on vomit, which could cause death by asphyxiation in a person who is not conscious.

You should also know that a person's BAC can continue to rise even while he or she is passed out. Even after a person stops drinking, alcohol in the stomach and intestine continues to enter the bloodstream and circulate throughout the body.

It is dangerous to assume the person will be fine by sleeping it off. Here are the signs you should watch out for. If anyone around you is drinking to the point of any of these symptoms, seek medical assistance (Figure 15).

If you suspect someone is having an alcohol overdose, call 911. Don't try to handle it on your own. An alcohol overdose can lead to irreversible brain damage. Rapid binge drinking (which often happens on a bet or a dare) is especially dangerous because the victim can ingest a fatal dose before even becoming unconscious (Figure 16).

Some people should never drink alcohol, even if their usage is considered low-risk. Low-risk does not mean no risk.

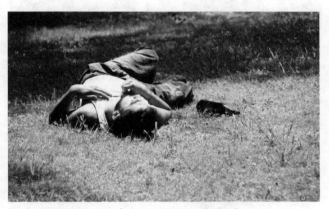

Figure 16. Passing out from drinking is always dangerous.

According to the US Dietary Guidelines, the following groups of people should not drink at all (Figure 17).

Alcohol and Sexual Activity

Any person of any gender or sexual orientation can be impacted by the combination of sex and alcohol. We frequently hear about sexual assault, particularly on college campuses and there are many factors to consider for everyone involved. When sex and alcohol are combined, there is an increased risk that you could make unwanted or unintended sexual advances toward someone, participate in unwanted or unintended sex, experience sexual assault, be accused of sexual assault, even if you thought it was consensual, have unprotected sex, leading to pregnancy or an STI or both, and have sex with multiple partners.

There are certain things you aren't legally allowed to do while you are drinking, such as get a tattoo, drive, or get married. There is a good reason for this—you're impaired and unable to make a rational decision on an important issue. Add sex to the list. If someone is drinking, they are not capable of making the decision about whether or not to engage in sexual activity safely, if at all. End of discussion. If they agree to it while intoxicated, they aren't really agreeing with their full awareness, and if you are also intoxicated, your ability to interpret their intentions is also compromised.

Drinking among College Students

College students and heavy alcohol use have coexisted for many years. When was the last time that you watched a movie about college life that didn't highlight at least some elements of the party life? There aren't many, and if they exist, they aren't very realistic. Your friend passed out on the floor of your apartment? That happens more often than we care to admit. College students are known for excessive drinking, particularly those at four-year universities.

Drinking at college has become a ritual that students often see as an integral part of their higher education experience (Figure 18). In fact, it has become so commonplace that we tend to normalize it or make light of it, which underestimates the severity of the issue. Many students come to college with established drinking habits, and the college environment can exacerbate the problem. According to a national survey, almost 60% of college students age 18–22 drank alcohol during any given month, and 2 in every 3 of those engaged in binge

drinking during that same timeframe.

Although the majority of students come to college already having some experience with alcohol, certain aspects of college life, such as unstructured time, the widespread availability of alcohol, inconsistent enforcement of underage drinking laws, and limited interactions with parents and other adults, can intensify the problem. In fact, college students have higher binge-drinking rates and a higher incidence of driving under the influence of alcohol than their non-college peers. The dangers of college drinking include the following annual statistics:

Death—About 1,825 college students between 18–24 die from alcohol-related, unintentional injuries, including motor vehicle crashes every year.

Assault—About 696,000 students between 18–24 are assaulted by another student who has been drinking every year.

Anyone under age 21

 People of any age who are unable to restrict their drinking to moderate levels

 Women who may become pregnant or who are pregnant

 People who plan to drive, operate machinery, or take part in other activities that require attention, skill, or coordination

 People taking prescriptions or over-the-counter medications that can interact with alcohol

Figure 17. Some groups of people should never drink alcohol.

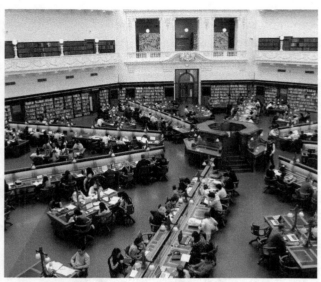

Figure 18. Drinking in college is almost as common as studying.

Sexual Assault—About 97,000 students between 18–24 report experiencing alcohol-related sexual assault or date rape every year.

Academic Problems—About 1 in 4 college students report academic consequences from drinking, including missing class, falling behind in class, doing poorly on exams or papers, and receiving lower grades overall, particularly those who binged.

Alcohol Use Disorder (AUD)—About 20% of college students meet the criteria for AUD.

Other Consequences—These include suicide attempts, health problems, injuries, unsafe sex, and driving under the influence of alcohol, as well as vandalism, property damage, and involvement with the police.

Women and Alcohol Use

An estimated 5.3 million women in the US regularly drink in a way that threatens their health, safety, and general well-being (Figure 19). Earlier in this chapter, you learned how the physiological differences between men and women impact their metabolism of alcohol. Between the lower muscle mass, differences in enzymes, and lower body water (lower body weight), women generally can (or should) consume less alcohol. Because of their physical make-up, a woman's brain and other organs are exposed to more alcohol and to more of the toxic byproducts that result when the body breaks down and eliminates alcohol. This makes them more at risk for motor vehicle crashes, other injuries, high blood pressure, liver damage, cardiovascular disease, brain injury, stroke, violence, suicide, and certain types of cancer.

Research suggests that as little as one drink per day can slightly raise the risk of breast cancer in some women, especially those who are postmenopausal or have a family history of breast cancer. It is not possible, however, to predict how alcohol will affect the risk for breast cancer in any one woman.

It's important to highlight that drinking makes young women more vulnerable to sexual assault and unsafe and unplanned sex. On college campuses, assaults, unwanted sexual advances, and unplanned and unsafe sex are all more likely among students who drink heavily on occasion. In general, when a woman drinks to excess, she is more likely to be a target of violence or sexual assault.

Alcohol Use and Pregnancy

There is no known safe amount of alcohol use during pregnancy or while trying to get pregnant. All types of alcohol are equally harmful, including all wines and beer. Women also should not drink alcohol if they are sexually active and do not use effective birth control. This is because a woman might get pregnant and expose her baby to alcohol before she knows she is pregnant. When a pregnant woman drinks alcohol (Figure 20), so does her baby.

These recommendations from the CDC may sound extreme, but the risks to an unborn child really are that high. Nearly half of all pregnancies in the US are unplanned. Most

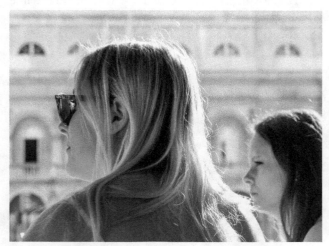

Figure 19. Women who may become pregnant should avoid drinking alcohol.

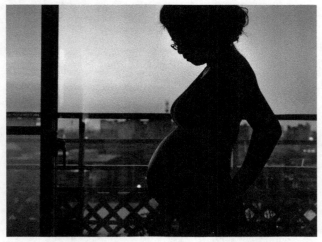

Figure 20. Women who are pregnant shouldn't drink at all.

women will not know they are pregnant for up to 4–6 weeks from the time of conception.

Alcohol in the mother's blood passes to the baby through their umbilical cord. Drinking alcohol during pregnancy can cause miscarriage, stillbirth, and a range of lifelong physical, behavioral, and intellectual disabilities. These disabilities are known as **fetal alcohol spectrum disorders** (FASDs). Children with FASDs may not present sypmtoms at birth, but they might have the following characteristics and behaviors later in life:

- Abnormal facial features, such as a smooth ridge between the nose and upper lip

- Small head size

- Smaller-than-average height and weight

- Poor coordination, memory, reasoning, and judgment skills

- Hyperactive behavior or difficulty with attention

- Difficulty in school (especially with math)

- Learning and intellectual disabilities or low IQ

- Speech and language delays

- Sleep and sucking problems as a baby

- Vision or hearing problems

- Problems with the heart, kidney, or bones

FASD is most likely to occur in infants whose mothers drank heavily (3 or more drinks per occasion or more than 7 drinks per week) and continued to drink heavily throughout pregnancy. It can also occur even with lesser amounts like moderate usage of one drink per day. If you find out you are pregnant and have been drinking, it is important to stop immediately, see your health care provider, and begin prenatal care.

Alcohol Abuse

Problem drinking that becomes severe is given the medical diagnosis of **alcohol use disorder**, or AUD. AUD is a chronic relapsing brain disease characterized by compulsive alcohol use, loss of control over alcohol intake, and a negative emotional state when not using.

An estimated 16 million people in the US have AUD. In 2015 alone, approximately 6.2%, or 15.1 million adults

ages 18 and older had AUD. This includes 9.8 million men and 5.3 million women. Adolescents can be diagnosed with AUD as well, and in 2015, an estimated 623,000 adolescents ages 12–17 had AUD.

Anyone meeting any two of the eleven criteria during the same 12-month period receives a diagnosis of AUD. The severity of AUD—mild, moderate, or severe—is based on the number of criteria met. To assess whether you or loved one may have AUD, here are some questions to ask (Figure 21).

If you have any of these symptoms, your drinking may already be a cause for concern. The more symptoms you have, the more urgent the need for change. A health care professional can conduct a formal assessment of your symptoms to see if AUD is present.

However severe the problem may seem, most people with AUD can benefit from treatment. Unfortunately, less than ten % of people with AUD receive any treatment. Ultimately, receiving treatment can improve an individual's chances of success in overcoming AUD.

Treatment for Alcohol Abuse

Many people struggle with controlling their drinking at some time in their lives. Millions of adults have AUD, and 1 in 10 children live in a home with a parent who has a drinking problem.

There's good news. No matter how severe the problem may seem, most people benefit from some form of treatment. Research suggests that about one-third of people who are treated for alcohol problems have no further symptoms 1 year later. Many others substantially reduce their drinking and report fewer alcohol-related problems.

It's not all 12-step programs or 28-day inpatient rehab any more. In fact, there are a variety of treatment methods currently available, thanks to significant advances in the field over the past 60 years. Ultimately, there is no one-size-fits-all solution, and what may work for one person may not be a good fit for someone else. Simply understanding the different options can be an important first step.

Behavioral treatments are aimed at changing drinking behavior through counseling. Mutual-support groups like Alcoholics Anonymous (AA) and other 12-step programs provide peer support for people quitting or cutting back on their drinking. Combined with treatment led by health professionals, mutual-support groups can offer a valuable added layer of support. In addition, there are 3 medications approved in the US to help people stop or reduce their drinking and prevent relapse. These are prescribed by a health care provider and may be used alone or in combination with counseling.

Overcoming an alcohol use disorder is an ongoing process, one that can include setbacks. Because an alcohol use disorder can be a chronic relapsing disease, persistence is key. It is rare that someone would go to treatment once and then never drink again. More often, people must repeatedly try to quit or cut back, experience recurrences, learn from them, and then keep trying. For many, continued follow-up with a treatment provider is critical to overcoming problem drinking, as are mental health services for those suffering from coexisting mental illness.

People with drinking problems are most likely to relapse during periods of stress or when exposed to people or places associated with past drinking. Just as some people with diabetes

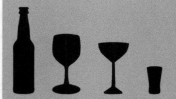

In the past year, have you:

Had times when you ended up drinking more, or longer than you intended?

More than once wanted to cut down or stop drinking, or tried to, but couldn't?

Spent a lot of time drinking? Or being sick or getting over the after effects?

Experienced craving — a strong need, or urge, to drink?

Found that drinking — or being sick from drinking — interfered with taking care of your home or family? Or caused job troubles? Or school problems?

Continued to drink even though is was causing trouble with your family or friends?

Given up or cut back on activities that were important or interesting to you, or gave you pleasure, in order to drink?

More than once gotten into situations while or after drinking that increased your chances of getting hurt (such as driving, swimming, using machinery, walking in a dangerous area,or having unsafe sex)?

Continued to drink even though it was making you feel depressed or anxious or adding to another health problem? Or after having a memory blackout?

Had to drink much more than you once did to get the effectyou want? Or found that your usual number of drinks hadmuch less effect than before?

Found that when the effects of alcohol were wearing off you had withdrawal symptoms, such as trouble sleeping, shakiness, irritability, anxiety, depression, restlessness, nausea, or sweating? Or sensed things that were not there?

Figure 21. If you answer yes to 2 or more of these questions, you may have AUD.

or asthma may have flare-ups of their disease, a relapse to drinking can be seen as a temporary set-back to full recovery and not a complete failure.

Seeking professional help can prevent relapse—behavioral therapies can help people develop skills to avoid and overcome triggers, such as stress, that might lead to drinking. Most people benefit from regular checkups with a treatment provider. Medications also can deter drinking during times when individuals may be at greater risk of relapse (e.g., divorce, death of a family member).

Alcohol Treatment Resources

- Al-Anon: www.al-anon.org/

- Center for Substance Abuse Treatment: www.samhsa.gov/about-us/who-we-are/offices-centers/csat or call 1-800-662-HELP (4357)

- Narconon: narconon.org/drug-rehab/alcoholic-family.html or call 1-888-391-7310

Tobacco and Nicotine

Tobacco use is the leading cause of preventable disease and death in the US, accounting for more than 480,000 deaths every year, or one of every five deaths. In 2015, about 15% of adults aged 18 years or older currently smoked cigarettes. This means an estimated 36.5 million adults in the US currently smoke cigarettes (Figure 22). With these numbers, it's not hard to imagine why more than 16 million Americans live with a smoking-related disease. Smoking causes many different cancers as well as chronic lung diseases, such as emphysema and bronchitis, heart disease, pregnancy-related problems, and many other serious health problems.

Tobacco is a leafy plant grown around the world. Four countries—China, Brazil, India, and the US—produce approximately two-thirds of the world's tobacco. Tobacco is currently grown in 16 US states. The largest tobacco-producing states are Kentucky and North Carolina. They account for 71% of all tobacco grown in the US.

Dried tobacco leaves can be consumed in several forms: shredded and smoked in cigarettes, cigars, and pipes, ground into snuff, which is sniffed through the nose, cured and made into chewing tobacco, moistened, ground, or shredded into dip, which is placed in the mouth between the lip and gum.

Each day, more than 3,200 people under 18 smoke their first cigarette, and approximately 2,100 youth and young adults become daily smokers. 9 out of 10 smokers start before the age of 18, and 98% start smoking by age 26. One in five adults and teenagers smoke. Men (16.7%) smoke more than women (13.6%). From 1964–2014, the proportion of adult smokers declined from 42.0% to 18.0%. Adults aged 25–44 smoke the most, followed closely by adults aged 45–64. American Indians and Alaskan Natives are more likely to smoke (21.9%) compared to whites and blacks (approximately 16%), Hispanics (10%), and Asians (7%). People in the Midwest are most likely to smoke (18.7%), followed by the South (15.3%), Northeast (13.5%), and West (12.7%). People living below the federal poverty level are among the highest population of smokers.

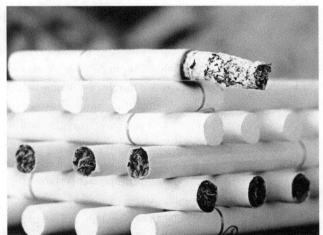

Figure 22. Cigarettes are a common source of nicotine.

Cigarette Content

Tobacco smoke contains a deadly mix of more than 7,000 chemicals. Around 93 are harmful and potentially harmful. These include nicotine, cadmium, lead, ammonia, carbon monoxide, arsenic, chromium, hydrogen cyanide, mercury, and formaldehyde. And these are just the chemicals that sounded familiar. Formaldehyde is commonly used by morticians as a preservative in the process of preparing bodies for burial—not something you should be looking to put in your body while you're still alive.

Some tobacco products also contain additives used to enhance their flavor. Menthol is a flavor additive widely used in consumer and medicinal products. However, its use in tobacco products is not currently regulated. It has a minty taste and aroma, and may have cooling or painkilling properties—which can reduce the irritation and harshness of smoking when used in cigarettes and may allow a person to breathe in more deeply. Studies suggest that it also reinforces smoking behaviors by making the side effects less bothersome and the process more rewarding.

The cocktail of both naturally occurring and added chemicals make for a perfect storm of potential carcinogens. **Carbon monoxide** (CO), for example, is a pollutant we've long associated with driving. In fact, our nation has worked hard to cut down on this form of pollution in our environment. Yet smokers inhale this with every puff. Breathing CO can cause headaches, dizziness, vomiting, and nausea. Exposure to moderate and high levels of CO over long periods of time has also been linked with increased risk of heart disease. CO interferes with the body's ability to absorb oxygen, which strains the heart and can cause suffocation. Someone who smokes a pack a day can have a 3–6% carboxyhemoglobin (COHb) level in the blood. This is a stable complex of CO. If they smoke two packs a day, the number is 6–10%. At three packs a day, it climbs as high as 20% COHb blood level.

Many of the chemicals are dangerous and problematic, but the big culprit that keeps people coming back for more, doing serious damage to their bodies, is nicotine.

Nicotine

The chemical **nicotine** makes tobacco an addictive substance and a very commonly abused one. Like heroin or cocaine, nicotine changes the way your brain works and causes you to crave more and more of it to achieve the same effect. This addiction to nicotine is what makes it so difficult to quit smoking other tobacco products. About 5% (by weight) of the tobacco plant is nicotine, a naturally occurring liquid alkaloid. An alkaloid is an organic compound made out of carbon, hydrogen, nitrogen, and sometimes oxygen, and it can have potent effects on the human body.

Nicotine absorbs into your bloodstream. Within 10 seconds of entering your body, the nicotine reaches your brain. It causes the brain to release adrenaline, creating a buzz of pleasure and energy. The buzz fades quickly though, and leaves you feeling tired, a little down, and wanting the buzz again. This feeling is what makes you light up the next cigarette. Since your body is able to build up a high tolerance to nicotine, you'll need to smoke more and more cigarettes in order to get nicotine's pleasurable effects and prevent withdrawal symptoms.

This up and down cycle repeats over and over, leading to addiction. Addiction keeps people smoking even when they want to quit. Cigarette makers know that nicotine addiction helps sell their products. Cigarettes today deliver more nicotine more quickly than ever before. Tobacco companies also use additives and chemicals to make them more addictive.

Nicotine addiction happens quickly and can be hard to kick. It's easy to relapse when trying to quit, especially if your social group contains a lot of others who smoke or you are experiencing a lot of stress. People also tend to have certain triggers that cause them to crave the tobacco. These can be emotional, physical, social, or pattern triggers.

When you stop smoking or cutback your tobacco use, your body begins to withdrawal. You may experience anxiety, irritability, headache, hunger, and cravings for cigarettes and other sources of nicotine. This does make it hard to quit. However, nicotine withdrawal is short-lived and symptoms pass in time, usually in less than a week. Withdrawal is the most uncomfortable part of quitting, but the real challenge is beating long-term cravings and staying away from tobacco.

Other Nicotine Delivery Systems

Pipes and **cigars** are very similar to cigarettes, except that people usually don't inhale. This means all the harmful chemicals in cigarettes linger in the mouth. Avid pipe and cigar smokers can expect to have discolored teeth, bad breath, and a high risk for developing oral cancer. They also still take in second-hand smoke.

Chewing tobacco—otherwise known as dip, chew, and snuff—contains more nicotine than cigarettes. These give you a more concentrated delivery system, one you can partake in nearly everywhere—no designated smoking area. You may not be as invasive to others in public as someone who smokes, but these products still pack an unhealthy punch. Holding an average-sized dip in your mouth for 30 minutes can give you as much nicotine as smoking three cigarettes. Using two cans of snuff a week gives you as much nicotine as someone who smokes one and a half packs of cigarettes a day.

Oral, esophageal, and pancreatic cancer are common among people who chew tobacco. Other regular problems include uncontrolled drooling and stained clothing, not to mentioned discolored teeth, bad breath, and dental issues. And

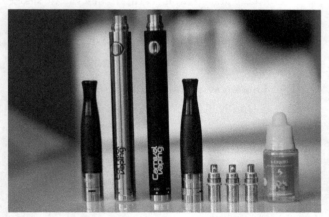

Figure 23. E-cigarettes or vaporizers are a relatively new and popular nicotine delivery system.

to make matters worse, almost no one will want to kiss you!

Smoking **cloves**, or kretek, smoking has an increased risk for acute lung injury, lung damage that can include a range of characteristics, such as decreased oxygen, fluid in the lungs, leakage from capillaries, and inflammation, especially among susceptible individuals with asthma or respiratory infections. Regular kretek smokers have 13–20 times the risk for abnormal lung function (e.g., airflow obstruction or reduced oxygen absorption) compared to nonsmokers.

Electronic cigarettes (e-cigarettes) or vaporizers are battery-operated products designed to turn nicotine and other chemicals into a vapor that you inhale (Figure 23). These products are often made to look like cigarettes, cigars, pipes, or pens in shape. Many people use e-cigarettes because they assume they are healthier than traditional ones. Others use them as a way of tapering their cigarette usage because they allow the person to still inhale nicotine without many of the other chemicals (in theory). Currently, there are no e-cigarettes approved by FDA for therapeutic uses so they cannot be recommended as a cessation aid.

E-Cigarettes may contain ingredients that are known to be toxic to humans. Because clinical studies about the safety of e-cigarettes have not been submitted to the US Food and Drug Administration (FDA), you have no way of knowing if they are safe, which chemicals they contain, or how much nicotine you could be inhaling.

Additionally, these products may be attractive to kids. They like electronic devices and with their colorful styles and shiny exterior, these have an added "cool" factor that traditional cigarettes don't. Since many adults use them as a transitional tool when trying to quit smoking, young people may be under the impression that they aren't harmful. However, they still contain nicotine. What's more, we don't yet know the side effects of the vaping process. Using e-cigarettes may also lead kids to try other tobacco products.

Effects of Tobacco on the Body

Smoking harms nearly every organ of the body. Some of these harmful effects are immediate and can become chronic (see below). One of the obvious short-term effects of smoking is the smell—whoever just smoked a cigarette is usually the worst-smelling person in the room. It permeates your clothing, hair, breath, fingernails, home, car, and anything it comes into contact with. Once the immediate smell dissi-

pates, the stale smell sets in and really becomes foul. But odor is the least of your worries. Other short-term effects include:

- Initial stimulation, then reduction in activity of brain and nervous system

- Increased alertness and concentration

- Feelings of mild euphoria

- Feelings of relaxation

- Increased blood pressure and heart rate

- Decreased blood flow to fingers and toes

- Decreased skin temperature

- Decreased appetite

- Dizziness

- Nausea, abdominal cramps and vomiting

- Headache

- Coughing due to smoke irritation

The sheer quantity of potential long-term effects of smoking should be enough to make people never light their first cigarette, and cause people who already smoke to quit. Nearly every vital organ and system in your body is impacted from cigarette smoke (Figure 24) and other forms of tobacco, including:

Your ears—Smoking reduces the oxygen supply to the cochlea, a snail-shaped organ in the inner ear. This may result in permanent damage and mild to moderate hearing loss.

Your eyes—Smoking causes physical changes in your eyes that can threaten your eyesight. Nicotine from cigarettes restricts the production of a chemical necessary for you to be able to see at night. Smoking also increases your risk of developing cataracts and macular degeneration (both can lead to blindness).

Your mouth—Smokers have more oral health problems than non-smokers, like mouth sores, ulcers, and gum disease. You are more likely to have cavities and lose your teeth at a younger age. You are also more likely to get cancers of the mouth and throat.

Your face—Smoking can cause your skin to be dry and lose its elasticity, leading to wrinkles and stretch marks. Your skin tone may become dull and grayish.

Your heart—Carbon monoxide from inhaled cigarette smoke contributes to a lack of oxygen, making the heart work harder. It also makes your blood thick and sticky, and increases your cholesterol levels, further straining your heart and increasing your risk of blood clots, heart disease, and heart attacks.

Your lungs—Smoking causes inflammation in the small airways and tissues of your lungs. Continued inflammation builds up scar tissue, which leads to physical changes to your lungs and airways that can make breathing hard. It can also lead to serious and potentially fatal lung diseases, such as emphysema, frequent respiratory infections, and lung cancer.

Your belly—People who smoke have bigger bellies and less muscle than non-smokers. They are more likely to develop Type 2 diabetes, even if they don't smoke every day. Smoking also makes it harder to control diabetes.

Female hormones—Smoking lowers estrogen levels in women, making it harder for them to become pregnant or have a healthy baby. Smoking can also lead to early menopause, which increases your risk of developing certain diseases (like heart disease).

Male sexual performance—Smoking increases the risk of erectile dysfunction in men—the inability to get or keep and erection. Toxins from cigarette smoke can also damage the genetic material in sperm, which can cause infertility in the father or genetic defects in the child.

Your immune system—When you smoke, the number of white blood cells in your body stays high. A high

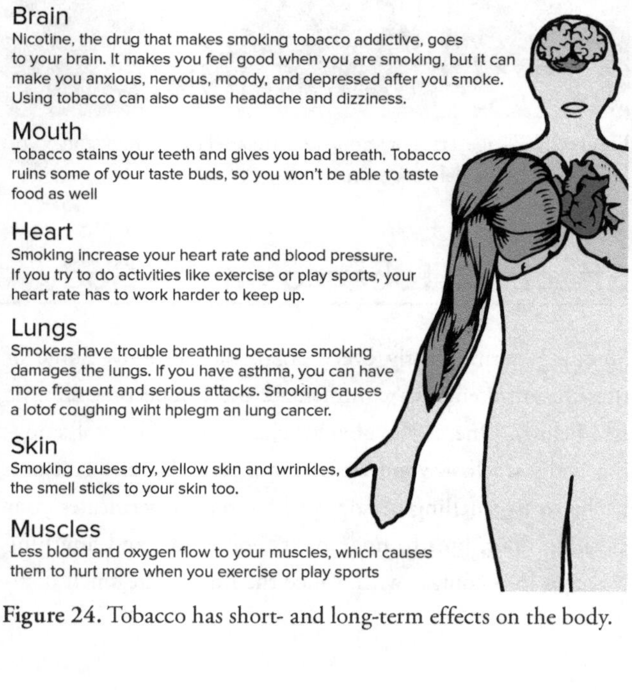

Brain
Nicotine, the drug that makes smoking tobacco addictive, goes to your brain. It makes you feel good when you are smoking, but it can make you anxious, nervous, moody, and depressed after you smoke. Using tobacco can also cause headache and dizziness.

Mouth
Tobacco stains your teeth and gives you bad breath. Tobacco ruins some of your taste buds, so you won't be able to taste food as well

Heart
Smoking increase your heart rate and blood pressure. If you try to do activities like exercise or play sports, your heart rate has to work harder to keep up.

Lungs
Smokers have trouble breathing because smoking damages the lungs. If you have asthma, you can have more frequent and serious attacks. Smoking causes a lotof coughing wiht hplegm an lung cancer.

Skin
Smoking causes dry, yellow skin and wrinkles, the smell sticks to your skin too.

Muscles
Less blood and oxygen flow to your muscles, which causes them to hurt more when you exercise or play sports

Figure 24. Tobacco has short- and long-term effects on the body.

white blood cell count is like a signal from your body, letting you know you've been injured. White blood cell counts that stay elevated for a long time are linked with an increased risk of heart attacks, strokes, and cancer. This means you're more likely to get sick.

Your healing ability—People who smoke also have difficulty healing. Nutrients, minerals, and oxygen are all supplied to the tissue through the blood stream. Nicotine causes blood vessels to tighten, which decreases levels of nutrients supplied to wounds. As a result, wounds take longer to heal. Slow wound healing increases the risk of infection after an injury or surgery and painful skin ulcers can develop, causing the tissue to slowly die.

Your muscles—Smoking reduces blood and oxygen flow to your muscles, making it harder to build muscle. The lack of oxygen also makes muscles tire more easily, giving you more muscle aches and pains than non-smokers.

Your bones—Ingredients in cigarette smoke also disrupt the natural cycle of bone health and impact bone density. Your body is less able to form healthy new bone tissue, and it breaks down existing bone tissue more rapidly. Over time, smoking leads to a thinning of bone tissue and loss of bone density, increasing your risk of bone fractures. Women who have gone through menopause and smoke have an increased risk and a higher chance of fractures.

Smoking During Pregnancy

Women who smoke may have a harder time getting pregnant. Smoking during pregnancy causes premature birth, low birth weight, certain birth defects, and ectopic pregnancy in which the fertilized egg implants somewhere in the abdomen other than the womb. Smoking during pregnancy also causes complications with the placenta, the organ through which nutrients pass from mother to fetus. These complications include placenta previa and placental abruption, conditions that jeopardize the life and health of both mother and child.

After birth, studies suggest there is an increased risk of SIDS (sudden infant death syndrome, also called "crib death") in babies born to women smokers, along with an increased risk of asthma, colic, and obesity for the child. Even emotional and behavioral problems in children can occur when the mother smokes while pregnant. These risks can be reduced if the woman quits within the first four months of pregnancy.

Women who are pregnant or who are planning a pregnancy should not smoke. It's important to encourage women to quit smoking before or early in pregnancy, when the most health benefits can be achieved, but cessation in all stages, even in late pregnancy, benefits maternal and fetal health.

Secondhand Smoke

So, why does it matter if you quit smoking? You're only hurting yourself, right? Among the more than 7,000 chemicals that have been identified in **secondhand** tobacco smoke, at least 250 are known to be harmful or cancerous, for example, hydrogen cyanide, carbon monoxide, ammonia, arsenic, benzene, butadiene (a hazardous gas), beryllium (a toxic metal), cadmium, chromium, ethylene oxide, nickel, polonium-210, vinyl chloride, formaldehyde, Benzo[a]pyrene, and toluene.

Secondhand smoke (also called **environmental tobacco smoke**, involuntary smoke, and passive smoke) is the combination of **sidestream** smoke (the smoke given off by a burning tobacco product) and **mainstream** smoke (the smoke exhaled by a smoker). In the US, most secondhand smoke comes from cigarettes, followed by pipes, cigars, and other tobacco products.

The amount of smoke created by a tobacco product depends on the amount of tobacco available for burning. The amount of secondhand smoke emitted by smoking one large cigar is similar to that emitted by smoking an entire pack of cigarettes.

Inhaling secondhand smoke causes lung cancer in nonsmoking adults. Approximately 3,000 lung cancer deaths occur each year among adult nonsmokers in the US as a result of exposure to secondhand smoke. The US Surgeon General estimates that living with someone who smokes increases a nonsmoker's chances of developing lung cancer by 20–30%. Risk even extends to your pets, which can be more prone to eye infections, allergies, lung and nasal cancer!

There is no safe level of exposure to secondhand smoke. Even low levels of secondhand smoke can be harmful. The only way to fully protect nonsmokers from secondhand smoke is to completely eliminate smoking in indoor spaces. Separating smoking from nonsmoking areas, cleaning the air, and ventilating buildings cannot completely eliminate exposure to secondhand smoke. There is a good reason why bars, restaurants, and hotels no longer permit smoking indoors—smoking and non-smoking sections simply don't work.

Secondhand Smoke Effects Children

Secondhand smoke causes numerous health problems in infants and children, including more frequent and severe asthma attacks, respiratory infections, ear infections, bronchitis, pneumonia, and sudden infant death syndrome (SIDS). It's so risky that smoking with children in the car (where they cannot even hope to distance themselves from the source) is illegal in some states (Figure 25). The impact can be significant, even fatal.

Parents can help protect their children from secondhand smoke by taking some simple precautions, such as not allowing anyone to smoke in or near your home, and definitely not in your car, even with the window down. Make sure your child's day care center and school are tobacco-free campuses. And choose restaurants and other venues of entertainment that don't allow smoking. "No smoking" sections don't protect you and your family from secondhand smoke. Sometimes you are still only a table away—the barrier is really an imaginary line.

Reducing Secondhand Smoke

Secondhand smoke can travel into buildings and drift hundreds of feet from a smoker, while still threatening the health of anyone who inhales it. Many states no longer have many public areas where smoking is allowed, but we do face challenges periodically. In outdoor event venues, for example, sometimes smoking has fewer restrictions. Casinos also tend to ignore the dangers of secondhand smoke in lieu of keeping smoking patrons parked in front of a slot machine (time is money). Here are a few things you can do to avoid smoke:

- Vote for legislation that bans public smoking

- Avoid businesses and venues that allow smoking. Let those businesses know that you choose not to frequent them as a consumer and why.

- Educate your children and set a good example. Don't rely on the school system to do this for you—they will learn first from you!

- Encourage your friends and family members to quit and be supportive. If you have children and do not want them around the smoke, be honest with your loved ones about why.

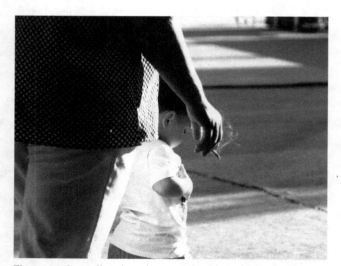

Figure 25. Secondhand smoke causes health problems for kids.

The Benefits of Quitting Smoking

Unlike the slow process of trying to reduce your body fat percentage, the minute you quit smoking, you begin to reap the benefits! After you quit, your body begins to heal within 20 minutes of your last cigarette. The nicotine leaves your body within three days. As your body starts to repair itself, you may feel worse instead of better, temporarily. Withdrawal can be difficult, but it's a sign that your body is healing.

There are plenty of long-term rewards, too. Quitting smoking can add years to your life. Smokers who quit before age 40 reduce their chance of dying early from smoking-related diseases by about 90%. Those who quit by age 45–54 reduce their chance of dying early by about 60%. You can take control of your health by quitting and staying smoke free. Over time, you'll greatly lower your risk of death from

NRT Type	How to Get Them	How to Use Them
Patch	Over the counter	Place on the skin. Gives a small and steady amount of nicotine.
Gum	Over the counter	Chew to release nicotine. Chew until you get a tingling feeling, then place between cheek and gums.
Lozenge	Over the counter	Place in the mouth like hard candy. Releases nicotine as it slowly dissolves in the mouth.
Inhaler	Prescription	Cartridge attached to a mouthpiece. Inhaling through the mouthpiece gives a specific amount of nicotine.
Nasal Spray	Prescription	Pump bottle containing nicotine. Put into nose and spray.

Figure 26. Nicotine replacement therapy types and availability.

lung cancer and other diseases such as heart disease, stroke, chronic bronchitis, emphysema, and at least 13 other kinds of cancer.

The efforts are well worth it. When a person quits smoking, their risks begin to drop right away. Within one year, the improvements to health are dramatic, the risks are cut in half, and even individuals who have previously had a heart attack have a significantly lower risk of having another. Within five years, a former smoker has almost the same risk as a non-smoker. The younger you are when you quit, the greater you increase your potential life span. Someone who quits when they are 30 years of age can add at least 10 years to their life compared to a smoker. By age 60, that number decreases to three years.

When you quit, you'll also protect your loved ones from dangerous secondhand smoke. You'll set a good example and show your family that a life without cigarettes is possible.

You've likely seen several ads or commercials for some form of smoking cessation product. You may have even tried one yourself. Smoking and tobacco use can be difficult to quit—many people try multiple times before succeeding long term. As with any area of wellness, it can help to set some SMART goals and some of these methods can help.

According to the CDC, most former smokers quit without using one of the treatments that scientific research has shown can work. However, the following treatments are proven to be effective for smokers who want help to quit.

Nicotine Replacement Therapy (NRT)

Nicotine replacement therapy (NRT) is the most commonly used type of medication to help you quit smoking. NRT reduces withdrawal feelings by giving you a small controlled amount of nicotine-but none of the other dangerous chemicals found in cigarettes. This small amount of nicotine helps satisfy your craving for nicotine and reduces the urge to smoke.

Health care providers and other medical experts think NRT is the one of the most helpful tools smokers can use to quit. Some smokers have mild to moderate side effects. However, research shows that NRT is safe and effective. NRT can be an important part of almost every smoker's strategy to quit. NRT products are sold over-the-counter (nicotine patch, gum, or lozenge) or by prescription (nicotine patch, inhaler, or nasal spray) (Figure 26).

NRT and other medications like bupropion SR (Zyban®) and varenicline tartrate (Chantix®) can't do all the work. It can help with withdrawal and cravings. But it won't completely take away the urge to smoke. Combining NRT with other strategies can improve your chances of quitting and staying quit. To give yourself the best chance for success, explore other quitting methods you can combine with medication (Figure 27).

Counseling and medication are both effective for treating tobacco dependence, and using them together is more effective than using either one alone. The American Lung Association also offers the following words of wisdom that can help you along the way:

It's never too late to quit. Earlier in life is better but quitting at any age will improve your quality of life.

Learn from past mistakes. If you've tried to quit before, consider what worked well and what didn't and adapt your approach.

You don't have to quit alone. Enlist support from friends and family or join a support group.

Use medication. Be sure to follow the directions. They don't work well if you aren't using them properly or long enough.

Every person can quit. It's just a matter of finding the right combination of approaches that work for you.

Community-Based Options

Community support is a major factor for whether or not a person will quit. Quitting can be more difficult, for example, if you are in an intimate relationship with someone who smokes but doesn't also want to quit. Other smokers, even good friends, are not reliable tools to help you quit. Anyone who has ever smoked knows how easy it is to get another smoker to give them a cigarette.

However, having a strong social support system can double your chances of quitting. Seeking counseling and support groups is a good start. You can also join groups, bringing you in contact with people who are less likely to smoke.

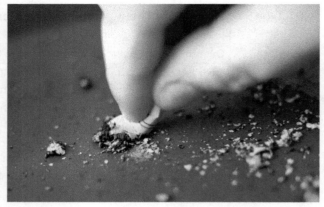

Figure 27. Cigarette smoke impacts more than just the smoker's health.

Smoking Prevention Policies in the US

Tobacco control programs aim to reduce disease, disability, and death related to tobacco use. A comprehensive approach—one that includes educational, clinical, regulatory, economic, and social strategies—has been established as the best way to eliminate the negative health and economic effects of tobacco use.

Federal laws, like the Family Smoking Prevention and Tobacco Control Act (Tobacco Control Act) are usually enforced through executive branch agencies, such as the Food and Drug Administration (FDA).

Laws can also be enacted at the state and local level to protect public health and make tobacco products less affordable, less accessible, and less attractive. For example, states may pass smoke-free indoor air laws and cigarette price increases, which have been proven to reduce cigarette use, prevent youth from starting to smoke, and encourage people to try to quit. The purpose of laws to eliminate smoking includes economic reasons, too. The total economic cost of smoking is more than $300 billion a year, including nearly $170 billion in direct medical care for adults, and more than $156 billion in lost productivity due to premature death and exposure to secondhand smoke.

Some good news is that prevention programs seem to be working. Among all current US adult cigarette smokers in 2015, nearly seven out of every ten (68.0%) reported that they wanted to quit completely. In fact, since 2002 the number of former smokers has been greater than the number of current smokers. According to a 2015 study, 55.4% of adult cigarette smokers reported stopping cigarettes for more than one day in an attempt to quit smoking (Figure 28).

The **Family Smoking Prevention and Tobacco Control Act** (FSPTCA), also known as the Tobacco Control Act, gives the Food and Drug Administration (FDA) the authority to regulate the manufacture, distribution, and marketing of tobacco products to protect public health. The Tobacco Control Act gave the FDA immediate authority to regulate cigarettes, cigarette tobacco, roll-your-own tobacco, and smokeless tobacco.

For other kinds of tobacco products, the statute authorizes the FDA to issue regulations "deeming" them to be subject to such authorities. Consistent with the statute, once a tobacco product is deemed sellable, the FDA may put in place "restrictions on the sale and distribution of a tobacco product," including age-related access restrictions as well as advertising and promotion restrictions, if the FDA determines the restrictions are appropriate for the protection of the public health.

This act is important because it has effectively taken control away from tobacco companies, who have shown a universal willingness to mislead the public on the universally negative effects of tobacco use, and is proven to be a major factor in the reduction of smoking and tobacco use throughout the US.

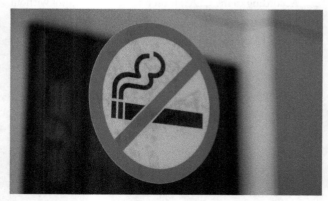

Figure 28. Public anti-smoking campaign.

Marijuana

In some parts of the US, you cannot drive two blocks with seeing a store (or three) that sells marijuana products. The signs outside these establishments read like those on a fast food restaurant, advertising discounts on pre-rolled marijuana cigarettes or and new bulk products. You've likely heard (or engaged in) arguments over marijuana's legalization for many years now. Advocates claim it can be used safely, or that it's even healthy, and not a gateway to other drugs. People against legalization claim the opposite. Regardless of its drawbacks or merits, marijuana continues to be one of the most commonly used substances in the US.

Marijuana is a green, brown, or gray mixture of dried, shredded leaves, stems, seeds, and flowers of the hemp, or *Cannabis sativa,* plant. It goes by many different names—pot, herb, weed, grass—and stronger forms include sinsemilla (sin-seh-me-yah), hashish (*hash* for short), and hash oil. It can be rolled up and smoked like a cigarette or cigar or smoked in a pipe. Sometimes people mix it in food (edibles) or inhale vaporized extracts such as resin or shatter in a vaporizer.

All forms of marijuana are psychoactive, changing how the brain works. Marijuana contains more than 400 chemicals, including **THC** (delta-9-tetrahydrocannabinol). Since THC is the main active chemical in marijuana, the amount of THC in marijuana determines its potency, or strength, and therefore its effects. The THC content of marijuana has been increasing over the past few decades.

Cannabinoids

The active ingredient of marijuana and the thing people seek from it are cannabinoids. There are two, specifically, that produce significant physiological and psychological effects—THC and Cannabidiol (CBD).

THC's chemical structure is similar to the brain chemical anandamide. Similarity in structure allows the body to recognize THC and to alter normal brain communication. Your body produces its own cannabinoids that function as neurotransmitters—they send chemical messages between nerve cells (neurons) throughout the nervous system. They affect brain areas that influence pleasure, memory, thinking, concentration, movement, coordination, and sensory and time perception.

Because of this similarity, THC is able to attach to molecules called cannabinoid receptors on neurons in these brain areas and activate them, disrupting various mental and physical functions and causing the brain areas listed above to be affected. The neural communication network that uses these cannabinoid neurotransmitters, known as the endocannabinoid system, plays a critical role in the nervous system's normal functioning, so interfering with it can have profound effects.

For example, THC is able to alter the functioning of the hippocampus and orbitofrontal cortex, brain areas that enable a person to form new memories and shift their focus. As a result, using marijuana causes impaired thinking and interferes with a person's ability to learn and perform complicated tasks.

THC also disrupts functioning of the cerebellum and basal ganglia, brain areas that regulate balance, posture, coordination, and reaction time. This is the reason people who have used marijuana may not be able to drive safely and may have problems playing sports or engaging in other physical activities. People who have taken large doses of the drug may experience an acute psychosis, which includes hallucinations, delusions, and a loss of the sense of personal identity.

THC activates the brain's reward system, which includes regions that govern the response to healthy pleasurable behaviors such as sex and eating (marijuana is well known to increase appetite). Like most other drugs that people misuse, THC stimulates the body's reward system to release dopamine at higher levels than normal. This flood of dopamine contributes to the pleasurable "high" that those use who recreational marijuana seek.

Organs in the body have fatty tissues that quickly absorb the THC in marijuana. In general, standard urine tests can detect traces of THC several days after use. In heavy marijuana users, however, urine tests can sometimes detect THC traces for weeks after use stops.

The amount of THC in marijuana has been increasing steadily over the past few decades. For a person who is new to marijuana use, this may mean exposure to higher THC levels with a greater chance of a harmful reaction. Higher THC levels may explain the rise in emergency room visits involving marijuana use. The popularity of edibles also increases the chance of harmful reactions. Edibles take longer to digest and produce a high. Therefore, people may consume more to feel the effects faster, leading to dangerous results. Higher THC levels may mean a greater risk for addiction if people are regularly exposing themselves to high doses.

Effects of Marijuana on the Body

Some people feel nothing at all when they smoke marijuana. Others may feel relaxed or "high." Some experience sudden feelings of anxiety and paranoid thoughts (even more likely with stronger varieties of marijuana). In the short-term, marijuana can cause problems with learning and memory, distorted perception (sights, sounds, time, touch), poor coordination, and increased heart rate.

Regular use of marijuana has also been linked to depression, anxiety, and a loss of drive or motivation, which means a loss of interest even in previously enjoyable activities. Its effects can be unpredictable (Figure 29), especially when mixed with other drugs.

We all know the stereotype (we've seen a movie or two)—the guy who grew up in the 1960s smoking lots of weed and continues to smoke for years. In the films, he sits in corners or in the back of his smoke-filled van, smiling and content, but he's slow to respond or react in any intelligent manner. While it may seem like fiction or exaggeration, we know a lot about how marijuana impacts the brain and how it affects cannabinoid receptors. Research suggests that the effects on memory, learning, and intelligence can be long-term and even permanent in people who begin using marijuana regularly as teens. Lost mental abilities might never fully return, even if a person quits using marijuana as an adult.

Someone who smokes marijuana regularly may also have many of the same breathing and lung problems that tobacco smokers do, such as a daily cough and a greater risk of lung infections like pneumonia. As with tobacco smoke, marijuana smoke has a toxic mixture of gases and tiny particles that can harm the lungs. Although we don't yet know if marijuana causes lung cancer, many people who smoke marijuana also smoke cigarettes, which do cause cancer—and smoking marijuana can make it harder to quit cigarette smoking.

Dangers of Smoking Marijuana

Sometimes people will say marijuana is "harmless," pointing to the idea that it is "natural" and that the active ingredient comes from a plant. This is faulty reasoning—cocaine and heroin also come from plants. Marijuana can be harmful if misused, like any medicine. Also, the primary method of ingesting marijuana is through smoking, which isn't safe.

Like tobacco smoke, marijuana smoke irritates the throat and lungs and can cause a heavy cough during use. It also contains levels of volatile chemicals and tar similar to tobacco smoke, raising concerns about risk for cancer and lung disease.

Marijuana smoking can inflame your airways, increase airway resistance, and hyperinflate your lungs. Those who smoke marijuana regularly report more symptoms of chronic bronchitis than those who do not smoke. One study found that people who frequently smoke marijuana had more outpatient medical visits for respiratory problems than non-smokers. Smoking marijuana may also reduce the respiratory system's immune response, increasing the likelihood of the person acquiring respiratory infections, including pneumonia.

Whether smoking marijuana causes lung cancer, as cigarette smoking does, remains an open question. Marijuana smoke contains carcinogenic combustion products. Because of how it is typically smoked (deeper inhale, held for longer), marijuana smoking leads to four times the deposition of tar compared to cigarette smoking. Studies are still inconclusive.

One complexity in comparing the lung-health risks of marijuana and tobacco concerns the very different ways the two substances are used. While people who smoke marijuana often inhale more deeply and hold the smoke in their lungs for a longer duration than is typical with cigarettes, marijuana's effects last longer, so people who use marijuana may smoke less frequently than those who smoke cigarettes. Additionally, the fact that many people use both marijuana and tobacco makes determining marijuana's precise contribution to lung cancer risk, if any, difficult to establish.

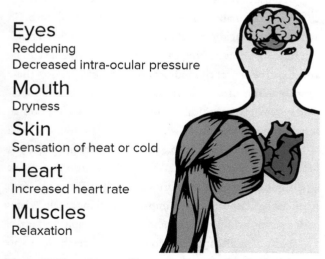

Eyes
Reddening
Decreased intra-ocular pressure

Mouth
Dryness

Skin
Sensation of heat or cold

Heart
Increased heart rate

Muscles
Relaxation

Figure 29. Cannabis use affects several parts of the body.

Marijuana During Pregnancy

Women who are pregnant should not smoke or consume marijuana. Marijuana use during pregnancy is linked to lower birth weight and increased risk of both brain and behavioral problems in babies. If a pregnant woman uses marijuana, the drug may affect certain developing parts of her fetus's brain. Challenges for the child may include problems with attention, memory, and problem-solving. Some research also suggests that moderate amounts of THC are excreted into the breast milk of nursing mothers. With regular use, THC can reach amounts in breast milk that could affect the baby's developing brain.

Marijuana's Impact on Mental Illness

Several studies have linked marijuana use to increased risk for psychiatric disorders, including psychosis (schizophrenia), depression, anxiety, and substance use disorders, but whether and to what extent it actually causes these conditions is not always easy to determine. The amount of drug used, the age at first use, and genetic vulnerability have all been shown to influence this relationship. Studies are still inconclusive.

Recent research has suggested that people who use marijuana and carry a specific variant of the AKT1 gene, which affects dopamine signaling in the striatum, are at increased risk of developing psychosis. The striatum is an area of the brain that becomes activated and flooded with dopamine when certain stimuli occur. One study found that the risk of psychosis among those with this variant was seven times higher for those who used marijuana daily compared with those who used it infrequently or used none at all.

Marijuana in the US

Marijuana is the most commonly used illicit drug in the US. In 2013, 7.5% of the US population over 12 years old (19.8 million people) reported using marijuana during the preceding month. In 2014, a total of 2.5 million persons over 12 years of age had used marijuana for the first time during the preceding 12 months, an average of approximately 7,000 new users each day.

During 2002–2014, the prevalence of marijuana use rose among adults, but not among those between 12–17 years old. The increase in adult usage is likely due to the drug's legalization in some states. In other words, even in states where recreational use is legal, it's still illegal for people under 21, so their numbers have not increased, while it has for legal adults. Among persons over 1 2 years old, studies also showed that their perception that the drug carried risk decreased—again, possibly due to relaxing laws on the substance.

The statistics on how many children use marijuana, however, may startle you. In 2016, 9.4% of 8th graders reported marijuana use in the past year and 5.4% in the past month. Among 10th graders, 23.9% had used marijuana in the past year and 14% in the past month. Rates of use among 12th graders were higher still—35.6% had used marijuana during the year prior to the survey and 22.5 % used in the past month. 6% said they used marijuana daily or near daily.

Medical emergencies related to marijuana use have also increased. The Drug Abuse Warning Network (DAWN) estimated that in 2011, there were nearly 456,000 drug-related emergency department visits in the US in which marijuana use was mentioned in the medical record (a 21% increase over 2009). About two-thirds of patients were male and 13% were between the ages of 12 and 17. It is unknown whether this increase is due to increased use, increased potency of marijuana (amount of THC it contains), or other factors. It should be noted, however, that mentions of marijuana in medical records do not necessarily indicate that these emergencies were directly related to marijuana intoxication.

Medical Marijuana and Therapeutic Theories

Marijuana has been a point of controversy for some time now. You could say that we have a love-hate relationship with it as a country. Many people fully support the idea that it has therapeutic value, while others focus on the negative effects and federal status as an illicit drug and theories that it can be a "gateway" to more harmful substances.

Despite this, some states have approved "medical marijuana" to ease symptoms of various health problems. The term medical marijuana refers to using the whole, unprocessed marijuana plant or its basic extracts to treat symptoms of illness and other conditions. The US Food and Drug Administration

(FDA) has not approved the marijuana plant as a medicine (Figure 30). However, there have been scientific studies of cannabinoids. This has led to two FDA-approved medicines containing THC. They treat nausea caused by chemotherapy and increase appetite in patients who have severe weight loss from HIV or AIDS.

Scientists are doing more research with marijuana and its ingredients to determine its potential to treat many diseases and conditions. A number of studies over the last two decades or more have investigated Cannabidiol (CBD) and its use to reduce seizures. Some case studies and anecdotal reports suggest that CBD may be effective in treating children with drug-resistant epilepsy. However, there have only been a few small, randomized clinical trials examining the efficacy of CBD as a treatment for epilepsy with significant flaws in both method and statistical analysis. Not many have been done with humans.

CBD has also been shown to have neuroprotective properties that may help with several neurodegenerative diseases, including Alzheimer's, stroke, glutamate toxicity, multiple sclerosis (MS), Parkinson's disease, and neurodegeneration caused by alcohol abuse. There have been multiple clinical trials demonstrating the efficacy of nabiximols (an extract of THC) on nerve pain, rheumatoid arthritis, and cancer pain. Research is inconclusive as to whether both THC and CBD have an impact or whether it is CBD alone.

In addition to the research on the use of cannabinoids in comfort treatments for cancer—reducing pain and nausea and increasing appetite—there are also several pre-clinical reports showing anti-tumor effects of CBD in lab tests. Reduced cell viability, increased cancer cell death, decreased tumor growth, and inhibition of metastasis may be due to the antioxidant

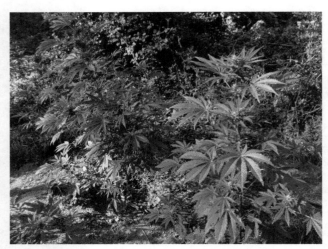

Figure 30. Marijuana grows in nature, but is still unsafe.

and anti-inflammatory effects of CBD.

Marijuana can produce acute psychotic episodes at high doses, and several studies have linked marijuana use to increased risk for chronic psychosis in individuals with specific genetic risk factors. Research suggests that these effects are prompted by THC, and it has been suggested that CBD may mitigate these effects.

CBD has shown therapeutic efficacy in a range of animal testing of anxiety and stress, reducing both behavioral and physiological (e.g., heart rate) measures of stress and anxiety. In addition, CBD has been shown to be effective in small human laboratory and clinical trials. CBD reduced anxiety in patients with social anxiety subjected to a stressful public speaking task. In a lab test designed to model post-traumatic stress disorders, CBD improved the ability to forget traumatic memories. Again, more research is needed.

Marijuana Use and Addiction

Marijuana use can lead to the development of problem use, known as a **marijuana use disorder**, which takes the form of addiction in severe cases. Recent data suggests that 30% of people who use marijuana may have some degree of marijuana use disorder. People who begin using marijuana before age 18 are 4–7 times more likely to develop a marijuana use disorder than adults.

Marijuana use disorders are often associated with dependence—the brain adapts to large amounts of the drug by reducing production of and sensitivity to its own endocannabinoid neurotransmitters. People who use marijuana frequently often report irritability, mood and sleep difficulties, decreased appetite, cravings, restlessness, and/or various forms of physical discomfort that peak within the first week after quitting and last up to 2 weeks.

Marijuana use disorder becomes addiction when the person cannot stop using the drug even though it interferes with many aspects of his or her life. In 2015, about 4 million people in the US met the diagnostic criteria for a marijuana use disorder, and 138,000 people voluntarily sought treatment for their marijuana use.

A Gateway Drug?

Long-term studies of drug use patterns indicate that most high school students who use other illegal drugs have tried marijuana first. However, many young people who use marijuana do not go on to use other drugs. To explain why some do, there are a few theories.

- Exposure to marijuana may affect the brain, particularly during development, which continues into users' early twenties. Effects may include changes to the brain that make other drugs more appealing. For example, animal research suggests that early exposure to marijuana makes opioid drugs (like Vicodin® or heroin) more pleasurable.

- Someone who is using marijuana is likely to be in contact with other users and sellers of other drugs, increasing the risk of being encouraged or tempted to try them.

- People at high risk of using drugs may use marijuana first because it is easy to get (like cigarettes and alcohol).

Legalization of Marijuana

Twenty-nine states and the District of Columbia have legalized marijuana for medical or recreational purposes. It is still a "Schedule I" drug at the federal level, which makes it a potential federal felony offense to possess and sell pot. There are a lot of reasons behind these state legislations—changing social attitudes, prisons overflowing with nonviolent drug offenders, and the potential state income taxing marijuana represents.

Whether this legalization will continue to other states and even a federal level remains to be seen. It also remains to be seen whether we will benefit from this legalization as a nation or begin seeing a host of problems related to marijuana usage. What is certain is that use of marijuana has increased in areas where it has been legalized recreationally (Figure 31).

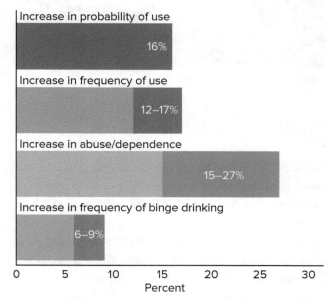

Figure 31. Marijuana use has grown since it became legalized for medical and recreational use in many states.

Opioids, Painkillers, and Prescriptions

Narcotic medications have psychoactive properties, so people commonly abuse them—that is, take them for reasons or in ways or amounts not intended by a health care provider, or take medications prescribed for someone else. In fact, prescription and over-the-counter (OTC) drugs are, after marijuana and alcohol, the most commonly abused substances in the US by people age 14 and older, with cough and cold remedies containing dextromethorphan being high on the list of abused medications (Figure 32).

You learned earlier about the different classes of psychoactive drugs. Of these, the most commonly misused and abused are opioid pain relievers (Vicodin and Oxycodone), stimulants for Attention Deficit Hyperactivity Disorder (Adderall and Ritalin), and CNS depressants for relieving anxiety (Valium and Xanax) (Figure 33).

People often think that prescription and over-the-counter drugs must be safer than illicit drugs. But they can be just as addictive and dangerous and put users at risk for other adverse health effects, including overdose—especially when taken with other drugs or alcohol. Before prescribing drugs, a health care provider considers a patient's health conditions, current and prior drug use, and other medicines to assess their risks and benefits.

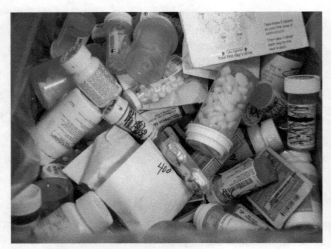

Figure 32. Various prescription drugs.

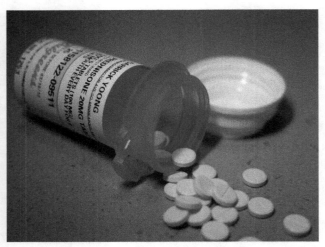

Figure 33. Prescriptions are carefully designed to treat medical conditions and should never be misused.

Prescription Drug Abuse

You've been studying for days for finals. You only have two exams to go, but exhaustion seems to have taken over. Your roommate offers you some Ritalin that she borrowed from a friend, claiming it will give you energy and improve your attention span. In desperation, you give it a try. This scenario is all too common, and is an example of how a seemingly innocent experiment can lead to prescription drug misuse and potential abuse.

Prescription and OTC drugs may be abused in one or more of the following ways:

Taking a medication that has been prescribed for somebody else. Unaware of the dangers of sharing medications, people often unknowingly contribute to this form of abuse by sharing their unused pain relievers with their family members.

Taking a drug in a higher quantity or in another manner than prescribed. Most prescription drugs are dispensed orally in tablets, but abusers sometimes crush the tablets and snort or inject the powder to hasten the effect.

Taking a drug for another purpose than prescribed. Many of the drugs mentioned can produce pleasurable effects at sufficient quantities, so taking them for the purpose of getting high is one of the main reasons people abuse them.

Taking a drug to improve your performance. ADHD drugs like Adderall and Ritalin are also often abused by students seeking to improve their academic performance. However, although they may boost alertness, there is little evidence they improve cognitive functioning for those without a medical condition.

Effects of Opioids and other Prescription Drugs on the Body

Taken as intended, prescription and OTC drugs safely treat specific mental or physical symptoms. But when taken in different quantities or when such symptoms aren't present, they may affect the brain in ways very similar to illicit drugs (Figure 34).

For example, stimulants such as Ritalin achieve their effects by acting on the same neurotransmitter systems as cocaine. Opioid pain relievers such as Oxycodone attach to the same cell receptors targeted by illegal opioids like heroin. Prescription depressants produce sedating or calming effects in the same manner as the club drugs GHB and Rohypnol. And when taken in very high doses, dextromethorphan acts on the same cell receptors as the club drugs PCP or ketamine, producing similar out-of-body experiences. All of these classes of drugs, when taken inappropriately, directly or indirectly cause a pleasurable increase in the amount of dopamine in the brain's reward pathway. Repeatedly seeking to experience that feeling can lead to addiction.

Opioids can produce drowsiness, cause constipation, and—depending upon the amount taken—depress breathing. The latter effect makes opioids particularly dangerous, especially when they are snorted or injected or combined with

Immediate effects

Rush of dopamine

Slowing respiratory system

Sense of calm

Blocking of pain

Euphoria

Sometimes nausea

Effects over time

Changes in brain stem

Strong cravings for drugs

Reduction of gray matter

Changes in limbic system and amygdala

Harder to feel pleasure without opiates

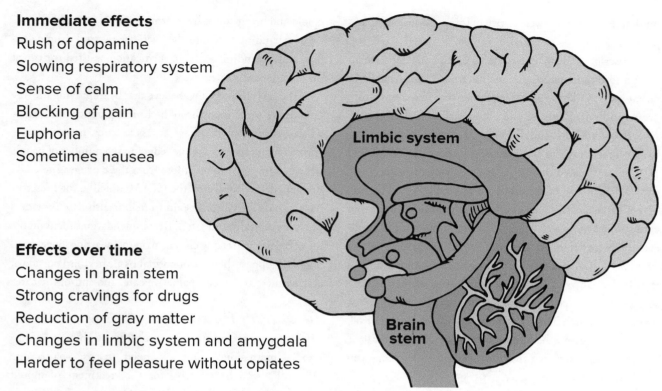

Figure 34. Opioid use has short- and long-term affects on the complex anatomy of the brain.

other drugs or alcohol.

While the relationship between opioid overdose and depressed respiration (slowed breathing) has been confirmed, researchers are also studying the long-term effects on brain function. Depressed respiration can affect the amount of oxygen that reaches the brain, a condition called hypoxia. Hypoxia can have short- and long-term psychological and neurological effects, including coma and permanent brain damage.

Researchers are also investigating the long-term effects of opioid addiction on the brain. Studies have suggested some deterioration of the brain's white matter due to heroin use, which may affect decision-making abilities, the ability to regulate behavior, and responses to stressful situations.

CNS depressants slow down brain activity and can cause sleepiness and loss of coordination. Continued use can lead to physical dependence and withdrawal symptoms if discontinuing use.

Dextromethorphan can cause impaired motor function, numbness, nausea or vomiting, and increased heart rate and blood pressure. On rare occasions, hypoxic brain damage—caused by severe respiratory depression and a lack of oxygen to the brain—has occurred due to the combination of dextromethorphan with decongestants often found in the medication.

All of these drugs have the potential for addiction, and this risk is amplified when they are abused. Also, as with other drugs, abuse of prescription and OTC drugs can alter a person's judgment and decision making, leading to dangerous behaviors such as unsafe sex and drugged driving.

The Opioid Epidemic in the US

More people die from overdoses of prescription opioids than from all other drugs combined, including heroin and cocaine. More than 2 million people in the US suffer from substance use disorders related to prescription opioid pain relievers. The terrible consequences of this trend include overdose deaths, which have more than quadrupled in the past decade and a half. The causes are complex, but they include over-prescription of pain medications. In 2013, 207 million prescriptions were written for prescription opioid pain medications.

Prescription drug abuse-related emergency department visits and treatment admissions have risen significantly in recent years. Other negative outcomes that may result from prescription drug misuse and abuse include falls and fractures in older adults, and, for some, initiating injection drug use with resulting risk for infections such as hepatitis C and HIV. It is estimated that the abuse of opioid analgesics costs the US $72 billion in medical costs annually.

What makes this such a challenging problem is that opioid abuse often begins with a legitimate prescription for painkillers. The potential for addiction to drugs like Oxycodone, for example, has practically become common knowledge and it can affect anyone. The idea that all drug addicts became so because they "chose" a way of life through partying just doesn't hold water. This could be an uncle who hurt his back on the job, your mother, grandparents, or siblings—a little bad luck may result in a treatment that turns someone you know into someone you don't.

Worse still, according to results from a 2014 study, 12.7% of new illicit drug users began with prescription pain relievers. Many opioid abusers often later develop problem usage of heroin, a problem the Department of Health and Human Services continues to investigate. When talking about prescription opioid abuse and deaths, we often discuss heroin at the same time.

Drug overdose deaths involving prescription opioid pain relievers have increased dramatically since 1999 (Figure 35). Combined federal and state efforts have been made to curb this epidemic. In 2011, the White House released an inter-agency strategy for Responding to America's Prescription Drug Crisis. Enacting this strategy, federal agencies have worked with states to educate providers, pharmacists, patients, parents, and youth about the dangers of prescription drug abuse and the need for proper prescribing, dispensing, use, and disposal.

Improvements have been seen in some regions of the country by decreasing the availability of prescription opioid drugs. Overdose deaths have declined in states with the most aggressive policies. However, since 2007, overdose deaths related to heroin have started to increase. The CDC counted 10,574 heroin overdose deaths in 2014, which represents more than a five-fold increase of the heroin death rate from 2002 to 2014.

In March of 2015, the Secretary of Health and Human Services announced the Secretary's Opioid Initiative, which aims to reduce addiction and mortality related to prescription opioid and heroin abuse by reforming opioid prescribing practices, expanding access to the overdose-reversal drug naloxone, and expanding access to medication-assisted treatment for opioid use disorder.

The DHHS and CDC believe that by improving the way opioids are prescribed through clinical practice guidelines, we can ensure patients have access to safer, more effective chronic pain treatment while reducing the number of people who misuse, abuse, or overdose from these drugs. The CDC developed and published the CDC Guideline for Prescribing Opioids for Chronic Pain to help health care providers prescribe ethically and safely. Recommendations focus on the use of opioids in treating chronic pain (pain lasting longer than 3 months or past the time of normal tissue healing) outside of active cancer treatment, palliative care, and end-of-life care.

Treatment for Abuse

Medications, including buprenorphine (Suboxone®, Subutex®), methadone, and extended release naltrexone (Vivitrol®), can be effective for the treatment of opioid use disorders. The World Health Organization refers to uprenorphine and methadone as "essential medicines." Medications like these should be combined with behavioral counseling for a holistic approach known as Medication Assisted Treatment (MAT).

MAT has been shown to decrease opioid use, opioid-related overdose deaths, criminal activity, and infectious disease transmission. For example, after buprenorphine became available in Baltimore, heroin overdose deaths decreased by 37%. Patients treated with medication have higher social participation in therapy and are more likely to remain in therapy compared to patients receiving MAT.

Treatment of opioid-dependent pregnant women with methadone or buprenorphine improves outcomes for their babies. MAT reduces symptoms of neonatal abstinence syndrome and the length of their hospital stay.

Unfortunately, less than half of privately-funded substance use disorder treatment programs offer MAT and only one-third of patients with opioid dependence at these programs actually receive it.

- The proportion of opioid treatment admissions with treatment plans that included receiving medications fell from 35% in 2002 to 28% in 2012.

- Nearly all US states do not have sufficient treatment capacity to provide MAT to all patients with an opioid use disorder.

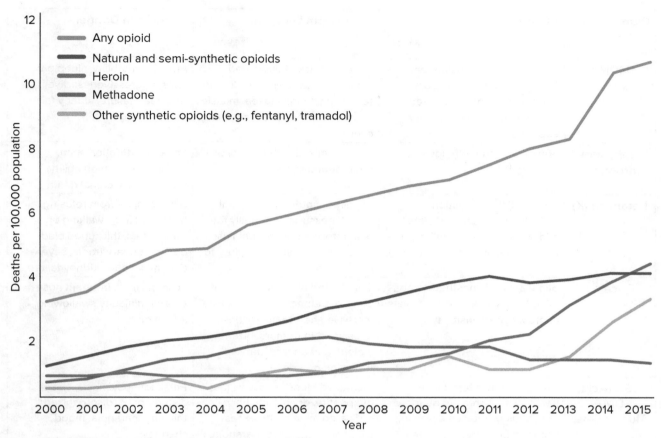

Figure 35. Opioid overdose is becoming increasingly common (Source: CDC).

Much of the hesitation to use medication assistance comes from social stigma—the belief that these medications swap one addictive substance for another. But drugs like methadone and buprenorphine do not work this way. When someone is treated for an opioid addiction, the dosage of medication used does not get them high—it helps reduce opioid cravings and withdrawal. These medications restore balance to the brain circuits affected by addiction, allowing the patient's brain to heal while working toward recovery.

If you or someone you care about has an opioid use disorder, ask a health care provider about available MAT options and about naloxone, an opioid antagonist that can reverse an opioid overdose. Many states allow you to get naloxone from a pharmacist without bringing in a prescription from a health care provider. This can be kept on hand to help save someone who may be overdosing on opioids.

Club Drugs

Club drugs are a group of psychoactive drugs that tend to be abused by teens and young adults at bars, nightclubs, concerts, and parties. Rohypnol, ketamine, cocaine, and LSD, as well as MDMA (Ecstasy) and methamphetamine are some of the drugs included in this group. They all have slightly different origins and effects. Some are natural, like cocaine, and others have synthetic versions.

These drugs are popular because they are relatively inexpensive to obtain, come in a variety of forms (making them easy to circulate), and their properties are believed to enhance the club experience. They are also notoriously easy to slip into someone's drink without their knowledge, so be wary of your cup when you're out on the town. These drugs most often provide a burst of energy and heightened sensitivity to sights and sounds. This heightened awareness also tends to apply to the user's sense of arousal. Yet despite their euphoric effects, they can be extremely dangerous (Figure 36).

Club Drugs	Effects	Short-Term Dangers	Long-Term Dangers
MDMA (Ecstasy)	Stimulant and hallucinogen: increased energy, pleasure, emotional warmth, distorted sensory and time perception, euphoria	Increased risk of unwanted sexual activity, chills, involuntary teeth clenching, nausea, muscle cramps, blurred vision, sweating, overdose	Anxiety, irritability, sleep problems, aggressiveness, liver failure, heart failure, kidney failure, addiction
Rohypnol (Roofies)	Sedative: extreme fatigue, memory loss	Lethal if mixed with alcohol or other depressants	Impaired attention span, decreased learning ability, memory loss, coma, death
Ketamine (K)	Anesthetic: dissociation, distorted perception of sight and sound, detachment, hallucinations, delirium, amnesia	Impaired motor function, high blood pressure, potentially fatal respiratory problems, painlessness causing traumatic injury to go untreated	Severe injury from refusing treatment (e.g., walking on a broken leg), thickened bladder and urinary tracts, severe abdominal pain, kidney failure
Cocaine	Stimulant and anesthetic: dopamine floods, extreme happiness, energy, hypersensitivity	Constricted blood vessels, irritability, extreme paranoia, nausea, increased heart rate, restlessness, muscle tremors, bizarre, violent, and unpredictable behavior, overdose	Lose of smell, frequent nosebleeds, difficulty swallowing, addiction
LSD (Acid, DMT, Mushrooms)	Hallucinogen: altered sensory perception, increased heart rate, nausea, intense emotion, changed perception of time	Increased blood pressure, loss of appetite, dry mouth, uncoordinated movement, excessive sweating, panic, paranoia, psychosis, poisoning, seizures, coma	Persistent psychosis, visual disturbances, disorganized thinking, paranoia, mood changes
Methamphetamine	Stimulant: dopamine floods, euphoria, increased wakefulness, excitement, decreased appetite	Rapid breathing and heartrate, increased body temperature, poisoning, overdose	Nerve damage, dopamine irregularity, sleep problems, anxiety, weight loss, dental problems, excessive itching, paranoia, hallucinations, loss of memory, addiction

Figure 36. Club drug use puts you at risk for many short- and long-term dangers to your health.

Club Drug Addiction Treatment

With most drugs, regardless of their nature, there are traditional methods for treatment. Most involve detoxification (the process by which the body rids itself of a drug), behavioral therapy, medication (similar to opioid, tobacco, or alcohol addiction), evaluation and treatment for co-occurring mental health issues such as depression and anxiety, contingency management or motivational incentives—providing rewards to patients who remain substance free, therapeutic communities—drug-free residences in which people in recovery from substance use disorders help each other to understand and change their behaviors, and long-term follow-up to prevent relapse.

A range of care with a tailored treatment program and follow-up options can be crucial to success. Treatment should include both medical and mental health services as needed. Follow-up care may include community- or family-based recovery support systems.

Caffeine

Ah, that morning cup of coffee—where would we be without it? None of us are strangers to caffeine use. We often consider it a common and necessary drug for daily functioning. Didn't sleep well? Have a cup of coffee (Figure 37). Hanging out with friends? Let's get coffee. Energy drinks are on the rise while typical sleep time is on the decline, particularly for college students. But what is it about caffeine that feeds our love and need for this drug?

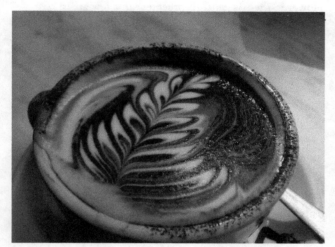

Figure 37. Though not as dangerous as illicit substances, caffeine is also a drug.

Caffeine is a stimulant that comes from a bitter substance that occurs naturally in more than 60 plants including coffee beans, tea leaves, kola nuts (used to flavor colas), and cacao pods (used to make chocolate). There are also synthetic (man-made) versions of caffeine that are added to some medicines, foods, and drinks. For example, some pain relievers, cold medicines, and over-the-counter products for alertness contain synthetic caffeine. So do energy drinks and "energy-boosting" gums and snacks.

Most people consume caffeine from drinks. The amounts of caffeine in different drinks can vary a lot, but the amount of caffeine in a drink generally is between 15–200mg (Figure 38).

Effects of Caffeine on the Body

Caffeine has many effects on your body's metabolism. It stimulates your central nervous system, making you feel more awake and giving you that boost of energy. It also acts like a diuretic, helping salt (and other bodily fluids) move through your system.

Not all of its effects are comfortable. It increases acid in the stomach leading to heartburn or a sour belly. And that jolt of energy you got? That increases your blood pressure. Within one hour of eating or drinking caffeine, it reaches its peak level in your blood. You may continue to feel the effects of caffeine for four to six hours.

For most people, it is not harmful to consume up to 400mg of caffeine a day. If you do eat or drink too much caffeine, it can cause health problems, such as restlessness and shakiness, insomnia, headaches, dizziness, dehydration, anxiety, and dependency.

How many times have you gotten a headache from *not* drinking caffeine? Probably plenty, even if you didn't realize it. Your body gets used to its daily fix. We don't often consider it as a drug from which we will withdrawal, but we do! If we go without it, we become more tired than usual, irritable, and even nauseous.

Beverage/Food	Serving Size	Caffeine
Tea	8 oz. (240 ml)	15-70 mg
Decaffeinated Tea	8 oz. (240 ml)	less than 12 mg
Roobios Tea	8 oz. (240 ml)	0 mg
Herbal Tea or Tisane	8 oz. (240 ml)	0 mg
Coffee	8 oz. (240 ml)	27-200 mg
Decaffeinated Coffee	8 oz. (240 ml)	2-12 mg
Espresso	1 oz. (30 ml)	29-120 mg
Decaffeinated Espresso	1 oz. (30 ml)	8 mg
Chocolate (Dark)	1 oz.	20 mg
Chocolate (Milk)	1 oz.	6 mg
Pepsi MAX	12 oz.	69 mg
Mountain Dew	12 oz.	54 mg
Coca-Cola Classic	12 oz.	34 mg
7-Up and Root Beers	12 oz.	0 mg
Rockstar Energy Drink	16 oz.	160 mg
Red Bull Energy Drink	8.4 oz.	80 mg

Figure 38. Amount of caffeine in common drinks.

Energy Drinks

Energy drinks are beverages that have added caffeine, sometimes a very ample amount—often as much as 5 times the amount in a cup of coffee. The amount of caffeine in energy drinks can vary widely, and sometimes the labels on the drinks do not give you the actual amount of caffeine in them. Energy drinks may also contain sugars, vitamins, herbs, and supplements.

Companies that make energy drinks claim that the drinks can increase alertness and improve physical and mental performance. This has helped make the drinks popular with American teens and young adults, but there's limited data to support these claims. But what we do know is that energy drinks can be dangerous because they have large amounts of caffeine. And since they have lots of sugar, they can contribute to weight gain and worsen diabetes.

Sometimes young people mix their energy drinks with alcohol, which can be a deadly cocktail. First, consuming high levels of caffeine with high levels of alcohol can be quite the shock to your organs. Caffeine can also interfere with your ability to recognize how drunk you are, which can lead you to drink more. This also makes you more likely to make bad decisions. In 2011, over 8,000 people ended up in the emergency room while combining energy drinks and alcohol and, of these, 8% were hospitalized.

Even without combining them with alcohol, energy drinks can be dangerous. According to the Drug Abuse Warning Network, the number of emergency room visits involving energy drinks among patients 12 years of age or older doubled between 2007–2011 (from 10,068 to 20,783). In 2011, 1 in 10 emergency room visits due to caffeine consumption resulted in a hospital admission.

Some people either cannot tolerate caffeine, consume way too much, or are at high risk for other reasons. Pregnant women, for example, are advised to limit caffeine usage to 200mg a day. It is a stimulant and can be passed to the child with negative effects (including while breastfeeding). People with anxiety, heart disease, high blood pressure, ulcers, migraines, and sleep disorders should also avoid it. Consider the reactions of caffeine on the body. If this is likely to interfere with an existing problem, you should keep consumption limited. For example, if you are already prone to headaches, and caffeine causes headaches, its usage would exacerbate the problem.

Caffeine's Impact on Sports Performance

Despite considerable research in this area, the role of caffeine as a performance enhancing drug is still controversial. Some of the data conflicts, which is in part due to how the experimental studies were designed and what methods were used. However, there is general agreement in a few areas:

- Caffeine may benefit short term, high intensity exercise (e.g., sprinting)
- Caffeine can enhance performance in endurance sports.

Glycogen is the principal fuel for muscles and exhaustion occurs when it is depleted. A secondary fuel, which is much more abundant, is fat. As long as there is still glycogen available, working muscles can utilize fat. Caffeine mobilizes fat stores and encourages working muscles to use fat as a fuel. This delays the depletion of muscle glycogen and allows you to prolong exercise. The first 15 minutes of exercise seems to be the key, during which caffeine has been shown to decrease glycogen utilization by as much as 50%. The glycogen saved is then available during the later stages of exercise. The exact method by which caffeine does this is still unclear.

Caffeine Overdose

The 2014 death of an Ohio high school senior caused by an overdose of powdered caffeine prompted the FDA to issue a safety advisory about caffeine powders. These products may be attractive to young people looking for added caffeine stimulation or for help losing weight, but they are extremely dangerous. Just a teaspoon of pure caffeine powder equals about 25 cups of coffee—a lethal amount. Besides death, severe caffeine overdose can cause fast and erratic heartbeat, seizures, vomiting, diarrhea, and disorientation—symptoms much more extreme than those of drinking too much coffee or tea or consuming too many sodas or energy drinks.

Although caffeine is generally safe at the dosages contained in popular beverages, caffeine powder is so potent that safe amounts cannot be measured with ordinary kitchen measuring tools, making it very easy to overdose on them even when users are aware of their potency. The FDA thus recommends that consumers avoid caffeine powder altogether and wishes to alert parents to the existence of these products and their hazards.

It isn't just powders that can be a concern. People often

consume too much or multiple sources at one time without thinking—coffee, energy drinks, diet pills that contain forms of caffeine that sound like herbs—there are many ways to overconsume.

Cutting Back on Caffeine

Most people don't need to eliminate caffeine from their diet. But, if you find that you have withdrawal symptoms from missing that cup of coffee, or are experiencing negative side effects from too much caffeine, it's probably time to cut back. Here are a few tips to help you do that:

Taper your usage—Don't go "cold turkey" unless you have instructions from your health care provider to immediately stop using it. Wean yourself off of it, consuming a bit less each day. This will help you avoid the really unpleasant side effects of withdrawal.

Keep tabs—Caffeine is in many substances, such as drinks and foods and medications that we may not be aware of. Keep track of where your caffeine comes from.

Go decaf—Decaffeinated drinks can help give you the same level of emotional comfort without the risk.

Conclusion

Your next steps should be to avoid substance abuse in all forms. If you drink alcohol, drink responsibly. If you consume caffeinated beverages, make sure that you aren't drinking an amount that harms your health. It's also worth examining your behaviors to notice any behavioral addictions that may be developing. Educating yourself and others about the risks associated with drug use is often the most effective deterrent to using drugs.

If you or someone you know has a substance abuse problem, getting help requires behavioral change. Review the stages of change theoretical model in Chapter 1 and look for information on addiction treatment in your area.

Reflection Questions

1. What is the difference between drug misuse, substance abuse, and addiction? How are they similar?

2. How, in your own words, can substance abuse impact the different dimensions of wellness? Identify at least three dimensions of wellness, and for each, give an example of how substance abuse might affect the dimension.

3. How does an addiction develop?

4. What are strategies a person could use for drinking responsibly?

5. In what ways can alcohol and tobacco affect women differently than men?

6. What options exist for quitting smoking? What strategies can help a person quit?

7. What do you think should be done on a public health level to reduce the prevalence of substance abuse in the US?

Chapter 12
Environmental Health

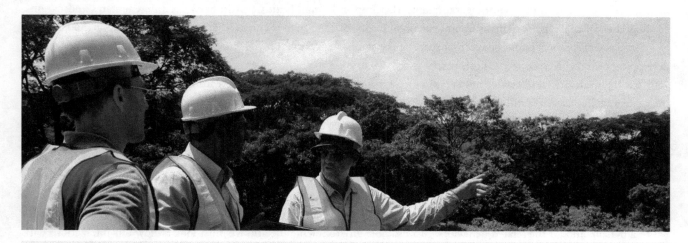

Learning Objectives

1. Describe the environmental impact of population growth.

2. Identify the six criteria air pollutants and discuss their potential effects on human health.

3. Identify the major sources of environmental contaminants.

4. Discuss climate change and the potential impact on the environment and human health.

5. Identify strategies for reducing air and water pollution, radioactivity, and noise.

For years, you've thought of yourself as a friend to the environment. You know everything there is to know about protecting Mother Earth and conserving her natural resources. You recycle like a champ, can sing along to the "reduce, reuse, recycle" song, drive an electric car, and wear your Earth Day shirt on any day you choose. You even compost! But did you know that it wasn't just the safety of the planet you were protecting?

Environmental health refers to all the ways our natural and man-made environment impact human health. It covers your home, workplace, and neighborhood. It covers the places you might go fishing, hunting, and camping. It covers the water you drink, the air you breathe, and the soil in which you grow your food. Human population growth has put environmental health at risk, but the situation can be improved by better managing the pollutants that people expel into the world.

This chapter defines environmental health and its importance to wellness. It then describes population growth and the concerns associated with unmanageable pollution levels. Finally, this chapter defines several types of pollution and makes suggestions to decrease your own pollution to contribute to better environmental health.

Defining Environmental Health

The environment plays a crucial role in each person's physical, mental, and social well-being. Despite significant improvements, major differences in environmental quality that impact human health remain between different states and nations. This can make it challenging to make improvements and control damage to the areas where people live, work, eat, and breathe.

Have you ever seen a photo taken from space of the smog over China? Or the amount of garbage piled on the shores of a developing country? Maybe you've noticed that when you drove into another state, you no longer had a place to easily recycle your plastic bottles? That's because not every country or state has the infrastructure required to protect the environment in the same way. But there are still many ways we can approach this problem. The complex relationships between environmental factors and human health should be seen in a broader spatial, socioeconomic, and cultural context.

Environmental health involves protection against environmental factors that may adversely impact human health or the ecological balances essential to long-term human health and environmental quality, whether in natural or man-made environments. We interact with the environment constantly. Our interactions and those of others around the globe impact our quality of life, the years of healthy life we'll live, and health disparities among different populations. The World Health Organization (WHO) defines **environment** as an element of health, citing "all the physical, chemical, and biological factors external to a person, and all the related behaviors." To promote environmental health, we must look at how our interactions with the environment can impact disease, injury, and disability and work to protect against negative effects to health and wellness.

Environmental Health Goals

The Healthy People 2020 environmental health objectives focus on 6 core themes, each of which highlights an element of environmental health:

Outdoor Air Quality — Poor air quality is linked to premature death, cancer, and long-term damage to respiratory and cardiovascular systems. Progress has been made to reduce unhealthy air emissions, but in 2008, approximately 127 million people lived in US counties that exceeded national air quality standards. Decreasing air pollution is an important step in creating a healthy environment.

Surface and Groundwater — Surface and groundwater quality concerns apply to both drinking water and recreational waters. Contamination by infectious agents or chemicals can cause mild to severe illness. Protecting water sources and minimizing exposure to contaminated water sources are important parts of environmental health.

Toxic Substances and Hazardous Wastes — The health effects of toxic substances and hazardous wastes are not yet fully understood. Research to better understand how these exposures may impact health is ongoing. Meanwhile, efforts to reduce exposures continue. Reducing exposure to toxic substances and hazardous wastes is fundamental to environmental health.

Homes and Communities — People spend most of their time at home, work, or school. Some of these environments may expose people to indoor air pollution, inadequate heating and sanitation, structural problems, electrical and fire hazards, or lead-based paint hazards. These hazards can impact health and safety. Maintaining healthy homes and communities is essential to environmental health.

Infrastructure and Surveillance — Preventing exposure to environmental hazards relies on many partners, including state and local health departments. Personnel, surveillance systems, and education are important resources for investigating and responding to disease, monitoring for hazards, and educating the public. Additional methods and greater capacity to measure and respond to environmental hazards are needed.

Global Environmental Health — Healthy People 2020 is concerned not just with issues in the US, but with worldwide issues. Many global problems overlap with our domestic ones. For example, water quality is an important global challenge. Diseases can be reduced by improving water quality and sanitation and increasing access to adequate water and sanitation facilities.

Creating healthy environments can be complex and relies on continuing research to better understand the effects of exposure to environmental hazards on people's health. We do know that globally, 23% of all deaths and 26% of deaths among children under age 5 are due to preventable environmental factors.

The reality is that the environment directly affects your quality of life much more than you may realize. Many things impact the degradation of the environment on a daily basis — air pollution, noise, chemicals, poor quality water, loss of natural areas, and even changing lifestyles may be contributing to substantial increases in rates of obesity, diabetes, cardiovascular and nervous system diseases, and cancer. Reproductive and mental health problems are also on the rise. Poor environmental quality has its greatest impact on children and people whose health status is already at risk. All of these are major public health concerns in the US.

The 6 Healthy People 2020 themes for environmental health focus on separate elements of the environment and their links to health. The field of environmental health continues to evolve and must address the societal and environmental factors that increase the likelihood of exposure and disease. While not all complex environmental issues can be predicted, some known emerging issues in the field include:

Climate change — This is projected to impact sea level, patterns of infectious disease, air quality, and the severity of natural disasters such as floods, droughts, and storms.

Disaster Preparedness — Preparing for the environmental impact of natural disasters, technological disasters, and those of human origin includes planning for human health needs and their impact on public infrastructure, such as water and roadways.

Nanotechnology — The potential impact of nanotechnology (the study and application of very tiny devices) is significant and offers possible improvements to disease prevention, detection, and treatment along with electronics, clean energy, manufacturing, and environmental risk assessment.

The Built Environment — Features of man-made spaces appear to impact human health — influencing behaviors, physical activity patterns, social networks, and access to resources.

Several major environmental health issues exist on a global scale, while others are relatively local in scope. Some issues are important in both, such as air quality. First, let's look at how some global trends in population growth, biodiversity, food supply, land degradation, water pollution, and energy consumption impact any discussion of environmental health. These are the major issues that affect us all and must be taken into account when describing environmental health.

Population Growth

Population growth and **density** are important factors to environmental health because their impact is cumulative. Each person produces waste that needs to be removed, increases the strain on already limited farmlands, and increases the number of pollutants in the air and water. You simply need to visit a major city and look around. What does the air look like or smell like? How much garbage do you see lying around? What kind of infrastructure is needed to keep sewage out of nearby waterways? These signs all represent the problems we face when populations grow (Figure 1).

The current world population of 7.3 billion people is expected to reach 8.5 billion by 2030, 9.7 billion in 2050, and 11.2 billion in 2100, according to a United Nations Department of Economic and Social Affairs (DESA) report. Most of the projected increase in the world's population can be attributed to a short list of high-fertility countries, mainly in Africa, or countries with already large populations. During 2015–2050, half of the world's population growth is expected to be concentrated in just 9 countries: India, Nigeria, Pakistan, the Congo, Ethiopia, Tanzania, the US, Indonesia and Uganda, listed according to the size of their contribution to the total growth.

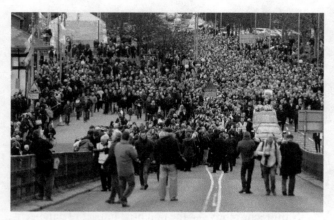

Figure 1. Populations are growing around the world.

Country	Total Fertility Rate (Children Born/Woman)
Niger	6.62 children born/woman
Chad	4.45 children born/woman
Somalia	5.89 children born/woman
Congo	4.53 children born/woman
India	2.45 children born/woman
Mexico	2.25 children born/woman
United States	1.87 children born/woman
Australia	1.77 children born/woman
Canada	1.6 children born/woman
China	1.6 children born/woman
Russia	1.61 children born/woman
Germany	1.44 children born/woman
Japan	1.41 children born/woman

Figure 2. Fertilty rates in countries around the world.

Human population can't just continue to grow indefinitely without it having a negative impact. Earth has limits to its life-sustaining resources. These limits are referred to as Earth's carrying capacity. The **carrying capacity** is the maximum number of individuals in a particular species that their environment can support indefinitely. Every species on Earth has one, including humans. Earth can only support a certain number of human beings comfortably, though it can be difficult for ecologists to determine a solid number for human carrying capacity. From culture to culture and nation to nation, people reproduce, consume resources, and treat their environment differently. Carrying capacity, therefore, must be estimated based on cultural and environmental trends, along with technological and economic development.

Global Trends

Part of this projection for carrying capacity includes estimating fertility rates around the world. This helps us anticipate the population burden of a particular region and consider how its inhabitants will deal with it. One method is to calculate the **total fertility rate (TFR)**, which compares the average number of children that would be born per woman if all women lived to the end of their childbearing years and bore children according to a given fertility rate at each age. TFR focuses more on birth potential rather than birth rate, which looks at past data. The highest TFR in the world, as of 2017, belongs to Niger, with almost seven births per woman. The lowest is in Singapore which averaged a little less than one birth per woman. The US average for 2017 was 1.87 births per woman (Figure 2).

TFR tracking facilitates planning. Imagine an area with already limited resources for farmland, water, and sewage processing, or an area that is already overflowing with people,

vehicles, and smog. Sudden population increases in these areas can be catastrophic, overloading the resource use, causing hunger or spreading infectious disease and waste that can be detrimental to the people there and in other areas around the globe.

Though the global population is still growing, the rates of growth have begun to slow. Globally, the TFR has dropped from 4.45 in 1970 to around 2.5 in 2014. If the rate keeps falling, the world population will eventually stop growing and may actually start shrinking towards the end of the 21st century.

A country's population is considered stable when its TFR is approximately 2.1 — the estimated replacement level needed to maintain a population. The replacement level considers multiple factors, such as children dying before they reach adulthood and mothers dying in childbirth.

With that in mind, many countries in the world now have a TFR below replacement level, including China, Russia, the US, much of Europe, Japan, Canada, and Australia, among others. This means that without immigration, all these countries will see long-term population decrease.

Yet the earth still has many years of rising population ahead. Human population growth has such a profound effect on Earth's environment and geology that some geologists have proposed we call the current geological era the Anthropocene (the age of humans) to reflect these impacts. Their claim is that our current geological age could be measured more by what we've contributed to the planet as humans than at any other point in history. Rather than nature doing its job to move, shift, and adapt the earth, humans have forced changes that would not have otherwise occurred.

Loss of Biodiversity

Biodiversity is the variety of life forms on the planet and within specific ecosystems. Scientists have tracked the loss of biodiversity on Earth for decades. The planet has always experienced the decline and even extinction of entire species. Many of these changes and losses are caused natural environmental change. Physical, geological, and biological data show that this is true. Why do people get so worried about species decline and extinction if this is a natural part of life and existence on this planet?

In short, the cause for worry is that this usually natural process is speeding up. It normally happens slowly, giving different species time to adapt or transition to new environments. For example, many humans are no longer born with wisdom teeth. Our species has slowly, over many centuries, learned that we do not need them. Many species adapt this way, or if they can't adapt to change, the species eventually disappears entirely. At first, much of the species loss in the twentieth century was attributed to these natural changes in biodiversity that occur in living ecosystems (natural selection). Scientists that study biodiversity now believe that we are seeing more than usual fluctuations and adaptations. Much of the current extinction levels in mammals, birds, and amphibians can be related to human activity. Human action, and not nature, is causing certain species to decline and potentially become extinct.

Humans have undoubtedly had a negative impact on biodiversity (Figure 3), particularly since the industrial revolution. We fish too much, hunt too much, and build too much, removing or destroying many animals' habitat. Our agricultural practice of introducing pollutants have forced pesticides, herbicides, and other toxic substances into the natural world. It is estimated that there are over 5,000 vertebrates, over 2,000 invertebrates, and an excess of 8,000 plants on the list of threatened species. The number of documented extinctions since 1500 BCE is now 784 species. Estimated extinction rates are now 50 to 500 times higher than previous estimated rates.

Food Supply

As food demand increases, nations have become more and more industrialized with food production (Figure 4). We've developed intensive farming techniques, artificial fertilization methods to replace nutrients stripped from the soil, and converted important natural biospheres into grazing land for cattle.

The demand for meat, which increases globally as more people enter the middle class in developing nations, creates environmental health problems. Industrial farming techniques, such as many of the factory farming methods used to meet the high demand, produces 9% of all the greenhouse

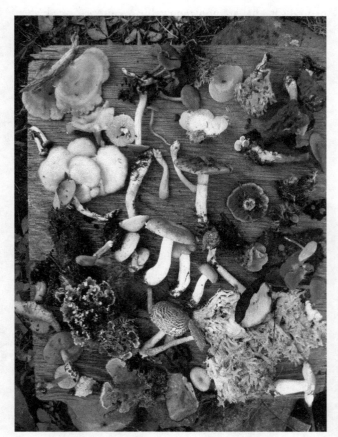

Figure 3. The variety of species is shrinking in areas of agriculture affected by overconsumption.

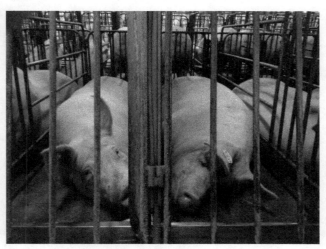

Figure 4. Factory farm conditions in the pork industry.

gases in the US and an enormous amount of fecal waste. A pig farm with 2,400 swine, for example, produces as much waste as 24,000 people. The vast quantity of waste produced by livestock has very few uses and often finds its way into the water supply. Livestock also require a massive amount of water to drink, not to mention the water used to water the plants used for their feed.

Food supply issues aren't limited to issues on land. The popularity of seafood has led to overfishing. This problem is compounded by toxic chemicals and fecal waste entering oceans, raising nitrogen levels, and creating huge "dead zones" that can't support most types of sea life. Popular types of edible fish have become increasingly rare. Combine this with the very manmade problem of plastic in our oceans (e.g., the Great Pacific Garbage Patch), and our marine life could continue to see a marked decline.

Land Degradation

People often underestimate the value of land, and we're not talking the price of a piece of property. Humans depend on the land for more than we may realize. It's uses for producing food and other needs is obvious, but land also contributes to our water systems, helping us manage droughts and floods. Land also provides an abundance of recreational activities.

The quantity and quality of land directly impacts food security around the world, safety, and overall quality of life. **Land degradation** is the decline in the quality of the land, largely due to human activities. It can be measured in terms of the loss of actual or potential productivity or utility. This can occur through natural factors, such as the way water causes soil erosion, or through the way we care for the land.

Land degradation has been a major global issue during the last century and will likely remain high on the international agenda. As populations grow, the resources that land provides become even more valuable for things like its growing capacity for food and space for housing. But population growth matters less than what that population does with the land. People can be a major asset in reversing any trends towards land degradation. However, their need to be healthy should be supported politically and economically by people motivated to care for the land. Too often, problems arise out of subsistence agriculture, where people farm land with only the motivation to feed as many people as possible in the moment, potentially damaging the land for the future. Poverty and lack of knowledge are important causes of land and environmental degradation.

Land degradation often leads to **desertification**, in which fertile irrigated land transforms into dry, dead desert that has lost its fertility and vegetation. According to the World Health Organization, weather extremes — particularly drought — and human activities that pollute or degrade land (including over-cultivation, overgrazing, and deforestation) convert farmable land into desert. As ecosystems change and deserts expand, food production diminishes, water sources dry up, and populations must relocate to more hospitable areas.

Increased Energy Consumption

The demand for energy worldwide will likely continue to grow over the next 30 years. Countries with high populations and large production industries, like China and India, account for more than half of the world's total projected increase in energy consumption. The US Energy Information Administration projects that world energy consumption will grow by 48% by the year 2040.

Energy sources can be grouped into two categories — fossil and non-fossil fuels. The US Department of Energy explains **fossil fuels** as energy sources, including oil, coal, and natural gas, that are **non-renewable** resources formed when prehistoric plants and animals died and gradually became buried by layers of rock. Over millions of years, different types of fossil fuels formed — depending on what combination of organic matter was present, how long it was buried and what temperature and pressure conditions existed as time passed. Today, fossil fuel industries drill or mine for these energy sources, burn them to produce electricity, or refine them for use as fuel for heating or transportation. Over the past 20 years, nearly three-fourths of human-caused emissions came from burning fossil fuels.

Non-fossil fuels, in contrast, are those that come from sources other than the dead dinosaurs we imagine. These sources of energy come from the sun, wind, water, and even from plants or waste (biofuel or biomass). Most are **renewable** in that they naturally regenerate or occur and most have fewer pollutants than fossil fuels. There are a few exceptions — the burning of trees or wood for fuel, for example.

We've long been concerned about the amount and type of energy needed to power the world while still reducing the impact of fossil fuel emissions on the environment. The high cost of oil has added to these concerns, driving the need for more cost-effective solutions. The push for non-fossil renewable energy sources and nuclear power have been accelerating,

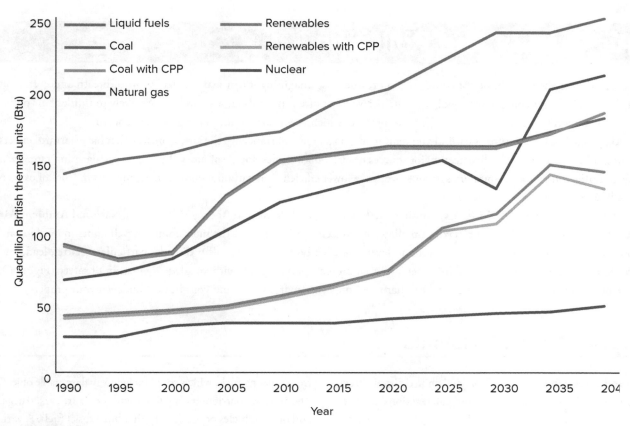

Figure 5. World energy consumption by source type.

making them some of the world's fastest-growing energy sources today. Renewable energy is expected to increase by an average 2.6% per year through 2040, nuclear power by 2.3% per year (Figure 5).

Even though non-fossil fuels will likely grow faster than fossil fuels, fossil fuels will still likely account for more than three-quarters of world energy consumption through 2040. The use of natural gas, which has a lower carbon intensity than coal and petroleum, continues to rise with consumption expected to increase by 1.9% per year. Liquid fossil fuels, mainly petroleum-based, still remain the largest energy source, but consumption is expected to fall 3% by 2040.

Coal has the reputation of being one of the dirtiest and most toxic forms of fuel, responsible for putting lots of soot and chemicals into the air — carbon monoxide, sulfur dioxide, lead, mercury, nitrous oxides, and even arsenic. The growth of coal as a fuel is predicted to slow in most areas as large coal consumers, like China and the US, work to reduce their carbon footprint.

Though the world has made some progress toward renewable energies that are less damaging to the air, soil, and wildlife, all forms of energy have some environmental impact.

Most energy sources still require land use and water use at minimum, in addition to any waste produced in the process. Moving toward clean energy is important, but humans will continue to leave a footprint, no matter how clean, for many years to come.

Pollution: The Greatest Threat to Environmental Health

You likely have noticed a consistent theme when it comes to population growth — as more people inhabit the planet, more of the natural environment declines or becomes negatively impacted. The pollution of our air, water, and land takes the largest toll on environmental health.

The rest of this chapter expands on the largest threats to us and our environment. All of these threats can be described as pollution of some kind. People produce a variety of pollutants that can be reduced on a personal and systemic level. Taking personal responsibility and helping to reduce pollution in your neighborhood, town, county, and state has far-reaching results. The trash you recycle each day, the water you conserve while brushing your teeth, and the days you bike to work instead of drive all have a cumulative positive impact.

Air Quality and Pollution

Most people fear the thought of not being able to breathe. Just imagining it can make us feel short of breath and even a bit panicked. But when it comes to the quality of our air, we don't often think about it — we're more likely to think of air pollution as an aesthetic issue. People need clean air to breathe, which is why air pollution is a growing concern.

Air pollution is a mixture of natural and man-made, poisonous substances in the air we breathe that have harmful effects on human health. People who live near major sources of air pollutants develop respiratory illnesses at an alarming rate. Even being in traffic causes your respiratory system to work at a lower efficiency, as carbon monoxide basically cuts in front of oxygen in the line to get into your bloodstream.

The **Clean Air Act of 1963 (CAA)** requires the Environmental Protection Agency (EPA) to set **National Ambient Air Quality Standards** (NAAQS) for maximum allowable concentrations of six of the most common pollutants in outdoor air, known as "criteria pollutants." These are ground-level ozone, carbon monoxide, sulfur dioxide, particulate matter, lead, and nitrogen dioxide. The standards establish a set level that protects public health with an adequate margin of safety (Figure 6). These pollutants can occur anywhere and can harm not only the environment (and your health) but even your property.

The Six Criteria Pollutants

Ground level ozone, or "bad" ozone is not emitted directly into the air. It's created by chemical reactions between oxides of nitrogen (NO_x) and volatile organic compounds in sunlight. Emissions from industrial facilities, electric utilities, motor vehicle exhaust, gasoline vapors, and chemical solvents offer some of the major sources of NO_x and volatile organic compounds. Breathing ozone (O_3) can trigger a variety of health problems, particularly for children, older adults, and people of all ages who have lung diseases such as asthma. Ground level ozone can also have harmful effects on sensitive vegetation and ecosystems.

Carbon monoxide (CO) is a colorless, odorless gas that can be harmful when inhaled in large amounts. CO comes from burning fuels, which could include any flammable object. The greatest contributors of CO to outdoor air are cars, trucks, and other vehicles or machinery that burn fossil fuels. A variety of items in your home — such as unvented kerosene and natural gas space heaters, leaking chimneys and furnaces, and gas stoves — also release CO and can affect air quality indoors.

Breathing air with a high concentration of CO reduces the amount of oxygen that can be transported in the blood stream to critical organs like the heart and brain. At very high levels, CO can cause dizziness, confusion, unconsciousness, and death.

Very high levels of CO aren't likely to occur outdoors, but even elevated levels can be concerning for people with some types of heart disease. These people already have difficulty getting

Pollutant	Sources	Effects
Ground level ozone (O_3)	Chemical reactions from nitrogen oxide emissions and volatile or-ganic compounds	Lung damage, particularly in children, older adults, and people with lung disease or asthma
Carbon Monoxide (CO)	Burned fuels	Reduced oxygen flow to the blood when inhaled
Sulfer Dioxide (SO_2)	Power plant emissions, burned fuels with high sulfur content	Impaired breathing
Particulate matter	Any source of dust, dirt, soot, or smoke	Impaired breathing
Lead	Lead smelters, lead building ma-terials, metal processors	Lead poisoning: impacting the nervous system, kidneys, immune system, reproductive and devel-opmental systems, and cardiovascular system; cognitive damage in children
Nitrogen Dioxide (NO_2)	Burned fuels	Impaired breathing, may cause asthma to develop

Figure 6. The six criteria pollutants' sources and their effects on humans.

oxygenated blood to their hearts in situations where the heart needs more oxygen than usual. They can be especially vulnerable to the effects of CO when exercising or under increased stress. In these situations, short-term exposure to elevated CO may result in reduced oxygen to the heart accompanied by chest pain.

The EPA's NAAQS for **sulfur dioxide** (SO_2) protect against exposure to the entire group of sulfur oxides (SO_x). SO_2 is the component of greatest concern and is used as the indicator for the larger group of gaseous sulfur oxides. Other gaseous sulfur oxides (such as SO_3) can be found in the atmosphere at concentrations much lower than SO_2.

Power plants and other industrial facilities are the largest sources of SO_2. Smaller sources of SO_2 emissions include: industrial processes such as extracting metal from ore; natural sources such as volcanoes; and trains, ships, and other vehicles and heavy equipment that burn fuel with a high sulfur content. Emissions that lead to high concentrations of SO_2 generally also lead to the formation of other SO_x. These chemicals can react with other compounds in the atmosphere to form small particles that contribute to particulate matter pollution.

Short-term exposures to SO_2 can harm the respiratory system and make breathing difficult. Children, older adults, and those who suffer from asthma are particularly sensitive to effects of SO_2.

Particulate matter (**PM**) pollution is the term for a mixture of solid particles and liquid droplets found in the air. Some particles, such as dust, dirt, soot, or smoke, can be large or dark enough to be seen with the naked eye. Others are so small they can only be detected using an electron microscope. They typically range in size from 2.5–10 micrometers, but they can be even smaller. To give you an idea of how small that is, one strain of human hair is 70 micrometers in diameter. This means you can inhale PM without even realizing it's happening.

These particles come in many sizes and shapes and can be made up of hundreds of different chemicals. Some are emitted directly from a source such as construction sites, unpaved roads, fields, smokestacks, or fires. Most particles form in the atmosphere as a result of complex reactions of chemicals such as sulfur dioxide and nitrogen oxides.

Inhaled PM can cause serious health problems. Particles less than 10 micrometers in diameter pose the greatest problems, because they can get deep into your lungs, and some may even get into your bloodstream. Fine particles (2.5 micrometers) are the main cause of reduced visibility (haze) in parts of the US, including many of our national parks and wilderness areas.

Sources of **lead** emissions vary from one area to another.

At the national level, most lead in the air comes from ore and metals processing and piston-engine aircraft operating on leaded aviation fuel. Other sources include waste incinerators, utilities, and lead-acid battery manufacturers. The highest air concentrations of lead are usually found near lead smelters. Lead pollutes more than just air. The lead in air pollution finds its way into soil and water, too.

We've learned more about the dangers of lead over the years and made changes as a result, removing it from gasoline and paint, among other products. Lead in the bloodstream distributes throughout the body and accumulates in the bones. Depending on the level of exposure, it can affect your nervous system, kidneys, immune system, reproductive and developmental systems, and the cardiovascular system. It impacts your blood's ability to carry oxygen. Infants and children are particularly sensitive to even low levels of lead, which can negatively impact their mental development including behavior and learning. People with cardiovascular diseases are also at a higher risk of problems from lead exposure.

As of 2017, approximately 4 million houses and buildings in the US with children living in them that still pose a risk for lead exposure. Nearly 500,000 children age 1–5 in the US have blood lead levels at or above 5 micrograms per deciliter ($\mu g/dL$), which is currently the reference level at which the CDC recommends public health actions be taken. Even blood lead exposure levels as low as 2 micrograms per deciliter ($\mu g/dL$) can affect a child's cognitive function. Since no safe blood lead level has been identified for children, any exposure should be taken seriously. However, since lead exposure often occurs with no obvious signs or symptoms, it often remains unrecognized.

Nitrogen Dioxide (NO_2) is one of a group of highly reactive gases known as oxides of nitrogen or nitrogen oxides (NO_x). NO_2 primarily gets in the air from the burning of fuel from cars, trucks and buses, power plants, and off-road equipment. NO_2, along with other NO_x, reacts with other chemicals in the air to form both particulate matter and ozone. Both of these are harmful when inhaled due to effects on the respiratory system.

That sounds bad enough, but it gets worse. NO_2 and other NO_x interact with water, oxygen, and other chemicals in the atmosphere to form acid rain. Acid rain harms sensitive ecosystems such as lakes and forests. The nitrate particles that result from NO_x make the air hazy and difficult to see through. If you've ever visited a major city during hot weather when it hasn't rained in a while, you've seen that reduced visibility in the air. That comes from NO_2 and other forms of air pollution, and you may be breathing in the same thing obstructing your view.

Air Quality Index Levels	Numerical Value	Color	Meaning
Good	0 to 50	Green	Air quality is considered satisfactory, and air pollution poses little or no risk.
Moderate	51 to 100	Yellow	Air quality is acceptable. However, for some pollutants, there may be a moderate health concern for a very small number of people who are unusually sensitive to air pollution.
Unnhealthy for Sensitive Groups	101 to 150	Orange	Members of sensitive groups may experience health effects. The general public is not likely to be affected.
Unhealthy	151 to 200	Red	Everyone may begin to experience health effects; members of sensitive groups may experience more serious health effects.
Very Unhealthy	201 to 300	Purple	Health alert: everyone may experience more serious health effects.
Hazardous	301 to 500	Maroon	Health warnings of emergency conditions. The entire population is more likely to be affected.

Figure 7. People with respiratory problems should consult AQI Ratings before going outside.

Breathing air with a high concentration of NO_2 can irritate airways in the human respiratory system. Such exposures over short periods can aggravate respiratory diseases, leading to coughing, wheezing, or difficulty breathing. For some, this means a trip to the emergency room. Longer exposures to elevated concentrations of NO_2 may contribute to the development of asthma and potentially increase susceptibility to respiratory infections. People with asthma, as well as children and older adults, are generally at greater risk for the health effects of NO_2.

Air Quality Index

The **Air Quality Index** (AQI) measures daily air quality. It tells you how clean or polluted your air is and what associated health effects might be a concern for you. The AQI focuses on the health effects that you may experience within a few hours or days after breathing polluted air (Figure 7). EPA calculates the AQI for five of the six major air pollutants, with the exception of lead. Ground-level ozone and airborne particles pose the greatest threat to human health in this country.

The higher the AQI value, the greater the level of air pollution and the greater the health concern. For example, an AQI value of 50 represents good air quality with little potential to affect public health, while an AQI value over 300 represents hazardous air quality. An AQI value of 100 generally corresponds to the national air quality standard for the pollutant set by the EPA. Above 100, air quality is considered to be unhealthy, at least for certain sensitive groups of people, then for everyone as AQI values get higher.

Indoor Air Quality

It seems like a safe assumption to think that once you're indoors, you're safe from pollution. Yet this may not be the case. **Indoor Air Quality** (IAQ) refers to the air quality within and around buildings and structures, especially as it relates to the health and comfort of building occupants.

It may come as a surprise to you that pollutants like carbon monoxide, nitrogen, and sulfur dioxide, lead, and other chemicals can live in and around your home. This is in addition to any cigarette smoke, animal dander, mold, or other elements that can cause breathing discomfort and health hazards. Your water supply, ventilation and air ducts, fireplaces, and the proximity of your home to pollution sources can put you at increased risk. Some problems may be made worse by an inadequate supply of air from outdoors or from the heating, cooling, or humidity conditions present indoors.

Exposure to some forms of indoor pollutant can cause immediate effects, such as irritation of the eyes, nose, and throat, or headache, dizziness, and fatigue. For people at higher risk like those with a chronic disease, this could aggravate or worsen their existing symptoms. These can be treated quickly if a pollutant is identified as the culprit and removed from the air. But too often, problems with IAQ can be difficult to identify. Certain immediate effects bear similarity to those from colds or flu and go unidentified.

Some people only become sensitive to biological or chemical pollutants or experience negative effects after repeated or high-level exposures. Some health effects may not appear until years after your exposure. These effects can be severely

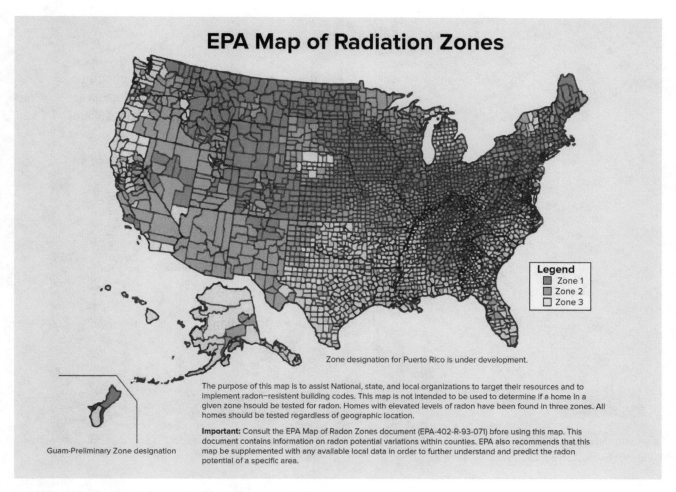

Figure 8. Radiation zones help shape public policy around radon.

debilitating or fatal, since they include some respiratory diseases, heart diseases, and cancers. You should try to be aware of and improve the indoor air quality in your home even if symptoms are not noticeable.

But how can you tell the IAQ is poor if you don't have symptoms? Some health effects can be useful indicators of an IAQ problem, especially if they appear after a person moves to a new residence, remodels or refurnishes a home, or treats a home with pesticides. If you think that you have symptoms that may be related to your home environment, discuss them with your doctor or your local health department. You may also want to consult a certified allergist or an occupational medicine specialist that can help answer your questions related to potential IAQ problems.

Another way to judge whether your home has or could develop indoor air problems is to identify potential sources of indoor air pollution. Under normal conditions, these potential sources are totally safe. But being aware of the type and number of potential sources can be an important step toward assessing the air quality in your home. Some potential sources include:

Combustion sources — oil, gas, kerosene, wood, and tobacco

Building materials (especially if deteriorating) — asbestos-containing insulation, lead paint, certain pressed wood products

Household, hobby, or home renovation materials — cleaners, solvents, air fresheners, pesticides, or paint thinners and strippers

Ventilation problems — smelly or stuffy air, moisture condensation on windows or walls, dirty central heating and air cooling equipment, areas where books, shoes, or other items become moldy

Proximity to outside air pollution — close proximity to utility sources like water treatment or electrical hubs, industrial areas, or construction sites

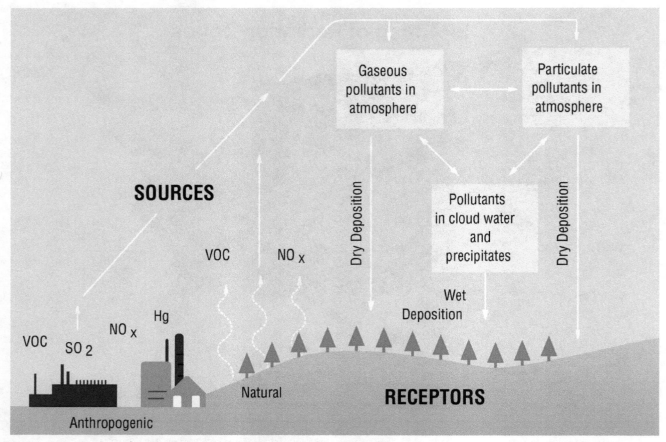

Figure 9. How acid rain forms in the air and is deposited.

Your nose, or the nose of a friend, can be a good barometer for some forms of air pollution. Leave the house (or suspected room) for a while. What do you smell when you come back in? What smells do your friends notice? If they smell strong or strange odors, you may have an indoor pollution source.

Radon

Radon forms when uranium in water, rocks, and soil begins to break down, releasing radioactive radon gas into the dirt beneath your home (Figure 8). This can seep in through cracks in walls, gaps in floors, spaces around pipes, fireplaces and furnaces, or water from a well. Contaminated air can even blow in through open windows. In the US, an estimated 21,000 people die from radon-related lung cancer every year. It is the second leading cause of lung cancer next to tobacco smoke and the primary cause for non-smokers.

The federal government recommends that you measure the level of radon in your home. Radon is colorless, odorless, and tasteless. Without measurements, there is no way to tell if radon is present. Inexpensive devices are available for measuring radon. Home test kits can be purchased or may be available for free in your area through state and local sources. Because radon is a significant source of lung cancer, the American Lung Association can help locate test kits.

The EPA indicates that numbers of 4 pCi/L (piocuries per liter) or above need attention. Experienced contractors can help you determine the radon's source of entry and ways to either prevent entry or mitigate radon levels within the home.

Acid Deposition (Acid Rain)

Acid rain, or acid deposition, is a broad term that includes any form of precipitation with acidic components, such as sulfuric or nitric acid that fall to the ground from the atmosphere in wet or dry forms. This can include rain, snow, fog, hail or even dust that is acidic.

Acid rain results when sulfur dioxide (SO_2) and nitrogen oxides (NO_x) are emitted into the atmosphere and transported by wind and air currents. The SO_2 and NO_x react with water, oxygen, and other chemicals to form sulfuric and nitric acids. These then mix with water and other materials before falling to the ground.

Acid rain is measured by its acidity and alkalinity using a pH scale. The lower a substance's pH level (less than 7), the higher the acidity. The higher a substance's pH (greater than 7), the more alkaline it is. Normal rain has a pH of about 5.6 — it is slightly acidic because carbon dioxide (CO_2) dissolves into it forming weak carbonic acid. Acid rain usually has a pH between 4.2 and 4.4.

There are two forms of acid rain — wet deposition and dry deposition. **Wet deposition** is what we most commonly think of as acid rain. The sulfuric and nitric acids formed in the atmosphere fall to the ground mixed with rain, snow, fog, or hail. Acidic particles and gases can also deposit from the atmosphere in the absence of moisture as **dry deposition**. The acidic particles and gases may deposit to surfaces (water bodies, vegetation, buildings) quickly, or they may form larger particles that can be harmful to human health if they get back into the air.

When the accumulated acids wash off a surface by during rain, this acidic water flows over and through the ground, and can harm plants and wildlife, such as insects and fish. The amount of acidity in the atmosphere that deposits to earth through dry deposition depends on the amount of rainfall an area receives. For example, in desert areas the ratio of dry to wet deposition is higher than an area that receives several inches of rain each year.

When acid deposition washes into lakes and streams, it can cause the water to become acidic (Figure 9). This sounds like it would burn your skin, but walking in acid rain, or even swimming in a lake affected by acid rain, is no more dangerous to humans than walking in normal rain or swimming in non-acidic lakes. For humans, it's the particles in the air that matter.

Acid rain has many ecological effects, but its impact on lakes, streams, wetlands, and other aquatic environments is the greatest. It increases acid levels in the water and causes them to absorb the aluminum that makes its way from soil into lakes and streams. Our water systems contain many creatures not suited to this acidic environment. For these creatures — like crayfish, clams, fish, and other aquatic animals — it becomes toxic.

Reducing Acid Rain

Reducing the amount of acid rain means first reducing the amount of sulfur dioxide in the air. Scientists are at work on new methods to solve the problem, like producing a coal that contains less sulfur, a method to "wash" coal to remove some of its sulfur, and forms of alternative energy like wind and solar power and technology like cleaner burning car engines. In fact, car manufacturers have been improving methods for reducing emissions for many years now. Some are now looking toward cleaner fuels and power sources as well, such as bio-fuels, natural gas, hydrogen, and electricity.

The Ozone Layer

The **ozone layer** is an important atmospheric layer in the stratosphere that protects Earth's surface (and everything on it) from harmful solar radiation. It's like the earth's sunscreen. Plants, animals, and humans all need protection from the sun. In areas of human population where ozone depletion has been more severe, instances of deadly skin cancers are much higher than normal. This is because ozone layer depletion increases the amount of ultraviolet A (UVA) and ultraviolet B rays (UVB) that reaches the earth's surface (Figure 10). Both types of UV rays have been linked to skin cancer, and UVB has also been linked to the development of cataracts, a clouding of the eye's lens.

Atmospheric ozone has two effects on the temperature balance of the earth. It absorbs solar ultraviolet radiation, which heats the stratosphere. It also absorbs infrared radiation

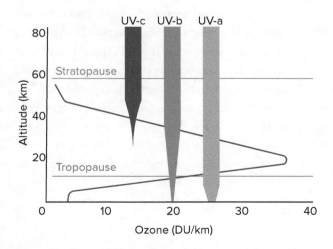

Figure 10. Ozone altitude UV graph (Source: EPA).

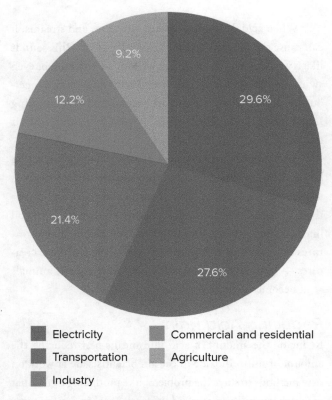

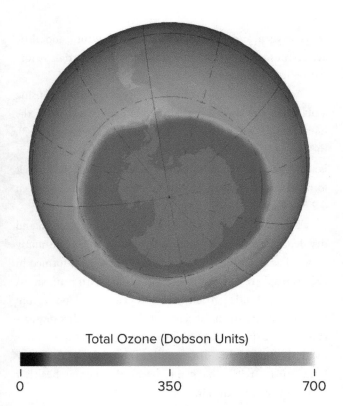

Total Ozone (Dobson Units)

0   350   700

Figure 11. Total US sources of greenhouse gas emissions (Source: EPA).

Figure 12. The hole in the ozone layer over the south pole.

emitted by the earth's surface, effectively trapping heat in the troposphere. Therefore, the climate impact of changes in ozone concentrations varies with the altitude at which these ozone changes occur.

The major ozone losses that have been observed in the lower stratosphere due to human-produced chlorine- and bromine-containing gases have a cooling effect on the earth's surface. On the other hand, the ozone increases that are estimated to have occurred in the troposphere (the lowest region) because of surface-pollution gases have a warming effect on the earth's surface, thereby contributing to the **"greenhouse" effect**. Most greenhouse gas emissions in the US come from utility and public works sources (Figure 11). Carbon dioxide concentrations also contribute significantly to this problem.

Chlorofluorocarbons (CFC's), chemicals found mainly in spray aerosols, are the primary culprits in ozone layer breakdown. When CFC's reach the upper atmosphere, they come into contact with ultraviolet rays. This causes them to break down into substances that include chlorine. The chlorine

reacts with the oxygen atoms in ozone and rips apart the ozone molecule. According to the EPA, one atom of chlorine can destroy more than a hundred thousand ozone molecules. In areas where the sun shines for significant parts of the day, such as the Antarctic, the ozone layer is very thin. This is the "hole in the ozone layer" you may have heard about (Figure 12).

Industrialized countries like the US and Europe create about 90% of CFC's currently in the atmosphere. These countries had banned CFC's by 1996, and the amount of chlorine in the atmosphere is now falling. Scientists estimate it will take another 50 years for chlorine levels to return to their natural levels. Meanwhile, other sources of greenhouse gases remain problematic (Figure 13). Not all the news is bad. Continued declines in ozone-depleting emissions are expected to result in a near complete recovery of the ozone layer near the middle of the twenty-first century. These substances take a long time to dissipate through natural processes, but we are seeing improvement.

Climate Change

Climate is the usual weather of a place, which depends on geography and season. **Climate change** is a change in the usual weather of a place. Weather changes rapidly, while climate takes many hundreds of years to change.

Earth-orbiting satellites and other technological advances have enabled scientists to see the big picture, collecting many different types of information about our planet and its climate on a global scale. This body of data, collected over many years, reveals the signals of a changing climate. Scientists know that the world is slowly but surely experiencing a **global warming**.

Climate change has become a bit of a controversial topic in recent years. There are a few reasons behind this. First, some climate change occurs from natural causes like the position of the sun to the earth, volcanic eruptions, and changes in the ocean. As a result, many people see climate change as a natural

part of the earth's evolution. Second, climate change is difficult to comprehend because it can take millions of years to occur. Many people use the evidence of a particularly cold winter to suggest that global warming is nothing more than a hoax.

But changes to climate don't only occur naturally. Much of the warming of the earth has been the result of human behavior, particularly pollution (Figure 14). The heat-trapping nature of carbon dioxide and other gases (the result of pollutants) has been known and well-documented since the nineteenth century. NASA has invested a great deal of time and resources into studying global gases, determined how these gases transfer energy, and compared current warming trends to those that would have happened thousands and even millions of years ago. Their determination is that no question remains that increased levels of greenhouse gases must cause Earth to warm.

U.S. GHG Emissions Flow Chart
Sector/IPCC Reporting category

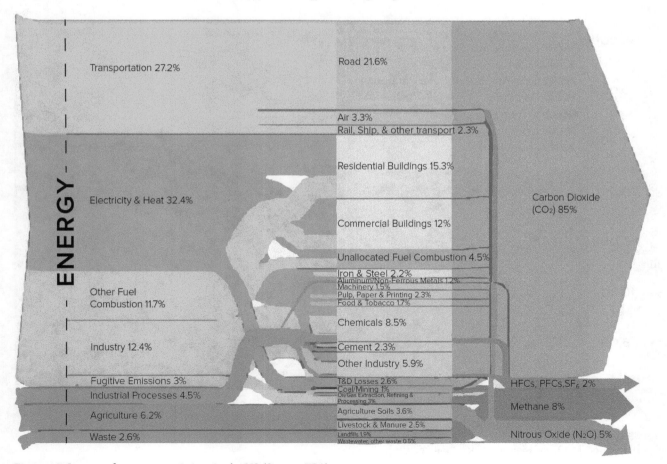

Figure 13. Sources of ozone gas emissions in the US (Source: EPA).

Scientists estimate that there is a greater than 95% probability that the current warming trend is the result of human activity since the middle of the twentieth century, and that the gas emissions that cause it are proceeding at an unprecedented rate (Figure 15). The planet's average surface temperature has risen about 2 degrees Fahrenheit since the late nineteenth century, a change driven largely by increased carbon dioxide and other man-made emissions into the atmosphere. Most of the warming occurred in the past 35 years, with 16 of the 17 warmest years on record occurring since 2001. Not only was 2016 the warmest year ever, but 8 of the 12 months that make up the year — from January through September, with the exception of June — were the warmest in history for those respective months.

Effects of Climate Change

Scientists have been monitoring the impact of climate change on the earth and its inhabitants for a long time and have watched many of their predictions surface. One effect is rising sea levels. The global sea level rose about eight inches in the last 100 years, and it continues to increase at a rapid

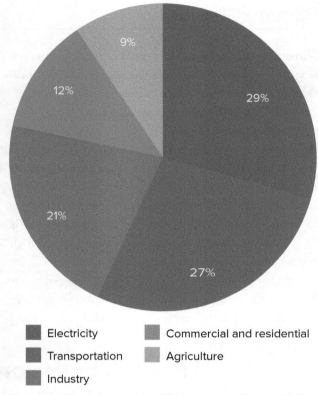

Figure 14. CO_2 emissions from different sources (Source: EPA).

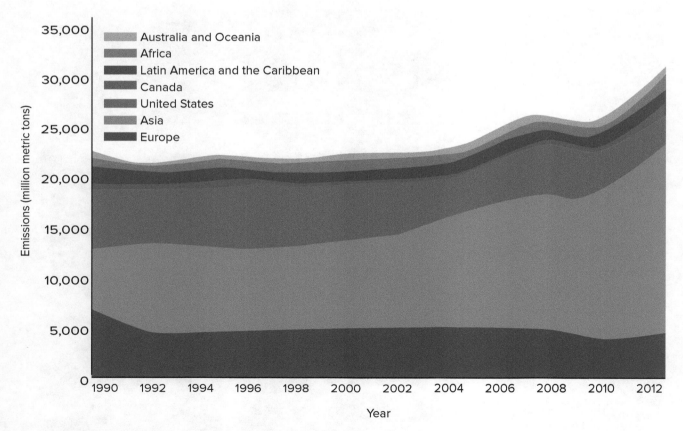

Figure 15. Global CO_2 emissions by region (Source: EPA).

pace. Earth's oceans have absorbed much of the increased heat caused by global warming, with the top 700 meters (about 2,300 feet) of ocean showing warming of 0.302 degrees Fahrenheit since 1969.

Much of the cause of the rising sea level is melting ice. As we all know, ice and heat don't mix very well, and the world's glaciers are certainly feeling it. The Greenland and Antarctic ice sheets, for example, have decreased in mass. Data from NASA shows Greenland lost 150 to 250 cubic kilometers of ice per year between 2002 and 2006, while Antarctica lost

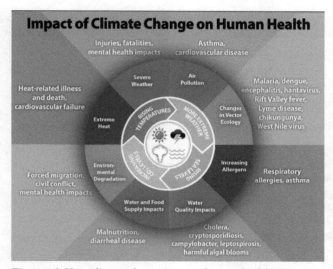

Figure 16. How climate change impacts human health (Source: CDC).

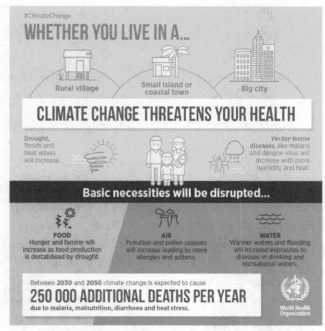

Figure 17. How climate change impacts the world (Source: World Health Organization).

about 152 cubic kilometers per year between 2002 and 2005. Glaciers are retreating almost everywhere around the world — including in the Swiss Alps, the Himalayas, the Andes, the Rocky Mountains, the Alaska Range, and the African Atlas Mountains.

Annual glacial melt and snow run-off are an important source of fresh water for drinking and agriculture. Long-term reduction of glaciers will lower the amount of water from annual melt. Without this melt, droughts are longer and more frequent. Satellite observations reveal that the amount of spring snow cover in the Northern Hemisphere has decreased over the past five decades and that the snow is melting earlier, which could have a similar impact over the long run.

Why does this matter? Changes in temperature and water sources creates a multiplying effect (Figure 16). Longer and more intense droughts and heat waves can occur that impact both agricultural food sources and wildlife. Drought can also lead to dangerous storm surges as higher levels of water push farther inland, creating problems with intense flooding. This leads to loss of property and life.

These changes have already resulted in a wide impact across every region of the country and many sectors of the economy. They have the potential to affect human health in a number of ways, too, according to the World Health Organization. The changing seasonal nature of our environment could encourage certain infectious diseases, disturb food-producing ecosystems, and increase the frequency of extreme weather events, such as hurricanes (Figure 17). More specifically, the WHO highlights the following concerns:

- Climate change affects the social and environmental determinants of health — clean air, safe drinking water, sufficient food, and secure shelter.

- Between 2030–2050, climate change is expected to cause approximately 250,000 additional deaths per year, from malnutrition, malaria, diarrhea, and heat stress.

- The direct health care costs, excluding costs in health-determining sectors such as agriculture and water and sanitation, is estimated to be between $2–4 billion/year by 2030.

- Areas with weak health infrastructure — mostly in developing countries — will be the least able to cope without assistance to prepare and respond. The costs for providing this assistance will be high, but can only get higher if preparations aren't made ahead of time.

If the world ignores these problems, we can expect the situation to get much worse. Scientists are confident that global temperatures will continue to rise for decades to come. The Intergovernmental Panel on Climate Change (IPCC), which includes more than 1,300 scientists from the US and other countries, forecasts a temperature rise of 2.5–10 degrees Fahrenheit over the next 100 years.

The magnitude of climate change beyond the next few decades depends primarily on the amount of heat-trapping gases emitted globally, and how sensitive the earth's climate is to those emissions. Because human-induced warming is imposed on an already naturally varying climate, the temperature rise has not been — and will not be — uniform or smooth across the country or over time. The largest impacts could happen suddenly.

Reducing the Threat of Global Warming

Climate change continues to be one of the most complex issues facing us today. It involves many dimensions — science, economics, society, politics, and moral and ethical questions. Controversies remain over what should be done (even whether it should be done at all), who should take responsibility, and how much of an impact can be made. This problem did not occur quickly, nor will it resolve overnight. Even if we stopped emitting all greenhouse gases today, global warming and climate change will continue to affect future generations. In this way, humanity is "committed" to some level of climate change.

How much climate change is now unavoidable? NASA indicates that will be determined by how our emissions continue and how our climate system responds to those emissions. Despite increasing awareness of climate change, emissions of greenhouse gases continue to rise. In 2013, the daily level of carbon dioxide in the atmosphere surpassed 400 parts per million for the first time in human history. The last time levels were that high was about 3–5 million years ago, during the Pliocene era.

Because we are already committed to some level of climate change, responding to climate change involves a two-pronged approach: reducing emissions and stabilizing the levels of heat-trapping greenhouse gases in the atmosphere ("mitigation"), and adapting to the climate change already in play ("adaptation").

Mitigation involves reducing the flow of heat-trapping greenhouse gases into the atmosphere, either by reducing sources of these gases (for example, the burning of fossil fuels for electricity, heat, or transport) or enhancing the "sinks" that accumulate and store these gases (such as the oceans, forests, and soil). The goal of mitigation is to avoid significant human interference with the climate system and stabilize levels to allow ecosystems to naturally adapt before food production becomes threatened.

Adaptation involves adjusting to actual or expected future climate. This means reducing our vulnerability to the harmful effects of climate change (like sea-level encroachment, more intense extreme weather events, or food insecurity). It also encompasses making the most of any potential beneficial opportunities associated with climate change (for example, longer growing seasons or increased yields in some regions).

Mitigation of air pollution is a significant step. In the US, we have the EPA, which sets standards that no state can drop below (and every state is welcome to exceed). But mitigation in the US alone is not nearly enough. Air pollution occurs all over the globe and the effects are far reaching — chemical and particulate matter in the air does not respect borders. For this reason, we have agreements and treaties with other nations to help curb emissions. These agreements have the following goals:

- Slowing depletion of the ozone layer

- Making changes in energy, transportation, and industrial practices

- Ending rapid deforestation (the destruction of animal and plant habitats for human use)

- Practicing sustainable development

Sustainable Development

In 2015, the United Nations and world leaders joined together to establish 17 sustainable development goals as part of their commitment to the protection of our planet and prosperity of its inhabitants. Their goals are focused on climate change, as well as fighting poverty and inequalities around the world.

The concept of **sustainability** revolves around using renewable resources and conserving the ones we have. That means choosing products and methods that don't contribute to the problem. For the United Nations, it means larger issues, such as a focus on how urban areas manage their infrastructure and transportation systems, the creation of jobs that do not strain the land and its resources, increasing green spaces, and working toward cleaner energies.

In your home and community, the concepts are the same. What can we do to lessen traffic and emissions? What can we do to preserve resources like water? How can we reduce waste and the harmful gases that arise from it?

For us, much of the issues come down to waste. We waste everything. We leave lights on in empty rooms, buy more food than we need, and throw away massive amounts of trash. Our waste means more production — of clothing, food, electricity, fuel, you name it! The more we manufacture and transport, the more resources our nation uses, and the more greenhouse gases are emitted.

Consider some of the many post-apocalyptic television shows you've watched in which people must learn to survive without the energy, technology, and conveniences of modern living. The scenarios are often the same — transportation, food, water, clothing, fuel, everything becomes scarce and they must learn to survive similarly to how people lived before the industrial revolution. In nearly every show, they begin to grow their own food, seek out renewable resources, and conserve. Waste is not an option. They become champions of the "reduce" and "reuse" portions of the 3 R's.

You're lucky — you don't have to adopt post-apocalyptic standards to make an impact. But try envisioning yourself with a need to conserve as you go through your day. Ask yourself — if this source of energy was limited, how would I handle this? Or, is the energy source I'm using clean and renewable? Could I be using a better source? Consider some of these simple methods from a United Nations list of tips for how you can help as an individual. These include methods of conserving water, paper, electricity, and food as well as being smart with how much you purchase.:

Things you can do from your couch:

Save electricity — Plug appliances into a power strip and turn them off completely when not in use, including your computer.

Save paper — Stop automated paper statements from utilities and banks and pay your bills online. No paper, no need for forest destruction.

Don't print — See something online you need to remember? Jot it down in a notebook or a digital post-it note and spare the paper.

Turn off the lights — Your TV or computer screen provides a cozy glow, so turn off other lights if you don't need them.

Things you can do from home:

Air dry — Let your hair and clothes dry naturally instead of running a machine. Make sure the load is full when you wash your clothes.

Take short showers — Bathtubs require gallons more water than a 5–10-minute shower.

Eat less meat, poultry, and fish — More resources are used to provide meat than plants.

Avoid pre-heating the oven — Unless you need a precise baking temperature, start heating your food right when you turn on the oven.

Replace old appliances — Find energy efficient models and light bulbs.

Things you can do outside your house:

Shop local — Supporting neighborhood businesses keeps people employed and helps prevent trucks from driving far distances.

Shop Smart — Plan meals, use shopping lists, and avoid impulse buys. Don't succumb to marketing tricks that lead you to buy more food than you need, particularly for perishable items. Though these may be less expensive per ounce, they can be more expensive overall if much of that food is discarded.

Buy funny fruit — Many fruits and vegetables are thrown out because their size, shape, or color are not "right." Buying these perfectly good funny fruit, at the farmer's market or elsewhere, utilizes food that might otherwise go to waste.

Eat sustainably — At restaurants ask if they serve sustainable seafood. Let your favorite businesses know that ocean-friendly seafood is a priority.

Cut back on fuel — Biking or walking to school or work is healthy and saves fuel. Take the bus or train which can reduce the number of vehicles on the road and often utilize cleaner forms of fuel.

Another way individuals can make an impact is to start thinking about the internal and external spaces they encounter on a regular basis and to what types of pollution they may expose themselves to regularly. For example, what is the air quality inside your home (Figure 18)? In your workplace? What steps could improve this quality?

Another thing to think about is how much time you spend outdoors and what you do while there. Many of us enjoy hunting, fishing, and hundreds of other outdoor activities. A person who is an avid hunter or who enjoys fishing has a vested interest in the quality of the water and land because contaminants have a nasty habit of making it into the flesh of the animals we eat.

When you're camping, hiking, or out for a run, think about what kinds of pollution negatively affect your experience. What sorts of litter do you see on the trail? How clean is the air? Even people who aren't that interested in the wilderness can ask the same questions about their own neighborhoods.

After thinking about it, you will find that you can make minor changes to your habits that end up having positive environmental and health effects. You can choose not to drive to locations that are less than a couple of miles away, for example, which will cut down on auto emissions while giving you necessary exercise. The list goes on, but you get the idea — a whole lot of people can do things that aren't really an inconvenience and make real, lasting changes (Figure 19).

For more tips on sustainable living, visit:

- www.epa.gov/greenerproducts
- www.un.org/sustainabledevelopment/takeaction

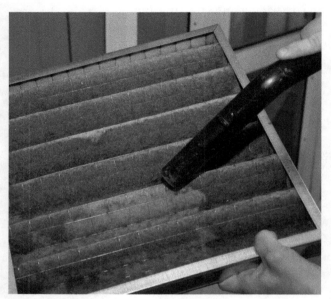

Figure 18. Cleaning your furnace filter can save money.

Ways to Reduce and Reuse	Impact	Benefits
Buy used	You can find everything from clothes to building materials at specialized reuse centers and consignment shops. Often, used items are less expensive and just as good as new.	Prevents pollution caused by reducing the need to harvest new raw materials
Look for products that use less packaging	When manufacturers make their products with less packaging, they use less raw material. This reduces waste and costs. These extra savings can be passed along to the consumer. Buying in bulk, for example, can reduce packaging and save money.	Saves energy
Buy reusable over disposable items	Look for items that can be reused; the little things can add up. For example, you can bring your own silverware and cup to work, rather than using disposable items.	Reduces greenhouse gas emissions that contribute to global climate change
Maintain and repair	Products like clothing, tires, and appliances can be repaired so that they won't have to be thrown out and replaced as frequently.	Helps sustain the environment for future generations
Borrow, rent, or share	Letting others use items that are used infrequently, like party decorations, tools, or furniture allows products to be used to their fullest extent.	Reduces the amount of waste that will need to be recycled or sent to landfills and incinerators

Figure 19. Even simple methods to reduce and reuse can have a big impact.

Water Quality and Pollution

When the water in our rivers, lakes, and oceans becomes polluted, it can endanger wildlife, make our drinking water unsafe, and threaten the waters where we swim and fish. Safe and readily available water is more important for public health than we realize, going far beyond the faucet in our homes. In the US, most people can take water safety for granted. Think about how many times each day you access water in some way. We use it for food production, drinking, showering, cleaning, recreation, and any number of things.

Water pollution is any contamination of water with chemicals or other foreign substances detrimental to human, plant, or animal health. These pollutants include fertilizers and pesticides from agricultural runoff; sewage and food processing waste; lead, mercury, and other heavy metals; chemical wastes from industrial discharges, and chemical contamination from hazardous waste sites.

Water pollution has a significant impact on environmental health and wellness. Worldwide, nearly 2 billion people drink contaminated water that could be harmful to their health. Over 151,000 public water systems provide drinking water to most Americans, and this is just a piece of the way water interweaves into every facet of our lives. The bottom line — water is a vital source of life for nearly every living thing on this planet.

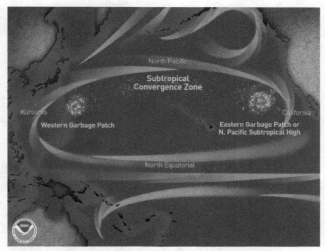

Figure 20. Ocean currents contribute to the Great Pacific Garbage Patch.

The Great Pacific Garbage Patch

Pollution types intersect with one another. Later in this chapter, you will learn more about land pollution. Unfortunately, much of our land pollution now resides in the ocean, lodged in gyres — circular currents driven by the earth's rotation. There are many gyres in our oceans, but the most famous (or notorious) has become home to the **Great Pacific Garbage Patch** (Figure 20). This spiral holds an inestimable amount of trash, much of it plastic. Plastic does not biodegrade — ever. It only breaks down into smaller pieces of plastic (microplastics). In the ocean, animals mistakenly feed on microplastics, consuming toxins and deadly objects that they can't rid from their systems. Ocean trash seriously threatens our ecosystems. To control this form of water pollution, we must first control land pollution.

Groundwater and Surface Water

The nation's freshwater supply — gathered by rainfall, snowmelt, runoff, and infiltration — distributes unevenly across the landscape, throughout the seasons, and from year to year. In many areas, people have grown concerned about the adequacy of the available ground and surface water supply and the quality of the water for its intended uses.

Groundwater lives and moves in the spaces in soil, sand, or cracks in the rocks known as **aquifers**. It supplies drinking water for 51% of the US population and 99% in rural areas. The largest portion of it is used to irrigate crops. **Surface water** is exactly that, water collected on the surface. This is water we can see in our lakes, streams, rivers, and reservoirs. Approximately 80% of all the water used in the US comes from surface water, to drink, irrigate crops, and support our power systems. Groundwater may become surface water if it seeps into streams, lakes, and oceans.

Aquifers are typically made up of gravel, sand, sandstone, or fractured rock, like limestone (Figure 21). Water can move through these materials because they have large connected spaces that make them permeable. The pace at which groundwater travels depends on the size of the spaces in aquifers. When people dig wells for their homes, for example, they dig into an aquifer to retrieve groundwater.

Threats to Groundwater

In areas where material above the aquifer is permeable, pollutants can easily sink into the groundwater supplies. Groundwater can be polluted by landfills, storage tanks, septic tanks, leaky underground gas tanks, factories, livestock farms, and from overuse of fertilizers and pesticides. This is referred to as **point source pollution**, which means that we can identify the source of the problem. If groundwater becomes polluted, it will no longer be safe to drink (Figure 22).

Nonpoint source pollution (NPS) generally results from land runoff, precipitation, atmospheric deposition, drainage, seepage, or hydrologic modification (alteration of stream flow by human activities). NPS pollution is caused by rainfall or snowmelt moving over and through the ground. As the runoff moves, it picks up and carries away natural and man-made pollutants (gasoline, oil, road salt, livestock waste), finally depositing them into lakes, rivers, wetlands, coastal waters, and ground waters (Figure 23).

Groundwater contamination is nearly always the result of human activity. In areas where population density is high and human use of the land is intensive, groundwater is especially vulnerable. Virtually any activity that releases chemicals or wastes into the environment, whether intentionally or accidentally, has the potential to pollute groundwater.

Dangers of Contaminated Groundwater

Contamination of groundwater can result in poor drinking water quality, loss of water supply, degraded surface water systems, high cleanup costs, high alternative water supply costs, and potential health problems. The consequences of contaminated groundwater or degraded surface water can be serious and impact large amounts of people and wildlife habitats. For example, estuaries that have been impacted by high nitrogen levels from groundwater sources have lost critical shellfish habitats.

In some instances, ground water contamination can be so severe that the water supply must be abandoned as a source of drinking water. In other cases, the groundwater can be cleaned up and used again, if the contamination is not too severe and if the municipality is willing to spend a good deal of money. Follow-up water quality monitoring is often required for many

Aquifers and wells

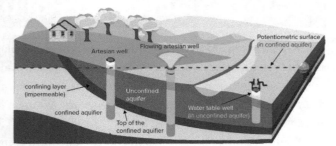

Figure 21. Different ways to access groundwater.

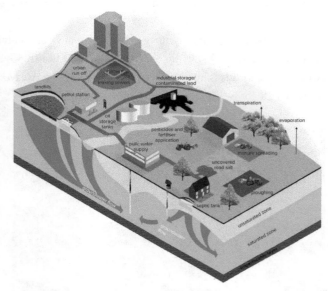

Figure 22. Hazards to clean water come from several sources.

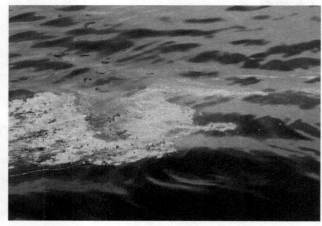

Figure 23. Water pollution isn't always visible on the surface.

years. Because groundwater generally moves slowly, contamination often remains undetected for long periods of time. This makes cleanup of a contaminated water supply difficult, if not impossible. Cleanup can cost thousands to millions of dollars.

A number of microorganisms and thousands of synthetic chemicals have the potential to contaminate ground water. Drinking water containing **bacteria and viruses** can result in illnesses such as hepatitis, cholera, or giardiasis (infection of the small intestine). Methemoglobinemia or "blue baby syndrome," an illness affecting infants, can be caused by drinking water that is high in **nitrates**. High levels of nitrate can enter the water through overuse of chemical fertilizers and improper disposal of human and animal waste. **Benzene**, a component of gasoline, is a known human carcinogen. It can leech into water systems from factories, gas storage tanks, and landfills. The serious health effects of **lead** are well known. It can cause learning disabilities in children; nerve, kidney, and liver problems; and pregnancy risks. Lead can enter drinking water through plumbing.

Concentrations in drinking water of these and other substances are regulated by federal and state laws. Hundreds of other chemicals, however, are not yet regulated, and many of their health effects are unknown or not well understood.

Overuse

Where surface water such as lakes and rivers are inaccessible, people use groundwater to meet their water needs (Figure 24). In the US, aside from being the main source of drinking water, groundwater is used for agricultural needs, consuming over 50 billion gallons per day. **Groundwater depletion**, a term often defined as long-term water-level decline caused by sustained groundwater pumping, is a key issue associated with groundwater use. Many areas of the US face problems with groundwater depletion.

The US Geological Survey has explained that water stored in the ground is comparable to money in a bank account. If you withdraw money at a faster rate than you deposit new

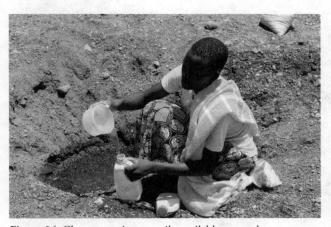

Figure 24. Clean water is not really available everywhere.

money, you will eventually start having supply problems (you'll go broke). Pumping water out of the ground faster than it is replenished over the long-term causes similar problems. The volume of groundwater in storage is decreasing in many areas of the US in response to pumping. Groundwater depletion is primarily caused by sustained groundwater pumping. Some of the negative effects of groundwater depletion include wells drying up, reduced water in streams and lakes, deterioration of water quality, increased pumping costs, and land subsidence (collapse of soil). The environment and our food supplies take a hit when water shortages occur, and so do we. Resources may decline, and the consumer's cost for water and products can increase.

Overuse leads to other problems than shortages. A major issue with water pollution is that individuals use too much water, contributing to waste and extra energy being spent on recycling water unnecessarily. When water goes into the sewer system, it winds up at a treatment plant, where it is processed until it is safe to reintroduce the water into the water supply. This process is expensive and consumes a lot of energy, which is why it is important to use water frugally. Another concern is that we currently use potable water in our toilets, to water our lawns, and for a variety of other purposes that can produce water waste.

Is My Tap Water Safe to Drink?

The US enjoys one of the world's most reliable and safest supplies of drinking water. **The Clean Water Act (CWA)** in 1974 established the basic structure for regulating discharges of pollutants into the waters of the United States and regulating quality standards for surface waters. Congress passed the **Safe Drinking Water Act (SDWA)** in 1974 to protect public health by regulating public water systems. This requires the EPA to establish and enforce standards that public drinking water systems must follow. These EPA standards require tap water to be safe to drink, and this is usually the case. Unfortunately, recent unethical practices in Flint, Michigan and the failure of Portland Public Schools to update their plumbing have cast very public doubts on the safety of tap water. Luckily, it is easy to conduct a test to check water safety.

There are a couple of factors that may lead to valid questions about the quality of your tap water. One factor is the age of the infrastructure through which the water travels and whether there are contaminants in the water. For example, an older home may be on a system that is newer, but the pipes leading from the water main to the house may be made of lead.

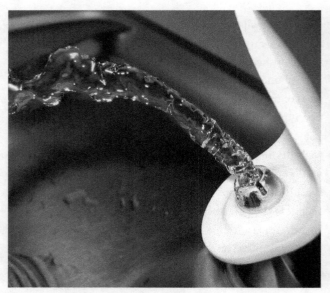

Figure 25. Water fountains are typically filtered for contaminants.

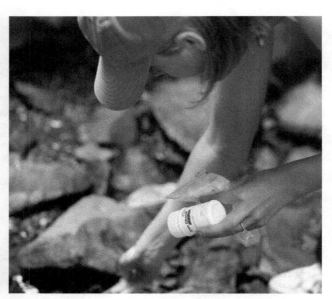

Figure 26. Well water users should test their water quality.

As we've already learned, no level of lead is safe in drinking water. Check for lead at the tap if you have old pipes.

If the lead test is clear, the water is safe to drink. You can usually request a test kit from your water utility provider. If you are still worried, you can buy a water filter. Water filters can improve flavor and, when used properly, keep potential contaminants like lead out of the water (Figure 25).

Some people think tap water is always unsafe and prefer to drink bottled water. The problem with that approach is that bottling water is often expensive and wasteful. Also, most concerns about tap water quality are wrong. Consumers of a public water system can contact their local water supplier and ask for information on contaminants in their drinking water, or they can request a copy of their Consumer Confidence Report. This report lists the levels of contaminants that have been detected in the water, including those by EPA, and whether the system meets state and EPA drinking water standards.

About 10 % of people in the US rely on water from private wells. Private wells are not regulated under the SDWA. People who use private wells need to take precautions to ensure their drinking water is safe (Figure 26). If you still have concerns, some tips on protecting your water supply can give you confidence that you can drink safely (Figure 27).

Establish a routine that protects our water:

Follow instructions for the use, storage, and disposal of household chemicals.

Check your vehicles for leaks; leaks can go unnoticed and contaminate groundwater.

Avoid using fertilizers and other chemicals in your yard. Consider less toxic or natural alternatives.

Avoid overwatering, especially after applying fertilizers and pesticides.

Landscape with native plants, which require little fertilizer, pesticides, and water.

Never pour household chemicals or used motor oil down storm drains or on ground.

Dispose of batteries properly to keep heavy metals out of the environment.

Check underground storage tanks for leaks; many older homes have underground heating oil tanks.

Report chemical spills and illegal dumping.

Dispose of pet waste.

Figure 27. Ways to protect groudwater at home.

Reducing Water Pollution

The EPA advocates a program they call P2 — **Pollution prevention**. This is any practice that reduces, eliminates, or prevents pollution at its source — source reduction. Have you ever heard the old expression "an ounce of prevention is worth a pound of cure?" P2 applies this approach to waste management. Reducing the amount of pollution produced means less waste to control, treat, or dispose. Less pollution means less hazards posed to public health and the environment, including our water supplies.

Preventative measures can be applied to all potential and actual pollution-generating activities. This includes every sector of our society including energy, agriculture, federal, consumer, and industrial. These practices help preserve wetlands, groundwater sources, and other critical ecosystems — areas in which we especially want to stop pollution before it begins.

In the energy sector, pollution prevention can reduce environmental damages from extraction, processing, transport and combustion of fuels. This can be accomplished by increasing efficiency in energy use and the using more environmentally friendly fuel sources (like renewable energies).

In the agricultural sector, approaches include reducing the use of water and chemical inputs, using less environmentally harmful pesticides, and cultivating crop strains with natural resistance to pests. It also includes protecting sensitive areas, such as wetlands, endangered or rare species' habitats, and areas close to water supplies.

The industrial sector can apply P2 practices in many areas and have a significant impact. Many businesses now work to modify production process to produce less waste and reuse materials such as drums and pallets rather than disposing of them as waste. They are encouraged to use non-toxic or less toxic chemicals as cleaners, degreasers, and other maintenance chemicals. Implementing water and energy conservation practices in the industrial sector means significant progress. The industrial sector in the state of Texas alone used 1.5–2 million gallons of water per day in 2015.

In homes and schools, examples of P2 practices include using reusable water bottles instead of disposable, automatically turning off lights when not in use, repairing leaky faucets and hoses, and switching to "green" cleaners.

Pollution prevention reduces both financial costs (waste management and cleanup) and environmental costs (health problems and environmental damage). Pollution prevention protects not only the environment by conserving and protecting natural resources, but also strengthens economic growth through more efficient production in industry and less need for households, businesses, and communities to handle waste.

You can reduce your waste and risk for pollution at home, too. Here are some ways you can target potential waste and pollution in different areas of your home:

Bathroom — Install a toilet dam or plastic bottle in your toilet tank. Install a water-efficient showerhead (2.5 gallons or less per minute). Take short showers and draw less water for baths. If you buy a new toilet, purchase a low-flow model. Check your toilet for "silent" leaks by placing a little food coloring in the tank and seeing if it leaks into the bowl. Turn off water while brushing your teeth and shaving.

Kitchen or Laundry — Compost your food scraps rather than using a garbage disposal in your sink. Keep a gallon of drinking water in the refrigerator rather than running the tap until the water gets cold. Always run your washing machine with a full load of clothes. Wash clothes with warm water instead of hot, and rinse them with cold water instead of warm. Wash with cold water when you can, and when it's warm enough, hang your clothes to dry.

Outdoors — Install a drip-irrigation water system for valuable plants. Use drought-tolerant plants and grasses for landscaping and reduce grass-covered areas. Cut your grass at least three inches high to shade the roots, making it more drought tolerant. Water grass and plants only in the evening or very early morning to minimize evaporation. If you have porous pavement (gravel) instead of asphalt for driveways and walkways, the rain can recharge groundwater supplies instead of running off and contributing to erosion. Use a broom instead of a hose to clean off your driveway or sidewalk. Wash your car less often, or wash it at a car wash where they clean and recycle the water. If you do wash your car at home, use a bucket of soapy water rather than running the hose. Keep a spring-loaded nozzle on the hose so no water is wasted when you're scrubbing.

Global Protection

The EPA is not the only agency hard at work. Agencies around the globe work to protect water supplies. These include the Convention on the Protection and Use of Transboundary Watercourses and International Lakes (Water Convention), the World Health Organization, the United Nations Economic Commission for Europe (UNECE), and the Global Environmental Facility (GEF). These agencies and others work together to implement improved systems, lobby for new regulation, coordinate research, protect public health, and implement systems aimed at cooperation among nations and agencies.

Land Pollution

Land pollution is the deterioration of the earth's land surfaces, often directly or indirectly as a result of human activities and their misuse of resources. We know what this looks like. In fact, this is probably one form of pollution that needs very little definition. Much of it comes from solid waste in some form or another. Waste from garbage, pesticides, fertilizers, household products, and so on. It comes from us at home, from energy producers, manufacturing plants, farms, and other forms of industry. We sometimes dispose of it improperly, and it ends up in the environment. We sometimes dispose of it properly, and it still ends up in the environment, if hopefully in a safer way. But this form of pollution is often right in front of our faces.

Solid Waste

Proper waste management is an essential part of society's public and environmental health. The Resource Conservation and Recovery Act of 1976, created the framework for America's hazardous and non-hazardous waste management programs. Materials regulated by this law are known as "solid wastes" and can also receive an additional classification of "hazardous" depending on the material.

Municipal solid waste (MSW) — more commonly known as trash or garbage — consists of everyday items we use and then throw away, such as product packaging, grass clippings, furniture, clothing, bottles, food scraps, newspapers, appliances, paint, and batteries. This comes from our homes, schools, hospitals, and businesses. This is our excess everything, and it almost always ends up in landfills (Figure 28).

Global solid waste generation, if left unchecked, could increase 70%, rising from more than 3.5 million tons per day in 2010 to more than 6 million tons per day by 2025. The waste from cities alone is already enough to fill a 3,000 miles-long line of garbage trucks every day. The global cost of dealing with all that trash is also rising. Global spending on garbage disposal services reached $205 billion in 2010,

a number expected to reach $375 billion by 2025, with the sharpest cost increases in developing countries.

In 2013, US residents generated about 254 million tons of trash and recycled and composted about 87 million tons of this material, equivalent to a 34.3% recycling rate. On average, we

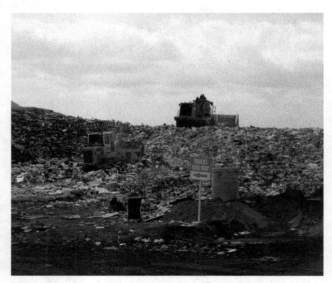

Figure 28. Managing waste is a major pollution issue.

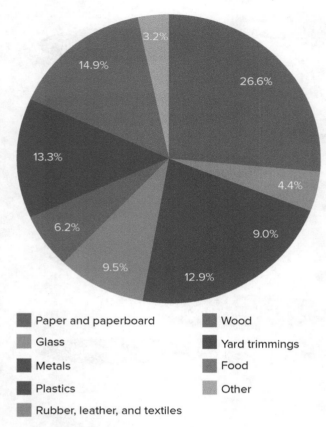

Figure 29. Most MSW can be recycled.

recycled and composted 1.51 pounds of our individual waste generation of 4.40 pounds per person per day. That means that the average person generates over 1600 pounds of garbage per year. If that same person lived to be 80 years old, they would generate over 64 tons of trash in their lifetime! Each person's trash can be broken down into types, with paper and food at the top of the list of most common trash items (Figure 29).

Do you know what happens to most of your 1600-pound gift to society? Have you ever seen a picture of a landfill or been to the dump? If you've never seen where your trash went, you can bet it isn't a pretty sight (or smell). Out of all the trash we generate, more than half ends up in landfills.

The US Love-Hate Relationship with Landfills

After the industrial revolution, the US saw an increase in the amount of garbage produced. We tried letting pigs eat the trash, but that wasn't very practical (or sanitary). We tried pil-

ing it up outside of town, but the smell was awful, and it was a breeding ground for disease. We tried burning it. That didn't work — we ended up with a lot of pollution and an inability to see the Los Angeles skyline. We went back to piling it up outside of town (or at least it used to be outside of town).

The landfills of today are different than the dumps of yesteryear. Landfills go through a careful process of construction and maintenance in an attempt to keep the trash right where it is and as "sanitary" as possible. Essentially, they bury it — dump it in a gigantic open area lined with several layers of protection and then carefully stack, level, and eventually cover the debris.

Landfills serve as the third-largest source of human-related methane emissions in the US, accounting for approximately 15.4 % of these emissions in 2015. At the same time, methane and other gas emissions from landfills can be used to generate energy. Landfill gas can be captured, collected, and used as a renewable form of energy by power plants. The US has over 400 plants utilizing this form of energy.

When MSW is first deposited in a landfill, it undergoes an aerobic (with oxygen) decomposition stage when little methane is generated. Then, typically within a year or less, anaerobic (without oxygen) conditions develop and methane-producing bacteria begin to decompose the waste and generate methane.

Landfills have their merits, at least in the US where we seem to have space, but they also have their drawbacks. Despite careful engineering, they can leak liquids into the groundwater that can be toxic. And just because we can harness some of the harmful gases for good use, it does not mean that all of the trash disappears or that all of the gas stays out of the atmosphere. Not all of the contents of the landfill completely degrade. The process they undergo to engineer the waste often serves to preserve much of it rather than facilitate breakdown.

We use landfills because we don't have a better solution, and for now, at least, we have the space. This will not always be the case. In many areas, we have lots of room. In others, like New York City, we don't. Some cities are forced to haul their trash long distances, even to other states for disposal. This means more gas emissions for transporting the garbage and more opportunity for waste to end up everywhere *but* where it is supposed to.

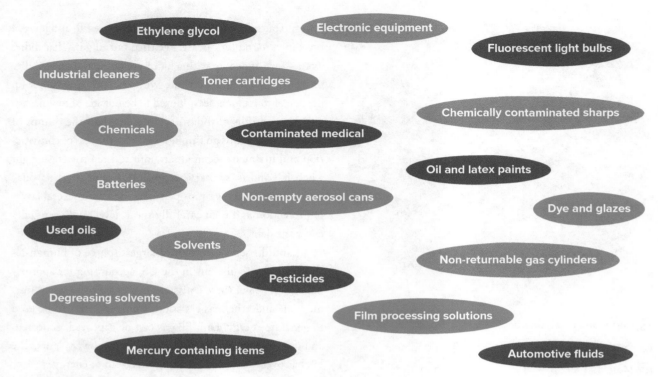

Figure 30. These common waste items are actually hazardous materials.

Hazardous Waste

Hazardous waste has properties that make it potentially dangerous or harmful to human health or the environment. The universe of hazardous wastes is large and diverse. Hazardous wastes can be liquids, solids, or contained gases. They can be the by-products of manufacturing processes, discarded used materials, or discarded unused commercial products, such as cleaning fluids (solvents) or pesticides. In regulatory terms, a hazardous waste is a waste that appears on one of the four RCRA hazardous wastes lists or that exhibits one of the four characteristics of a hazardous waste — ignitability, corrosivity, reactivity, or toxicity (Figure 30).

The EPA developed a regulatory definition and process that identifies specific substances known to be hazardous and provides objective criteria for including other materials in the regulated hazardous waste universe. This identification process can be very complex, so they encourage generators of waste to approach the issue using a series of questions designed to prevent misplacement (Figure 31).

Chemical wastes require special disposal methods because they present an immediate and long-term threat to public health. Some sites in the US have experienced significant toxic threats and have had to be closed down for clean-up. In 1980, Congress established the Comprehensive Environmental Response, Compensation and Liability Act to fund

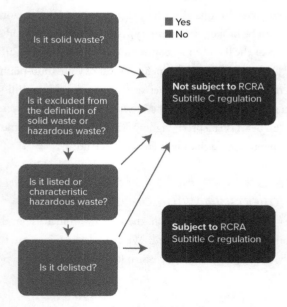

Figure 31. Flowchart used to identify hazardous waste.

and implement cleanup of these area. These are called **Superfund** sites.

A **Superfund site** is any land in the US that has been contaminated by hazardous waste and identified by the EPA as a candidate for cleanup because it poses a risk to human health and/or the environment. These sites are placed on the National Priorities List (NPL). EPA's Superfund program is responsible for cleaning up some of the nation's most contaminated land and responding to environmental emergencies, oil spills, and natural disasters. The goal is to return these places to livable, workable areas.

Electronic Waste

Do you want to replace your phone right now? Again? Of course you do. We all do. After all, there's a new one out each year and amazingly your old one just won't work as well as it used to. The problem is similar with computers, televisions, printers, and every other type of electronic gadget we own. They don't make them to last, and technology is advancing at such a rapid pace that people want the new and improved items. In fact, your phone doesn't need to last because you will replace it anyway. But what happens to these electronics at the end of their lifecycle?

E-waste is a popular, informal name for electronic products nearing the end of their "useful life." Many of these products can be reused, refurbished, or recycled. Certain components of some electronic products contain materials that render them hazardous, depending on their condition and density (Figure 32).

E-waste is an emerging problem given the sheer volume of e-waste being generated and the content of both toxic and valuable materials in these products. Over the past two decades, the global market of electrical and electronic equipment has continued to grow exponentially, while the typical life span of those products has become shorter and shorter. Predictably, the number of electronic devices will continue to increase on the global scale, and microprocessors will be used in ever-increasing numbers in more and more daily-use objects.

We can't dispose of our e-waste in the same way as our MSW. If we do, not only are we throwing away precious metals — such as silver, gold, and palladium — that are used in the product, but we are also throwing toxic chemicals into the environment. It's important to dispose of your e-waste properly. Done the right way, you might even get a little money back in the process. Here are some ways to reduce your e-waste:

Reuse and donate your electronics. Preventing waste in the first place is preferable to any waste management option, including recycling. Donating used (but still operating) electronics for reuse extends the lives of valuable products and keeps them out of the waste stream for a longer period of time. Donating electronics allows schools, nonprofit organizations and lower-income families to obtain equipment that they otherwise could not afford. Businesses can also take advantage of tax incentives for donated computer equipment. Some places will even give you cash or store credit for your old electronics.

Recycle your electronics. If donation for reuse or repair is not a viable option, households and business can send their used electronics for recycling. Recycling electronics helps reduce pollution that would be generated while manufacturing a new product and the need to extract valuable and limited virgin resources.

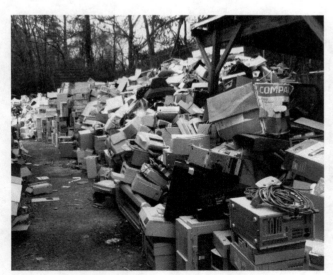

Figure 32. E-waste is common as new tech created.

Electronic recycling also reduces the energy used in new product manufacturing.

Buy green electronics. Environmentally responsible electronics use involves not only proper end-of-life disposition of obsolete equipment, but also purchasing new equipment that has been designed with environmentally preferable attributes. Green electronics contain fewer toxic components. The use of recycled materials in new products promotes many benefits: they are more energy efficient, are more easily upgraded or disassembled, and use less wasteful packaging.

The 3 "R's" for Resource Conservation

If you attended elementary school in the last few decades, you probably learned some version of the "Reduce, Reuse, Recycle" song. The EPA's strategy for resource conservation basically mirrors the song (Figure 33). Many areas of the country promote the importance of recycling. Recycling and composting prevented 87.2 million tons of material from being thrown away in 2013, up from 15 million tons in 1980. This prevented the release of approximately 186 million metric tons of carbon dioxide equivalent into the air in 2013 — equivalent to taking over 39 million cars off the road for a year (Figure 34).

This is great progress, but we can always do more! There are a lot of ways to minimize waste and a good first step is to avoid creating trash in the first place. This is what we call source reduction — starting at the very beginning of the chain of waste — and stopping it before it starts.

The 3 R's aren't just about the waste itself — they lead to a reduction in the use of resources. Every time we buy a new product, it takes resources to create it, ship it, and dispose of it at the end of its life. Each and every step consumes valuable resources and contribute to pollution. The 3 R's asks us to consider which steps we can alter to lower our negative impact to the environment.

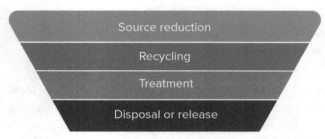

Figure 33. Environmental protection pollution prevention hierarchy.

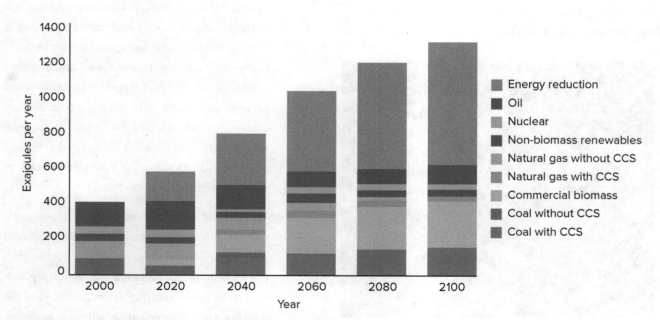

Figure 34. Environmental goals looking into the future (Souce: EPA).

Reduce

Making a new product requires a lot of materials and energy — raw materials must be extracted from the earth, and the product must be fabricated then transported to wherever it will be sold. You, the consumer, can only do so much to control that step. For manufacturers, there are ways that reduction can take place. When was the last time you ordered something online and it came in a box six times too big? Or, even worse, a box inside a box filled with non-recyclable packaging materials like packing foam? The companies that make your products do have the ability to reduce significantly.

So how do you play a role in reducing waste? You can often break your link in the chain with common sense and practicality. Consider some of these basic approaches:

Buy what you need — Check your pantry and make a shopping list before you buy

Buy what you can use — Don't buy in bulk if you cannot or will not use something before it expires

Buy smart — Many products are flimsy and cheap, not likely to last. Avoid products that you will only be able to use a few times before throwing them away.

Be thrifty — If you have six scarves that you never wear, do you need another?

Speak up — Tell manufacturers what you think about their wasteful packaging. If they don't get the point, use a different vendor.

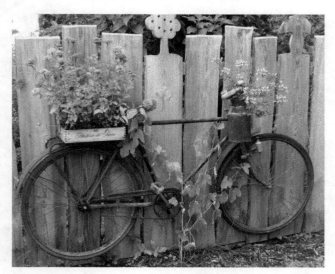

Figure 35. Finding new ways to reuse old items can be fun.

Reuse

This is a broad term with no one distinct definition. There are many ways that an item can be reused depending on the context. At home, there are some common items that frequently pose a problem and some easy ways to handle them:

Buy reused or recycled products when you can. This keeps the 3R chain intact and the waste chain from growing.

Donate your old items. Local churches, community centers, thrift stores, schools, and nonprofit organizations accept lightly used items as donations. Many may accept a variety of donated items, including used books, working electronics, and unneeded furniture (some will even buy them from you).

Repurpose your unwanted items. Consider how you might utilize an item as something else. Empty coffee cans, for example, make good storage containers. Empty pie tins and take-out containers make great greenhouses for plants (Figure 35). Many forms of "trash" can be repurposed.

Limit use of plastic shopping bags. Carry your own reusable shopping bags to the store to eliminate the need for paper or plastic.

Recycle

Recycling is the process of collecting and processing materials that would otherwise be thrown away as trash and turning them into new products. Familiar items that can be recycled include paper, cardboard, aluminum, tin, glass, and most plastic.

Recycling includes the three steps, which create a continuous loop, represented by the familiar recycling symbol:

Step 1: Collection and Processing — There are several methods for collecting recyclables, including curbside collection, drop-off centers, and deposit or refund programs. After collection, recyclables are sent to a recovery facility to be sorted, cleaned and processed into materials that can be used in manufacturing. Recyclables are bought and sold just like raw materials would be, and prices go up and down depending on supply and demand in the United States and the world.

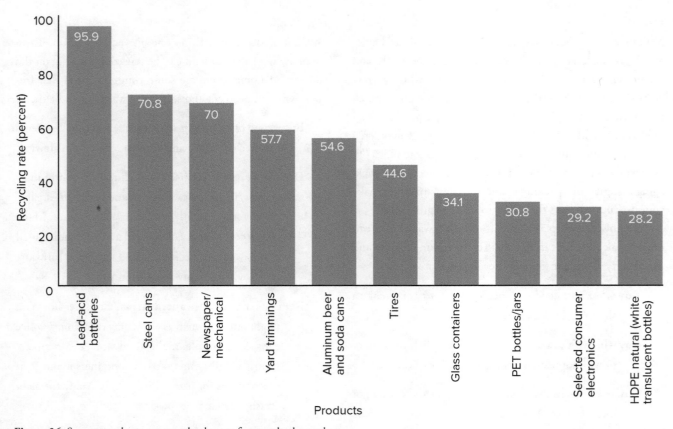

Figure 36. Some prooducts are recyclyed more frequently than others.

Step 2: Manufacturing — More and more of today's products are being manufactured with recycled content. Common household items that contain recycled materials include paper, plastic, aluminum, and glass (many of the things we turn in curbside). Recycled materials can also be used in new ways such as recovered glass in asphalt to pave roads or recovered plastic in carpeting and park benches.

Step 3: Purchasing New Products Made from Recycled Materials — You help close the recycling loop by buying new products made from recycled materials. As mentioned above, there are thousands of products that contain recycled content. When you go shopping, look for products that can be easily recycled, or are made from recycled content (Figure 36).

Refuse

Recycling consumes fewer natural resources and has less damage to the environment, but it still has some impact — some materials take energy to transport and convert to other products. For this reason, many people offer a fourth "R" — refuse. How many times do you accept a plastic bag at the grocery store when you don't need it? How many times to you accept a silly give-away freebie, some gimmick from someone pushing their products? Your closets and drawers might be littered with free t-shirts, magnets, calendars, toys, and bobble-heads that you didn't really want. How many times have you taken home your leftovers from a restaurant in a plastic container only to throw them away in a few days? Consider this before bringing home any new item. Ask yourself — what value will this have and where will it eventually end up? If enough people start refusing the freebies that no one really wants or needs, companies will stop producing them, and they'll stop ending up in landfills across the country.

Food Waste

Most people don't realize how much food they throw away every day — from uneaten leftovers to spoiled produce. About 95% of the food we throw away ends up in landfills or combustion facilities. In 2014, people disposed of more than 38 million tons of food waste. By managing food sustainably and reducing waste, businesses and consumers can save money, provide a bridge in our communities for those who do not have enough to eat, and conserve resources for future generations.

As mentioned earlier, one easy way is to plan ahead. Plan a menu for the week, check your pantry, and make a list. Plan your menu to use the leftovers from each meal for another meal, perhaps one you can freeze. Avoid buying items in bulk that you've never tried before or that you know you can't consume, even if it's cheaper. The goal is to buy only what you need.

Make use of your leftovers and food that's about to go bad. If your bananas are about to rot, make banana bread or

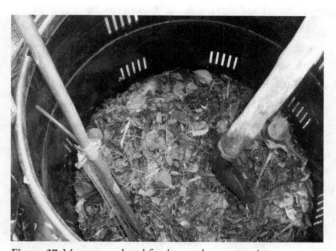

Figure 37. Manage yard and food waste by composting.

put them in the freezer for smoothies. Have leftover pot roast? Make soup! Think before you put something in the trash.

Composting

Compost is organic material that can be added to soil to help plants grow. Food scraps and yard waste currently make up 20 to 30 % of what we throw away and can be composted instead. Making compost keeps these materials out of landfills where they take up space and release methane (Figure 37).

All composting requires three basic ingredients:

Browns — This includes materials such as dead leaves, branches, and twigs.

Greens — This includes materials such as grass clippings, vegetable waste, fruit scraps, and coffee grounds.

Water — Having the right amount of water, greens, and browns is important for compost development.

Your compost pile should have an equal amount of browns to greens. You should also alternate layers of organic materials of different-sized particles. The brown materials provide carbon for your compost, the green materials provide nitrogen, and the water provides moisture to help break down the organic matter.

Composting is a good way to be sustainable. The scraps from the fruits and vegetables you consume, for example, can create fertilizer to help you grow more. But it does take a little time and know-how to get started. Look online for tutorials on how to compost well. If you don't have the discipline to compost on your own, many waste companies offer composting services. All you need to do is save the waste and put it in the proper bin at the curb. They'll do the rest.

Energy Recovery from Waste

Energy recovery from the combustion of municipal solid waste is a key part of the non-hazardous waste management hierarchy, which ranks various management strategies from most to least environmentally preferred. Energy recovery ranks below source reduction and recycling/reuse but above treatment and disposal.

Confined and controlled burning, known as combustion,

can not only decrease the volume of solid waste destined for landfills, but can also recover energy from the waste burning process. This generates a renewable energy source and reduces carbon emissions by offsetting the need for energy from fossil sources and reduces methane generation from landfills.

At an MSW combustion facility, the waste is placed into a combustion chamber to be burned. The heat released from burning converts water to steam, which is then sent to a turbine generator to produce electricity. The remaining ash is collected and taken to a landfill where a high-efficiency baghouse filtering system captures particulates. As the gas stream travels through these filters, more than 99% of particulate matter is removed. The facility transports the ash residue to an enclosed building where it is loaded into covered, leak-proof trucks and taken to a landfill designed to protect against groundwater contamination. Ash residue from the furnace can be processed for removal of recyclable scrap metals.

Other Environmental Health Concerns

Since we have learned the environmentally damaging effects of our industrial practices and started seeking solutions, we have often had to proceed to new practices with caution. Will the technology that saves us from toxic air today be the problem we need to solve tomorrow? This question is often raised when we talk about nuclear power.

Nuclear Power

Many power plants, including **nuclear power** plants, use water to produce energy (Figure 38). Nuclear power plants use steam from heated water to spin large turbines that generate electricity. They do this through a process called nuclear fission.

In **nuclear fission**, atoms split apart to form smaller atoms, releasing energy. Fission takes place inside the reactor of a nuclear power plant. At the center of the reactor is the core, which contains uranium fuel. The uranium fuel is formed into ceramic pellets. Each ceramic pellet produces roughly the same amount of energy as 150 gallons of oil. These energy-rich pellets are stacked end-to-end in 12-foot metal fuel rods. A bundle of fuel rods, sometimes containing hundreds, is called a fuel assembly. A reactor core contains many fuel assemblies.

The heat produced during nuclear fission in the reactor core is used to boil water into steam, which turns the turbine blades. As the turbine blades turn, they drive generators that make electricity. Afterward, the steam is cooled back into water in a separate structure at the power plant called a cooling tower. The water can then be reused.

Nuclear power plants have generated about 20% of US electricity since 1990. The US has 99 nuclear reactors at 61 operating nuclear power plants located in 30 states. We generate more nuclear power than any other country. Of the 31 countries in the world that have commercial nuclear power plants, the US has the most nuclear capacity and generation. France has the second-highest nuclear electricity generation and obtains about 75% of its total electricity from nuclear energy. Fifteen other countries generate more than 20% of their electricity from nuclear power.

Unlike fossil fuel-fired power plants, nuclear reactors do not directly produce air pollution or carbon dioxide while operating. However, the processes for mining and refining uranium ore and making reactor fuel all require large amounts of energy. Nuclear power plants also have large amounts of metal and concrete, which require large amounts of energy to manufacture. If fossil fuels are used for mining and refining uranium ore, or if fossil fuels are used when constructing the nuclear power plant, then the emissions from burning those fuels could be associated with the pollution that nuclear power plants generate.

The primary environmental concern related to nuclear power is the creation of **radioactive wastes** such as uranium

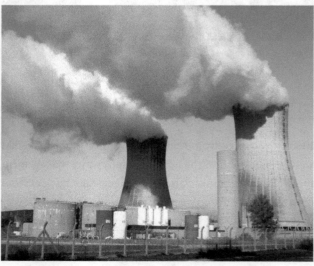

Figure 38. Steam rising from cooling nuclear power plants.

mill tailings, and spent (used) reactor fuel, among others. These materials can remain radioactive and dangerous to human health for thousands of years. Radioactive wastes are subject to special regulations that govern their handling, transportation, storage, and disposal to protect human health and the environment.

The radioactivity of nuclear waste decreases over time through a process called radioactive decay. The amount of time it takes for the radioactivity of material to decrease to half its original level is called its radioactive half-life. Radioactive waste with a short half-life is often stored temporarily before disposal to reduce potential radiation doses to workers who handle and transport the waste. This storage system also reduces the radiation levels at disposal sites.

By volume, most of the waste related to the nuclear power industry has a relatively low level of radioactivity. High-level radioactive waste consists of irradiated or spent nuclear reactor fuel, such as the fuel rods mentioned earlier. These radioactive spent reactor fuel assemblies must be stored in specially designed pools of water. The water cools the fuel and acts as a radiation shield. Spent reactor fuel assemblies can also be stored in specially designed dry storage containers. An increasing number of reactor operators now store their older spent fuel in dry storage facilities using special outdoor concrete or steel containers and air cooling. The US doesn't currently have a permanent disposal facility for high-level nuclear waste. In many ways, we can look at nuclear waste as yet another form of trash that we can't get rid of — one that can be very dangerous.

When a nuclear reactor stops operating, it must be decommissioned. Decommissioning involves safely removing from service the reactor and all equipment that has become radioactive. The radioactivity must be reduced to a level that permits other uses of the property. This is largely where controversy arises. Once a reactor is decommissioned, what do we do with it? Are there harmful effects to the neighborhoods near these radioactive plants? Is the waste at risk?

Nuclear Reactor Safety and Security Features

An uncontrolled nuclear reaction inside a reactor could result in widespread contamination of air and water. The risk of this happening at nuclear power plants in the US is considerably small because of the diverse and redundant barriers and numerous safety systems in place at nuclear power plants, the training and skills of the reactor operators, testing and maintenance activities, and the regulatory requirements and oversight of the US Nuclear Regulatory Commission. A large area surrounding nuclear power plants is restricted and guarded by armed security teams. US reactors also have containment vessels designed to withstand extreme weather events and earthquakes.

Despite this, we have seen other countries sustain catastrophic damage due to problems with their reactors. This combined with controversy over whether or not people living near the reactors are exposed to any level of radioactivity makes them a hot topic of debate. When decommissioned reactors sit idly, people get nervous. The future of nuclear energy will likely depend on how the nation decides to store and protect waste long-term and how comfortable they can make the community.

Radiation

This may be surprising, but we are exposed to naturally-occurring radiation in the environment every day, some of which has an effect on our health. Energy emitted from any source is generally referred to as **radiation**. Examples include heat or light from the sun, microwaves from an oven, X rays, and gamma rays from radioactive elements.

Ionizing radiation can cause concern. The World Health Organization defines **ionizing radiation** as radiation with enough energy so that during an interaction with an atom, it can remove tightly bound electrons from the orbit of an atom, causing the atom to become charged or ionized. This type of radiation has sufficient energy to cause chemical changes in cells and

damage them. Some cells may die or become abnormal, either temporarily or permanently. By damaging the genetic material contained in the body's cells, radiation can cause cancer. Fortunately, our bodies are extremely efficient at repairing cell damage.

A very large amount of radiation exposure (acute exposure) can cause sickness or even death within hours or days. Such acute exposures are extremely rare.

Radioactive Material in the Earth and in Our Bodies

Uranium and thorium naturally found in the earth are called primordial (existing since the formation of the solar system).

Trace amounts of uranium, thorium, and their decay products can be found everywhere. Traces of radioactive materials can be found in the body, mainly naturally occurring potassium-40. Potassium-40 is found in the food, soil, and water we ingest, allowing it to be absorbed into our bodies.

48% of the average American's dose of radiation, however, comes from medical procedures. This total does not include the dose from radiation therapy used in the treatment of cancer, which is typically many times larger.

Chronic and Acute Exposure

In general, the amount and duration of radiation exposure affects the severity or type of health effect. There are two broad categories of health effects — chronic (long-term) and acute (short-term).

Chronic exposure is continuous or intermittent exposure to radiation over a long period of time. With chronic exposure, there is a delay between the exposure and the observed health effect. These effects can include cancer, benign tumors, cataracts, and potentially harmful genetic changes. Current studies are not yet clear about whether doses of low-level radiation cause cancer. Experts disagree over the exact definition and effects of "low dose." US radiation protection standards are based on the premise that any radiation dose carries some risk, and that risk increases directly with each dose.

Background radiation is present on Earth at all times. The majority of background radiation occurs naturally from minerals, and only a small fraction comes from man-made elements such as nuclear weapons testing and medical procedures. Naturally occurring radioactive minerals in the ground, soil, water, and your body produce background radiation, as does cosmic radiation from outer space. In fact, people at higher altitudes are exposed to more cosmic radiation.

Acute exposure means short-term, like what we receive during an x-ray. Repeated x-rays, for example, could result in chronic exposure. Acute exposure can be serious if the source is a significant dose of radiation. Survivors of atomic bomb blasts or nuclear power plant disasters can experience acute radiation syndrome. The severity and symptoms depend on the nature of the exposure. They often begin with nausea, vomiting, and diarrhea that last for several days. After this, the person may develop more long-lasting problems with bone marrow, cardiovascular, central nervous, or gastrointestinal systems. Some of these issues will resolve. For some, acute radiation syndrome is fatal.

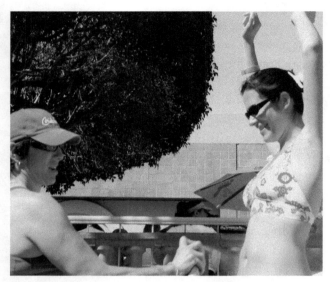

Figure 39. Always apply sunscreen to avoid UV radiation.

Ultraviolet Radiation

Ultraviolet radiation is ubiquitous in sunlight and comes in three main types: UV-A, UV-B, and UV-C. Our atmosphere protects us from UV-C, which quickly damages cells.

UV-A causes premature skin aging, damages cells at the genetic level, and causes melanin release, which is the body's relatively ineffective defense against sun exposure. UV-A damage is what causes a suntan. People who purposefully expose themselves to UV-A via tanning beds are 75% more likely to develop melanoma, a skin cancer which metastasizes quickly.

UV-B causes sunburn, which is a defense response to UV-B damage, similar to what happens with an open wound. The body reacts to UV-B damage as if it is an infection, which is why the skin becomes inflamed and puffy — blood and white blood cells rush to the surface of the skin.

The best defense against UV-A and UV-B radiation damage is to minimize exposure to the sun by staying out of it, wearing sun-protective clothing, and by correctly applying broad spectrum sunscreen with a 30+ SPF rating. If the label on the sunscreen does not indicate it is broad spectrum, then it will only protect against UV-B radiation.

SPF

Sun Protection Factor (SPF) is a measure of how much solar energy (**UV radiation**) is required to produce sunburn on protected skin (i.e., in the presence of sunscreen) relative to the amount of solar energy required to produce sunburn on unprotected skin. As the SPF value increases, sunburn protection increases (Figure 39).

Generally, a sunburn takes less time to occur if you're exposed to the same amount of solar energy at midday compared to early morning or late evening because the sun is more intense at this time. Solar intensity also relates to geographic location, with greater solar intensity occurring at lower latitudes. Because clouds absorb solar energy, solar intensity is generally greater on clear days than cloudy days.

In addition to solar intensity, a number of other factors influence the amount of solar energy that a consumer is exposed to:

Skin type — Fair-skinned individuals absorb more solar energy than dark-skinned under the same conditions.

Amount of sunscreen applied — The amount and SPF of sunscreen impact the level of exposure to UV radiation.

Reapplication frequency — Sunscreens wear off and become less effective with time, so the frequency of reapplication of sunscreen is critical to limiting absorption of solar radiation. Sweat, water, and physical activity can wash or rub sunscreen away. In general, more frequent reapplication is associated with decreased absorption of solar radiation.

SPF does not inform consumers about the time that can be spent in the sun without getting sunburn. Rather, SPF is a relative measure of the amount of sunburn protection provided by sunscreens. It allows consumers to compare the level of sunburn protection provided by different sunscreens. For example, consumers know that SPF 30 sunscreens provide more sunburn protection than SPF 8 sunscreens.

Noise Pollution

"Turn that noise down!" How many times have you heard someone from an older generation refer to music as noise? To them, loud thrashing music or thumping beats are a kind of pollution — an unwelcome, unwanted sound that disturbs their peace. The traditional definition of noise is "unwanted or disturbing sound." Sound becomes unwanted if it either interferes with normal activities, such as sleeping and conversation, or it disrupts or diminishes one's quality of life.

The fact that you can't see, taste, or smell noise may help explain why it has not received as much attention as other types of pollution, such as air or water pollution. Yet the air around us is constantly filled with sounds, even if we've grown a bit deaf to them. For some of us, the persistent and escalating sources of sound can often be considered an annoyance. This "annoyance" can have major consequences, primarily to one's overall health (Figure 40).

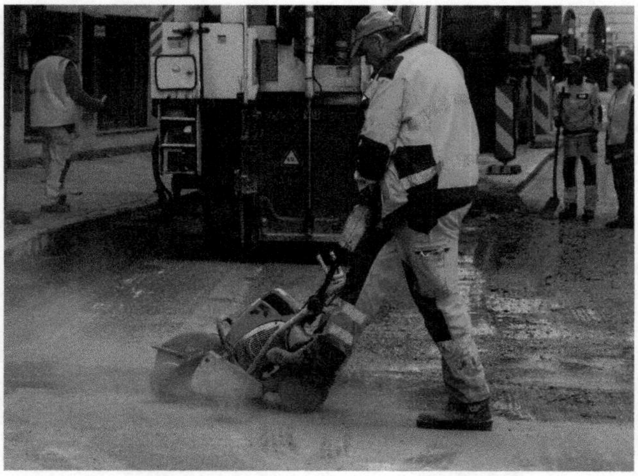

Noise pollution adversely affects the lives of millions of people. Studies have shown that there are direct links between noise and health. Problems related to noise include stress related illnesses, high blood pressure, speech interference, hearing loss, sleep disruption, and lost productivity.

Noise Induced Hearing Loss (NIHL) is the most common effect of noise pollution on health. NIHL can make it hard to understand speech in noisy environments, such as restaurants. NIHL can be caused by a one-time exposure to an intense "impulse" sound, such as an explosion, or by continuous exposure to loud sounds over an extended period of time, such as noise generated in a woodworking shop.

Recreational activities can also put you at risk for NIHL. Examples include target shooting and hunting, snowmobile riding, listening to MP3 players at high volume through earbuds or headphones, playing in a band, and attending loud concerts. Harmful noises at home may come from sources including lawnmowers, leaf blowers, and woodworking tools.

Sound is measured in units called decibels. Sounds of less than 75 decibels, even after long exposure, are unlikely to cause hearing loss. However, long or repeated exposure to sounds at or above 85 decibels can cause hearing loss. The louder the sound, the shorter the amount of time it takes for NIHL to happen. Note the average decibel ratings of some

Figure 40. Noise pollution can be a real problem at work.

Noise Type	Decibels
A humming refrigerator	45
Normal conversation	60
Noise from heavy city traffic	85
A motorcycle	95
An MP3 player at maximum volume	105
Sirens	120
Firecrackers and firearms	150

Figure 41. Average decibel levels of common sounds.

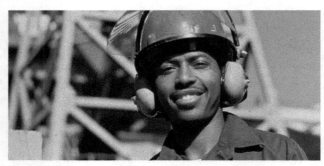

Figure 42. Always wear ear protection in loud environments.

familiar sounds, and consider whether you are continuously exposed to sounds above 85 decibels either from this list or comparable sounds (Figure 41).

NIHL is associated with increased aggression, decreased helpful behavior, reduced motivation and task performance, and even impaired cognitive development in children. Think about it this way — when you have to ask someone to repeat themselves more than once, don't you get agitated? Maybe you even give up trying to understand them. When you try to watch a movie but can't hear it for some reason (maybe your friend won't stop talking), don't you become annoyed? This is similar to what happens with people who experience hearing loss.

Noise Pollution at Work

According to the CDC, noise pollution is especially prominent in the workplace. An estimated 16 million people work in manufacturing, which is about 13% of the US workforce. According to the Bureau of Labor Statistics, occupational hearing loss is the most commonly recorded occupational illness in manufacturing (17,700 cases out of 59,100 cases), accounting for 1 in 9 recordable illnesses. These numbers are particularly disturbing considering that a person's hearing loss must be determined to be work-related — and the hearing loss must be severe enough that the worker has become hearing impaired — in order to be considered recordable. Many more workers could have measurable occupational hearing loss but may not yet have become hearing impaired.

Protecting Your Hearing

If you know you are going to be in a high-decibel environment, use ear protection. Earplugs and sound-canceling earmuffs are inexpensive and easy to keep on hand (Figure 42). Adequate hearing protection is that which reduces noise exposure to below 85 decibels over the course of an average work shift of eight hours. Some people won't wear hearing protection because they think it makes them look silly. That's a silly reason to permanently damage your ears.

Conclusion

This chapter discussed the different types of pollution, their effects on the health of the environment and the population, and ways that you can help reduce your exposure to pollution. Your next steps should be to assess the ways you can reduce your individual pollutants and encourage others around you — at work and in your community — to reduce overall pollution and improve environmental health for all people. Think about why it is important to you to be environmentally aware, and consider strategies that you could use to reduce, reuse and recycle to make a personal impact on the planet.

Reflection Questions

1. How concerned are you about issues related to environmental health? Please explain your reasoning.

2. Identify one of the criteria air pollutants and discuss its main sources and possible health effects.

3. What is climate change, and how can it affect health?

4. What do you think should be the role of government in environmental health and pollution reduction? Please explain your thoughts.

5. What is noise pollution, and how can it impact health?

6. What is one behavior change you could make to improve your environmental wellness? Why do you think this might be important? How willing are you to adopt this strategy?

Text Acknowledgments

Chapter 1

This chapter reuses content from the following openly licensed sources:

Our World in Data (https://ourworldindata.org/life-expectancy/).

HE 250: Personal Health, Portland Community College (https://www.oercommons.org/authoring/14221-he-250-personal-health-portland-community-college/view).

This chapter reuses content in the Public Domain from the following US Government sources:

Centers for Disease Control and Prevention (https://www.cdc.gov).

Office of The Assistant Secretary for Planning and Evaluation (https://aspe.hhs.gov).

Healthy People 2020 (https://www.healthypeople.gov).

Eunice Kennedy Shriver National Institute of Child Health and Human Development (https://www.nichd.nih.gov).

US Department of Health and Human Services (https://www.hhs.gov).

This chapter reuses content under fair use from the following international non-profit organizations:

World Health Organization (http://www.who.int/about/mission/en/).

Chapter 2

This chapter reuses content in the Public Domain from the following US Government sources:

Centers for Disease Control and Prevention (https://www.cdc.gov).

National Center for Biotechnology Information (https://www.ncbi.nlm.nih.gov).

Office of Disease Prevention and Health Promotion (www.health.gov).

National Institute of Diabetes and Digestive and Kidney Diseases (https://www.niddk.nih.gov).

Oregon Department of Education (www.oregon.gov/ODE).

National Weather Service (http://www.nws.noaa.gov).

Environmental Protection Agency (www.epa.gov).

National Institutes of Health (http://www.nih.gov).

This chapter reuses content under fair use from the following national non-profit organizations and scholarly sources:

Medicine & Science in Sports and Exercise (http://journals.lww.com/acsm-msse/Abstract/2011/07000/Quantity_and_Quality_of_Exercise_for_Developing.26.aspx).

American College of Sports Medicine (http://www.acsm.org/public-information/articles/2016/10/07/basic-injury-prevention-concepts).

Asthma and Allergy Foundation of America (http://www.aafa.org/page/exercise-induced-asthma.aspx).

Chapter 3

This chapter reuses content in the Public Domain from the following US Government sources:

National Heart, Lung, and Blood Institute (https://www.nhlbi.nih.gov/health/health-topics/topics/phys/benefits).

Centers for Disease Control and Prevention (https://www.cdc.gov).

National Center for Biotechnology Information (https://www.ncbi.nlm.nih.gov).

Office of Disease Prevention and Health Promotion (www.health.gov).

National Cancer Institute (https://training.seer.cancer.gov/anatomy/cardiovascular/).

US National Library of Medicine (https://medlineplus.gov).

National Institutes of Health (http://www.nih.gov).

This chapter reuses content under fair use from the following national non-profit organizations and scholarly sources:

American Lung Association (http://www.lung.org/lung-health-and-diseases/lung-disease-lookup/copd/living-with-copd/physical-activity.html).

Harvard Health Publishing at Harvard Medical School (http://www.health.harvard.edu/blog/resting-heart-rate-can-reflect-current-future-health-201606179806).

National Academy of Sports Medicine (http://blog.nasm.org/weight-loss-specialist/myths-of-weight-management-you-have-to-exercise-at-a-low-intensity-to-burn-fat/).

American College of Sports Medicine (http://www.acsm.org/about-acsm/media-room/news-releases/2011/08/01/acsm-issues-new-recommendations-on-quantity-and-quality-of-exercise).

American College of Sports Medicine (https://www.acsm.org/docs/brochures/high-intensity-interval-training.pdf).

Chapter 4

This chapter reuses content in the Public Domain from the following US Government sources:

National Cancer Institute (https://training.seer.cancer.gov/anatomy/muscular/).

US Department of Health and Human Services (https://www.hhs.gov/fitness/).

Social Security Administration (https://www.ssa.gov/planners/retire/1943.html).

National Center for Biotechnology Information (https://www.ncbi.nlm.nih.gov).

National Institute on Alcohol Abuse and Alcoholism (https://pubs.niaaa.nih.gov/publications/arh27-4/317-324.htm).

National Human Genome Research Institute (https://www.genome.gov/dnaday/q.cfm?aid=5905&year=2006).

Centers for Disease Control and Prevention (https://www.cdc.gov).

Office of Disease Prevention and Health Promotion (www.health.gov).

National Institutes of Arthritis and Musculoskeletal and Skin Diseases (https://www.bones.nih.gov/health-info/bone/bone-health/exercise/exercise-your-bone-health).

National Institute on Aging (https://www.nia.nih.gov/research/intramural-research-program/dynamics-health-aging-and-body-composition-health-abc).

US National Library of Medicine (https://medlineplus.gov).

National Institute on Drug Abuse (https://www.drugabuse.gov).

Office on Women's Health (https://womenshealth.gov).

Office of Dietary Supplements (https://ods.od.nih.gov).

This chapter reuses content under fair use from the following national non-profit organizations and scholarly sources:

PubChem Open Chemistry Database (https://pubchem.ncbi.nlm.nih.gov/compound/creatine).

PT Direct Tools for Personal Training Success (http://www.ptdirect.com/training-design/anatomy-and-physiology/skeletal-muscle-roles-and-contraction-types).

Therapeutic Advances in Cardiovascular Disease (http://journals.sagepub.com/doi/pdf/10.1177/1753944708089701).

American College of Sports Medicine (http://acsm.org/about-acsm/media-room/news-releases/2011/08/01/acsm-issues-new-recommendations-on-quantity-and-quality-of-exercise).

American College of Sports Medicine (https://www.acsm.org/docs/brochures/resistance-training.pdf).

Chapter 5

This chapter reuses content in the Public Domain from the following US Government sources:

Centers for Disease Control (https://www.cdc.gov).

Office of Disease Prevention and Health Promotion (www.health.gov).

National Center for Biotechnology Information (https://www.ncbi.nlm.nih.gov).

National Institute of Neurological Disorders and Stroke (https://www.ninds.nih.gov/Disorders/Patient-Caregiver-Education/Fact-Sheets/Low-Back-Pain-Fact-Sheet).

National Institute on Aging (https://go4life.nia.nih.gov/exercises/flexibility).

US National Library of Medicine (https://medlineplus.gov).

National Institutes of Arthritis and Musculoskeletal and Skin Diseases (https://www.niams.nih.gov/health-topics/kids/healthy-joints).

National Institutes of Health (https://newsinhealth.nih.gov).

Genetic and Rare Diseases Information Center (https://rarediseases.info.nih.gov/diseases/2081/ehlers-danlos-syndrome-hypermobility-type).

US Department of Veterans Affairs (https://www.move.va.gov/docs/NewHandouts/PhysicalActivity/P33_SampleFlexibilityProgramForBeginners.pdf).

This chapter reuses content under fair use from the following national non-profit organizations and scholarly sources:

Harvard Health Publishing at Harvard Medical School (http://www.health.harvard.edu/staying-healthy/exercising-to-relax).

American College of Sports Medicine (http://www.acsm.org/about-acsm/media-room/news-releases/2011/08/01/acsm-issues-new-recommendations-on-quantity-and-quality-of-exercise).

Chapter 6

This chapter reuses content in the Public Domain from the following US Government sources:

National Institute of General Medical Sciences (https://publications.nigms.nih.gov/insidelifescience/fats_do.html).

National Heart, Lung, and Blood Institute (https://www.nhlbi.nih.gov/health/health-topics/topics/obe/causes).

National Center for Biotechnology Information (https://www.ncbi.nlm.nih.gov).

Centers for Disease Control (https://www.cdc.gov).

US National Library of Medicine (https://medlineplus.gov/ency/article/007199.htm).

Center for Clinical Interventions (http://www.cci.health.wa.gov.au/docs/set%20point%20theory.pdf).

National Institute on Aging (https://www.nia.nih.gov/health/what-menopause).

Surgeon General's Report (https://www.surgeongeneral.gov/library/reports/50-years-of-progress/sgr50-chap-10.pdf).

National Institute of Diabetes and Digestive and Kidney Diseases (https://www.niddk.nih.gov/health-information/weight-management/bariatric-surgery/types).

National Institute of Mental Health (https://www.nimh.nih.gov/health/statistics/prevalence/eating-disorders-among-children.shtml).

US National Library of Medicine (https://medlineplus.gov).

Office on Women's Health (https://womenshealth.gov).

Federal Trade Commission (https://www.consumer.ftc.gov/articles/0261-dietary-supplements).

This chapter reuses content under fair use from the following national non-profit organizations and scholarly sources:

University of Hawai'I Windward Community College (http://krupp.wcc.hawaii.edu/BIOL100L/nutrition/energy.pdf).

National Eating Disorders Collaboration (http://www.nedc.com.au/body-image).

Bradley University (https://www.bradley.edu/sites/bodyproject/male-body-image-m-vs-f/).

Academy of Nutrition and Dietetics (http://www.eatright.org/resource/health/weight-loss/fad-diets/staying-away-from-fad-diets).

Academy of Nutrition and Dietetics (http://www.eatright.org/resource/health/weight-loss/your-health-and-your-weight/healthy-weight-gain).

The Center for Eating Disorders (https://eatingdisorder.org/eating-disorder-information/osfed/).

Chapter 7

This chapter reuses content in the Public Domain from the following US Government sources:

US Department of Health and Human Services (https://www.hhs.gov/fitness/).

Office of Disease Prevention and Health Promotion (www.health.gov).

Choose MyPlate (https://www.choosemyplate.gov/nutrition-nutrient-density).

Centers for Disease Control (https://www.cdc.gov).

National Institute on Aging (https://www.nia.nih.gov/health/smart-food-choices-healthy-aging).

US Department of Agriculture (https://www.usda.gov/).

US National Library of Medicine (https://medlineplus.gov).

National Institute of Diabetes and Digestive and Kidney Diseases (https://www.niddk.nih.gov/health-information/digestive-diseases/celiac-disease/eating-diet-nutrition).

Food and Drug Administration (https://www.accessdata.fda.gov/scripts/InteractiveNutritionFactsLabel/factsheets/Dietary_Fiber.pdf).

National Institutes of Health (https://newsinhealth.nih.gov).

Australian Government Department of Health (https://www.eatforhealth.gov.au/food-essentials/fat-salt-sugars-and-alcohol/fat).

National Center for Complementary and Integrative Health (https://nccih.nih.gov/health/antioxidants/introduction.htm).

Office of Dietary Supplements (https://ods.od.nih.gov/factsheets/VitaminC-HealthProfessional/).

US Geological Survey (https://water.usgs.gov/edu/propertyyou.html).

National Heart, Lung, and Blood Institute (https://www.nhlbi.nih.gov/files/docs/public/heart/dash_brief.pdf).

This chapter reuses content under fair use from the following national non-profit organizations and scholarly sources:

Harvard Health Publishing at Harvard Medical School (https://www.health.harvard.edu/staying-healthy/the-truth-about-fats-bad-and-good).

Harvard School of Public Health (https://www.hsph.harvard.edu/nutritionsource/gluten/).

Harvard School of Public Health (https://www.hsph.harvard.edu/nutritionsource/carbohydrates/added-sugar-in-the-diet/).

Harvard School of Public Health (https://www.hsph.harvard.edu/nutrition-source/2017/04/24/removing-trans-fats-from-restaurant-menus-associated-with-drop-in-heart-attacks-and-strokes/).

Oregon State University Linus Pauling Institute Micronutrient Information Center (http://lpi.oregonstate.edu/mic/minerals).

Chapter 8

This chapter reuses content in the Public Domain from the following US Government sources:

National Institute of Mental Health (https://www.nimh.nih.gov/health/publications/stress/index.shtml).

Centers for Disease Control (https://www.cdc.gov).

National Center for Complementary and Integrative Health (https://nccih.nih.gov/health/stress).

National Center for Biotechnology Information (https://www.ncbi.nlm.nih.gov).

Substance Abuse and Mental Health Services Administration (https://www.samhsa.gov/samhsaNewsLetter/Volume_22_Number_3/working_with_anger/).

State of New Hampshire Employee Assistance Program (https://das.nh.gov/wellness/Docs/Percieved%20Stress%20Scale.pdf).

This chapter reuses content under fair use from the following national non-profit organizations and scholarly sources:

Harvard Health Publishing at Harvard Medical School (https://www.health.harvard.edu/staying-healthy/understanding-the-stress-response).

American Psychological Association (http://www.apa.org/monitor/2011/01/stressed-america.aspx).

American Psychological Association (http://www.apa.org/news/press/releases/stress/2015/snapshot.aspx).

American Psychological Association (http://www.apa.org/topics/anger/control.aspx).

American Psychological Association (http://www.apa.org/topics/personality/).

American Psychological Association (http://www.apa.org/news/press/releases/stress/2013/sleep.aspx).

Anxiety and Depression Association of America (https://adaa.org/living-with-anxiety/women/facts).

Anxiety and Depression Association of America (https://adaa.org/understanding-anxiety/related-illnesses/other-related-conditions/stress/physical-activity-reduces-st).

University of New Mexico Open Library College Success (http://open.lib.umn.edu/collegesuccess/chapter/10-5-stress/).

Chapter 9

This chapter reuses content in the Public Domain from the following US Government sources:

Centers for Disease Control (https://www.cdc.gov).

National Heart, Lung, and Blood Institute (https://www.nhlbi.nih.gov).

National Institute of Neurological Disorders and Stroke (https://www.ninds.nih.gov/Disorders/All-Disorders/Cerebral-Arteriosclerosis-Information-Page).

National Cancer Institute (www.cancer.gov).

National Institute of Diabetes and Digestive and Kidney Diseases (https://www.niddk.nih.gov/health-information/diabetes/overview/what-is-diabetes).

US National Library of Medicine (https://medlineplus.gov).

This chapter reuses content under fair use from the following national non-profit organizations and scholarly sources:

American Heart Association (http://www.heart.org/HEARTORG/Conditions/HeartAttack/WarningSignsofaHeartAttack/Angina-in-Women-Can-Be-Different-Than-Men_UCM_448902_Article.jsp#.WepxpBNSwlJ).

World Health Organization (http://www.who.int/tobacco/quitting/benefits/en/).

Harvard Health Publishing at Harvard Medical School (http://www.health.harvard.edu/blog/mild-high-blood-pressure-in-young-adults-linked-to-heart-problems-later-in-life-201506238100).

Harvard Health Publishing at Harvard Medical School (http://www.health.harvard.edu/heart-health/race-and-ethnicity-clues-to-your-heart-disease-risk).

Harvard Health Publishing at Harvard Medical School (https://www.health.harvard.edu/blog/should-kids-have-their-cholesterol-checked-201112224020).

Harvard Health Publishing at Harvard Medical School (https://www.health.harvard.edu/heart-health/11-foods-that-lower-cholesterol).

Chapter 10

This chapter reuses content in the Public Domain from the following US Government sources:

Centers for Disease Control (https://www.cdc.gov).

National Center for Biotechnology Information (https://www.ncbi.nlm.nih.gov).

US National Library of Medicine (https://medlineplus.gov).

National Institute of Allergy and Infectious Diseases (https://www.niaid.nih.gov).

Health and Human Services Secretary's Minority AIDS Initiative Fund (https://www.hiv.gov/hiv-basics/overview/about-hiv-and-aids/what-are-hiv-and-aids).

This chapter reuses content under fair use from the following national non-profit organizations and scholarly sources:

American Association of Retired Persons (https://www.aarp.org/home-family/sex-intimacy/info-03-2013/sexually-transmitted-infections-should-you-worry.html).

Kaiser Family Foundation (https://www.kff.org/global-health-policy/fact-sheet/the-global-hivaids-epidemic/).

Trust for America's Health (http://healthyamericans.org/assets/files/Final%20Outbreaks%202014%20Report.pdf).

American Academy of Pediatrics (https://www.healthychildren.org/English/health-issues/conditions/infections/Pages/Overview-of-Infectious-Diseases.aspx).

American Academy of Family Physicians (http://www.aafp.org/afp/2015/0501/p652.html).

Chapter 11

This chapter reuses content in the Public Domain from the following US Government sources:

Centers for Disease Control (https://www.cdc.gov).

National Institute on Drug Abuse (https://www.drugabuse.gov).

US National Library of Medicine (https://medlineplus.gov).

National Center for Biotechnology Information (https://www.ncbi.nlm.nih.gov).

National Institute on Alcohol Abuse and Alcoholism (https://pubs.niaaa.nih.gov/publications/aa35.htm).

Department of Health and Human Services (https://betobaccofree.hhs.gov/about-tobacco/Smoked-Tobacco-Products/index.html).

Food and Drug Administration (https://www.fda.gov/TobaccoProducts/Labeling/RulesRegulationsGuidance/ucm297786.htm).

United Kingdom Smokefree National Health Service (https://www.nhs.uk/smokefree/help-and-advice/e-cigarettes).

National Cancer Institute (www.cancer.gov).

National Institutes of Health Office of Disease Prevention (https://prevention.nih.gov/tobacco-regulatory-science-program/about-the-FSPTCA).

This chapter reuses content under fair use from the following national non-profit organizations and scholarly sources:

Substance Abuse and Mental Health Services Administration (https://www.samhsa.gov/prescription-drug-misuse-abuse).

American Lung Association (http://www.lung.org/stop-smoking/i-want-to-quit/five-secrets-for-quitting-smoking.html).

Rice University (http://www.rice.edu/~jenky/sports/caffeine.html).

Brown University (https://www.brown.edu/campus-life/health/services/promotion/alcohol-other-drugs-alcohol/alcohol-and-your-body).

Chapter 12

This chapter reuses content in the Public Domain from the following US Government sources:

European Environment Agency (https://www.eea.europa.eu/soer/synthesis/synthesis/chapter5.xhtml).

Office of Disease Prevention and Health Promotion (https://www.healthypeople.gov).

United Nations Department of Economic and Social Affairs (http://www.un.org/en/development/desa/news/population/2015-report.html).

National Institute on Deafness and Other Communication Disorders (https://www.nidcd.nih.gov/health/noise-induced-hearing-loss).

Central Intelligence Agency World Factbook (https://www.cia.gov/library/publications/the-world-factbook/rankorder/2127rank.html).

Environmental Protection Agency (https://www.epa.gov).

National Center for Biotechnology Information (https://www.ncbi.nlm.nih.gov).

National Resources Conservation Service (https://www.nrcs.usda.gov/wps/portal/nrcs/detail/soils/use/?cid=nrcs142p2_054028).

National Institute of Environmental Health Sciences (https://www.niehs.nih.gov/health/topics/agents/water-poll/index.cfm).

US Energy Information Administration (https://www.eia.gov).

US Global Change Research Program (http://www.globalchange.gov/climate-change).

National Aeronautics and Space Administration (https://climate.nasa.gov).

Food and Drug Administration (https://www.fda.gov/aboutfda/centersoffices/officeofmedicalproductsandtobacco/cder/ucm106351.htm).

US Geological Survey (https://water.usgs.gov/edu/wusw.html).

Portland Water Bureau (https://www.portlandoregon.gov/water/article/32978).

California Department of Toxic Substances Control (http://www.dtsc.ca.gov/HazardousWaste/upload/HWMP_DefiningHW111.pdf).

CalRecycle (http://www.calrecycle.ca.gov/electronics/whatisewaste/).

This chapter reuses content under fair use from the following national non-profit organizations and scholarly sources:

World Health Organization (http://www.who.int/ionizing_radiation/about/what_is_ir/en/).

World Health Organization (http://www.who.int/topics/climate/en/).

World Population History (http://worldpopulationhistory.org/carrying-capacity/).

Wheeling Jesuit University Center for Educational Technologies (http://ete.cet.edu/gcc/?/bio_loss_of_diversity_humact/).

United Nations (http://www.un.org/sustainabledevelopment/takeaction/).

University of Delaware Office of Campus and Public Safety (http://www1.udel.edu/ehs/waste/chemical-waste-management.html).

Image Acknowledgments

Chapter 1

Figure 0. "Push ups" by skeeze is in the Public Domain (https://pixabay.com/en/push-ups-exercise-fitness-workout-888024/).

Figure 1. "Multnomah falls" by AirHaake is licensed under CC BY 2.0 (https://www.flickr.com/photos/80519348@N02/33861704144/).

Figure 5. "Football Children" by Sasint is in the Public Domain (https://pixabay.com/en/football-children-sports-action-1807520/).

Figure 7. "Family Jump" by Evil Erin is licensed under CC BY 2.0 (https://www.flickr.com/photos/evilerin/3565026821).

Figure 9. "Meditation" by Maxlkt is in the Public Domain (https://pixabay.com/en/meditate-theravada-buddhism-monk-2105143/).

Figure 15. "Improvements to Vaccines" by CDC Global is licensed under CC BY 2.0 (https://www.flickr.com/photos/cdcglobal/8190819133/).

Figure 16. "Health Care Provider" by travisdmchenry is in the Public Domain (https://pixabay.com/en/nurse-military-child-1796924/).

Figure 17. "Tokyo Infinity and Houses in a Woody Valley" by Jens Lelie and Pawel Nolbert is in the Public Domain (https://unsplash.com/photos/4u2U8EO9OzY and https://unsplash.com/photos/vIBkCjlYp3o).

Figure 26. "Brussels Marathon Runners" by Martins Zemlickis is licensed under CC BY 4.0 (https://unsplash.com/photos/NPFu4GfFZ7E).

Figure 27. "Fruits, Veggies, and Whole Grains " by dbreen is in the Public Domain (https://pixabay.com/en/carrot-kale-walnuts-tomatoes-1085063/).

Figure 29. "Meditation" by Marcos Moraes is licensed under CC BY 4.0 (https://unsplash.com/photos/LQ-n5xBg1rs).

Figure 30. "Sleep" by claudioscott is in the Public Domain (https://pixabay.com/en/woman-girl-bella-read-sleep-2197947/).

Figure 33. "Critical Thinking About Health Care" by Ilmicrofono Oggiono is licensed under CC BY 2.0 (https://www.flickr.com/photos/115089924@N02/16256199615/).

Figure 34. "Friends" by Anna Vander Stel is licensed under CC BY 4.0 (https://unsplash.com/search/friends?photo=zimQNLdnKp0).

Figure 36. "Calendar, desk, table, and wood" by Rawpixel is in the Public Domain (https://unsplash.com/photos/ZMMXSRMSoI8).

Chapter 2

Figure 0. "Active" by Josh Marshall is in the Public Domain (https://unsplash.com/search/active?photo=BDI3NS0kZOM).

Figure 1. "Sneaker, stair, climb, and exercise" by Bruno Nascimento is in the Public Domain (https://unsplash.com/photos/PHIgYUGQPvU).

Figure 2. "Freedom" by Dino Reichmuth is in the Public Domain (https://unsplash.com/search/freedom?photo=1tFd-Bb1pxk).

Figure 4. "Yoga" by Dave Rosenblum is licensed under CC BY 2.0 (https://www.flickr.com/photos/daverose215/9707554768/sizes/l).

Figure 10. "Pilates" by UptownFitness is in the Public Domain (https://pixabay.com/en/weights-pilates-girls-1948837/).

Figure 11. "Skill-Related Fitness" by Skeeze is in the Public Domain (https://pixabay.com/en/high-jump-track-field-competition-695308/).

Figure 14. "Cyclist and Swimmer" by Dave Hosford is licensed under CC BY 2.0 and Public Domain (https://www.flickr.com/photos/baltimoredave/4715256656/sizes/l and https://pixabay.com/en/swimming-swimmer-female-race-78112/).

Figure 16. "Hiking and Park Life" by Adam Bautz and Stan V Peterson is licensed under CC BY 2.0 and Public Domain (https://www.flickr.com/photos/130811041@N04/19824324090/sizes/l and https://pixabay.com/en/park-life-park-people-walking-life-2251981/).

Figure 17. "Running Shoes Display" by MarkBuckawicki is in the Public Domain (https://commons.wikimedia.org/wiki/File:Running_shoes_display.JPG).

Figure 22. "Smoggy day" by Alex Gindin is in the Public Domain (https://unsplash.com/photos/ifpBOcQlhoY).

Figure 24. "RPG wounded Iraq veteran exercising" by Virginia Reza is in the Public Domain (https://commons.wikimedia.org/wiki/File:RPG_wounded_Iraq_veteran_exercising_Army-dot-mil-2007-02-07-103140.jpg).

Figure 27. "Adaptive Kompressionsbandage, Farrow wrap" by Enter is licensed under CC BY-SA 4.0 (https://commons.wikimedia.org/wiki/File:Adaptive_Kompressionsbandage,_Farrow_wrap.JPG).

Chapter 3

Figure 0. "Cardio Exercise" by hardloperhans is licensed under CC BY 2.0 (https://www.flickr.com/photos/hardloperhans/3648376652/).

Figure 5. "Blood Pressure Cuff" by Morgan is licensed under CC BY 2.0 (https://www.flickr.com/photos/meddygarnet/3489151194/).

Figure 8. "Cardio Exercise" by ThomasWolter is in the Public Domain (https://pixabay.com/en/relay-race-competition-stadium-655353/).

Figure 10. "Ready, set, go" by William Stitt is in the Public Domain (https://unsplash.com/photos/YadCgbsLHcE).

Figure 19. "Bicyclist" by Skeeze is in the Public Domain (https://pixabay.com/en/bicyclist-bicycling-biking-bike-569279/).

Chapter 4

Figure 1. "Paddle Boarding" by Don DeBold is licensed under CC BY 2.0 (https://www.flickr.com/photos/ddebold/19130073248/).

Figure 2. "Climbing" by Terry Robinson is licensed under CC BY-SA 2.0 (https://www.flickr.com/photos/suburbanadventure/4472605204/).

Figure 8. "Endurance activity" by cellue communication is licensed under CC BY SA 2.0 (https://www.flickr.com/photos/131350192@N03/19270296086/).

Figure 10. "Might As Well Jump" by istolethetv is licensed under CC BY 2.0 (https://www.flickr.com/photos/istolethetv/3484450808/sizes/l).

Figure 13. "Big Bay Boot Camp 2012" by Port of San Diego is licensed under CC BY 2.0 (https://www.flickr.com/photos/portofsandiego/7244618416/).

Figure 15. "Rock Climbing and Woman Standing Up Paddle Surfing" by U.S. Army and Bill Ebbesen is licensed under CC BY 3.0 (https://www.flickr.com/photos/soldiersmediacenter/6162645413/ and https://commons.wikimedia.org/wiki/File:Woman_stand_up_paddle_surfing.jpg).

Figure 20. "Planking" by ThoroughlyReviewed is licensed under CC BY 2.0 (https://thoroughlyreviewed.com).

Figure 23. "Weight Machines" by janeb13 is licensed under CC0 Creative Commons (https://pixabay.com/en/gym-room-fitness-sport-equipment-1178293/).

Figure 24. "Weight Lifting" by Eric Astrauskas is licensed under CC BY 2.0 (https://www.flickr.com/photos/121183998@N08/26502758192/).

Figure 25. "Strength Movements" by Pexels and Clem Onojeghuo is in the Public Domain (https://pixabay.com/en/exercise-fitness-lateral-lunges-1845759/ and https://unsplash.com/search/photos/workout?photo=n6gnCa77Urc).

Figure 30. "Protein" by Kennejima is licensed under CC BY 2.0 (https://www.flickr.com/photos/kennejima/29542075312/).

Chapter 5

Figure 0. "Cold Weather" by stocksnap is in the Public Domain (https://pixabay.com/en/cold-weather-winter-jacket-2557515/).

Figure 1. "Stretching Flexibility" by tee1036 is in the Public Domain (https://pixabay.com/en/stretching-flexibility-fitness-2307890/).

Figure 2. "Christine Merrill UCSD Tritons" by SD Dirk is licensed under CC BY 2.0 (https://www.flickr.com/photos/dirkhansen/7674548308/).

Figure 9. "Gout" by James Heilman is licensed under CC BY-SA 3.0 (https://commons.wikimedia.org/wiki/File:Gout2010.JPG).

Figure 11. "Swing Away!" by Zach Dischner is licensed under CC BY 2.0 (https://www.flickr.com/photos/zachd1_618/4683150851/).

Figure 15. "PNF Technique" by Itskelvs is licensed under CC BY-SA 3.0 (https://commons.wikimedia.org/wiki/File:PNF_Technique.JPG).

Figure 17. "Group Stretching" by Rose Physical Therapy is licensed under CC BY 2.0 (https://www.flickr.com/photos/damonbowe/33931712626/sizes/l).

Figure 19. "Abdominal Exercise Fitness" by Keifit is in the Public Domain (https://pixabay.com/en/abdominal-exercise-fitness-gym-1203880/).

Chapter 6

Figure 6. "Meditation" by Balint Foldesi is licensed under CC BY 2.0 (https://www.flickr.com/photos/balintfoeldesi/11752252314/).

Figure 7. "Suburb view on a foggy morning" by Artur Posukin is in the Public Domain (https://unsplash.com/photos/fhR_60xEv0Q).

Figure 8. "Lunch at DC Public Schools" by DC Centural Kitchen is licensed under CC BY 2.0 (https://www.flickr.com/photos/dccentralkitchen/8071512999/).

Figure 9. "Food deserts in the US 2010" by Bldavis2 is licensed under CC BY-SA 4.0 (https://commons.wikimedia.org/wiki/File:Food_Deserts_in_US_(2010).jpg).

Figure 15. "Photos" by Angelina Litvin and Mídia NINJA is licensed under CC BY-NC-SA 2.0 (https://unsplash.com/photos/jrcrJWDywI4 and https://www.flickr.com/photos/midianinja/29259052693/).

Figure 16. "Sprinting in Vienna" by Alexander Redl is in the Public Domain (https://unsplash.com/photos/d3bYmnZ0ank).

Figure 26. "Underwater Weighing" by Sarah Grace Spann is licensed under CC BY 3.0 (https://www.youtube.com/watch?v=Pylv0ushj5s).

Figure 27. "Skinfold Measurement" by Fernando Alacid is licensed under CC BY 3.0 (https://www.youtube.com/watch?v=21vZFgmEcA0).

Chapter 7

Figure 0. "Produce Market" by Patrick Feller is licensed under CC BY 2.0 (https://www.flickr.com/photos/nakrnsm/3815441846/).

Figure 5. "Breads" by FotoshopTofs is in the Public Domain (https://pixabay.com/en/breads-cereals-oats-barley-wheat-1417868/).

Figure 6. "Danish Pancake with Raspberry" by Vegan Feast Catering is licensed under CC BY 2.0 (https://www.flickr.com/photos/veganfeast/5108221092/).

Figure 11. "Avocado" by Chad Miller is licensed under CC BY-SA 3.0 (https://www.flickr.com/photos/chadmiller/69170988/).

Figure 19. "Berries" by Tomasz Stasiuk is licensed under CC BY-SA 2.0 (https://www.flickr.com/photos/zstasiuk/5317397606/).

Figure 20. "Spam Can Nutritional Label" by Lhe3460 is licensed under CC BY-SA 4.0 (https://commons.wikimedia.org/wiki/File:Spam_Can_Nutritional_Label.jpg).

Figure 32. "Celery" by 821292 is in the Public Domain (https://pixabay.com/en/celery-vegetables-vegetable-green-692867/).

Figure 33. "Peaches" by Celine Nadeau is licensed under CC BY-SA 2.0 (https://www.flickr.com/photos/celinet/4962398284/).

Figure 34. "Yellow and red onions" by Alexis Lamster is licensed under CC BY 2.0 (https://www.flickr.com/photos/amlamster/6608862125).

Figure 35. "Milk, beans, soy, and soya" by Rawpixel is in the Public Domain (https://unsplash.com/photos/PKWA8Pei3-c).

Figure 37. "Cooking" by congerdesign is in the Public Domain (https://pixabay.com/p-1013631/?no_redirect).

Chapter 8

Figure 0. "Relax" by Sole Treadmill is licensed under CC BY 2.0 (https://www.flickr.com/photos/149902454@N08/35507035266/sizes/l).

Figure 4. "Study girl writing" by AdinaVoicu is in the Public Domain (https://pixabay.com/en/study-girl-writing-notebook-1231393/).

Figure 8. "Learning" by CollegeDegrees360 is licensed under CC BY-SA 2.0 (https://www.flickr.com/photos/83633410@N07/7658284016/).

Figure 19. "East Hollywood Art Cycle" by SupportPDX is licensed under CC BY 2.0 (https://www.flickr.com/photos/rocketboom/4432507224/sizes/l).

Figure 22. "Depression" by Ryan_M651 is licensed under CC BY 2.0 (https://www.flickr.com/photos/120632374@N07/13974181800/sizes/l).

Figure 25. "Angst" by braerik is licensed under CC BY-SA 2.0 (https://www.flickr.

com/photos/braerik/25022496121/sizes/l).

Figure 27. "Schedule" by fo.ol is licensed under CC BY-SA 2.0 (https://www.flickr.com/photos/forresto/488853222/sizes/l).

Figure 30. "Covey's Task Prioritizer" by Steven Covey is used by permission of Steven Covey.

Figure 32. "Yoga Fitness Program" by Fort Meade is in the Public Domain (https://www.flickr.com/photos/ftmeade/7551022750/sizes/l).

Figure 33. "The Fall Salad" by organicboi is licensed under CC BY 2.0 (https://www.flickr.com/photos/141471286@N06/34854933566/).

Chapter 9

Figure 0. "Colon Biopsy" by Ed Uthmen is licensed under CC BY 2.0 (https://www.flickr.com/photos/euthman/4771852848/).

Figure 10. "Chest Pain" by Pexels is in the Public Domain (https://pixabay.com/en/adult-affection-chest-chest-pain-1846050/).

Figure 15. "Blood Pressure Monitor" by geraldoswald62 is in the Public Domain (https://pixabay.com/en/blood-pressure-monitor-bless-you-1749577/).

Figure 19. "Sunbathing Newlyweds" by Mike Schinkel is licensed under CC BY 2.0 (https://www.flickr.com/photos/mikeschinkel/288584045/).

Figure 22. "Insulin Screening Kit" by Alisha Vargas is licensed under CC BY 2.0 (https://www.flickr.com/photos/alishav/3534216143/).

Figure 23. "Family" by funkblast is licensed under CC BY 2.0 (https://www.flickr.com/photos/funkblast/103936734/).

Figure 25. "Runway Couple" by United States Army is licensed under CC BY 2.0 (https://www.flickr.com/photos/armymedicine/13452149373/).

Figure 26. "Bowl of Granola" by Marco Verch is licensed under CC BY 2.0 (https://www.flickr.com/photos/30478819@N08/35094200403/).

Figure 27. "Depressed" by Sander van der Wel is licensed under CC BY-SA 2.0 (https://www.flickr.com/photos/jar0d/4649749639/).

Figure 28. "Angry Woman" by LARA SCHNEIDER is licensed under CC BY 2.0 (https://commons.wikimedia.org/wiki/File:Angry_woman.jpg).

Figure 29. "A Multigenerational Slice of Life in Mumbai" by Dion Hinchcliffe is licensed under CC BY-SA 2.0 (https://www.flickr.com/photos/dionhinchcliffe/22090447908/).

Chapter 10

Figure 3. "Hi shaking hands friendship" by Jackmac34 is in the Public Domain (https://pixabay.com/en/hi-shaking-hands-friendship-2292499/).

Figure 4. "Chase coughing" by Ryan Boren is licensed under CC BY 2.0 (https://www.flickr.com/photos/ryanboren/2899151607/).

Figure 7. "Clean Hands" by Arlington County is licensed under CC BY-SA 2.0 (https://www.flickr.com/photos/arlingtonva/4314530838/).

Figure 12. "Throat Warts and Spinaliom" by GalliasM and Klaus M Peter is licensed under CC BY-SA 4.0 International (https://commons.wikimedia.org/wiki/File:Throat_Warts_-_HPV.jpg and https://commons.wikimedia.org/wiki/File:Spinaliom3.jpg).

Figure 15. "24 Weeks" by Sara Neff is licensed under CC BY 2.0 (https://www.flickr.com/photos/97725616@N06/14241752215/).

Figure 18. "Pregnant" by Jerry Lai is licensed under CC BY-SA 2.0 (https://www.flickr.com/photos/jerrylai0208/14281758292/).

Figure 19. "AIDSVu Map of 2015 Rate of Adults and Adolescents Living With an HIV Diagnoses" by A1dsVU is licensed under CC BY-SA 4.0 (https://commons.

wikimedia.org/wiki/File:AIDSVu_Map_of_2015_Rate_of_Adults_and_Adolescents_Living_With_an_HIV_Diagnoses.png).

Figure 22. "Analisi Urina" by Federico Candoni is licensed under CC BY-SA 4.0 (https://commons.wikimedia.org/wiki/File:20150120_Analisi_Urina_1.jpg).

Figure 23. "HIV Testing" by Marcello Casal is licensed under CC BY 3.0 BR (https://commons.wikimedia.org/wiki/File:Oraquick.jpg).

Figure 24. "Diseased Livers" by Wellcome is licensed under CC BY 4.0 International (https://commons.wikimedia.org/wiki/File:Diseased_livers;_hepatitis,_syphilis,_angioma,_pylephlebitis_Wellcome_V0010282EL.jpg).

Figure 25. "Empty Rolled Condom" by Empcon54 is licensed under CC BY-SA 4.0 International (https://commons.wikimedia.org/wiki/File:Empty_rolled_condom.JPG).

Figure 26. "Female condoms" by Anqa is in the Public Domain (https://pixabay.com/en/female-condoms-condom-contraception-849411/).

Chapter 11

Figure 2. "Emergency Room Ambulance" by ArtisticOperations is in the Public Domain (https://pixabay.com/en/emergency-room-ambulance-ems-emt-3326156/).

Figure 10. "Alcohol Hangover Event" by Jarmoluk is in the Public Domain (https://pixabay.com/en/alcohol-hangover-event-death-drunk-428392/).

Figure 14. "ISC Integration Party Fall 2011" by Jirka Matousek is licensed under CC BY 2.0 (https://www.flickr.com/photos/jirka_matousek/8437433279).

Figure 16. "Drunk Man" by Mario Antonio Pena Zapatería is licensed under CC BY-SA 2.0 (https://commons.wikimedia.org/wiki/File:Drunk_man.jpg).

Figure 18. "Library" by andrew_t8 is in the Public Domain (https://pixabay.com/en/library-la-trobe-study-students-1400312/).

Figure 19. "Women" by Susanne Nilsson is licensed under CC BY-SA 2.0 (https://www.flickr.com/photos/infomastern/34262951724/).

Figure 20. "31 Weeks Pregnant" by Jerry Lai is licensed under CC BY-SA 2.0 (https://www.flickr.com/photos/jerrylai0208/15514557255/).

Figure 22. "Cigarettes" by Klimkin is in the Public Domain (https://pixabay.com/en/cigarette-smoking-ash-habit-1642232/).

Figure 23. "E-Cigarette Starter Kit" by Ecig Click is licensed under CC BY-SA 2.0 (https://www.flickr.com/photos/ecigclick/16581902047/).

Figure 25. "What's Wrong With This Picture?" by alex yosifov is licensed under CC BY-SA 2.0 (https://www.flickr.com/photos/sashomasho/718292525/).

Figure 27. "Only the Last Time" by Morgan is licensed under CC BY 2.0 (https://www.flickr.com/photos/meddygarnet/4170136164/).

Figure 28. "No Smoking Sign" by smartSign is licensed under CC BY 2.0 (https://www.flickr.com/photos/smartsignbrooklyn/10213459946/).

Figure 30. "DSC_0124" by USFS Region 5 is licensed under CC BY 2.0 (https://www.flickr.com/photos/usfsregion5/4888965362/).

Figure 33. "P1130349C" by Thirteen of Clubs is licensed under CC BY-SA 2.0 (https://www.flickr.com/photos/thirteenofclubs/5520512981/).

Figure 37. "Coffee Feathering" by Vivian Evans is licensed under CC BY-SA 2.0 (https://www.flickr.com/photos/vivevans/4106191761/).

Chapter 12

Figure 1. "Huge Crowds Gather in the Bogside" by Sinn Fein is licensed under CC BY 2.0 (https://www.flickr.com/photos/sinnfeinireland/33511256992/).

Figure 3. "Fungi of Saskatchewan" by Sasata is licensed under CC BY-SA 3.0 (https://commons.wikimedia.org/wiki/File:Fungi_of_Saskatchewan.JPG).

Figure 4. "Undercover Investigation at Manitoba Pork Factory Farm" by Mercy for Animals Canada is licensed under CC BY 2.0 (https://www.flickr.com/photos/mercyforanimalscanada/8250109079).

Figure 13. "US GHG Emissions Flow Chart" by World Resources Institute is in the Public Domain (http://www.wri.org/resources/charts-graphs/us-greenhouse-gas-emissions-flow-chart).

Figure 17. "Climate Change Threatens Your Health" by World Health Organization is in the Public Domain (http://www.who.int/globalchange/climate/infographics/en/).

Figure 18. "Stacken" by Janwikifoto is licensed under CC BY-SA 3.0 (https://commons.wikimedia.org/wiki/File:Stacken_0c149d_1755.jpg).

Figure 21. "Aquifers and Wells" by USGS is in the Public Domain (https://water.usgs.gov/edu/earthgwaquifer.html).

Figure 22. "Groundwater Pollution" by Foundation of Water Research is in the Public Domain (http://www.euwfd.com/assets/images/Groundwater-pollution02.jpg).

Figure 24. "Digging for Drinking Water in a Dry Riverbed" by DFID - UK Department for International Development is licensed under CC BY 2.0 (https://commons.wikimedia.org/wiki/File:Digging_for_drinking_water_in_a_dry_river-bed_(6220146368).jpg).

Figure 25. "Water Fountain 3" by joshme17 is licensed under CC BY 2.0 (https://www.flickr.com/photos/joshme17/1751994184/).

Figure 26. "Water Quality Testing Activity" by Shenandoah National Park is in the Public Domain (https://www.flickr.com/photos/snpphotos/36589911655/).

Figure 32. "E-Waste" by Curtis Palmer is licensed under CC BY 2.0 (https://www.flickr.com/photos/techbirmingham/345897594/).

Figure 35. "Rust Bike Garden" by Alex123456 is in the Public Domain (https://pixabay.com/en/rust-bike-garden-fence-261167/).

Figure 37. "Composting in the Escuela Barreales" by Diego Grez is in the Public Domain (https://commons.wikimedia.org/wiki/File:Composting_in_the_Escuela_Barreales.jpg).

Figure 38. "Eurodif Nuclear Power Plant, Tricastin, France" by IAEA is licensed under CC BY-SA 2.0 (https://www.flickr.com/photos/iaea_imagebank/8168889853/).

Figure 39. "Sunscreen" by Maggiejumps is licensed under CC BY 2.0 (https://www.flickr.com/photos/38494596@N00/443642299/sizes/l/).

Figure 40. "Asphalt" by PxHere is in the Public Domain (https://pxhere.com/en/photo/1012613).

CPSIA information can be obtained
at www.ICGtesting.com
Printed in the USA
FSHW02n2338010918
51543FS

9 781943 536443